One Health: Human, Animal, and Environment Triad

One Health

Human, Animal, and Environment Triad

Edited by Meththika Vithanage and Majeti Narasimha Vara Prasad

WILEY

Published by John Wiley & Sons, Inc., Hoboken, New Jersey.
Published simultaneously in Canada.

Library of Congress Cataloging-in-Publication Data
Names: Vithanage, Meththika, editor. | Prasad, M. N. V. (Majeti Narasimha Vara), 1953– editor.
Title: One Health : human, animal, and environment triad / edited by Meththika Vithanage, Majeti Narasimha Vara Prasad.
Description: Hoboken, NJ : Wiley, 2023. | Includes bibliographical references and index.
Identifiers: LCCN 2022056911 (print) | LCCN 2022056912 (ebook) | ISBN 9781119867302 (cloth) | ISBN 9781119867319 (adobe pdf) | ISBN 9781119867326 (epub)
Subjects: LCSH: One Health (Initiative) | World health–Case studies. | World health–Environmental aspects–Case studies. | Environmental health–Case studies. | Communicable diseases–Prevention–Case studies. | Zoonoses–Prevention–Case studies.
Classification: LCC RA441 .O535 2023 (print) | LCC RA441 (ebook) | DDC 362.1–dc23/eng/20230106
LC record available at https://lccn.loc.gov/2022056911
LC ebook record available at https://lccn.loc.gov/2022056912

Cover design: Wiley
Cover image: © dptro/Shutterstock

Set in 9.5/12.5pt STIXTwoText by Straive, Pondicherry, India
Printed and bound by CPI Group (UK) Ltd, Croydon, CR0 4YY

C9781119867302_200623

Contents

List of Contributors

N.P.M. Abeysinghe
Department of Export Agriculture
Faculty of Agricultural Sciences
Sabaragamuwa University of Sri Lanka
Belihuloya, Srilanka

Dipo Aldila
Department of Mathematics
University of Indonesia
Depok, Indonesia

Prasada Rao Allu
Department of Horticulture
Sikkim Central University
Gangtok, Sikkim, India

Nimroth Ambanpola
Department of Chemistry
Faculty of Science
University of Kelaniya
Kelaniya, Sri Lanka

Lakshmi Badrinarayanan
Department of Nanobiotechnology
Vision Research Foundation
Sankara Nethralaya, Chennai
Tamil Nadu, India

Johannes A.C. Barth
GeoZentrum Nordbayern
Friedrich-Alexander University Erlangen-Nürnberg (FAU)
Erlangen, Germany

Tanushree Basumatary
Bioremediation Technology Research Group
Department of Botany
Bodoland University
Kokrajhar, Assam, India

Jayanta Kumar Biswas
Enviromicrobiology
Ecotoxicology and Ecotechnology Research Laboratory
(3E-MicroToxTech Lab)
Department of Ecological Studies
University of Kalyani, Kalyani
West Bengal, India

International Centre for Ecological Engineering
University of Kalyani, Kalyani
West Bengal, India

Shermila M. Botheju
Department of Indigenous Medical Resources
Faculty of Indigenous Health Sciences and Technology
Gampaha Wickramarachchi University
of Indigenous Medicine
Yakkala, Sri Lanka

Rohana Chandrajith
Department of Geology
Faculty of Science
University of Peradeniya
Peradeniya, Sri Lanka

GeoZentrum Nordbayern
Friedrich-Alexander University Erlangen-Nürnberg (FAU)
Erlangen, Germany

Mitali Chetia
Department of Zoology
Nanda Nath Saikia College
Titabar, Assam, India

Reshma Choudhury
Department of Biotechnology
Royal Global University
Guwahati, Assam, India

Neehasri Kumar Chowdhury
Department of Zoology
Gauhati University
Guwahati, Assam, India

Nalika R. Dayananda
Department of Indigenous Medical Resources
Faculty of Indigenous Health Sciences and Technology
Gampaha Wickramarachchi University
of Indigenous Medicine
Yakkala, Sri Lanka

Department of Chemistry
Faculty of Science
University of Kelaniya
Kelaniya, Sri Lanka

Peninna Deberdt
CIRAD, UPR HortSys
Montpellier, France

CIRAD, HortSys
Univ Montpellier
Montpellier, France

Jean-Philippe Deguine
CIRAD, UMR PVBMT
Can Tho University
Can Tho City, Vietnam

Saranga Diyabalanage
Instrument Centre
Faculty of Applied Sciences
University of Sri Jayewardenepura
Nugegoda, Sri Lanka

Ecosphere Resilience Research Center
Faculty of Applied Sciences
University of Sri Jayewardenepura
Nugegoda, Sri Lanka

Sailaja V. Elchuri
Department of Nanobiotechnology
Vision Research Foundation
Sankara Nethralaya, Chennai
Tamil Nadu, India

Marina E. Eremeeva
Jiann-Ping Hsu College of Public Health
Georgia Southern University
Statesboro, GA, USA

G.A.H. Galahitigama
Department of Export Agriculture
Faculty of Agricultural Sciences
Sabaragamuwa University of Sri Lanka
Belihuloya, Srilanka

Naleen Chaminda Ganegoda
Department of Mathematics
University of Sri Jayewardenepura
Nugegoda, Sri Lanka

Bhoirob Gogoi
Bioremediation Technology Research Group
Department of Botany
Bodoland University
Kokrajhar, Assam, India

Viraj Gunarathne
Laboratory of Soil- and Groundwater-Management
Water- and Waste-Management
Institute of Foundation Engineering
School of Architecture and Civil Engineering
University of Wuppertal
Wuppertal, Germany

Yasodhara Gunasekara
Department of Veterinary Public Health and Pharmacology
Faculty of Veterinary Medicine and Animal Science
University of Peradeniya
Peradeniya, Sri Lanka

H. Harischandra
Genetics and Molecular Biology Unit
Faculty of Applied Science
University of Sri Jayewardenepura
Nugegoda, Sri Lanka

Narayanan Janakiraman
Department of Nanobiotechnology
Vision Research Foundation
Sankara Nethralaya, Chennai
Tamil Nadu, India

Randika Jayasinghe
Faculty of Technology
University of Sri Jayewardenepura
Nugegoda, Sri Lanka

Nimanthi Jayathilaka
Department of Chemistry
Faculty of Science
University of Kelaniya
Kelaniya, Sri Lanka

Luhan Jiang
Department of Obstetrics and Gynecology
Li Ka Shing Faculty of Medicine
The University of Hong Kong
Hong Kong SAR, China

Rasika Jinadasa
Department of Veterinary Pathobiology
Faculty of Veterinary Medicine & Animal Science
University of Peradeniya
Peradeniya, Sri Lanka

Ruwani Kalupahana
Department of Veterinary Public Health and Pharmacology
Faculty of Veterinary Medicine and Animal Science
University of Peradeniya
Peradeniya, Sri Lanka

V. Kantono
Department of Environmental Management
College of Agriculture and Environmental Sciences
Makerere University
Kampala, Uganda

Niwantha Kanuwana
Department of Indigenous Medical Resources
Faculty of Indigenous Health Sciences and Technology
Gampaha Wickramarachchi University of Indigenous Medicine
Yakkala, Sri Lanka

M. Kaziro
Department of Zoology
Entomology and Fisheries Sciences
College of Natural Sciences
Makerere University
Kampala, Uganda

Suranga P. Kodithuwakku
Department of Obstetrics and Gynecology
Li Ka Shing Faculty of Medicine
The University of Hong Kong
Hong Kong SAR, China

Department of Animal Science
Faculty of Agriculture
University of Peradeniya
Peradeniya, Sri Lanka

Institute of Veterinary Medicine and Animal Sciences
Estonian University of Life Sciences
Tartu, Estonia

Pabasari Arundathi Koliyabandara
Faculty of Technology
University of Sri Jayewardenepura
Nugegoda, Sri Lanka

Sanda Kottawatta
Department of Veterinary Public Health and Pharmacology
Faculty of Veterinary Medicine and Animal Science
University of Peradeniya
Peradeniya, Sri Lanka

J. Kyayesimira
Department of Biological Sciences
Faculty of Science
Kyambogo University
Kampala, Uganda

Kai-Fai Lee
Department of Obstetrics and Gynecology
Li Ka Shing Faculty of Medicine
The University of Hong Kong
Hong Kong SAR, China

Shen Zhen Key Laboratory of Fertility Regulation
The University of Hong Kong-Shenzhen Hospital
Shenzhen, China

H.M.S.P. Madawala
Department of Botany
Faculty of Science
University of Peradeniya
Peradeniya, Sri Lanka

Dhammika N. Magana-Arachchi
Molecular Microbiology and Human Diseases Unit
National Institute of Fundamental Studies
Kandy, Sri Lanka

Thibaud Martin
CIRAD, UPR HortSys
Montpellier, France

CIRAD, HortSys
Univ Montpellier
Montpellier, France

F. Muheirwe
Department of Educational Foundation and Psychology
Faculty of Science
Mbarara University of Science and Technology
Mbarara, Uganda

Progya Mukherjee
Enviromicrobiology
Ecotoxicology and Ecotechnology Research Laboratory
(3E-MicroToxTech Lab)
Department of Ecological Studies
University of Kalyani, Kalyani
West Bengal, India

Bhagya Nallaperuma
Department of Indigenous Medical Resources
Faculty of Indigenous Health Sciences and Technology
Gampaha Wickramarachchi University
of Indigenous Medicine
Yakkala, Sri Lanka

R.M. Nalwanga
Department of Zoology
Entomology and Fisheries Sciences
College of Natural Sciences
Makerere University
Kampala, Uganda

J. Nattabi
Department of Zoology
Entomology and Fisheries Sciences
College of Natural Sciences
Makerere University
Kampala, Uganda

S.U. Nimalratna
Centre for Biotechnology
Faculty of Applied Sciences
University of Sri Jayewardenepura
Nugegoda, Sri Lanka

Thilini Nisansala
Faculty of Veterinary Medicine
Universiti Malaysia Kelantan
Kota Bharu, Kelantan, Malaysia

Sandun J. Perera
Department of Natural Resources
Faculty of Applied Sciences
Sabaragamuwa University of Sri Lanka
Belihuloya, Sri Lanka

Majeti Narasimha Vara Prasad
School of Life Sciences
University of Hyderabad, Hyderabad
Telangana, India

Rupika S. Rajakaruna
Department of Zoology
University of Peradeniya
Peradeniya, Sri Lanka

Sanchayita Rajkhowa
Department of Chemistry
The Assam Royal Global University
Guwahati, Assam, India

Tharaka Ranathunge
Department of Zoology
Faculty of Science
Eastern University of Srilanka
Chenkaladi, Sri Lanka

Alain Ratnadass
CIRAD, UPR Aïda
Réunion, France

CIRAD, Aïda
Univ Montpellier
Montpellier, France

Dhanashree Ratra
Shri Bhagwan Mahavir Department of Vitreo
Retinal Services
Medical Research Foundation
Sankara Nethralaya, Chennai
Tamil Nadu, India

Jörg Rinklebe
Laboratory of Soil- and Groundwater-Management
Water- and Waste-Management
Institute of Foundation Engineering
School of Architecture and Civil Engineering
University of Wuppertal
Wuppertal, Germany

Hemen Sarma
Bioremediation Technology Research Group
Department of Botany
Bodoland University
Kokrajhar, Assam, India

Jyotirmoy Sarma
Department of Chemistry
Assam Don Bosco University
Guwahati, Assam, India

Kapila N. Seneviratne
Department of Chemistry
Faculty of Science
University of Kelaniya
Kelaniya, Sri Lanka

Mathilde Sester
CIRAD, Aïda
Univ Montpellier
Montpellier, France

CIRAD, UPR Aïda
Institut Technologique du Cambodge
Phnom Penh, Cambodia

Suprity Shyam
Bioremediation Technology Research Group
Department of Botany
Bodoland University
Kokrajhar, Assam, India

B.G.D.N.K. de Silva
Centre for Biotechnology
Faculty of Applied Sciences
University of Sri Jayewardenepura
Nugegoda, Sri Lanka

Genetics and Molecular Biology Unit
Faculty of Applied Sciences
University of Sri Jayewardenepura
Nugegoda, Sri Lanka

Ayona Silva-Fletcher
Department of Veterinary Clinical Sciences
The Royal Veterinary College
University of London, United Kingdom

T.M.A.H. Tennakoon
Department of Pathology
Faculty of Medicine
University of Peradeniya
Peradeniya, Sri Lanka

Lahiru Udayanga
Department of Bio-Systems Engineering
Faculty of Agriculture & Plantation Management
Wayamba University of Sri Lanka
Kuliyapitiya, Sri Lanka

Meththika Vithanage
Ecosphere Resilience Research Centre
Faculty of Applied Sciences
University of Sri Jayewardenepura
Nugegoda, Sri Lanka

Rasika P. Wanigatunge
Department of Plant and Molecular Biology
Faculty of Science
University of Kelaniya
Kelaniya, Sri Lanka

Karunia Putra Wijaya
Mathematical Institute
University of Koblenz
Koblenz, Germany

Jithya Wijesinghe
Department of Indigenous Medical Resources
Faculty of Indigenous Health Sciences and Technology
Gampaha Wickramarachchi University
of Indigenous Medicine
Yakkala, Sri Lanka

Novil Wijeskara
Humphrey Fellowship Program
Department of Global Health
Rollins School of Public Health
Emory University
Atlanta, GA, USA

Disaster Preparedness and Response Division
Ministry of Health
Colombo, Sri Lanka

K.K. Wijesundera
Department of Veterinary Pathobiology
Faculty of Veterinary Medicine and Animal Science
University of Peradeniya
Peradeniya, Sri Lanka

Ewa Wiśniowska
Department of Sanitary Networks and Installations
Częstochowa University of Technology
Częstochowa, Poland

Preface

One Health is a multi-sectoral and trans-disciplinary strategy comprising local, national, regional, and international cooperative efforts to achieve optimal health for humans, animals, and the environment, which are interrelated. A significant change in the global health system is needed to maintain the well-being of people, animals, and the environment through cooperative problem resolution on a local, national, and international level. Various chapters in this book talk about this paradigm shift.

Many nations will expand investment in this field as society develops, particularly in light of the COVID-19's effects on the nation's present public health systems. It is encouraged by the fact that scientists from many disciplines and various professions collaborate to address major issues. Various health and illness issues can be resolved through this field of study. Issues that affect individuals and improve our capacity to tackle taking real-world health issues to a new level.

1) The Need for One Health Approach at the Recent Anthropocene
2) Emergence and Re-emergence of the Emerging Infectious Diseases (EIDs): Looking at "One Health" Through the Lens of Ecology
3) Environmental interfaces for One Health
4) Zoonoses: The Rising Threat to Human Health
5) Microplastics in Soil and Water: Vector Behavior
6) Cyanotoxin in Hydrosphere and Human Interface
7) Contributions to One Health Approach to Solve Geogenic Health Issues
8) Disasters: Health and Environment Interphase
9) Role of Microorganisms in Bioavailability of Soil Pollutants
10) Per- and Polyfluoroalkyl Substances (PFAS) Migration from Water to Soil–Plant Systems, Health Risks, and Implications, for Remediation
11) One Health Relationships in Microbe–Human Domain
12) Biomedical Waste During COVID-19: Status, Management, and Treatment
13) Spatiotemporal Dynamics of Disease Transmission: Learning from COVID-19 Data
14) Organic Farming: The Influence on Soil Health
15) Chronic Kidney Disease with Uncertain Etiology in Sri Lanka: Selected Case Studies
16) Waste in One Health: Building Resilient Communities Through Sustainable Waste Management
17) One Health Approach for Eye Care: Is It a Boon or Hype?
18) Waste in One Health: African Perspective
19) Endocrine Disruptors and Female Reproductive Health: A Problem to Tackle with One Health Perspective
20) Emerging and Re-emerging Zoonoses in South Asia: Challenges of One Health
21) Impacts of Crop Protection Practices on Human Infectious Diseases: Agroecology as the Preferred Strategy to Integrate Crop Plant Health Within the Extended "One Health" Frameworks
22) Tackling Antimicrobial Resistance Needs One Health Approach
23) Eco-epidemiology of Tick-Borne Pathogens: Role of Tick Vectors and Host Animal Community Composition in Their Circulation and Source of Infections
24) Natural Enemies Against Dengue: Opportunities and Constraints on Biological Control of Dengue Vectors in Sri Lanka
25) Planetary Health: Rethinking Health
26) SARS-CoV-2 and Other Pathogenic Organisms in Food and Water: Health Implications and Environmental Risk
27) Modifying the Anthropocene Equation with One Health Concept
28) Bioavailability of Trace Elements in Soils
29) "Light" as an Environmental Factor for the Well-Being of the "Plant, Animal, and Human Triad"

This book, with its diverse chapters enumerated supra vide, is needed for a variety of reasons – continuous changes in the environment, climate change, and people are more interested in the environment and health. The diversity can be observed in the word cloud map (Figure 1).

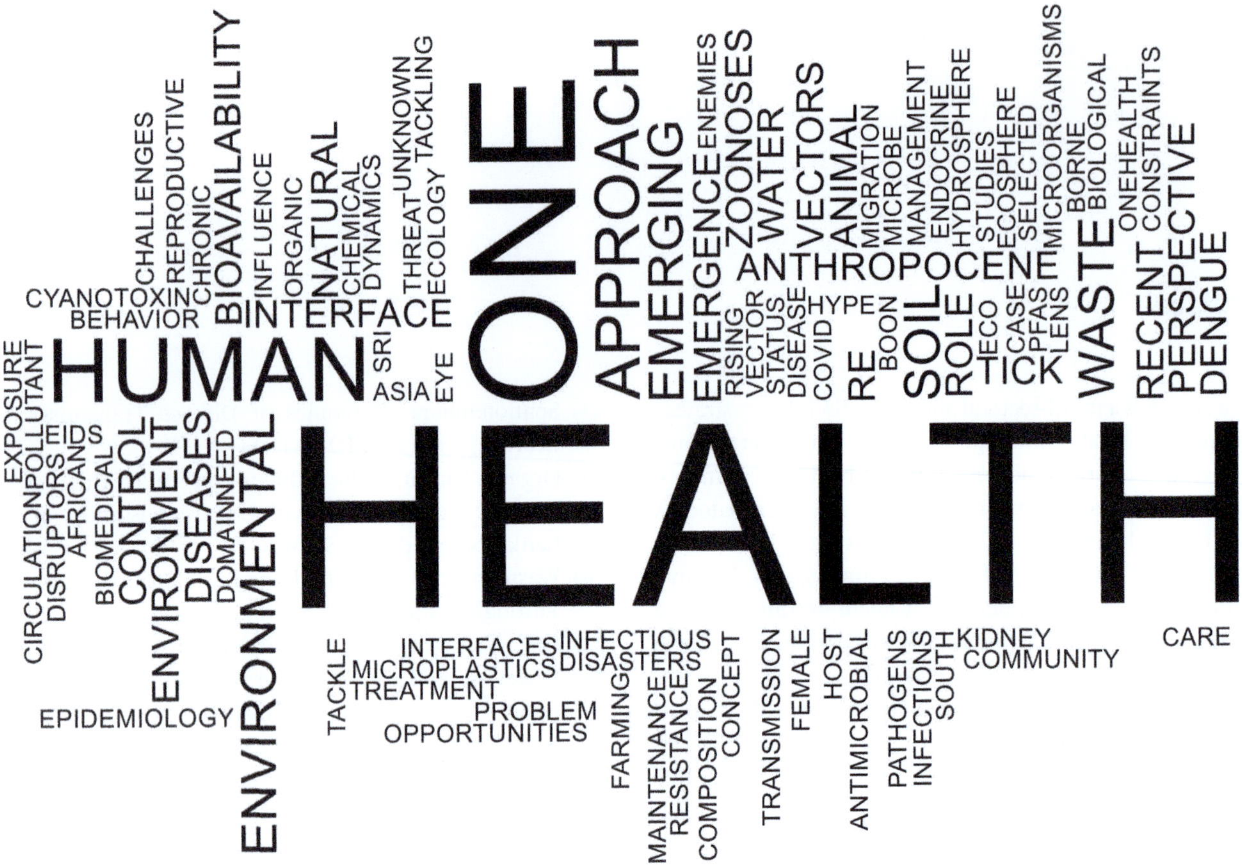

Figure 1 Word cloud map for the book chapters in the One Health book.

Section I

One Health Approach

1

The Need for One Health Approach at the Recent Anthropocene

Novil Wijeskara

Humphrey Fellowship Program, Department of Global Health, Rollins School of Public Health, Emory University, Atlanta, GA, USA
Disaster Preparedness and Response Division, Ministry of Health, Colombo, Sri Lanka

1.1 Anthropocene

Humans have become closer to both the environment and other life forms. In the early stages of our civilization, extraction of natural resources by humans resulted in minimal impacts on the ecosystem. Nevertheless, over the years, humanity thrived on natural resources, alleviating poverty with improving access to safe water and sanitation, hygiene, and housing (Deaton 2015). Developments in preventive and curative healthcare contributed toward reduction of both communicable and non-communicable diseases (Pinker 2020). Life expectancy at birth has increased, and under-five mortality has declined to unprecedented levels (Haines et al. 2019).

However, subsequently, our relationships with the ecosystem components have been more competitive than collaborative to a large extent. As a result, severe negative impacts have been had on the environment. Rising economic and population growth demanded an escalation of the use of natural resources for housing, agriculture, and industry (Steffen et al. 2015). Indiscriminate use of fossil fuels has become unsustainable (Steffen et al. 2015). It is estimated that the current extinction rates of species are 1000 times higher than the natural background rates of extinction, whereas the future rates would be 10,000 times higher (De Vos et al. 2015). A myriad of environmental conflicts such as ocean acidification, pollution, and overfishing have resulted in the meantime (Jackson 2010). The period in the history of the earth where the impacts of human beings have been so fast, profound, and far-reaching has been named the Anthropocene. The Working Group on the Anthropocene has agreed that the mid-twentieth century to be the starting point of the Anthropocene (Zalasiewicz et al. 2017).

1.2 Infectious Diseases: Animals to Humans

One of the necessary evils of humans becoming more and more closer to animals, both domesticated and wild, has increased the exposure of humans to infectious diseases. For example, 60% of known infectious diseases in humans and 70% of emerging infectious diseases (EIDs) have been caused by zoonotic pathogens (Woolhouse and Gowtage-Sequeria 2005; Taylor and Habibi 2020). It has also been found that zoonotic pathogens are two times more associated with emerging and reemerging infectious diseases than non-zoonotic pathogens (Woolhouse and Gowtage-Sequeria 2005). The evolution of the One Health Concept is closely linked to the infectious diseases in domesticated and wild animals that could infect humans or cause zoonoses. A zoonosis is any disease or infection that is naturally transmissible from vertebrate animals to humans (WHO 2020). We will commence this chapter by reviewing emerging and reemerging infectious diseases (RIDs), with a focus on zoonosis.

1.3 Emerging and Reemerging Infectious Diseases

EIDs and RIDs are used to signal the absolutely or relatively new risks of infectious diseases in each area or community. Thus, the definition of EIDs and RIDs takes the time and place into consideration. EIDs signal new infectious disease risks, whereas RIDs indicate older risks that are reappearing. Table 1.1 summarizes the definitions of EIDs and RIDs. A third category has been identified as deliberately emerging infectious diseases (DID), indicating those used with

One Health: Human, Animal, and Environment Triad, First Edition. Edited by Meththika Vithanage and Majeti Narasimha Vara Prasad.

Table 1.1 Definition of emerging and reemerging infectious diseases.

Emerging Infectious Diseases (EIDs)	
Description	**Example(s)**
Diseases that have not occurred in humans before	COVID-19[a]
Diseases that have occurred previously but affected only a small numbers of people in isolated places	AIDS, Ebola hemorrhagic fever
Diseases that have occurred throughout human history but have only recently been recognized as distinct diseases due to an infectious agent	Lyme diseases, gastric ulcers
Reemerging infectious Diseases (RIDs)	
Diseases that once were major health problems globally or in a particular country and then declined dramatically but are again becoming health problems for a significant proportion of the population	Malaria, tuberculosis
Deliberately Emerging Infectious Diseases (DIDs)[b]	
Diseases occurring due to pathogens that have been developed by man, usually for nefarious use	Anthrax
Accidently Emerging Infectious Diseases (AIDs)	Epizootic vaccinia, Transmissible vaccine-derived polioviruses

[a] The example of COVID-19 was added by the chapter authors.
[b] The definition of DID was adapted from (Morens et al. 2004).
Source: (Tabish 2009)

malicious intentions. Figure 1.1 shows the global examples of diseases belonging to these three categories.

An EID is a disease of which the prevalence has recently increased considering the timeframe of 20 years, and this rise may continue in the near future (Verma n.d.). Under EID, three categories of diseases could be identified.

The first category involves newly emerging infectious diseases in humans for the first time, such as HIV/AIDS (1981), Nipah virus (1999), SARS (2002), MERS (2012), and COVID-19 (2019).

The second category has historically been known to infect humans, but they appear in new locations (e.g. West Nile in the United States and Russia in 1999) or in more resistant forms (e.g. methicillin-resistant *Staphylococcus aureus*).

The third category includes diseases that have affected human beings over time but only have recently been identified as being due to an infective agent (e.g. Lyme diseases, gastric ulcer) (Tabish 2009).

RID is used to indicate infectious diseases that were once a significant health problem in an area, declined in their occurrence considerably, and are now reoccurring as a problem (e.g. malaria, tuberculosis) (Tabish 2009).

DID occurs due to the use of pathogenic organisms to cause human suffering (e.g. anthrax) (Morens et al. 2004). Accidentally emerging infectious disease (AID) occurs due to unintentional human errors (e.g. epizootic vaccinia and transmissible vaccine-derived polioviruses).

In addition to the categories mentioned earlier, some infections become endemic in areas where they were once newly emerging infections.

EIDs occur due to the complex interaction between many factors. An extensive list of factors has been identified in relation to the human, animal, and environmental interphases. We have summarized factors from literature on the subject in Table 1.2 (Church 2004; Health [US] and Study 2007; Morens et al. 2004; Morens and Fauci 2020; Tabish 2009).

As shown in Table 1.2, a range of factors operating at underlying, intermediate, and immediate level could be identified as contributing to the rise of EID, RID, DID, and AID. Underlying factors such as population growth, globalization, urbanization, and industrialization explain how, over time, a more favorable environment for the emergence of such diseases has evolved at the global level. In the meantime, political instability, social injustice, and inequality are contributing to the increased risk of such diseases. Further, climate change, which is anthropogenic and resulting from a combination of underlying factors, is also contributing to the rise of diseases.

Under intermediate factors, population mobility is considered. The movement of people within and between countries has contributed to the introduction of new diseases to new locations very quickly. The COVID-19 pandemic is the best example of this from the recent past. In addition, along with population growth and economic development, the demand for meat production has increased not only for food, but also for proteins. Hence the need for modern food production has increased, including food production in strictly regulated

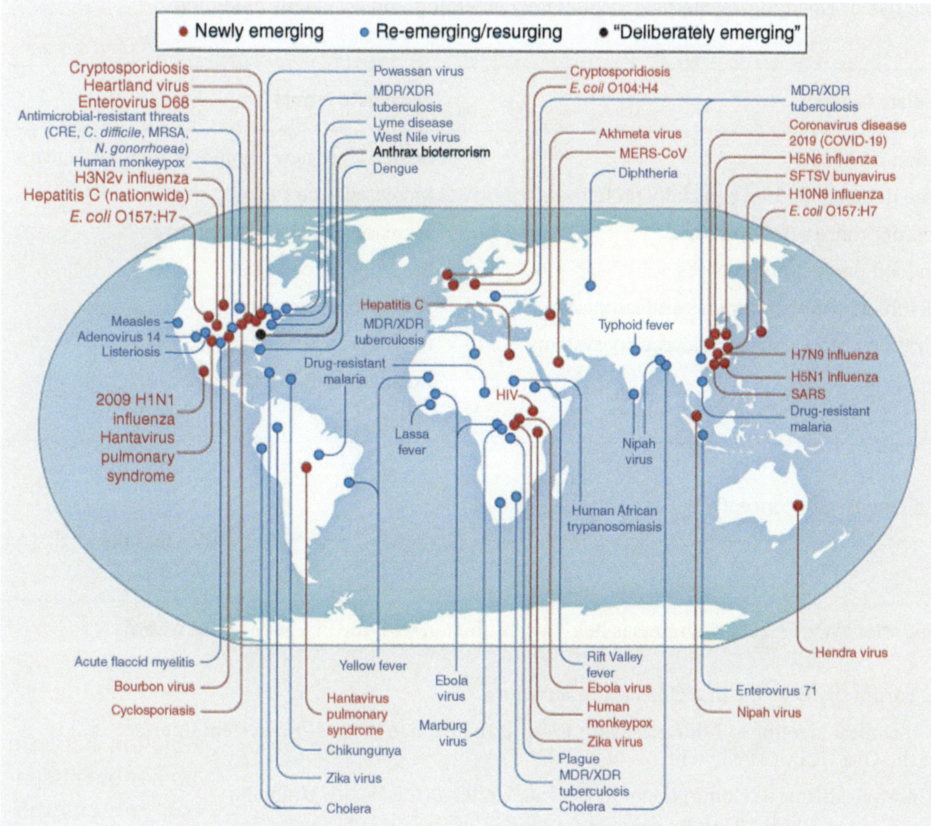

Figure 1.1 Map of emerging, re-emerging and deliberately emerging infectious diseases (Morens and Fauci 2020).

environments. Cross-border transportation of food, including meat and meat products, became a necessity, increasing the risk of EID and RID. Irrational use of antibiotics, not only for human health but also in animal husbandry, increased the risk of immediate risk factors such as antimicrobial resistance (AMR). The deterioration of biosafety and biosecurity systems, backed by global political instability as an underlying factor, contributed to the rise of DID and AIDs.

The interplay of the underlying and intermediate factors gives rise to the immediate factors for the emergence of EID, RID, DID, and AID. New or more virulent forms of known pathogens could rapidly arise. Increasing vector density could rapidly transmit the disease to humans. Humans being in close contact with the vectors could increase the spread. Breaches of food security will also increase the risk of food-borne diseases. Poor immunity of humans to such new organisms, coupled with increased exposure, could increase the risk of human infections. Breakdown of health services could hamper surveillance, early detection, and management of newly emerging diseases. AMR could further deteriorate the situation by making the available antibiotics effective against the pathogens.

When considering the contributory factor framework mentioned earlier, the emergence of EID, RID, DID, and AID cut across humans, animals, and the environment. Therefore, one discipline alone cannot engage all stakeholders, agencies, and organizations. One Health is an approach aimed at engaging the whole range of stakeholders from human health, animal health, and environmental health to address the complex problems of EIDs. This has been a concept that has been in evolution probably from the beginning of human civilization. The Greek physician Hippocrates, in the fifth or fourth century BCE, in his book *Airs, Waters, and Places*, explored the causal relationship between human disease and the environment (Miller 1962). Table 1.3 summarizes the historical evolution of the One Health concept. The core of the approach as enshrined in its definition, as well as the historical narrative, is that consorted efforts are needed to ensure the health of people, animals, and the environment instead of the compartmental and fragmented approach to addressing the health of each component separately.

Table 1.2 Factors contributing to the rise of emerging, reemerging, deliberately emerging, and accidently emerging infectious diseases.

Underlying factors	Intermediate factors	Immediate factors
Population growth	Population mobility	Evolution of new or more virulent organisms
Globalization	Increased demand for food especially protein	Increased vector breeding
Urbanization	Cross-border transportation of food	Increased exposure to pathogens
Industrialization	Modern food production practices	Breaches of food safety
Political instability	Antimicrobial misuse in humans and animals	Poor human immunity
Social injustice	Deterioration of biosafety and biosecurity systems	Antimicrobial resistance
Inequity		Breakdown of health services
Climate change		

Table 1.3 Historical evolution of the One Health concept.

Year	Events
2013	• The Second International One Health Congress is held in conjunction with the Prince Mahidol Award Conference
2012	• The Global Risk Forum sponsors the first One Health Summit
2011	• The High-Level Technical Meeting to Address Health Risks at the Human-Animal-Ecosystem Interface Builds Political Will for the One Health Movement
2010	• The European Union Reaffirms its Commitment to Operate Under a One Health Umbrella • The United Nations and the World Bank Recommend Adoption of One Health Approaches • Experts Identify Clear and Concrete Actions to Move the Concept of One Health from Vision to Implementation • The Hanoi Declaration, Which Recommends Broad Implementation of One Health, is Adopted Unanimously
2009	• Key Recommendations for One World, One Health™ are Developed • USAID Establishes the Emerging Pandemic Threats Program • The One Health Office is Established at CDC
2008	• One Health Becomes a Recommended Approach and a Political Reality • Food and Agriculture Organization of the United Nations (FAO), OIE, and WHO Collaborate with UNICEF, UNSIC, and the World Bank to develop a Joint Strategic Framework in Response to the Evolving Risk of Emerging and Re-emerging Infectious Diseases
2007	• The One Health Approach is Recommended for Pandemic Preparedness • The American Medical Association Passes the One Health Resolution Promoting Partnership Between Human and Veterinary Medicine
2004	• The Wildlife Conservation Society Publishes the 12 Manhattan Principles
1927–2006	• Calvin Schwabe Coins the Term "One Medicine" and calls for a Unified Approach Against Zoonoses That Uses Both Human and Veterinary Medicine
1947	• The Veterinary Public Health Division is Established at CDC
1849–1919	• William Osler, Father of Veterinary Pathology
1821–1902	• Virchow Recognizes the Link Between Human and Animal Health

Source: Adapted from (CDC 2022b)

1.4 Definition of One Health

Several definitions of One Health could be found, probably showcasing the focus of the agency that has created it in relation to the concept. A narrow and a broader approach to One Health have been described. The narrow approach had a biomedical focus, largely combining human and animal health through human and veterinary medicine. The WHO and Organization for Animal Health (WOAH, founded as OIE) definitions are examples of such narrow approaches addressing One Health. The broader definitions have been put forward by the One Health Commission and One Health Global Network. Hence, all definitions have some large overlaps; however, each has its own uniqueness, which probably would have contributed to the creation of yet another definition (Figure 1.2). Three definitions of One Health are considered in Table 1.4.

The broader scope of One Health could be shown using the following umbrella diagram by the One Health Initiative (Gibbs and Paul 2014; One Health Initiative 2019).

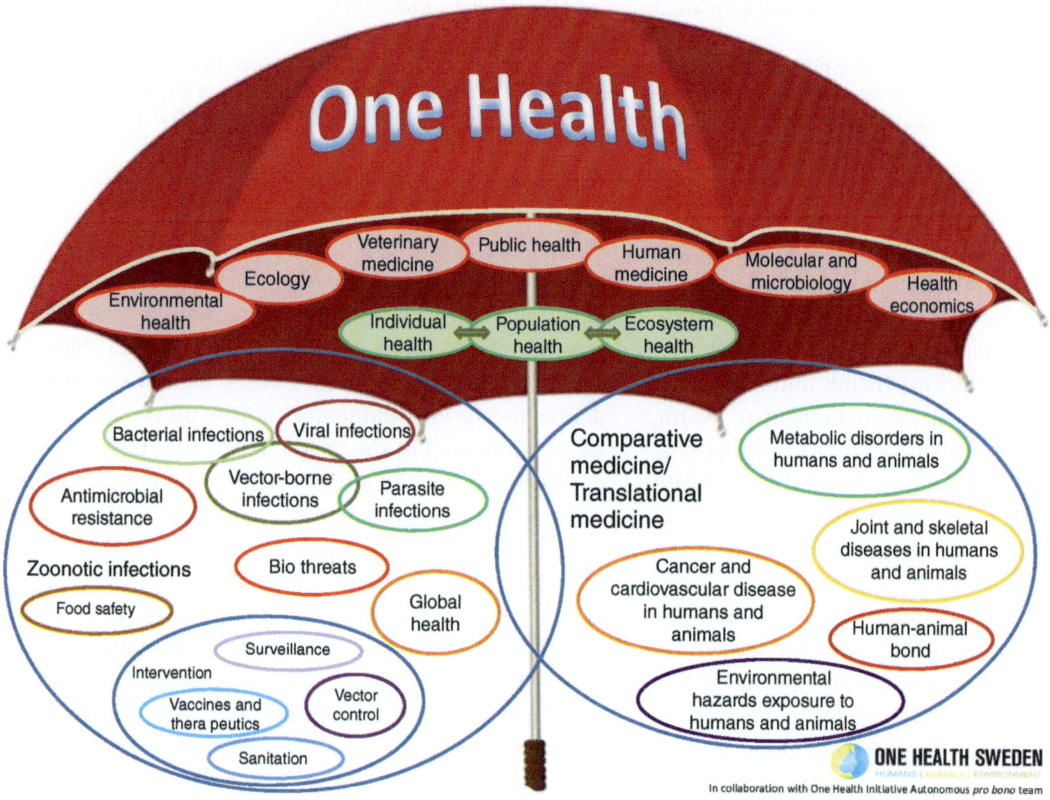

Figure 1.2 The One Health Umbrella. Source: One Health Initiative.

Table 1.4 Definitions of One Health.

WHO definition

An approach to designing and implementing programs, policies, and legislation and research in which multiple sectors communicate and work together to achieve better public health outcomes (WHO 2017).

Organization for Animal Health (WOHA, Founded as OIE) definition

A collaborative global approach to understand risks for human and animal health (including both domestic animals and wildlife) and ecosystem health as a whole.

US CDC and One Health Commission definition

One Health is a collaborative, multisectoral, and trans-disciplinary approach – working at local, regional, national, and global levels – to achieve optimal health (and well-being) outcomes recognizing the interconnections between people, animals, plants, and their shared environment (One Health Commission n.d.).

Food and Agriculture Organization definition

"A collaborative, international, cross sectoral, multidisciplinary mechanism to address threats and reduce risks of detrimental infectious diseases at the animal-human-ecosystem interface."

One Health Global Network – Aim of One Health

Aim of One Health is to "improve health and wellbeing through the prevention of risks and the mitigation of effects of crises that originate at the interface between humans, animals and their various environments."

One Health Initiative definition

A worldwide strategy for expanding interdisciplinary collaborations and communications in all aspects of health care for humans, animals, and the environment (Monath et al. 2010).

(*Continued*)

Table 1.4 (Continued)

Joint Tripartite (FAO, OIE, WHO) and United Nations Environmental Program (UNEP)
One Health is an integrated, unifying approach that aims to sustainably balance and optimize the health of people, animals, and ecosystems.
It recognizes the health of humans, domestic and wild animals, plants, and the wider environment (including ecosystems) are closely linked and inter-dependent.
The approach mobilizes multiple sectors, disciplines, and communities at varying levels of society to work together to foster well-being and tackle threats to health and ecosystems, while addressing the collective need for clean water, energy and air, safe and nutritious food, taking action on climate change, and contributing to sustainable development (WHO 2021; Panel [OHHLEP] et al. 2022).

The broader definition of One Health proposed by the One Health initiative involves disciplines such as environmental health, ecology, veterinary medicine, public health, human medicine, molecular microbiology, and health economics (Gibbs and Paul 2014; One Health Initiative 2019). It explores the relationship between individual health, population health, and ecosystem health. Two overlapping domains could be identified under the broad One Health umbrella: Zoonotic infections and comparative medicine/translational medicine. The former explores the spread and control of infectious diseases between humans, animals, and the environment, both naturally and intentionally. The comparative/translational medicine uses the One Health approach that uses animal models to explore cancer and therapeutics such as medicines and vaccines for human use.

An important feature of the WHO definition of One Health is its obvious focus on public health, while it calls for different tiers of action, namely programmatic, legislative, policy, and research. The OIE definition sheds light on both domestic and wild animals while emphasizing ecosystem health. The Joint Tripartite and UNEP definitions show a unification of the focus on human, animal, and environmental health while introducing the concept of sustainability.

1.5 Other Paradigms to One Health

It should be noted that in addition to One Health, at least two other paradigms also have arisen to address similar yet overlapping issues in the intersection of human, animal, and environmental health. They are Eco Health and Planetary Health.

"Eco health can be defined as systemic, participatory approaches to understanding and promoting health and wellbeing in the context of social and ecological interactions. (Waltner-Toews 2009)" The six pillars of Eco-Health approach are systems thinking, trans disciplinarity, participation, gender and social equity, sustainability, and knowledge to action (Lisitza and Wolbring 2018).

Planetary Health is defined as "the achievement of the highest attainable standard of health, wellbeing, and equity worldwide through judicious attention to the human systems – political, economic, and social – that shape the future of humanity and the Earth's natural systems that define the safe environmental limits within which humanity can flourish. Put simply, planetary health is the health of human civilization and the state of the natural systems on which it depends" (Whitmee et al. 2015). The core of Planetary Health is the balance between two systems: the human systems and natural systems.

The similarities and differences of One Health, Eco Health, and Planetary Health have been discussed extensively (Lerner and Berg 2017). The advantages of these approaches based on the differences in their foci have been acknowledged in this research while pointing out the challenges of these overlapping approaches competing for a limited number of resources available to address them meaningfully.

1.6 One Health Fundamentals

The implementation of One Health calls for a range of activities across human health, animal health, and wildlife health. Following actions are recommended by CDC, to ensure that One Health is in Action (Figure 1.3).

One Health approach calls for people who protect human, animal, and environmental health and other partners to get together. They would coordinate, collaborate, and communicate to achieve the best health outcomes for people, animals, plants, and the environment (CDC 2022c).

The intersectoral and interdisciplinary nature of One Health demands the engagement of professionals from diverse backgrounds in its implementation (Table 1.5).

In addition, coordination between different levels, from the global level to the community level, is essential for the effective implementation of the One Health approach. We will examine two of the global collaborative mechanisms

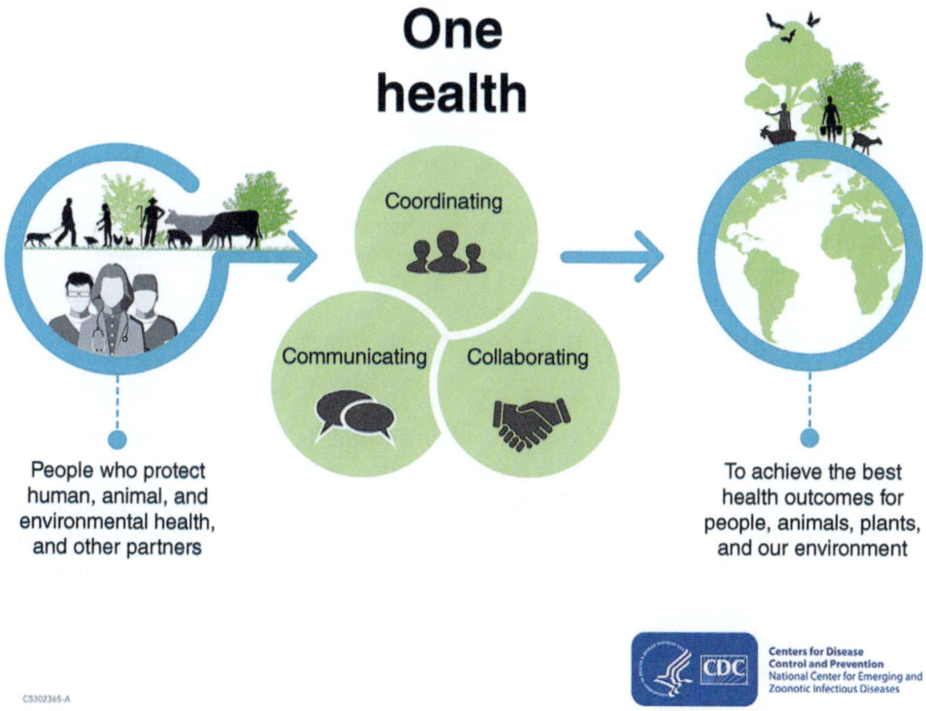

Figure 1.3 The foundations of One Health (https://www.cdc.gov/onehealth/basics/index.html) (*Source:* Centers for Disease Control and Prevention).

Table 1.5 Multistakeholder professional engagement for One Health approach.

Human health	Doctors, nurses, public health practitioners, and epidemiologists
Animal health	Veterinarians, paraprofessionals, and agricultural workers
Environment	Ecologists and wildlife experts
Other areas of expertise	Law enforcement, policymakers, agriculture, communities, and even pet owners

and platforms available that could be used for the implementation of the One Health approach (Table 1.6).

1.7 International Health Regulations and Its Evaluation Mechanisms

International Health Regulations (IHR) (2005) provides an overarching legal framework that promotes cross-border mobility of both humans and goods while minimizing public health threats. The IHR is part of an international law that is legally binding in 196 countries, including 194 WHO member states. It provides the criteria to determine an event as a "public health emergency of international concern" (WHO 2016). Zoonotic events

Table 1.6 International Health Regulations core capacities and Global Health Security Agenda action packages.

IHR core capacities	Global Health Security Agenda action packages
Legislation and policy	Antimicrobial resistance
Coordination	Biosecurity and biosafety
Surveillance	Immunization
Response	Laboratory systems
Preparedness	Legal preparedness
Risk communication	Surveillance
Human resources	Sustainable financing
Laboratory	Workforce development
Points of entry	Zoonotic diseases
Zoonotic events	
Food safety	
Chemical events	
Radio nuclear emergencies	

have been considered one of the IHR core capacities that a country has to develop. Other capacities too are linked to One Health indicating the public health risks across the human, animal, and environmental interphases. Several mechanisms are in place for the monitoring and evaluation of the implementation of IHR, such as State Party Self Reporting, Joint External Evaluation, After Action Review and Simulation Exercise. These mechanisms could be used to advocate for the implementation of the One Health approach at the country level (WHO 2016, 2022). In addition, the WOAH (Founded as OIE) has developed the Performance of Veterinary Services (PVS) Pathway, a capacity building platform for the sustainable improvement of national Veterinary Services. Efforts are on the way for connecting the IHR and PVS approaches as a part of global One Health efforts (World Organisation for Animal Health, 2019).

1.8 Global Health Security Agenda

The Global Health Security Agenda (GHSA) is a coalition of over 70 countries, international organizations and non-government organizations, and private sector companies working together to achieve the vision of a world safe and secure from global health threats posed by infectious diseases (Global Health Security Agenda 2014). GHSA has developed a framework to evaluate the health security of countries. Out of the action packages of GHSA, zoonotic diseases, AMR, and biosafety and biosecurity could be directly linked to the One Health approach, while all other action packages could be useful in promoting the One Health approach.

One key aspect that we need to address in the One Health concept is the interrelationships that operate between human health, animal health, and environmental health. A disease in one sector can jump into another and vice versa. Thus, it is important that we bring professionals from all sectors and communities together under the concept of One Health, for both disease surveillance and disease determinants and control. For example, good surveillance of the animals could help contain a potential disease before it could jump to humans. Thus, sharing surveillance data among different sectors, in turn, could increase not only the efficiency of surveillance in total but also the control across all sectors.

Another application of the One Health approach is the unity and clarity that it could bring to risk communication with the general public. The need to communicate uniform and coherent information by human and veterinary health authorities has sometimes been called the "One Communication" concept (Cipolla et al. 2015). In the absence of such a communication approach, it is likely that the human, animal, and wildlife professionals would provide contradictory messages. Let us take an example of a disease that has the potential to spread through cow's milk. With prevention in mind, public health professionals would say that drinking milk should be stopped, whereas wildlife and animal health professionals would say that it is ok to consume boiled or cooked milk. Thus, it could be very challenging and confusing for the general public to comprehend, digest, and act upon. In contrast, if professionals from all three sectors get together, discuss, come to a consensus based on facts, and then deliver the unanimous risk communication messages, it is likely that the general public will have less confusion and will be more likely to take action.

Table 1.7 One Health issues.

1) Zoonotic diseases
2) Antimicrobial resistance
3) Food safety and food security
4) Vector-borne diseases
5) Environmental contamination
6) Health threats on humans (chronic disease, mental health, injury, occupational health, and non-communicable diseases)
7) Health threats on animals
8) Health threats on the environment

Several issues have been identified that need to be addressed using the One Health approach, where the intersection between human, animal, and environmental health becomes significant (Table 1.7).

Some of the One Health issues listed in Table 1.7 are discussed in detail in the following sections.

1.8.1 Zoonotic Diseases

Zoonoses are infectious diseases that could be transmitted from animals, either domestic or wild, to humans or from humans to animals. In contrast to anthroponosis, which can be transmitted between humans, the spillover from the animal to the human or human to the animal is the whole mark feature of zoonosis.

Out of 1415 species of infectious organisms known to be pathogenic to humans, 868 (61%) are found to be zoonotic. In addition, out of the pathogenic organisms, 175 species are considered to be emerging. It has been found that zoonotic pathogens are more likely to be associated with emerging diseases than non-emerging ones. When considering the emerging infections, 75% were found to be zoonotic. Further, it was found that zoonotic pathogens were twice as likely to be associated with EIDs as non-zoonotic pathogens (Taylor et al. 2001).

The One Health approach is essential for the early identification of diseases with zoonotic potential in animals through surveillance. Sharing the results of such surveillance with the human health institution could contribute to the prevention of spillover to humans. In addition,

Case Study – Identification of West Nile Fever Outbreak in New York City

It was observed that many birds, starting with American crows to Chilean Flamingos and snowy owls, were dying unusually in New York in 1999. In the meantime, an unusual outbreak of equine encephalitis was also observed on Long Island. A human outbreak of encephalitis was also found simultaneously. The human outbreak was initially thought to be due to St. Louis encephalitis virus. However, subsequently, it was found that the avian, equine, and human infections were due to West Nile fever virus (WNV). The introduction of WNV to the USA was a clear example of the need for the One Health approach in the surveillance and management of emerging zoonotic infectious diseases (Nash et al. 2001).

uniform messages, agreed upon by health, animal, and environmental professionals, could help launch community awareness and engagement projects targeting the prevention and control of zoonoses.

1.8.2 Antimicrobial Resistance

AMR in bacteria arises when changes in bacteria lead the medications used to treat infections to become less effective. AMR will soon escalate to be one of the most serious public health issues of the twenty-first century. It is predicted that by 2050, 10 million lives will be lost per year due to antibacterial resistance in the world. In the meantime, the cumulative economic costs for the same period would be 100 trillion US dollars, accounting to 2.5–3.0% loss of Gross Domestic Product (GDP) globally (O'Neil 2014). It was estimated that in 2019, 1.27 million deaths (95% uncertainty interval [UI] 0.911–1.71) were directly attributable to resistance, while 4.95 million deaths (3.62–6.57) were associated with bacterial AMR globally for the same year (Murray et al. 2022). As per the Antibiotic Resistance Threat Report in 2019 by the CDC, it was found that more than 2.8 million antibiotic-resistant infections occur in the United States, with over 35,000 people dying as a result. In addition, nearly 223,900 people in the United States required hospitalization for *Clostridium difficile*, and at least 12,800 died as a result of the infection in 2017 (CDC 2022a).

Antibacterial resistance can occur due to several reasons. In the human health field, over-prescription of antibiotics by healthcare professionals and incomplete use of antibiotics by patients contribute to antibacterial resistance. In the animal health sector, overuse of antibiotics in livestock and fish farming has been identified. There have been arguments on which sector is responsible for this phenomenon, human health or animal health. These arguments have contributed to challenges in addressing this rising global concern.

One Health approach could help bring human health, animal health, and environmental health professionals under one umbrella for the shared analysis of the problem as well as the planning, implementation, and evaluation of effective interventions (McEwen and Collignon 2018). Human health and animal health have to agree upon best practices for the rational use of antibiotics. Infection prevention and control become essential in both human and animal health settings. General hygiene measures need to be adhered to by people, while such practices should be implemented in animal husbandry and fish farming settings. This means improving our practices with infection control, hygiene, and animal husbandry. We need to improve the development and delivery of effective and safe vaccines for humans and animals to reduce the need for antibiotics. The environmental health professional could help in ensuring access to safe water, which in turn could reduce infections and subsequently the need for antibiotic use. Further, environmental health professionals could assist in the surveillance of antibacterials in the environment, for example in surface water and sewerage. In addition, they could assist in designing methods for the removal of these substances from the ecosystem when the concentrations go beyond the critical levels. All these measures should be coupled with public awareness on the rational use of antibiotics as well as their disposal through uniform messages that have been agreed upon by professionals from all sectors (McEwen and Collignon 2018; Collignon and McEwen 2019; Langbehn et al. 2021).

It should be clear by now that without a multistakeholder coordination and collaboration mechanism like One Health, these complex issues could not be addressed by one sector alone effectively.

1.8.3 Food Safety and Food Security

Food safety is central to One Health (Boqvist et al. 2018). Many, but not all, of these zoonotic pathogens can be found in food (Abebe et al. 2020). Bovine spongiform encephalopathy (BSE) and *Escherichia coli* outbreaks are examples of food-related zoonoses. However, food safety concerns can extend beyond infectious organisms. Dioxin and melamine pollution are two examples. The absence of cross-sectoral collaboration across the food supply chain, including those from the animal health, food control, and human health sectors, has been one of the primary concerns in food safety (Wielinga and Schlundt 2012).

By 2050, the global human population is predicted to reach 9.7 billion people (United Nations, Department of Economic and Social Affairs, Population Division 2022). To meet demand, food demand is expected to rise by 35–56% by 2050 compared to 2010 (van Dijk et al. 2021). In addition to food quantity, food composition will shift toward more animal-based proteins, driven by economic development and urbanization. For example, protein consumption per capita has increased worldwide over the last 50 years, growing from 61 g per person per day in 1961–1973 to 80 g per person per day in 2009–2011 (Henchion et al. 2017).

As shown in Figure 1.4, global meat production is rising fastest in Asia, with some rise seen in Africa and South America as well. Over the period of 2010–2018, meat consumption seems to be quite stable in Europe, North America, Central America, and Oceania (Ritchie and Roser 2017).

As per Figure 1.5, it is clear that the total meat production in China has risen well passing that of the USA since the 1990s and is continuing to rise (Ritchie and Roser 2017).

Natural disasters can also have restrained food security. Further, animal and plant disease outbreaks could have serious impacts on food production. Transboundary

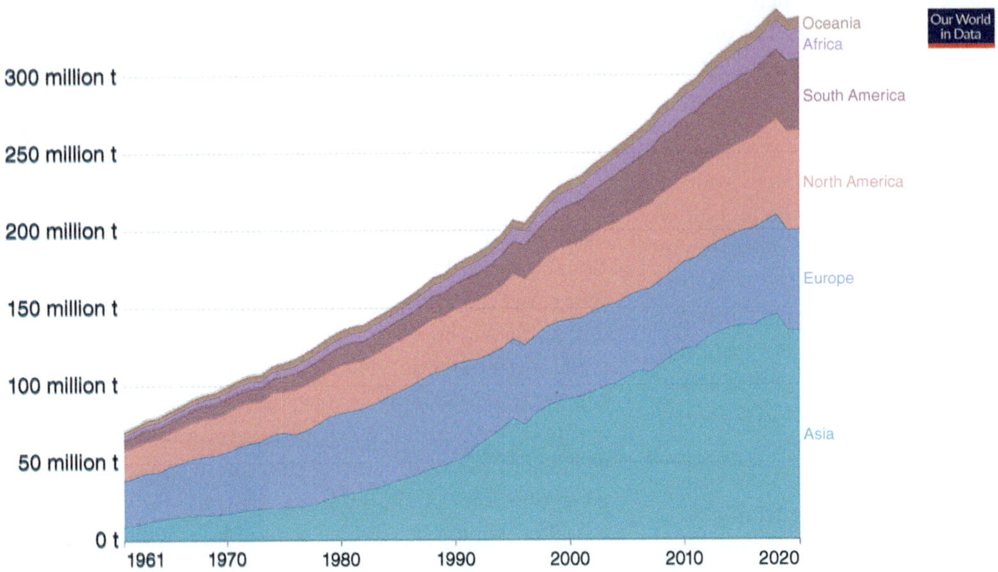

Figure 1.4 Global meat production 1961–2020 (*Source:* Ritchie and Roser 2017 and Food and Agriculture Organization of the United Nations/CC BY 4.0).

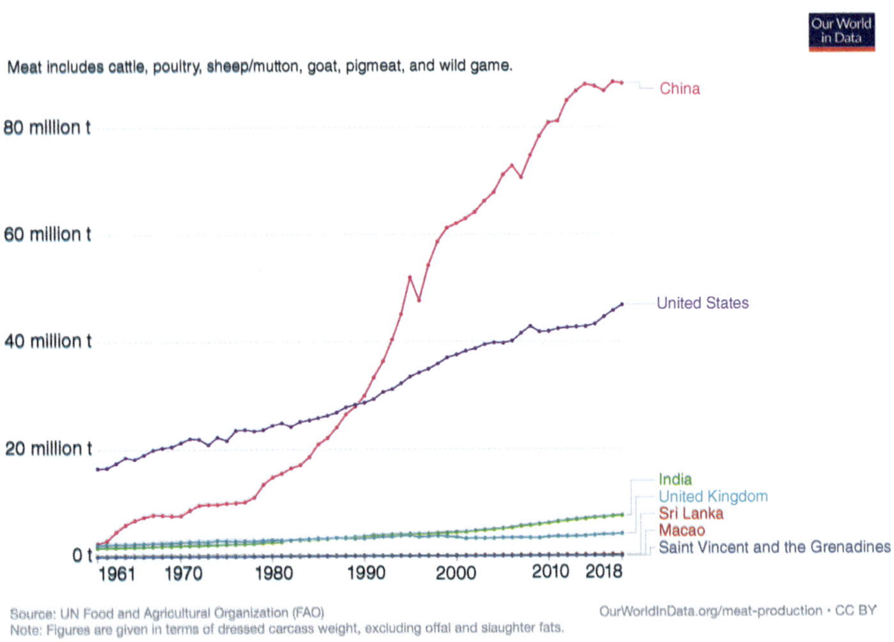

Figure 1.5 Meat production, 1961–2018.

Table 1.8 Transboundary diseases.

Transboundary diseases that can affect animals	Transboundary diseases that can affect both animals and humans
Foot-and-mouth disease	Brucellosis
Peste des petits ruminants	Bovine tuberculosis
Classical or African swine fevers	Parasitic illnesses
	Anthrax
	Bovine spongiform encephalopathy (BSE) and certain strains of influenza viruses

animal illnesses need special mention in this regard. Transboundary animal diseases are highly contagious epidemic diseases that can spread quickly across country borders. They cause high rates of animal death and disease, which can have serious impacts on food security, in addition to their socioeconomic and occasional human health impacts (Clemmons et al. 2021) (Table 1.8).

As much as for adequate safety, food security also demands close coordination of different sectors such as agriculture, animal husbandry, fish farming, and also human health, especially with regard to transboundary diseases that could affect human beings.

1.8.4 Vector-Borne Disease

As discussed earlier, zoonotic diseases are primarily diseases that exist in animals but are transmitted from animals to humans. A vector-borne disease on the other hand is transmitted by vectors such as mosquitoes or fleas. They carry pathogenic agents such as bacteria, viruses or parasites to healthy humans from infected humans, animals or vectors themselves. Therefore, some diseases could be classified as zoonotic vector-borne diseases (Table 1.9).

Table 1.9 Relationship between zoonotic and vector-borne diseases.

Zoonotic diseases but not vector-borne	Zoonotic and vector-borne	Not zoonotic but vector-borne
Brucellosis	Leishmaniasis	Chickungunya
Emerging coronaviruses	Lyme disease	Dengue
Leptospirosis	Lymphatic filarisis (*Brugia malayi*)	Lymphatic filariasis (Wucheraris brancofti)
Salomonella	Plague	Malaria
Rabies	Typhus (Flea-borne, endemic)	Zika
Tuberculosis	Rift valley fever	
	West Nile Fever	
	Yellow fever	

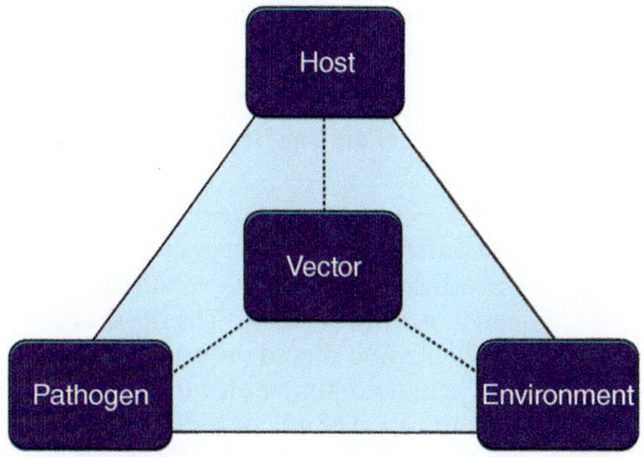

Figure 1.6 Epidemiological triad.

From Table 1.9, it is clear that certain diseases could be transferred from animals to humans without a vector, while the others could not. In addition, some can be transmitted from an infected person to another without an animal as an intermediate. The epidemiological triad has been used to describe the relationship between the vector, host, agent, and the environment (Figure 1.6).

The vector plays a critical role in connecting the host with the pathogen and the environment (CDC 2021). Therefore, any activities aimed at the prevention and control of vector-borne diseases, especially with a zoonotic host, call for coordinated action by the human, animal, and environmental health sectors for their control, which is the essence of the One Health approach.

1.8.5 Environmental Contamination

One Health approach has been used traditionally to address infectious diseases. However, it has been proven that the same approach could be used to address environmental contamination, which spreads across the boundaries of humans, animals, and the environment. The same epidemiological methods, as well as the disease control measures, could be used with the participation of human, animal, and environmental health authorities in addressing such environmental contamination issues.

Three examples of environmental contamination issues that were addressed through a One Health approach are summarized in Table 1.10.

1.9 COVID-19 and One Health

SARS-CoV-2 isolates from humans are genetically similar to coronaviruses obtained from bat populations, notably bats of the genus Rhinolophus. SARS-CoV, the virus that caused the 2003 SARS outbreak, is also closely linked to coronaviruses recovered from bats. These close genetic

Table 1.10 Example of environmental contamination issues addressed through One Health approach.

Year	Country	Summary of the One Health approach used
2004	Kenya	An outbreak of jaundice was investigated, which pointed out an environmental etiology. The deaths of chickens who shared the same food as the jaundiced humans led to the identification of aflatoxin-contaminated maize as the causative agent (Probst et al. 2007).
2009	Bangladesh	A disease was observed among the children in Bangladesh in the Dhmrai Subdistrict of Dhaka, Bangladesh. Infectious agents were excluded. Sudden deaths of calves and puppies in and close to the affected villages signaled an environmental etiology. The clinical signs in humans and animals signaled a cholinesterase inhibitor pesticide as the environmental etiology. Carbofuran, a carbamate-type pesticide, was revealed as the likely etiological agent (Mandour 2013).
2008	USA	Harmful algal blooms are a common occurrence in Florida, USA. A toxic dinoflagellate *Karenia brevis*. *K. brevis* produces a neurotoxin named as Brevotoxin. This neurotoxin can contaminate coastal aerosols or sea spray, giving rise to the neurotoxic shellfish poisoning. Susceptible individuals could report upper and lower respiratory tract irritation and measurable changes in pulmonary function. An integrated Ocean Observation System (IOOS) has been established with real-time reporting from lifeguards on the amount of dead fish, apparent levels of respiratory irritation among the people on the beach, and observation of the water color, surf condition, and beach warnings used (Pierce and Henry 2008).

relationships imply that they all originated in bat populations (WHO 2020).

The Huanan Wholesale Seafood Market in Wuhan City was directly linked to a major proportion of the initial cases in late December 2019 and early January 2020. The virus could have entered the human population through an animal or an infected human (Worobey et al. 2022).

Subsequently, the first human cases of SARS-CoV-2 infection have been identified as early as 1 December 2019, but these cases did not have a connection with the animal market. Additional studies are ongoing to determine whether unrecognized infections in humans may have happened earlier through contact with undetected cases.

At this time, it is not possible to pinpoint how individuals in China became infected with SARS-CoV-2. All known information, however, suggests that SARS-CoV-2 is of natural animal origin and is not a modified or engineered virus. The SARS-CoV-2 virus's ecological reservoir is most likely bats.

SARS-CoV-2, the virus that causes COVID-19, is a zoonotic virus, which means it can pass between humans and animals. As more animals are found to be infected with the COVID-19 virus, it becomes evident that a One Health strategy is critical to addressing new disease threats that affect both humans and animals. The worldwide geographical distribution of SARS-CoV-2 outbreaks in animals compiled by Food and Agricultural Organization (FAO) is shown in Figure 1.7.

The first case of SARS-CoV-2 in animals was officially reported to the (WOAH, Founded as OIE) by Hong Kong (SARC) on 29 February 2021 in a dog. The occurrence of the disease has been reported from 35 countries in the Americas, Africa, Asia, and Europe in 19 different animal species (cats, dogs, mink, otter, pet ferrets, lions, tigers, pumas, snow leopards, gorillas, white-tailed deer, fishing cat, Binturong, South American coati, spotted hyena, Eurasian lynx, Canada lynx, hippopotamus, and hamster) (World Organization for Animal Health 2022).

As per the evidence so far, animals do not appear to play a substantial role in the virus's spread among humans. Nevertheless, investigations using the One Health approach as well as animal surveillance are critical for evaluating the transmission between humans and animals. Such rigorous surveillance is essential since it will enhance our knowledge of the animals that can be infected as well as the hazards of the virus establishing new hosts and reservoirs where it can hide, evolve, and potentially reemerge as a new variation in the human population. The CDC's One Health Office is aiming to support One Health efforts and increase cross-sector collaboration. It is essential to strengthen the existing surveillance system, including that for animal and environmental health, as well as rapidly establish such systems in locations where they do not exist. National and sub-national surveillance and reporting systems for laboratory and epidemiological data on SARS-CoV-2 disease are critical components of putting One Health principles into practice.

The need for unified risk communication from professionals from all three sectors becomes extremely important during this phase, where outbreaks are occurring not only in humans but also in animals. Messaging for humans engaging with animals during the pandemic, including preventive measures, as well as steps to follow if their animals show symptoms of COVID-19 are so vital. In an

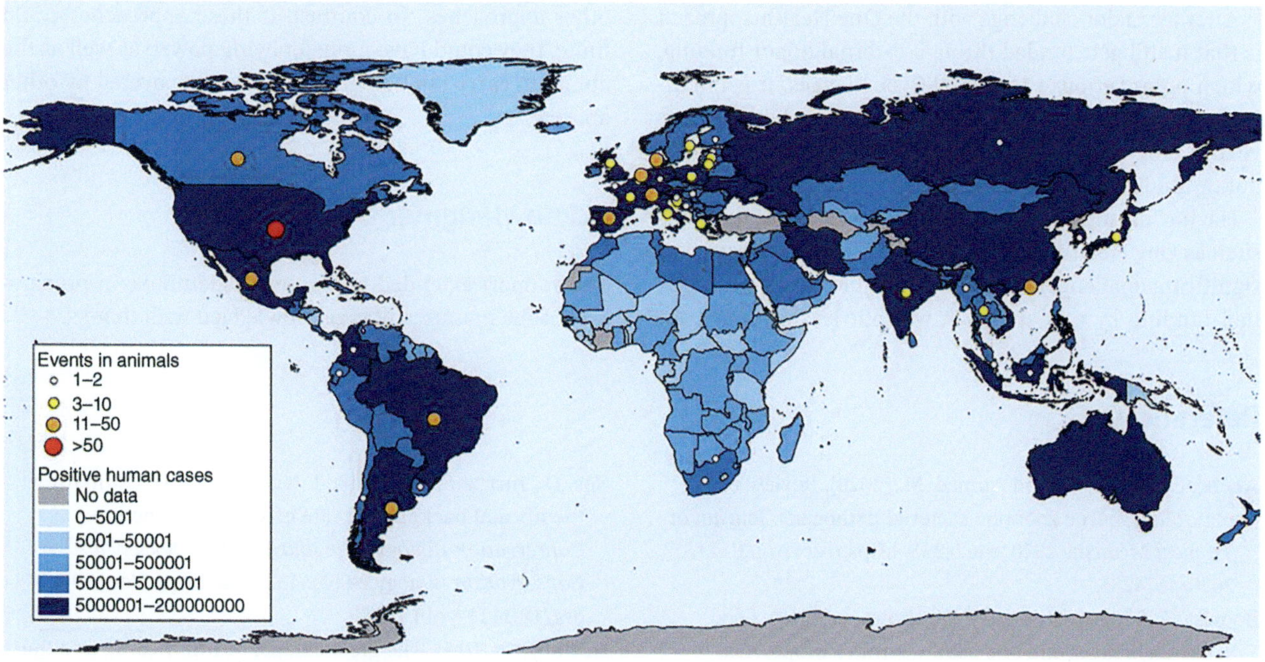

Figure 1.7 Map of published SARS-CoV-2 events in animals up to 6 December 2022 at national level, over a cumulative COVID-19 human cases background map.

environment of the rule of misinformation among the pandemic, such simple yet practically useful verified shared information from the professionals from all three disciplines cannot be over-emphasized.

1.10 Road Map for One Health

The One Health approach aims to sustainably balance and optimize the health of people, animals, and ecosystems through an integrated and unified approach. To achieve this goal, a road map for One Health calls for coordinated and collaborative approaches among the whole range of stakeholders involved, coupled with effective communication and capacity building.

The 10-Fold One Health Road Map calls for an increase in collaboration between the human, animal, and environmental health sectors and disciplines at the global, national, sub-national, and community level.

1) To advocate for the need of One Health approach and resource allocation for One Health to health and non-health decision makers.
2) To establish One Health Communities of Practice with clear channels of communication between each level and a governance structure.
3) To carryout collaborative basic and applied research to increase understanding of the interplay between healthy humans, healthy animals, and healthy ecosystems.
4) To strengthen surveillance and early-warning systems to pick up and act upon signals of diseases and contributory factors.
5) To innovate solutions to prevent and control health threats, including new medications and vaccines.
6) To increase intra- and inter-sectoral and disciplinary capacity building.
7) To effectively communicate risk to communities about threats to health.
8) To ensure rational and sustainable use of antimicrobial drugs.
9) To ensure the inclusivity of all segments of society including those who are most vulnerable, in One Health planning, implementation, monitoring, and evaluation while ensuring the equity and access.
10) To develop a joint One Health Results Based Monitoring and Evaluation Framework that is linked to other global frameworks such as Sustainable Development Goals, IHR, and Planetary Health.

1.11 Challenges of One Health Approach

Despite being a powerful concept, One Health still faces many implementation challenges. Even though conceptually One Health calls for all professionals to act together, in practice wider engagement of stakeholders still needs to be improved.

Another major challenge with the One Health approach is that it still gets funded through external donor funding, which poses serious sustainability challenges. It is important that domestic funding is allocated so that the One Health program continues even in the absence of external donor funding.

Having multiple overlapping and competing concepts such as One Health, Eco Health, and Planetary Health is a significant challenge. This situation could exhaust the limited funding by one approach without leaving much for other approaches. In contrast, if these approaches could unite, they could have more lobbying power, as well as the ability to carry out activities that are not covered by other approaches.

Acknowledgment

The support extended by Banura Nadathilake in preparation of the manuscript is acknowledged with thanks.

References

Abebe, E., Gugsa, G., and Ahmed, M. (2020). Review on major food-borne zoonotic bacterial pathogens. *Journal of Tropical Medicine* 2020: e4674235. https://doi.org/10.1155/2020/4674235.

Boqvist, S., Söderqvist, K., and Vågsholm, I. (2018). Food safety challenges and one health within Europe. *Acta Veterinaria Scandinavica* 60 (1): 1. https://doi.org/10.1186/s13028-017-0355-3.

CDC (2021). Principles of epidemiology|lesson 1 – section 8. https://www.cdc.gov/csels/dsepd/ss1978/lesson1/section8.html (accessed 17 August 2022).

CDC (2022a). Antibiotic resistance threat report. *Centers for Disease Control and Prevention.* https://www.cdc.gov/drugresistance/biggest-threats.html (accessed 6 August 2022).

CDC (2022b). History|one health|CDC. https://www.cdc.gov/onehealth/basics/history/index.html (accessed 23 July 2022).

CDC (2022c). One health in action|one health|CDC. https://www.cdc.gov/onehealth/in-action/index.html (accessed 31 July 2022).

Church, D.L. (2004). Major factors affecting the emergence and re-emergence of infectious diseases. *Clinics in Laboratory Medicine* 24 (3): 559–586. https://doi.org/10.1016/j.cll.2004.05.008.

Cipolla, M., Bonizzi, L., and Zecconi, A. (2015). From 'one health' to 'one communication': the contribution of communication in veterinary medicine to public health. *Veterinary Sciences* 2 (3): 135–149. https://doi.org/10.3390/vetsci2030135.

Clemmons, E.A., Alfson, K.J., and Dutton, J.W. (2021). Transboundary animal diseases, an overview of 17 diseases with potential for global spread and serious consequences. *Animals: An Open Access Journal from MDPI* 11 (7): 2039. https://doi.org/10.3390/ani11072039.

Collignon, P.J. and McEwen, S.A. (2019). One health-its importance in helping to better control antimicrobial resistance. *Tropical Medicine and Infectious Disease* 4 (1): E22. https://doi.org/10.3390/tropicalmed4010022.

Vos, D., Jurriaan, M., Joppa, L.N. et al. (2015). Estimating the normal background rate of species extinction. *Conservation Biology: The Journal of the Society for Conservation Biology* 29 (2): 452–462. https://doi.org/10.1111/cobi.12380.

Deaton, A. (2015). The great escape: health, wealth, and the origins of inequality. In: *Economics Books*, 1ee, 73–78. Princeton University Press.

van Dijk, M., Morley, T., Rau, M.L., and Saghai, Y. (2021). A meta-analysis of projected global food demand and population at risk of hunger for the period 2010–2050. *Nature Food* 2 (7): 494–501. https://doi.org/10.1038/s43016-021-00322-9.

Gibbs, E. and Paul, J. (2014). The evolution of one health: a decade of progress and challenges for the future. *Veterinary Record* 174 (4): 85–91. https://doi.org/10.1136/vr.g143.

Global Health Security Agenda (2014). Global Health Security Agenda. *Global Health Security Agenda.* https://ghsagenda.org (accessed 31 July 2022).

Haines, A., Scheelbeek, P., and Abbasi, K. (2019). Challenges for health in the anthropocene epoch. *BMJ* 364: https://doi.org/10.1136/bmj.l460.

Health (US), National Institutes of, and Biological Sciences Curriculum Study (2007). *Understanding Emerging and re-Emerging Infectious Diseases.* National Institutes of Health (US).

Henchion, M., Hayes, M., Mullen, A.M. et al. (2017). Future protein supply and demand: strategies and factors influencing a sustainable equilibrium. *Foods* 6 (7): 53. https://doi.org/10.3390/foods6070053.

Jackson, J.B.C. (2010). The future of the oceans past. *Philosophical Transactions of the Royal Society B: Biological Sciences* 365 (1558): 3765–3778. https://doi.org/10.1098/rstb.2010.0278.

Langbehn, R.K., Michels, C., and Soares, H.M. (2021). Antibiotics in wastewater: from its occurrence to the biological removal by environmentally conscious technologies. *Environmental Pollution (Barking, Essex: 1987)* 275: 116603. https://doi.org/10.1016/j.envpol.2021.116603.

Lerner, H. and Berg, C. (2017). A comparison of three holistic approaches to health: One Health, EcoHealth, and Planetary Health. *Frontiers in Veterinary Science* 4: 163. https://doi.org/10.3389/fvets.2017.00163.

Lisitza, A. and Wolbring, G. (2018). EcoHealth and the determinants of health: perspectives of a small subset of Canadian academics in the EcoHealth community. *International Journal of Environmental Research and Public Health* 15 (8): 1688. https://doi.org/10.3390/ijerph15081688.

Mandour, R.A. (2013). Environmental risks of insecticides cholinesterase inhibitors. *Toxicology International* 20 (1): 30–34. https://doi.org/10.4103/0971-6580.111556.

McEwen, S.A. and Collignon, P.J. (2018). Antimicrobial resistance: a one health perspective. *Microbiology Spectrum* 6 (2): https://doi.org/10.1128/microbiolspec.ARBA-0009-2017.

Miller, G. (1962). 'Airs, waters, and places' in history. *Journal of the History of Medicine and Allied Sciences* 17 (1): 129–140.

Monath, T.P., Kahn, L.H., and Kaplan, B. (2010). Introduction: one health perspective. *ILAR Journal* 51 (3): 193–198. https://doi.org/10.1093/ilar.51.3.193.

Morens, D.M. and Fauci, A.S. (2020). Emerging Pandemic Diseases: How We Got to COVID-19. *Cell* 182, (5): 1077–1092. ISSN 0092-8674, https://doi.org/10.1016/j.cell.2020.08.021. (https://www.sciencedirect.com/science/article/pii/S0092867420310126)

Morens, D.M., Folkers, G.K., and Fauci, A.S. (2004). The challenge of emerging and re-emerging infectious diseases. *Nature* 430 (6996): 242–249. https://doi.org/10.1038/nature02759.

Murray, C.J., Ikuta, K.S., Sharara, F. et al. (2022). Global burden of bacterial antimicrobial resistance in 2019: a systematic analysis. *The Lancet* 399 (10325): 629–655. https://doi.org/10.1016/S0140-6736(21)02724-0.

Nash, D., Mostashari, F., Fine, A. et al. (2001). The outbreak of West Nile virus infection in the New York city area in 1999. *New England Journal of Medicine* 344 (24): 1807–1814. https://doi.org/10.1056/NEJM200106143442401.

One Health Commission (n.d.). What is one health? https://www.onehealthcommission.org/en/why_one_health/what_is_one_health (accessed 20 July 2022).

One Health Initiative (2019). The one health umbrella. *One Health Initiative*. https://onehealthinitiative.com/the-one-health-umbrella (accessed 31 July 2022).

O'Neil, J. (2014). *Antimicrobial Resistance: Tackling a Crisis for the Health and Weatlh of Nations - The Review on Antimicrobial Resistance Chaired by Jim O'Neil*.

Panel (OHHLEP), One Health High-Level Expert, Adisasmito, W.B., Almuhairi, S. et al. (2022). One health: a new definition for a sustainable and healthy future. *PLoS Pathogens* 18 (6): e1010537. https://doi.org/10.1371/journal.ppat.1010537.

Pierce, R.H. and Henry, M.S. (2008). Harmful algal toxins of the Florida red tide (Karenia brevis): natural chemical stressors in South Florida coastal ecosystems. *Ecotoxicology (London, England)* 17 (7): 623–631. https://doi.org/10.1007/s10646-008-0241-x.

Pinker, S. (2020). Enlightenment now, the case for reason, science, humanism, and progress. *Revista Española de Investigaciones Sociológicas (REIS)* 170 (170): 163–167.

Probst, C., Njapau, H., and Cotty, P.J. (2007). Outbreak of an acute Aflatoxicosis in Kenya in 2004: identification of the causal agent. *Applied and Environmental Microbiology* 73 (8): 2762–2764. https://doi.org/10.1128/AEM.02370-06.

Ritchie, H. and Roser, M. (2017). *Meat and Dairy Production*. Our World in Data. OurWorldInData.org. https://ourworldindata.org/meat-production [Online Resource].

Steffen, W., Richardson, K., Rockström, J. et al. (2015). Planetary boundaries: guiding human development on a changing planet. *Science* 347 (6223): 1259855. https://doi.org/10.1126/science.1259855.

Tabish, S.A. (2009). Recent trends in emerging infectious diseases. *International Journal of Health Sciences* 3 (2): V–VIII.

Taylor, A. and Habibi, R. (2020). *The Collapse of Global Cooperation under the International Health Regulations at the Outset of COVID-19*. The American Society of International Law, ASIL Insights.

Taylor, L.H., Latham, S.M., and Woolhouse, M.E. (2001). Risk factors for human disease emergence. *Philosophical Transactions of the Royal Society B: Biological Sciences* 356 (1411): 983–989. https://doi.org/10.1098/rstb.2001.0888.

United Nations, Department of Economic and Social Affairs, Population Division. 2022. *World Population Prospects 2022: Ten Key Messages*.

Verma, V. (n.d.). A brief note on classification and treatment of emerging infectious diseases. *Journal of Infectious Diseases & Diagnosis* 6 (S3) NO: 1000003: 2.

Waltner-Toews, D. (2009). Eco-health: a primer for veterinarians. *The Canadian Veterinary Journal* 50 (5): 519–521.

Whitmee, S., Haines, A., Beyrer, C. et al. (2015). Safeguarding human health in the Anthropocene epoch: report of the Rockefeller Foundation–lancet commission on planetary health. *The Lancet* 386 (10007): 1973–2028. https://doi.org/10.1016/S0140-6736(15)60901-1.

WHO (2016). *International Health Regulations (2005)*, 3e. Geneva, Switzerland: WHO.

WHO (2017). One health. https://www.who.int/news-room/questions-and-answers/item/one-health (accessed 31 July 2022).

WHO (2020). *Origin of SARS-CoV-2*. WHO.

WHO (2021). Tripartite and UNEP support OHHLEP's definition of 'one health. https://www.who.int/news/item/01-12-2021-tripartite-and-unep-support-ohhlep-s-definition-of-one-health (accessed 31 July 2022).

WHO (2022). Indicator metadata registry details. https://www.who.int/data/gho/indicator-metadata-registry/imr-details/4824 (31 July 2022).

Wielinga, P.R. and Schlundt, J. (2012). Food safety: at the Center of a one health approach for combating Zoonoses. *One Health: The Human-Animal-Environment Interfaces in Emerging Infectious Diseases* 366: 3–17. https://doi.org/10.1007/82_2012_238.

Woolhouse, M.E.J. and Gowtage-Sequeria, S. (2005). Host range and emerging and reemerging pathogens. *Emerging Infectious Diseases Journal* 11 (12): https://doi.org/10.3201/eid1112.050997.

World Organization for Animal Health (2022). *SARS-COV-2 IN ANIMALS – SITUATION REPORT 12.*

World Organisation for *Animal* Health (2019). OIE Tool for the Evaluation of Performance of Veterinary Services SeventhEdition. https://www.woah.org/app/uploads/2021/03/2019-pvs-tool-final.pdf.

Worobey, Michael, Joshua I. Levy, Lorena Malpica Serrano, Alexander Crits-Christoph, Jonathan E. Pekar, Stephen A. Goldstein, Angela L. Rasmussen, Moritz U. G. Kraemer, Chris Newman, Marion P. G. Koopmans, Marc A. Suchard, Joel O. Wertheim, Philippe Lemey, David L. Robertson, Robert F. Garry, Edward C. Holmes, Andrew Rambaut, and Kristian G. Andersen. 2022. "The Huanan seafood wholesale market in Wuhan was the early Epicenter of the COVID-19 pandemic." *Science* 0(0):abp8715. https://doi.org/10.1126/science.abp8715.

Zalasiewicz, J., Waters, C.N., Summerhayes, C.P. et al. (2017). The working group on the Anthropocene: summary of evidence and interim recommendations. *Anthropocene* 19: 55–60. https://doi.org/10.1016/j.ancene.2017.09.001.

2

Emergence and Re-emergence of Emerging Infectious Diseases (EIDs)

Looking at "One Health" Through the Lens of Ecology

Jayanta Kumar Biswas[1,2], *Progya Mukherjee*[1], *Meththika Vithanage*[3], *and Majeti Narasimha Vara Prasad*[4]

[1] *Enviromicrobiology, Ecotoxicology and Ecotechnology Research Laboratory (3E-MicroToxTech Lab), Department of Ecological Studies, University of Kalyani, Kalyani, West Bengal, India*
[2] *International Centre for Ecological Engineering, University of Kalyani, Kalyani, West Bengal, India*
[3] *Ecosphere Resilience Research Centre, Faculty of Applied Sciences, University of Sri Jayewardenepura, Nugegoda, Sri Lanka*
[4] *School of Life Sciences, University of Hyderabad, Hyderabad, Telangana, India*

2.1 Introduction

In the twenty-first century, we are living in the luxury of well-furnished homes, sweet-smelling toilets, and sterilized food with the mundane idea of nirvana from the plethora of diseases that seemed to have plagued the human society ever since the beginning of human civilization centuries ago, but this imaginative bubble was brutally pricked by the advent of SARS-CoV-2, which ravaged the human society through and through ever since its advent in late December 2019 with an increased frequency of severe pneumonia cases in Wuhan, Hubei Province, China (Zhou et al. 2020), taking the shape of a global pandemic by 11 March 2020. The menacing effects of COVID-19 have brought everyone to the mercy of nature; the human supremacy has been shaken to some extent, indicating uncertainties in the future. The emerging infectious diseases (EID) have repeatedly reshaped the course of civilization, creating new norms and ways to start afresh. It is high time for us to view the Earth through the lens of ecology and to develop a better understanding of the deterioration of the ecological barrier that has led to the emergence and re-emergence of infectious diseases since prehistoric times. The advent of the Anthropocene era, which marked the dawn of the realization that human activity was indeed changing the Earth on a scale comparable with some of the major events of the ancient past. Human beings bring about permanent changes on the Earth's surface due to the unprecedented population growth from less than a billion to about eight billion in the present day. This exponential rise in population has led to the vast expense of fossil fuels, bringing about the industrial revolution coupled with rapid growth of urbanization. Mechanizing agricultural fields to feed billions of mouths propelled by the increasing economic growth and energy consumption has led to land use changes. Consequently higher magnitude of long-term erosion has heavily modified the soils of our fields, and the polluted water bodies, bringing about chemical and biological effects, that include the changes in the concentrations of carbon dioxide (CO_2), methane (CH_4), and other greenhouse gases. Today, the rise in CO_2 level to over a third above preindustrial levels has been demonstrated beyond reasonable doubt: by systematic measurement since the 1950s. According to the IPCC (2021) AR6, atmospheric CO_2 concentrations were higher in 2019 than at any time in at least 2 million years, and concentrations of CH_4 and N_2O were higher than at any time in at least 800,000 years. Since 1750s increases in CO_2 (47%) and CH_4 (156%) concentrations far exceed, and increases in N_2O (23%) were similar to the natural multi-millennial changes between glacial and interglacial periods over at least the past 800,000 years. Thus clearly the increased human dominance has outcompeted the natural processes to a great extent putting the ecosystem, biodiversity, and the overall safety of the planet at stake, which is evident through the creation of the halocarbon-induced ozone hole, increased acid rain, and the drastic land use changes. As a result 30–50% of the land surface of the world has been transformed, bringing double the land area under cultivation and declining the forest cover by about 20%. The coastal areas have also been affected, declining the mangrove population, worsening the ecosystem health, opening the floodgates of numerous EIDs, evolving the host–pathogen relationships driven by the constant arms race between microbial pathogens

One Health: Human, Animal, and Environment Triad, First Edition. Edited by Meththika Vithanage and Majeti Narasimha Vara Prasad.

and their hosts. The pathogens invade the host and to evade its defense, they develop drug resistance, adapt to the changing host environmental conditions more favorable for the r-selected species, and evolve virulence and transmission from one host to another breaking the boundary.

2.2 Emerging Infectious Diseases

An important principle of disease ecology is that population, society, and environment (both physical and biological) exist in dynamic equilibrium, and stress on this equilibrium can result in a cascade of emerging and re-emerging diseases. Like wars and famines infectious diseases have appeared as major challenges for centuries to humanity's sustenance and progress and remain the leading causes of death and disability worldwide. Against a constant background of established infections, epidemics of new and old infectious diseases emerge periodically, significantly increasing the global burden of infections. Studies of these emerging infections reveal the evolutionary properties of pathogenic microorganisms and the pathogenicity triad, i.e. the dynamic relationships between microorganisms, their hosts, and the environment (Morens et al. 2004). While discussing emerging diseases, it is essential to have a clear idea about its definition as the use of the word "emerging" has been ambiguous. In 1992, the US Institute of Medicine defined "emerging" as subsuming three things: (i) established infectious diseases undergoing increased incidence, (ii) newly discovered infections, and (iii) newly evolving (newly occurring) infections (McMichael 2004). EIDs can be defined as infections that have newly appeared in a population or have existed but are rapidly increasing in incidence or geographic region. Among recent examples are HIV/AIDS, hantavirus pulmonary syndrome (HPS), Lyme disease, and hemolytic uremic syndrome (a foodborne infection caused by certain strains of *Escherichia coli*) (Morse 2001). Our point of interest is the changing environment and the various physicochemical factors that potentiate the emergence of these infectious diseases. The initiation of this environmental event is marked by physical contact between humans and the potential infection (pathogens) that is controlled by a number of anthropogenically driven factors including (i) demographic characteristics and processes, human mobility, etc.; (ii) land use, other environmental changes, and encroachment on new environments; (iii) consumption behaviors (eating, drinking, and, more generally, culinary culture); (iv) other behaviors (sexual contact, drug use, hospital procedures, etc.); and (v) host conditions (malnutrition, diabetes, immune status, etc.).

2.3 Genesis of EIDs: Tracing from Natural History

While tracing the origin of infectious diseases, we date back to 50,000–100,000 years ago that marks the beginning of interpopulational contact, conflict leading to cultural evolution propelled by transition in the human ecology and interpopulational interactions, leading to major transitions between *Homo sapiens* and the natural world comprising both biotic and abiotic, which further leads to the emergence of infectious diseases. The transitions are as follows: (i) *prehistoric transition:* Dated million years ago from tree dwelling to savannahs, parasite fauna (bacteria, virus, protozoa, etc.) was found in the hunter-gatherer higher apes due to change in social relationships, family structure, tribal groupings, and increased movement in unfamiliar environment leading to change in patterns of day-to-day interaction (Dobson and Carper 1996; McMichael 2004). The direct life cycle of macroparasites, i.e. they do not require vectors for transmission, such as pinworms, ascaris, lice, and ticks were probably also common in hunter-gatherer societies, as were sexually transmitted diseases, which sustain in low-density host populations. The changes in social relationship and interactions and human behavior patterns led to three great transitions in human–microbe relationship, occurring in increasingly large scale and was recognizable following the emergence of agriculture and livestock herding. These transitions were first described by historian William McNeill (1976) as "Historic Transition." (ii) *First historic transition:* 50,000–100,000 years ago, during early human settlement enabled the enzootic pathogens to enter the *H. sapiens* (Weiss 2001) through the advent of many mutant urban species like rodents, flies, and pests from herd animals, most of them have failed but some of them like the HIV/AIDS, Nipah virus (NiV), and SARS virus have survived and prospered in the human body. (iii) *Second historic transition:* 1500–3000 years ago, during the early Eurasian civilization, there was swapping of infectious germ pool among Russia, China, and Mediterranean region that led to disastrous results, e.g. Justinian Plague of 542 CE that devastated Constantinople and the Roman Empire. The historical record is evident that China suffered a series of massive epidemics during these times (McNeill 1976). (iv) *Third historic transition:* Marked by European exploration and imperialism, beginning ca. 1500 CE and continuing over the past five centuries causing the trans-ocean shift of lethal infections, devastating impact of the repertoire of infections taken to the Americas by the Spanish conquistadores is well known; such infections mainly occurred during European explorations of the Asia-Pacific region, with European settlement in Australia and with the trans-Atlantic slave trade (McMichael 2004).

(v) *Fourth historic transition:* We are presently living in the fourth historic transition, characterized by changes occurring on every front – economic, demographic, social, environmental, cultural, and technological changes. The economic globalization culture, the rapidity of distant contact, the spread and intensification of urbanization, and our increasing reliance on either intricate or massive technology are reshaping the relations between humans and microbes, leading to changing human ecology, ecosystem stability, and evolutionary trajectory.

Environmental changes through deforestation, forest fragmentation, intensive agriculture, road and canal construction, and other development activities result in significant alterations of local ecosystems and ecological interactions. By extension, the disease is affected through changes in density, distribution, breeding places, and incubation period of vectors and pathogens. Modification and/or destabilization of ecosystem make the environment fit for r-selected species, that is, those small opportunistic species that (in contrast to the larger K species such as humans) live on footloose, rolling stone strategy, reproduce rapidly, invest in prodigious output rather than intensive parenting, and have mechanisms to efficiently disperse their offspring. Parasites are of the r-species, living in the world of increasing opportunity. Climate change is one of the most significant global events leading to the emergence of infections due to induced environmental changes (McMichael 2004). The increased sedentary habits of agriculture led to incidence of macroparasites like *Ascaris* sp. mainly because of the increasingly successful transmission of the long-lived free-living stages, while water supplies became pathogenical contaminated due to protozoan and bacterial infections.

Pathogens shared with wild or domestic animals cause more than 60% of infectious diseases in humans. Such pathogens and diseases include leptospirosis, cysticercosis and echinococcosis, toxoplasmosis, anthrax, brucellosis, rabies, Q fever, Chagas disease, type A influenza, Rift Valley fever, severe acute respiratory syndrome (SARS), Ebola hemorrhagic fever, and the original emergence of HIV. Transmission of pathogens into human populations from other species is a natural product of our relation and interaction with animals and the environment. The dynamics of zoonotic disease transmission are deeply embedded in the ecology and evolutionary biology of their hosts. A zoonosis entails interaction between at least three species: one pathogen and two host species, with people and another animal species acting as the reservoir of the infection. For vector-borne zoonoses, the ecology is complicated because the ecology of numerous other vector and reservoir host species can change transmission dynamics. Directly transmitted zoonoses can also have several reservoir hosts, potentially serving different roles in pathogen dynamics, such as amplification or transmission to human beings. The emergence of newly emerging, re-emerging, and historical kind of zoonoses can be considered as a coherent consequence of pathogens ecology and evolution, as microbes exploit new niches and adapt to new hosts. The underlying causes that create or provide access to these new niches seem to be mediated by anthropogenic activities including changes in land use, exploitation of natural resources, animal production systems, anti-microbial medicines use, current transportation, and international travel and trade. The advent and prevalence of EIDs over time is represented in Table 2.1.

Table 2.1 Advent and geographical prevalence of EIDs over the temporal scale.

Time	Disease	Infectious disease	Causative microorganism	Death	Affected countries/ regions
165–180	Plague of Athens	Small pox or measles Bubonic plague bacteria on rat flea	*Variola major, V. minor* *Morvillivirus* sp. *Yersinia pestis*	5–10 million	Roman empire
541–750	Plague of Justinian	Bubonic plague Small pox	*Yersinia pestis* *Variola major, V. minor*	25–100 million	Egypt, Constantinople
1346–1353	Black Death	Cocoliztli	Possibly *Salmonella enterica*	75–200 million	Worldwide
1518–1520	Small pox	Small pox	*Variola major, V. minor*	5–8 million	Dominican Republic, Haiti, Mexico
1545–1548	Cocoliztli	Cholera	*Vibrio cholera*	5–15 million	Mexico
Seventeenth to eighteenth century	Small pox	Small pox	*Variola major, V. minor*	90% Native Americans	North America
1816–1993	Several phases	Influenza A	Virus H3N8	±2–3 million	

(*Continued*)

Table 2.1 (Continued)

Time	Disease	Infectious disease	Causative microorganism	Death	Affected countries/ regions
1889–1890	Russia flu			1 million	India, China, Europe, Uzbekistan, North America
1918–1920	Spanish flu	Influenza A	Virus H1N1	20–100 million	Worldwide
1918–1922	Russia typhus	Typhus	Bacteria *Rickettsia prowazekii*	2–3 million	Russia
1957–1958	Asian flu	Influenza A	Virus H2N2	2–4 million	China, worldwide
1968–1970	Hong Kong flu	Influenza A	Virus H3N2	1–4 million	Hong Kong, worldwide
2009	H1N1	Influenza A	Virus H1N1	575 thousand	Asia, Africa, worldwide
1976–present	HIV/AIDS	HIV/AIDS	Virus	37.9 million+	Worldwide
2002–2004	SARS	SARS-CoV	Coronavirus	774	Southeast Asia, Egypt
2012–present	MERS	MERS-CoV	Coronavirus	941+	Worldwide
2019–present	COVID-19	SARS-CoV-2	Coronavirus	4.5 million+	Worldwide

2.4 Global Trends of EIDs

Anthropogenic activities have mostly served as the driver for the emergence and re-emergence of EIDs, that has frequently shaped the human society bringing about changes in the ecological systems. Nava et al. (2017) termed this as the "rivers of ecosystem change" defined as "a complex web of interactions between humans and their surroundings as humans seek to satisfy their basic needs and improve their wellbeing." Thus, EIDs pose significant burden on global economics and public health, driven by socioeconomic, environmental, and ecological factors (Jones et al. 2017). In the history of global human population, 335 infectious diseases between 1940 and 2004 have caused innumerable miseries and deaths in the human society, peaking in 1980s and early 1990s with ominous development like recognition of HIV/AIDS epidemic and the re-emergence of tuberculosis, having significant impacts on public health and global economics (Morens et al. 2004), often recognized as global killers and having surpassed the Black Death of the fourteenth century and the influenza pandemic of the years 1918–1921, causing death of about 50 million people in the world. Similar to AIDS minor cases of monkeypox imported into the United States (Illinois, Indiana, and Wisconsin, 2003) and some severe cases like that of SARS that had emerged in the same year caused widespread effects (Morens et al. 2004) in around 2003.

The global map of EIDs clearly furnishes their geographical distribution and prevalence (Figure 2.1; www.http://en.wikipedia.org/wiki/Emerging_infectious_disease#/media/File:Global_Examples_of_Emerging_and_Re-Emerging_Infectious_Diseases.jpg). The majority of pathogens involved in EIDs are bacteria or rickettsia (~53.5%), comprising mainly the drug-resistant strains of bacteria like the vancomycin-resistant *Staphylococcus aureus* and viral or prion cases comprising 25.4% of EID cases. The percentage of causative agents or pathogens of EIDs is found to be 10.7% for protozoa, 6.3% for fungi, and 3.3% for helminths; 60.3% of EIDs are caused due to zoonotic pathogens of which 70.8% are of wildlife origin – for example, the emergence of Nipah virus in Perak, Malaysia, and SARS in Guangdong Province, China. Infections from wildlife origin have risen significantly in the recent decade and constitute 52.0% of EID events; therefore, emphasis must be put on understanding the contact between humans and wildlife. Further, due to the changing global climatic conditions, the emergence of vector-borne diseases has increased with the climate change factors bringing about vectors that are sensitive to environmental and climatic changes like high temperature, heavy rainfall, and severe weather events (Patz et al. 2005). It has been observed that the environmental conditions like temperature and precipitation influence the occurrence of EIDs to some extent; therefore, lower latitudes tend to promote the transmission of diseases to a great extent. It is hypothesized that to drive this pattern, the EID events are mainly concentrated per million square kilometers of land in the latitude between 30° and 60° north and between 30° and 40° south, with the main hotspots in the northeastern United States, western Europe, Japan, and southeastern Australia. The other driving factors including socioeconomic factors like

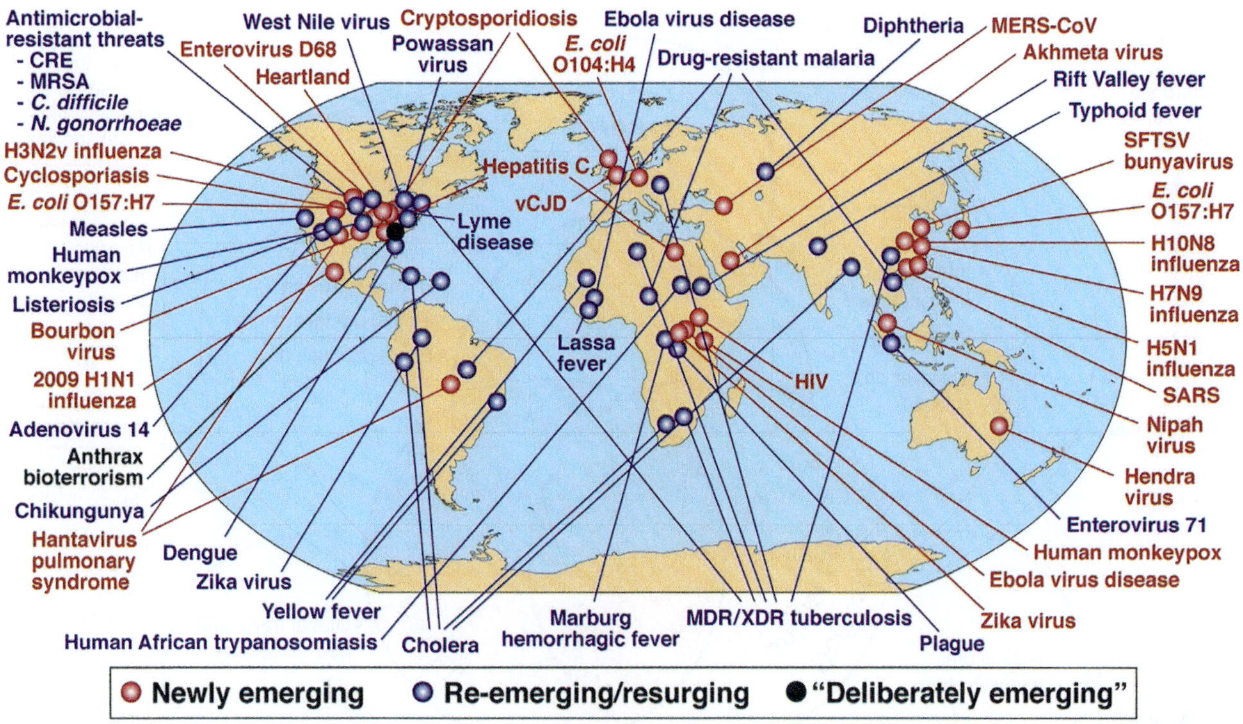

Figure 2.1 Global map of the distribution and prevalence of the newly emerging, re-emerging/resurging, and deliberately emerging infectious diseases. On one hand, developments such as globalization of trade and travel, exploding population growth, unchecked urbanization, and current climatic change cause spread of EIDs from local to global scale. On the other hand, the control of these diseases is facilitated by several modern advances comprising genome sequencing for virus identification, smart and rapid diagnostics, and novel approaches to vaccines and therapeutic design.

population density, antibiotic drug use, agricultural practices, zoonotic pathogens, and wildlife biodiversity have been hypothesized to influence the EID events.

2.5 Changes in Pathogen, Vector, and Human Ecology: A Faustian Bargain for EIDs

Anthropogenic drivers make maximum contributions toward the increased frequency of floods and drought increasing the severity of EIDs, posing threat to wild species responsible for pest prevalence; the global trade and travel cause the movement of parasite species and their establishment in new locations (Daszak et al. 2000; Kilpatrick and Randolph 2012). Human beings impact EIDs not only by the movement of hosts, parasites, and vectors but also by agriculture, urbanization, hunting, habitat fragmentation, and climate change. All these activities ultimately affect the ecosystem structure impacting infectious diseases and also affect the evolutionary dynamics of the diseases.

The emergence and spreading of EIDs among humans, domestic animals, and wildlife are not distinct and isolated events but a closely linked, overlapping, and integrated epidemiological phenomenon in the "One Health" world forming a trinity of EIDs that is subject to a host of dominant drivers, forcing factors and disease determinants that influence the sets of host and pathogen traits (Figure 2.2). EIDs can rightly be described as a fallout of land use changes and development. Human beings have altered their local and regional environment since the beginning of human civilization and have become a force of increasing global importance with magnification of anthropogenic impacts over the past decades (Burney and Flannery 2005). Land alteration includes a wide range of activities comprising deforestation, rangeland expansion, urbanization/suburbanization, infrastructure development (railroad, road, power lines), hydrological alteration (dams, irrigation, canal construction), agricultural development (crops, livestock), and natural resource extraction/depletion (mining, logging, hunting) (Foley et al. 2005). Diseases have often come out of the woods and wildlife and found their way into human populations – plague and

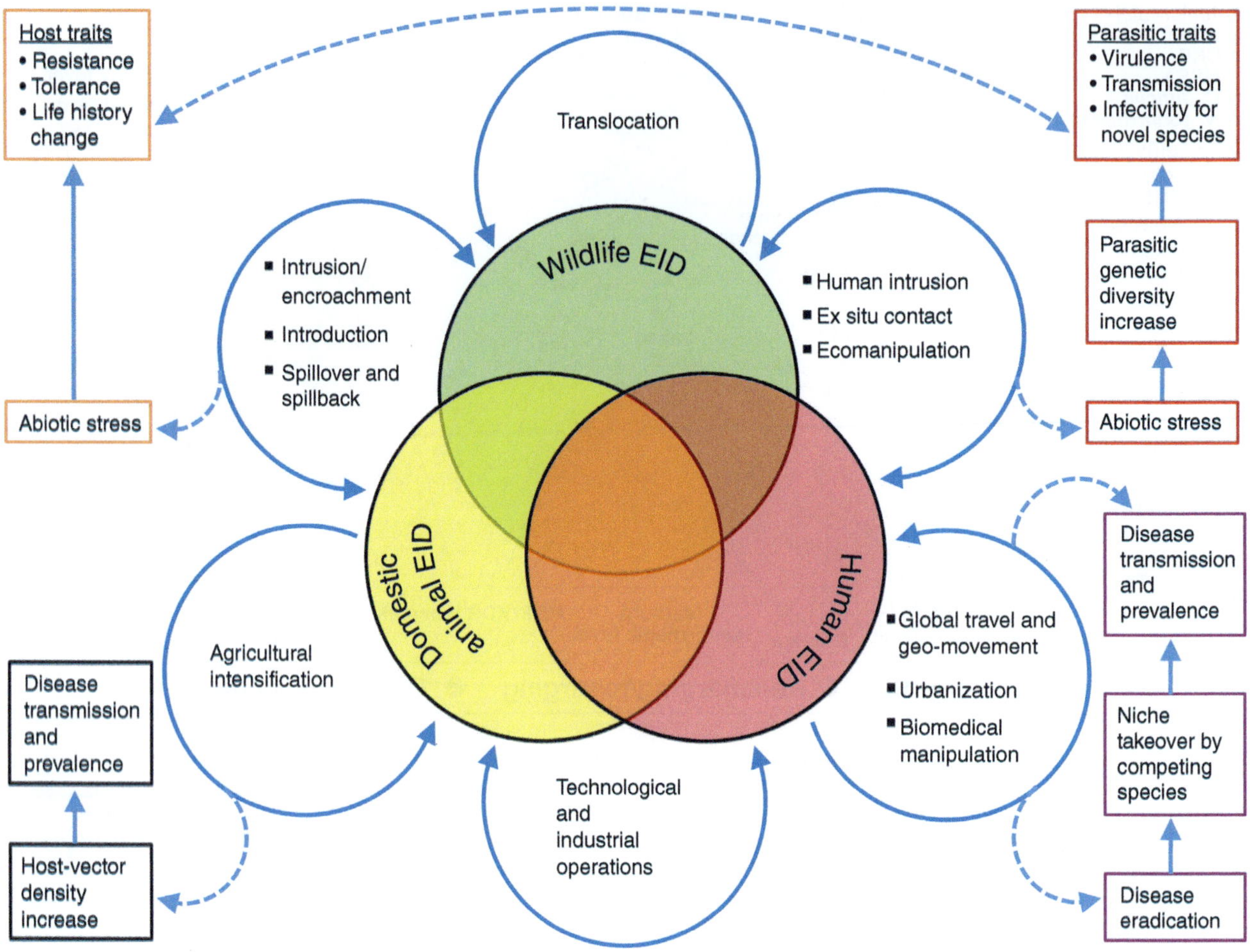

Figure 2.2 Linkages between EIDs of humans, domestic animals, and wildlife in the "One Health" world. Emergence and/or resurgence of EIDs are interdependent and integrated epidemiological phenomena being subjected to a host of dominant drivers, forcing factors, and disease determinants, which influence the sets of host and pathogen traits.

malaria are two examples. But emerging diseases have quadrupled in the past half-century, mainly due to increasing human encroachment into habitat, especially in disease "hotspots" around the globe, in general, and in the tropical regions in particular. And with modern air travel and a robust market in wildlife trafficking, the potential for a serious outbreak in large population center is enormous. Parasites associated with agriculture and animal husbandry can spill over into wild species as well as humans. Domestic hosts can also serve as "stepping stones" for parasites, which can move from wild to domestic species. Often, the stepping stones act ecologically (increasing parasite population sizes and/or transmission opportunities), allowing a parasite to move into a new species without evolutionary change. However, these systems also make it more likely that a genetic mutation will arise in the parasite that will allow it to successfully spill over into a novel host. The anthropogenic land use change is a dynamic process, negatively impacting the ecological integrity and biological diversity by disrupting food web structure and function, altering terrestrial and aquatic biogeochemical cycles, shifting equilibrium of the ecosystem, and continued changes until an equilibrium state is reached. This leads to the introduction of non-native species and pathogens into the existing population (Matson et al. 1997; Tilman 1999; Foley et al. 2005); changes in the level of disease transmission, and changes in the basic functioning of the ecosystem. These changes can be represented as follows:

The change in the ecosystem structure has severe impacts on the host–pathogen interaction, by change in the demography, behavior, and immune response contact between host species and vectors, as well as altering host community composition, leading to the emergence of infectious diseases in humans, domestic animals, and wildlife. A marked increase in EID cases since 1970s has been observed indicating the increased land use changes. The most commonly studied mechanism for the transmission of infectious diseases is altered niches for the vector, host, or pathogen; changes in community structure (e.g. species diversity or species composition); behavioral changes in hosts or vectors; nutrition; immunity; and altered coinfections. The alteration in the ecosystem processes leads to the alteration of the nutrients further due to the alteration in food resources for hosts and vectors. There are complex feedbacks between host nutrition and immunity, leading to nutritional deficiency causing immunity impairment, making the host susceptible to pathogens. These pathogens can further decrease host condition, resulting in positive feedbacks, creating "vicious circles" between nutrition and disease transmission (Beldomenico and Begon 2010). Different studies show changes in the pathogen–vector response according to the anthropogenic changes, and different parasites such as intestinal helminths and bacteria may interact with the immune system to increase host susceptibility to or transmission of microparasites (Telfer et al. 2010). Diverse anthropogenic activities bring about changes in the tripartite interactions among hosts, vectors, and their pathogens as well as transmission of diseases (Gottdenker et al. 2014; Table 2.2)

Along with the pathogen and vector ecology, changes in human ecology are responsible for the speed of transmission

Table 2.2 Causative factors, pathogens, and transmission mechanisms of the emerging infectious diseases.

Pathogen	Pathogen type	Transmission mechanism	References
Modified niche			
Malaria	Vector-borne protozoan	Increase in cattail cover in wet areas associated with cyanobacterial mats for *Anopheles cruciens* and decreased light for *Anopheles vestipennis* has led to an observed increase in anopheline mosquito vectors in areas of sugarcane development.	Grieco et al. (2006)
		A meta-analysis of anopheline mosquito vectors of malaria shows that mosquito's preference to sunlight, not niche width, is associated with increased malaria vector densities in areas of deforestation and agricultural development	Yasuoka and Levins (2007)
Ehrlichiosis	Tick-borne zoonotic bacteria	Greater numbers of *Ehrlichia chafeensis*-infected tick nymphs in areas of invasive honeysuckle; they prefer vegetation of the white-tailed deer host	Allan et al. (2010)
Bluetongue virus	Vector-borne virus of ungulates	With increased wastewater lagoons, suitable for *Culicoides* vector, that led to increased bluetongue virus in livestock	Mayo et al. (2012)
Riberoia ondatrae	Trophically (snail)-transmitted trematode of amphibians	Aquatic eutrophication, with increase in density of intermediate snail hosts, snail trematode production, and trematode infection intensity and reduced survivorship of amphibians	Johnson et al. (2007)
Changes in community composition			
Leishmaniasis	Vector-borne protozoan	Irrigation of desert lands led to dominance of *Phlebotomus papatisi*, a highly competent vector for visceral leishmaniasis	Eliseev et al. (1991)
Chagas disease	Vector-borne protozoan	Decreased wild mammal species richness in fragmented habitats associated with higher seroprevalence of the Chagas disease parasite in small mammal reservoir hosts	Vaz et al. (2007)

(*Continued*)

Table 2.2 (Continued)

Pathogen	Pathogen type	Transmission mechanism	References
Hantavirus	Directly transmitted zoonotic virus	Hantavirus seroprevalence in mammal reservoirs increased in areas of decreased rodent diversity	Suzán et al. (2008)
Change in spatial relationships			
Nipah virus	Directly transmitted zoonotic virus	In Malaysia, large-scale swine production facilities near mango orchards where fruit bats roost believed to be a driver of Nipah virus transmission from fruit bat reservoirs to pigs and eventual spillover into humans	Pulliam et al. (2012)
Change in movement or behavior of vectors and hosts			
Hendra virus	Directly transmitted zoonotic virus	Urban habituation of fruit bat reservoirs of henipavirus leading to increased contact between bats, humans, and domestic animals, and decreased migration potentially associated with reduced population immunity to hendravirus in urbanized bat populations	Plowright et al. (2017)
Malaria	Vector-borne protozoan	Deforestation associated with increased biting rate of anopheline (*Anopheles darlingi*) mosquito vectors of malaria	Vittor et al. (2006)
E. coli	Directly transmitted bacteria	Agricultural activity at the edge of Ugandan forest fragments inciting crop raiding behavior by primates, allowing for increased pathogen (enteric bacterial) exchange between human and non-human primates	Goldberg et al. (2008)
Socioeconomic factors			
American cutaneous leishmaniasis	Vector-borne protozoan	Poor, socially marginalized populations living close to forests are more susceptible to cutaneous leishmaniasis infection risk in areas of deforestation	Chaves et al. (2008)
Malaria	Vector-borne protozoan	Poor socioeconomic status has led to increased malaria risk in irrigated areas	Klinkenberg et al. (2004)
Pathogen pollution			
Toxoplasma gondii	Directly and trophically transmitted protozoan	Agricultural runoff contaminated with *Toxoplasma gondii*-infected cat feces and taken up by bivalves causes toxoplasmosis in sea otters by ingestion of *T. gondii*-contaminated bivalves	Miller et al. (2008)
Giardia sp.	Directly transmitted protozoan	Howler monkey *Giardia* sp. prevalence in a rural area higher compared to remote forests and villages due to increased contamination of water with livestock	Kowalewski et al. (2011)
Changes in host immunity, nutritional condition, or stress			
Lizard hemogregarine parasites	Vector-borne protozoa	In degraded oak forests, female lizards had higher parasite loads and lower body condition than lizards in undisturbed area	Amo et al. (2007)

of zoonotic diseases across the globe. Construction of roads and dams in recently cleared forest areas and rapid urbanization often bring people, especially migrant populations that are immunologically naive, in close contact with pathogens. The spread and persistence of chikungunya serves as a classic example of how immunologically naive populations can sustain an infectious disease. The fever is transmitted by *Aedes* mosquito. Chikungunya is thought to have originated in Africa, where the virus is maintained in a sylvatic cycle, between forest-dwelling mosquitoes and non-human primates. Outbreaks among humans have been observed to be sporadic and short-lived. In urban centers across Africa and Asia, the virus is sustained by immunologically naive human hosts. Recently an outbreak of chikungunya happened in Kenya in 2004 and spread to several Indian Ocean islands, India, and Southeast Asia. The outbreak started in India in 2006, and during the epidemic, the virus spread from India to Italy through travelers. It was then introduced into the local species of Aedes mosquitoes and sustained in a mosquito–human–mosquito transmission cycle in the Mediterranean country. Increased speed and scope of mobility due to globalization has amplified the extent of zoonoses. Proximity to forests or close contact with animal vectors or reservoirs is no longer a limiting constraint on the reach of a pathogen. The case of SARS exemplifies the situation. The SARS virus originated in wild animals in southern China. The virus mutated to adapt to nearby human settlements and jumped to humans in a few closely located towns and villages and then spread to the urban area of Guangzhou. The crowded region facilitated development of the disease into an epidemic in late 2002. In early 2003, the virus spread to Hong Kong that became the hub for a global pandemic. The SARS pandemic then spread within a few months to over 20 countries across the Americas, Europe, and Asia.

2.6 Forests and Emerging Infectious Diseases: Unleashing the Beast Within

Human beings are always dependent on forests in every perspective for their livelihoods. Woodlands provide food, fodder, fuel, fiber, building materials, and medicinal plants. People who live inside forests are often hunter-gatherers or shifting cultivators, and people living near forests are usually involved in agriculture outside the forest and regularly use forest products partly for their own subsistence purposes. However, urban dwellers are mainly concerned about commercial activities, for example the paper and pulp industries and timber production, that have led to land use changes primarily due to deforestation having major implications for ecosystem function and biodiversity conservation, thus being major components of the environmental changes. Deforestation and forestation degradation have contributed directly and indirectly to the steep increase in the rate of extinction among wild animals in the past few decades. The demise of species due to anthropogenic activities can have a cascading effect that threatens biodiversity, which is known to act as a buffer against the spread of pathogens because in a diverse ecosystem the concentration of reservoir species diminishes. The erosion of biodiversity results in a potential flourishing of the reservoir species, which, in turn, implies an increase in disease risk.

Tropical forests are the hotspots of biodiversity, providing humans with essential ecosystem services. On the other hand, deforestation can lead to the emergence of potential life-threatening diseases. Due to increased human activities, some forest ecosystems are lost forever, as highlighted, for instance, by the Amazon rainforest that has been decimated by widespread fires and logging (Carvalho et al. 2019; Lizundia-Loiola et al. 2020). Needless to say, the Earth's forested area and its varied biodiversity are becoming increasingly scarce and remain under pressure due to resource extraction and land conversion. This new anatomy creates novel conditions for pervasive risks to emerge and interact in the longer term; these changing environmental conditions have shown to reasonably impact the current and future zoonotic vector-borne emerging infections (Gottwalt 2013; Nava et al. 2017). The world has grappled with more than 300 zoonoses in the past eight decades, taking the world hostage as they spread in epidemic proportions.

2.6.1 Forest-Derived Human Infections

Macroecology shows large-scale patterns of relationships between pathogens and hosts, including humans, and their vectors or reservoirs. For example, the Ebola virus outbreak in Central and West Africa is due to deforestation on the biodiversity hotspot, causing disturbance and local community changes – possibly including reservoirs of pathogens, further enhancing the risk of new infections in human communities close to the forest margins (Rulli et al. 2017). One of the main effects of forest perturbation due to deforestation and habitat fragmentation leading to biodiversity loss is changes in the biological interaction between host and pathogens. This process is especially pronounced in tropical forest regions, which are biodiversity hotspots. Host–pathogen interactions are fundamentally important in forested ecosystems. Deforestation and habitat loss lead to an increase in pathogen infections from wildlife as a result of higher exposure due to human visits to these places for the extraction of mineral resources, harvest of nature resources, encroachment and implementation of new settlements, etc. (Hosseini et al. 2017).

In general, to understand the spread of zoonotic infection, it is necessary to understand the distribution of pathogenic species and host–pathogen interaction varying with changing conditions throughout the globe. It has been observed that the richness of observed human pathogen species peaks at equatorial latitudes and between the tropics, where large forest domains mainly occur; thus, human pathogen species mainly peaks in regions characterized by warm, wet, and more seasonally occurring conditions and decreases with colder and drier conditions. In terms of emergence, a greater diversity of potential zoonotic diseases and their mammal species is concentrated in northern latitudes, especially rodent-borne infections in Europe (Han et al. 2016); it can be concluded that tropical forests are the cradle for myriads of enzootic, zoonotic, and sapronotic microbes. The rapid anthropogenic interference has led to the spillover of microbes in the human society. The microbial hazards from forest clearing, fragmentation, and agricultural land uses are related to a boost in hantavirus reservoir species abundance and hantavirus prevalence in tropical areas, increasing the risk of *hantavirus cardiopulmonary syndrome* (HCPS). There is a higher risk of cutaneous leishmaniasis, attributed to insect bites in Amazonia (De Castro 2007; Herndon et al. 2009). Kala-azar (*visceral leishmaniasis*) is a deadly disease caused by the parasitic protozoa *Leishmania donovani* and transmitted to humans by the bite of infected female phlebotomine sand fly.

In summary, the pathogen spillovers and outbreaks are related to: (i) land use change, notably through deforestation for timber production, agriculture development, and land transformation for needed infrastructure development and (ii) increase of human populations living in or beneath core forests, who have contributed to the modification of the natural, sylvatic equilibrium between microbial forms, their reservoirs/hosts and vectors, and the human intruders, leading to the perturbation of host reservoirs, promoting the proliferation of zoonotic and sapronotic diseases (Guégan et al. 2020). Some of the forest-derived EIDs are discussed in the following sections.

2.6.1.1 Kyasanur Forest Disease

It broke out around the Kyasanur forest near Karnataka as a result of increased deforestation, forest logging, and human encroachment, infecting non-human primates in 1957. The causative agent of Kyasanur Forest disease (KFD) is Kyasanur Forest disease virus (KFDV), a highly pathogenic member of the family Flaviviridae that was first isolated in sick monkeys in Kyasanur forest of Shimoga district. The KFDV is maintained by tick, mammals, and bird cycles. KFD is a zoonotic disease, usually spreads by the bites of infected ticks (*Haemaphysalis spinigera*). Other than *H. spinigera*, there are 16 other tick species where KFDV has been isolated, especially in their nymphal stages, and they remain infected their entire life. The KFDV also circulates through small animals such as rodents, shrews, and birds, thus transmission from rodents to humans occurs. People exposed to rural or outdoor settings (e.g. hunters, herders, forest workers, and farmers) in these districts are potentially at the risk of being infected if they come in contact with infected ticks.

2.6.1.2 Nipah Virus

The spread of NiV occurs due to deforestation, foraging behavior of the reservoir hosts, and habitat loss leading to changes in the ecosystem structure and food resources availability. Several studies have suggested a link between forest land use changes, agricultural practices, and NiV emergence; fruit bats of the *Pteropus* genus have been identified as the reservoir of the NiV, and its emergence occurred in Malaysia in 1999 (Chua et al. 2002); in the deforested areas of Philippines, the outbreak of NiV virus affected 14 people and 10 horses in 2014. Habitat destruction can force species to venture into urban locales in search of food. In the first outbreak of encephalitis in Malaysia, fruit bats, which act as vectors for NiV, were displaced from their natural forested habitat due to severe deforestation and fires associated with the 1998 El Nino event. The bats relocated to pig farms nearby, where they fed on fruit trees. People who contracted the disease were closely associated with pigs, which were infected through contact with bats and bat feces.

2.6.1.3 Hantavirus

It is named after a river in South Korea where an early outbreak was observed. It has a natural reservoir in murid rodents. The virus causes hemorrhagic fever with renal syndrome in many parts of Asia and HPS in America. The infection spreads through bite, scratch, or fecal aerosols of rodents carrying the virus. Host species, in which pathogens multiply rapidly to high levels providing an important source of infection for vectors, are generalist species that invest less in immunity and more on adaptability to a wide variety of habitats and food sources. Contrarily, specialist species, which act as buffers against pathogen proliferation, are highly adapted only to one specific habitat and food type but invest heavily in their immune systems. Loss of biodiversity due to change in the habitat often results in simplification of the environment through elimination of specialist species and overpopulation of generalist species. Murid rodents that carry the hantavirus are generalist and can adapt to varied and changing ecosystems. Habitat change due to forest fragmentation has been linked with the emergence of HPS. The increase in local distribution and abundance of hantavirus reservoir species can be attributed to the change in the environment due to deforestation in tropical areas.

In areas with compromised biodiversity, the prevalence of pathogens in the blood of reservoir species was found to increase several folds compared to undisturbed habitats.

2.6.1.4 *Mycobacterium ulcerans*/Buruli Ulcer

This occurs due to deforestation, complex food web structure, shifts in trophic interactions, and modifications of trophic networks. *M. ulceran* is a slow-growing bacillus that causes a rare, neglected tropical disease in humans and is found in floodplains and wetland areas in tropical Africa, Central and South America, and Southeast Asia. Research shows that its aquatic persistence is due to complex food web interactions between various environmental biotic and abiotic factors; further explanations suggest that in sites of human perturbation, hosts flourish due to the reduction of predator species and could incidentally recover and concentrate the naturally persistent microbes, thus leading to the freshwater food web collapse and its consequence on *M. ulcerans* load in the more perturbed sites due to human intervention (Guégan et al. 2020).

2.6.1.5 HIV/AIDS

Forest logging and mining actions are to blame for the emergence of HIV/AIDS. The virus of AIDS usually spreads from infected chimpanzees and gorillas in Central Africa and those infecting sooty mangabeys in West Africa (D'arc et al. 2015); the main factors behind this increased exposure are demonstrated by the increase of bushmeat hunting and butchering, forest logging, and mining in West Central Africa since the early years of the twentieth century, leading to increased transmission from human to human and an increase in the probability of virus adaptation to the human population (Chitnis et al. 2000).

2.6.1.6 Malaria

A potentially fatal infectious human disease caused by protozoan parasites, due to increased deforestation and loss of forest cover. Plasmodium species that infect humans originate from primates and are transmitted to humans through the bite of infected mosquitoes of the genus *Anopheles*. Forest habitat destruction, opening of forest tracks, logging practices, and increased fire frequencies at forest edges (Chua et al. 2002) result in habitat modification of mosquito species communities, with the creation of new breeding sites and the development of favorable conditions for the expansion of efficient vectors for parasite transmission (Yasuoka and Levins 2007; Vittor et al. 2009).

2.6.1.7 Lyme Disease

Habitat fragmentation and biodiversity loss have been implicated in the emergence and transmission of novel diseases, such as Lyme disease, in the United States and Europe, to humans. The disease is caused by a bacterial pathogen, *Borrelia burgdorferi*. White-footed mice and white-tailed deer have been identified as natural reservoir species for the bacterium, which is transmitted by tick bites. Diminishing biodiversity and the lack of large predators have helped Lyme disease to be the most prevalent vector-borne disease in the United States.

2.7 Humans as the Dominant Driver of Emergence and Resurgence of EIDs

Human beings are considered as the dominant drivers of EIDs because their actions influence the ecological and evolutionary host–parasite dynamics, which may impose strong selective pressures on one another. The complex ecological and evolutionary interactions led to the emergence of the recent infectious diseases as the ecoevolutionary drivers of the play. Humans have contributed to the increased frequency and severity of EIDs, which pose a significant threat to wild and domestic species, as well as human health. Humans influence parasitism by altering (co)evolutionary interactions between hosts and parasites on ecological timescales. Human actions significantly increase the dispersal of host, parasite, and vector species, enabling a greater frequency of infection in naive host populations and host switches. Very dense host populations resulting from urbanization and agriculture can drive the evolution of more virulent parasites and, in some cases, more resistant host populations. Anthropogenic activities that reduce host genetic diversity or impose abiotic stress can impair the ability of hosts to adapt to disease threats. Besides, evolutionary responses of hosts and parasites can thwart disease management and biological control measures.

The human impacts can be summarized as follows:

i) *Novel species association:* Novel species associations are resulted from human activities, mainly due to global trade and travel, creating a world where the species are more closely connected than ever before (Kilpatrick and Randolph 2012). The anthropogenic activities indirectly alter associations of hosts, parasites, and vectors, primarily, by land use change and climate change, for example increased temperature at higher altitudes allow parasites and their vectors to expand their range into communities where hosts are naive; further the agricultural activities and animal husbandry practices led to the infection of novel host, causing spillover into wild species as well as humans, in other words allowing a parasite to move into a new species without evolutionary change; however, genetic mutation is likely to occur in the novel species for the spillover to occur in novel host, thus all these strongly impact EIDs.

ii) *Changes in host and/or vector density and diversity:* Urbanization and industrialization activities have huge impact on the increase in population density that further impacts host and vector population densities that can play an important role in both ecological and evolutionary dynamics affecting parasite prevalence (Rogalski et al. 2017). The potential of epidemic increases, with increased host population, increasing the likelihood of disease transmission, thus ultimately increasing the prevalence (Wilcox and Gubler 2005). Developed land has more host density, leading to increased parasite prevalence, for example, prevalence of West Nile virus is strongly associated with both urban and agricultural land use in North America. The parasite virulence is often related to transmission rates as parasites that co-opt more host resources produce more transmission stages and are also more virulent (de Roode et al. 2008) than the ones with low transmission rate. Agricultural activities, animal husbandry, and fish farming support host densities well above the natural population, which promote the evolution of more virulent parasites (Jones et al. 2013; Kennedy et al. 2016), increasing the susceptibility to major threats. Additionally, because higher host diversity often correlates with higher parasite diversity (Gollan et al. 2007), altered biodiversity might also influence cross-species transmission.

iii) *Changes in the abiotic environment:* When stressors come into play, the coevolutionary dynamics between hosts and parasites become complex. Human beings have altered the abiotic environmental conditions, changing the ecology of hosts and parasites. Coping with altered conditions has thus put stress on plants and animals, diverting resources from fighting parasites (Morley and Lewis 2014). The global climate change increases the temperature that affects the physiology of organisms, impacting a parasite's ability to develop and a host's ability to resist or tolerate parasites (Rohr et al. 2013). The parasites that have higher temperature optima than hosts are more virulent at higher temperatures. Exposure to pesticides also alters the host–parasite interactions.

iv) *Genetic diversity:* Human beings strongly impact genetic diversity through habitat fragmentation, over harvesting monocultures, etc., as the ability of the parasite to adapt depends on the genetic diversity of the host (Irving et al. 2012); losses of diversity should increase host vulnerability to parasite outbreaks. Habitat fragmentation and harvesting natural population reduces the gene flow by reducing the population size, changing the dynamics of sexual selection, and imposing selection directly via selective harvesting (Kreft and Jetz 2007; Kuparinen and Festa-Bianchet 2017).

v) *Intentional intervention:* When the parasites threaten human health, humans directly intervene with their evolutionary trajectory. One of the ways of intervention is vaccination, which is a successful means by which humans intervene in disease systems, especially when vaccination induces perfect lifelong immunity in the host, but on the other hand leaky vaccine or imperfect vaccine fails to provide the host perfect protection, as it does not entirely prevent the parasite from replicating within the host and transmitting to other individuals (Gandon et al. 2001). As parasites can still replicate in vaccinated hosts, leaky vaccines may actually result into increased virulence by altering the trade-off between virulence and transmission (Gandon et al. 2001). It can be said that leaky vaccines alleviate the infectious period.

vi) *Eradication of infectious disease*: Eradication of infectious diseases strongly impacts the host population, likely to dramatically alter the selective environment for the host. If the eradicated parasites interacted with other parasites, this might lead to dramatic changes in their infection prevalence, which might increase the strength of selection from those parasites (Rogalski et al. 2017).

2.8 Global Warming and EIDs

The planetary (earth) system consists of complex interacting systems namely the atmosphere, hydrosphere, biosphere, and lithosphere (IPCC 2021). Since the origin and evolution of life, temperature has been playing a very crucial role for the sustenance of life on the planet. Temperature gradually falls from higher to optimum, and many lower to higher life-forms, namely, prokaryotes, eukaryotes (unicellular as well as multicellular), different archaebacteria, and many unclassified infectious agents such as viruses, prions, and viroids, originated. They play specific roles for the maintenance of the stability of the ecosystem. These organisms sustain their lives as autotrophs or heterotrophs in various kinds of relationship as commensal, mutualistic, symbiotic, xenobiotic, parasitic, etc.

However, fossil fuel burning due to increased industrialization and urbanization has led to excessive emission of greenhouse gases, bringing about the phenomenon of global warming. The Earth's temperature has increased with an average of 0.3–0.7 °C since 1900, and by the end of twenty-first century it is predicted to increase by 1.1–5.8 °C (IPCC 2021). It is an average increase in the atmospheric temperature near the surface of the Earth and troposphere layer, which can influence climatic patterns at global scale. Climate plays a crucial role in the determination of health, control of infection and outbreak of pathogens, intensity of diseases, etc. The environmental changes due to enhanced global warming have caused emergence of several new diseases and also the re-emergence of older diseases in newer and different places. it can be concluded that the change and unstable climate have caused the global emergence, resurgence, and redistribution of infectious diseases. As an evidence in the past 30 years more than 30 emerging diseases have been recorded (Bhatia and Narain 2010). Among them foodborne, food poisoning, waterborne, water toxicities, algal bloom, vector-borne illness like malaria, Japanese encephalitis, Kyasanur forest disease, West Nile disease, and dengue are to name a few. Climate change as a consequence of global warming may trigger an ecological invasion evolving a sorting process that brings genetic adjustment with evolution of new disease agents or complexes. This continuous shift from the natural ecology, from the equilibrium state, leads to the emergence of new diseases.

Climate change is likely to have a *cascade effect*, primarily impacting agriculture and livestock, secondarily impacting livelihood and food security, further bringing about alterations in the poverty level including adaptation and coping mechanisms, and ultimately resulting in demographic and production shifts. In turn, these shifts will have a primary impact on host/pathogen interactions, including susceptibility and infectiousness, and, ultimately, the emergence/re-emergence and geographical spread of human and animal disease (Heffernan 2018).

2.8.1 Interactions Between Climate Change and Pathogens

The change in the atmospheric conditions under the climate change regime have led to changes in the pathogenic life cycle and the overall disease ecology in favor of the vectors and respective pathogens. The climate change events have created conducive environment for the cluster of insects and pathogens as well as rodents and pathogens that pose immense threat to public health. The depletion of the ozone layer has led to increased impingement of the harmful ultraviolet radiations leading to lead to alteration in the human immune system thereby causing stress and making an individual prone to malnutrition (Sakai et al. 2001; Mas-Coma et al. 2008; Bhatia and Narain 2010). The factors of malnutrition and climatic pressure on agriculture, ledads to uncertainty in the population as a whole, making them susceptible to rising infection trends with changing global temperature and climate change events. as a result of mMultiple determinants factors such as biological as well as human and ecological, causes increase in sea surface temperature and sea level, leading to higher incidences of water borne illnesses and algal toxin related infections (Bezirtzoglou et al. 2011). Flooding due to heavy rainfall and surface run-off cause high incidence of waterborne diseases, due to *Giardia* and *Cryptosporidium* (Curriero et al. 2001), and these conditions are raised mainly because of the contamination of water supply sources (Frumhoff et al. 2007).

The increased temperature conditions have led to the diffusion of wide spectrum of zoonotic diseases and pathogens. The increased temperature exerts an increasing selection pressure leading to a change in the biodiversity of pathogenic agents and the epidemiology of infections; for instance, many bacteria have developed mechanisms to survive and grow in unfavorable stress conditions over a long period of time e.g. *E. coli*, which can survive in pH 2 after its earlier exposure to pH 5; genetic transfer between related and unrelated species followed by environmental adaptation leads to the evolution of new microbes, e.g. nontoxigenic *Vibrio cholerae* strains acquired the genes encoding cholera toxin from bacteriophage and also the emergence of methicillin-resistant *S. aureus* (MRSA) (Mirski et al. 2012).

Further, increased CO_2 (carbon dioxide) concentration has led to the stimulation of microbial growth, higher humidity favors microorganisms to be more invasive in the host inducing development of the disease (Mirski et al. 2012), higher temperature leads to increased fungal growth and mycotoxin formation (Lacetera et al. 2003; Dhama 2013), and increased sea level led to increased flooding conditions leading to zoonoses. Further, increased El Nino cycle led to increased rainfall and crop production that ultimately led to an increase in the rodent population and rodent-borne zoonoses like hantavirus infection (Engelthaler et al. 1999). Changing temperature conditions leads to changes in the bird migration patterns leading to disease transmission from migratory water birds as avian influenza (Dhama et al. 2008; Gilbert et al. 2008). The suite of factors catalyzed by global warming and climate change have increased vector population, increased transmission period, reduced duration of growth, increased egg production amount, and increased invertebrate metabolic rates, leading to emergence of infectious diseases (Dhama 2013). The wide range of diseases caused by environmental changes is enlisted in Table 2.3.

Table 2.3 Major infectious diseases and their causative agents, associated vectors, and areas of risk.

Sl. no.	Name of the disease	Causative agent and vector	Areas at risk
1	Chikungunya	Chikungunya virus, insects	Temperate climatic regions
2	Crimean Congo hemorrhagic fever	Nairo virus, tick	Asia, Europe, Africa
3	Dengue	Flavivirus, mosquito	Asia, Africa, Caribbean Territories
4	Filariasis/Elephantiasis	*Wucheria bancrofti*, mosquitoes	Tropical countries
5	Japanese encephalitis	Flavivirus, mosquito	Japan, tropical countries
6	Leishmaniasis, Kala-Azar	*Leishmania donovani*	Africa, tropical countries
7	Leptospirosis	*Leptospira* spp., flood induced or waterborne infection	Rio de Janeiro, New Zealand, tropical countries
8	Lyme disease	*Borrelia burgdorferi*, ticks	United States
9	Malaria	*Plasmodium* spp., mosquitoes	Tropical countries
10	Murray river encephalitis	Flavivirus, mosquito	Australian regions
11	Plague	*Yersinia pestis*, rat flea	United States and others
12	Tick-borne encephalitis	Flavivirus/tick	Asia, Africa, Europe
13	West Nile Fever	Flavivirus, mosquito	United States and others
14	Hantavirus pulmonary syndrome	Hantavirus, rodents	United States, Central and South America
15	Trypanosomiasis	*Trypanosoma cruzei*, *Trypanosoma brucei*, tsetse fly or bugs	Central America and Africa
16	Yellow fever	Flavivirus, mosquito	Africa and America
17	Cholera	*Vibrio cholerae*, waterborne illness	Poland, India, Hungary, and Germany
18	Cryptosporidiosis	*Cryptosporidium parvums*, waterborne	North America, Texas, Europe
19	Amnesic shell fish poisoning (ASP), red tides and neurotoxicity (NSP)	Water toxicity due to excessive toxin release by diatoms and dinoflagellates	Europe, Africa, and North and South America
20	Respiratory illness, hepatitis, brown tides, and harmful algal blooms (HAB)	Cyanobacterial algal bloom toxicity	European countries, North Queensland, Brazil

2.9 COVID-19: The Latest Avatar of the EID

The advent of COVID-19 is like a pin that brutally pricked our mundane world of luxury and sweet-smelling toilets, where we considered ourselves supreme, making us realize that we are nothing but mere components of the ecosystem, fragile and helpless before the wrath of nature. According to Morens et al. (2004), "We have created a global, human-dominated ecosystem that serves as a playground for the emergence and host-switching of animal viruses." The advent of novel coronavirus (SARS-CoV-2) is basically attributed to the disturbance of natural habitats that can result in zoonotic pathogens being dislodged from their ecological niches and infect human populations; from research it has been observed the 96% of the coronavirus genes were obtained from wild bats (Honigsbaum and Méthot 2020). The epidemiologic information clearly implicates the SARS-CoV-2 is of bat origin, infecting unidentified animal species sold in China's live-animal markets. The very first case of COVID-19 was report on 31 December 2019, Wuhan City, Hubei Province, China. The etiology of the virus was different from the previous two coronaviruses – the severe acute respiratory syndrome coronavirus (SARS-CoV) outbreak in 2002 and the Middle East respiratory syndrome coronavirus (MERS-CoV) outbreak in 2012. The SARS-CoV-2 is the third coronavirus to emerge in the human population. The disease rapidly spread internationally, raising global public health concerns, and was subsequently termed coronavirus disease 19 (COVID-19) (Xu et al. 2020). The World Health Organization declared COVID-19 as a pandemic on 11 March 2020.

The SARS-CoV-2 belongs to *Sarbecovirus subgenus*, *Betacoronavirus* genus of the subfamily *Orthocoronavirinae* in the family *Coronaviridae* of the suborder *cornidovirineae* of the order Nidovirales (Zhou et al. 2020). The clinical manifestations are similar to those of SARS-CoV and MERS-CoV. Patients with 2019-nCoV have high fever, dry cough, dyspnea, and bilateral ground-glass opacities on chest CT scan. They rarely show obvious upper respiratory signs and symptoms (such as snot, sneezing, or sore throat), indicating that the virus primarily infects the lower respiratory tract (Huang et al. 2020); 20–25% of the patients show intestinal symptoms and signs (such as diarrhea). Similar to MERS-CoV or SARS-CoV (Huang et al. 2020), severe COVID-19 cases include acute respiratory distress syndrome, septic shock, metabolic acidosis, and bleeding and coagulation dysfunction. It is noted that severe and critically ill patients develop moderate to low fever during the course of the disease. The incubation period is about 10 days for the symptoms to surface. The worst aspect of the disease is that the transmission might occur even before the manifestation of the clinical symptoms in an infected person. The transmission routes mainly include transmission through droplets, close contact, aerosol, and maybe fecal-oral transmission, and patients in the incubation period can transmit the virus to other persons. The SARS virus is spread person to person through contact, respiratory droplets, fomites, and contaminated surfaces. There are several other factors that control the transmission of the virus that include the environment in buildings and human behavior, the exposure routes maybe through finger contact with virus-contaminates surfaces (fomites) and subsequent finger contact with facial membranes, inhalation of the virus carried in airborne particles (inhalable or respirable particles) exhaled from cough or vocalization, and droplet spray, the direct projection of the virus carried in particles exhaled from cough or vocalization onto the facial membranes; therefore, it is evident that the control of the environmental factor and human behavior are important for controlling the spread of SARS-CoV-2 (Azuma et al. 2020).

COVID-19 has devastated the health of world population and is continuing to do the same; in some parts, it has altered the fundamental daily activities around the world. To reduce the increasing infection risks, the exposure scientists have designed scientific mitigation strategies. The basic recommendation for individual actions we can take to protect ourselves from SARS-CoV-2 are fundamentally grounded in basic principles of exposure science. Physical distancing is the principal strategy based on the concept of particle fate and transport. Other strategies like the use of face masks, masks, and gloves hinge on the degree to which viruses can penetrate various materials, proper fit of personal protective equipment (PPE), and how PPE usage influences personal behavior. The most effective control is isolating oneself, substitution of usual behaviors with different ones will reduce exposures, engineered controls include the use of alcohol-based hand sanitizer that is active against COVID-19, administrative controls include social distancing in the workplace, limiting building occupancy can also be used to minimize risk, and the PPE is the last resort.

As there were no pre-existing COVID vaccines, researchers around the world have been racing to develop COVID-19 vaccines. The urgent need for vaccine has compressed the development timeline from 10 to 15 years to one to two years (Lurie et al. 2020), with overlapping preclinical, clinical, and scale-up manufacturing processes occurring in parallel. Due to the accelerated development process, the interim data from ongoing clinical and preclinical vaccine studies are being published almost in real time. The evolution process of vaccine preparation will continue over the next few years until more clinical trials are completed, additional vaccine strategies are evaluated, and host defense against SARS-CoV-2, including postinfection immunity, is better understood, until the global mass immunization is a reality (Jayanathan et al. 2020).

After the discovery of effective COVID vaccine, India carried out world's largest vaccination campaign against COVID-19, with a population of 1.38 billion. In the initial phase of the COVID-19 vaccination program, India aimed at vaccinating 300 million people by August 2021, including 30 million health workers and frontline workers (e.g. police and soldiers) and 270 million elderly people (i.e. aged over 50 years) and people with comorbidities (Bagcchi 2021). COVID-19 vaccination in India was initiated with two types of vaccines: Covishield (by Serum Institute of India Ltd.) and Covaxin (by Bharat Biotech International Ltd.) according to the press bureau information. For the cause of the largest vaccination drive "More than a lakh [i.e. 100,000] vaccinators were trained; multiple mock exercises were conducted; a pan-India national exercise was also conducted to hammer out the slightest glitches," said Harsh Vardhan, the Indian health minister (Bagcchi 2021).

2.10 Mitigation

From the above discussion it is evident that anthropogenic activities that include increased international mobility, poor public health systems, and microbial adaptations are some of the main drivers of EIDs. For effectively combating EIDs, the government and the scientific communities need to put efforts for the better understanding of the spread and detection of pathogens and surveillance of pathogens, with the potential to cause outbreaks, epidemics, and even pandemics. The real challenge for the identification of the pathogens is their huge diversity in nature.75% of the emerging diseases are zoonotic in nature, too often based on limited knowledge of the origin, pathogenicity, and basic biology of the wild host and pathogen coupled with poor communication among relevant stakeholders (Andersen et al. 2020); therefore, it is essential to understand the new potential infection in humans. Early detection of EIDs based upon the surveillance of the pathogens and their circulation in the human population would be a good strategy. Special attention is to be paid to the direct transmission of diseases that forms the basis of an epidemic. Many advancements and developments have already been made in the developed countries. Thus once the etiological agent is identified, conduits to stop the transmission chain can easily be established based on the transmission mode of the then pathogenic infection. On the whole, the optimal response to EID outbreak warrants (i) global surveillance for early detection of disease eruption, (ii) transparency and communication, (iii) infrastructural development and capacity building at domestic, national, and international levels; (iv) conducting basic and clinical research in a coordinated and collaborative manner; (v) involvement of all stakeholders of public health including the afflicted communities in policy decisions; (vi) pursuit, perfection, adoption, and diffusion of adaptable platform technologies for vaccines, diagnostics, and therapeutics; and (vii) adequate funding.

2.11 Conclusion

EIDs have always been an "unchartered territory," i.e. a territory that has never been explored, with no vaccine or specialized treatment. They are much like unpleasant surprises to humankind. In this era of rapid development, the nature is always trying out new genetic variations. As the ecological niches open and close, the human society wax and wane to deal with the challenges that abruptly change its course. Thus, viewing EIDs through ecological lens, it is understood that they are not independent events. It is based on the complex interactions between various factors that include environmental and ecological change, local pollutants, the widespread loss of top predators, economic and social changes, and international travel, which drive a great movement of hosts, and continues to change the profile of infectious disease occurrence, affecting pathogens across a wide taxonomic range of animals and plants. The entire system seems to be like an entangled string. One wrong step can result in the total entanglement that will require long time to be detangled again, similar to a destabilized ecosystem that attempts to attend stability. The pandemic is a stark reminder of how global mobility for travel and trade has rapidly increased the extent to which humans can act as carriers of deadly diseases. Diseases born in forests are no longer restricted to forests. As forests have been modified to suit their needs, many organisms in forests have also adapted to humans. Human mobility provides these organisms gateways to uncharted territories.

Human actions significantly increase dispersal of host, parasite, and vector species, enabling greater frequency of infection in naive host populations and host switches. Very dense host populations resulting from urbanization and agriculture can drive the evolution of more virulent parasites and, in some cases, more resistant host populations. Human activities that reduce host genetic diversity or impose abiotic stress can impair the ability of hosts to adapt to disease threats. Further, evolutionary responses of hosts and parasites can thwart disease management and biocontrol efforts. Finally, in rare cases, humans influence evolution by eradicating an infectious disease. Coping with unprecedented rise of pandemics and epidemics requires a holistic approach to medicine that treats human health as a part of environmental health. Although with the advent of modern tools such as satellite remote sensing, geographical information system (GIS), and mathematical modeling for better understanding of epidemiology of emerging diseases, it is possible to detect and identify ecological niche at finer resolutions and map and project the present and potential risk of the diseases having ecology-driven epidemiology. With increasing anthropogenic influence, humanity is striding toward the uncharted territory of fatal diseases that seems to put our existence at stake, evident through the history of EIDs to the present COVID-19 pandemic. Therefore, it is essential for us to realize that we are at the mercy of our mother nature, mere components of the ecosystem playing our individual roles, and a certain destabilization can lead us to ravaging consequences. The world is so intertwined that a problem in one place today will be a problem in another place tomorrow. Emerging infectious diseases are giving us a wake-up call to create a global community. If we do not, we may be facing the new Armageddon. Understanding the ecological and evolutionary processes involved, particularly the phenotypic traits that enable parasites and hosts to (co)evolve, will help not only to improve our understanding of human influences on EIDs but also aid in combating or wiping out parasites. To address zoonotic outbreaks and emergence and re-emergence of infectious diseases, there must be a proactive approach to restore wildlife health and habitat and to adopt coordinated, multidisciplinary, and multi-institutional efforts with close monitoring of how the increasing ecological footprint of humans is affecting health and disease dynamics.

References

Allan, B.F., Dutra, H.P., Goessling, L.S. et al. (2010). Invasive honeysuckle eradication reduces tick-borne disease risk by altering host dynamics. *Proceedings of the National Academy of Sciences* 107 (43): 18523–18527.

Amo, L., Lopez, P., and Martín, J. (2007). Habitat deterioration affects body condition of lizards: a behavioral approach with *Iberolacerta cyreni* lizards inhabiting ski resorts. *Biological Conservation* 135 (1): 77–85.

Andersen, K.G., Rambaut, A., Lipkin, W.I. et al. (2020). The proximal origin of SARS-CoV-2. *Nature Medicine* 26 (4): 450–452.

Azuma, K., Kagi, N., Kim, H., and Hayashi, M. (2020). Impact of climate and ambient air pollution on the epidemic growth during COVID-19 outbreak in Japan. *Environmental Research* 190: 110042.

Bagcchi, S. (2021). The world's largest COVID-19 vaccination campaign. *The Lancet. Infectious Diseases* 21 (3): 323.

Beldomenico, P.M. and Begon, M. (2010). Disease spread, susceptibility and infection intensity: vicious circles? *Trends in Ecology & Evolution* 25 (1): 21–27.

Bezirtzoglou, C., Dekas, K., and Charvalos, E. (2011). Climate changes, environment and infection: facts, scenarios and growing awareness from the public health community within Europe. *Anaerobe* 17 (6): 337–340.

Bhatia, R. and Narain, J.P. (2010). The challenge of emerging zoonoses in Asia Pacific. *Asia-Pacific Journal of Public Health* 22 (4): 388–394.

Burney, D.A. and Flannery, T.F. (2005). Fifty millennia of catastrophic extinctions after human contact. *Trends in Ecology & Evolution* 20 (7): 395–401.

Carvalho, W.D., Mustin, K., Hilário, R.R. et al. (2019). Deforestation control in the Brazilian Amazon: a conservation struggle being lost as agreements and regulations are subverted and bypassed. *Perspectives in Ecology and Conservation* 17 (3): 122–130.

Chaves, L.F., Cohen, J.M., Pascual, M., and Wilson, M.L. (2008). Social exclusion modifies climate and deforestation impacts on a vector-borne disease. *PLoS Neglected Tropical Diseases* 2 (2): e176.

Chitnis, A., Rawls, D., and Moore, J. (2000). Origin of HIV type 1 in colonial French Equatorial Africa? *AIDS Research and Human Retroviruses* 16 (1): 5–8.

Chua, K.B., Chua, B.H., and Wang, C.W. (2002). Anthropogenic deforestation, El Niiio and the emergence of Nipah virus in Malaysia. *Malaysian Journal of Pathology* 24 (1): 15–21.

Curriero, F.C., Patz, J.A., Rose, J.B., and Lele, S. (2001). The association between extreme precipitation and waterborne disease outbreaks in the United States, 1948–1994. *American Journal of Public Health* 91 (8): 1194–1199.

D'arc, M., Ayouba, A., Esteban, A. et al. (2015). Origin of the HIV-1 group O epidemic in western lowland gorillas. *Proceedings of the National Academy of Sciences* 112 (11): E1343–E1352.

Daszak, P., Cunningham, A.A., and Hyatt, A.D. (2000). Emerging infectious diseases of wildlife – threats to biodiversity and human health. *Science* 287 (5452): 443–449.

De Castro, E.V. (2007). The crystal forest: notes on the ontology of Amazonian spirits. *Inner Asia* 9 (2): 153–172.

De Roode, J.C., Yates, A.J., and Altizer, S. (2008). Virulence-transmission trade-offs and population divergence in virulence in a naturally occurring butterfly parasite. *Proceedings of the National Academy of Sciences* 105 (21): 7489–7494.

Dhama, K. (2013). Avian/bird flu virus: poultry pathogen having. *Journal of Medical Sciences* 13 (5): 301–315.

Dhama, K., Mahendran, M., and Tomar, S. (2008). Pathogens transmitted by migratory birds: threat perceptions to poultry health and production. *International Journal of Poultry Science* 7 (6): 516–525.

Dobson, A.P. and Carper, E.R. (1996). Infectious diseases and human population history. *Bioscience* 46 (2): 115–126.

Eliseev, L.N., Strelkova, M.V., and Zherikhina, I.I. (1991). The characteristics of the epidemic activation of a natural focus of zoonotic cutaneous leishmaniasis in places with a sympatric dissemination of *Leishmania major*, *L. turanica* and *L. gerbilli*. *Meditsinskaia Parazitologiia I Parazitarnye Bolezni* 3: 24–29.

Engelthaler, D.M., Mosley, D.G., Cheek, J.E. et al. (1999). Climatic and environmental patterns associated with hantavirus pulmonary syndrome, Four Corners region, United States. *Emerging Infectious Diseases* 5 (1): 87.

Foley, J.A., DeFries, R., Asner, G.P. et al. (2005). Global consequences of land use. *Science* 309 (5734): 570–574.

Frumhoff, P.C., McCarthy, J.J., Melillo, J.M. et al. (2007). *Confronting Climate Change in the US Northeast: Science, Impacts, and Solutions*. Union of Concerned Scientists (UCS).

Gandon, S., Mackinnon, M.J., Nee, S., and Read, A.F. (2001). Imperfect vaccines and the evolution of pathogen virulence. *Nature* 414 (6865): 751–756.

Gilbert, M., Slingenbergh, J., and Xiao, X. (2008). Climate change and avian influenza. *Revue Scientifique et Technique (International Office of Epizootics)* 27 (2): 459.

Goldberg, T.L., Gillespie, T.R., Rwego, I.B. et al. (2008). Forest fragmentation as cause of bacterial transmission among nonhuman primates, humans, and livestock, Uganda. *Emerging Infectious Diseases* 14 (9): 1375.

Gollan, T.H., Fennema-Notestine, C., Montoya, R.I., and Jernigan, T.L. (2007). The bilingual effect on Boston Naming Test performance. *Journal of the International Neuropsychological Society* 13 (2): 197–208.

Gottdenker, N.L., Streicker, D.G., Faust, C.L., and Carroll, C.R. (2014). Anthropogenic land use change and infectious diseases: a review of the evidence. *EcoHealth* 11 (4): 619–632.

Gottwalt, A. (2013). Impacts of deforestation on vector-borne disease incidence. *The Columbia University Journal of Global Health* 3 (2): 16–19.

Grieco, J.P., Johnson, S., Achee, N.L. et al. (2006). Distribution of *Anopheles albimanus*, *Anopheles vestitipennis*, and *Anopheles crucians* associated with land use in Northern Belize. *Journal of Medical Entomology* 43 (3): 614–622.

Guégan, J.F., Ayouba, A., Cappelle, J., and De Thoisy, B. (2020). Forests and emerging infectious diseases: unleashing the beast within. *Environmental Research Letters* 15 (8): 083007.

Han, B.A., Kramer, A.M., and Drake, J.M. (2016). Global patterns of zoonotic disease in mammals. *Trends in Parasitology* 32 (7): 565–577.

Heffernan, C. (2018). Climate change and multiple emerging infectious diseases. *Veterinary Journal (London, England: 1997)* 234: 43.

Herndon, C.N., Uiterloo, M., Uremaru, A. et al. (2009). Disease concepts and treatment by tribal healers of an Amazonian Forest culture. *Journal of Ethnobiology and Ethnomedicine* 5 (1): 1–22.

Honigsbaum, M. and Méthot, P.O. (2020). Introduction: microbes, networks, knowledge - disease ecology and emerging infectious diseases in time of COVID-19. *History and Philosophy of the Life Sciences* 42 (3): 1–9.

Hosseini, P.R., Mills, J.N., Prieur-Richard, A.H. et al. (2017). Does the impact of biodiversity differ between emerging and endemic pathogens? The need to separate the concepts of hazard and risk. *Philosophical Transactions of the Royal Society, B: Biological Sciences* 372 (1722): 20160129.

Huang, C., Wang, Y., Li, X. et al. (2020). Clinical features of patients infected with 2019 novel coronavirus in Wuhan, China. *The Lancet* 395 (10223): 497–506.

IPCC (2021). Summary for policymakers. In: *Climate Change 2021: The Physical Science Basis. Contribution of Working Group I to the Sixth Assessment Report of the Intergovernmental Panel on Climate Change* (ed. V. Masson-Delmotte, P. Zhai, A. Pirani, et al.). Cambridge University Press (In Press). https://www.ipcc.ch/report/ar6/wg1.

Irving, H., Riveron, J.M., Ibrahim, S. et al. (2012). Positional cloning of rp2 QTL associates the P450 genes CYP6Z1, CYP6Z3 and CYP6M7 with pyrethroid resistance in the malaria vector *Anopheles funestus*. *Heredity* 109 (6): 383–392.

Jeyanathan, M., Afkhami, S., Smaill, F. et al. (2020). Immunological considerations for COVID-19 vaccine strategies. *Nature Reviews Immunology* 20 (10): 615–632.

Johnson, P.T., Chase, J.M., Dosch, K.L. et al. (2007). Aquatic eutrophication promotes pathogenic infection in amphibians. *Proceedings of the National Academy of Sciences* 104 (40): 15781–15786.

Jones, B.A., Grace, D., Kock, R. et al. (2013). Zoonosis emergence linked to agricultural intensification and environmental change. *Proceedings of the National Academy of Sciences* 110 (21): 8399–8404.

Jones, B.A., Betson, M., and Pfeiffer, D.U. (2017). Eco-social processes influencing infectious disease emergence and spread. *Parasitology* 144 (1): 26–36.

Kennedy, D.A., Kurath, G., Brito, I.L. et al. (2016). Potential drivers of virulence evolution in aquaculture. *Evolutionary Applications* 9 (2): 344–354.

Kilpatrick, A.M. and Randolph, S.E. (2012). Drivers, dynamics, and control of emerging vector-borne zoonotic diseases. *The Lancet* 380 (9857): 1946–1955.

Klinkenberg, E., Konradsen, F., Herrel, N. et al. (2004). Malaria vectors in the changing environment of the southern Punjab, Pakistan. *Transactions of the Royal Society of Tropical Medicine and Hygiene* 98 (7): 442-449.

Kowalewski, M.M., Salzer, J.S., Deutsch, J.C. et al. (2011). Black and gold howler monkeys (*Alouatta caraya*) as sentinels of ecosystem health: patterns of zoonotic protozoa infection relative to degree of human–primate contact. *American Journal of Primatology* 73 (1): 75–83.

Kreft, H. and Jetz, W. (2007). Global patterns and determinants of vascular plant diversity. *Proceedings of the National Academy of Sciences* 104 (14): 5925–5930.

Kuparinen, A. and Festa-Bianchet, M. (2017). Harvest-induced evolution: insights from aquatic and terrestrial systems. *Philosophical Transactions of the Royal Society, B: Biological Sciences* 372 (1712): 20160036.

Lacetera, N., Scalia, D., Bernabucci, U., and Ronchi, B. (2003). in vitro assessment of the immunotoxicity of mycotoxins in goats. *Immunology Letters* 87: 323–324.

Lizundia-Loiola, J., Pettinari, M.L., and Chuvieco, E. (2020). Temporal anomalies in burned area trends: satellite estimations of the Amazonian 2019 fire crisis. *Remote Sensing* 12 (1): 151.

Lurie, N., Saville, M., Hatchett, R., and Halton, J. (2020). Developing Covid-19 vaccines at pandemic speed. *New England Journal of Medicine* 382 (21): 1969–1973.

Mas-Coma, S., Valero, M.A., and Bargues, M.D. (2008). Effects of climate change on animal and zoonotic helminthiases. *Revue Scientifique et Technique* 27 (2): 443–457.

Matson, P.A., Parton, W.J., Power, A.G., and Swift, M.J. (1997). Agricultural intensification and ecosystem properties. *Science* 277 (5325): 504–509.

Mayo, C.E., Gardner, I.A., Mullens, B.A. et al. (2012). Anthropogenic and meteorological factors influence vector abundance and prevalence of bluetongue virus infection of dairy cattle in California. *Veterinary Microbiology* 155 (2–4): 158–164.

McMichael, A.J. (2004). Environmental and social influences on emerging infectious diseases: past, present and future. *Philosophical Transactions of the Royal Society of London. Series B: Biological Sciences* 359 (1447): 1049–1058.

McNeill, J. (1976). The taxonomy and evolution of weeds. *Weed Research* 16 (6): 399–413.

Miller, M.A., Miller, W.A., Conrad, P.A. et al. (2008). Type X *Toxoplasma gondii* in a wild mussel and terrestrial carnivores from coastal California: new linkages between terrestrial mammals, runoff and toxoplasmosis of sea otters. *International Journal for Parasitology* 38 (11): 1319–1328.

Mirski, T., Bielawska-Drózd, A., and Bartoszcze, M. (2012). Impact of climate change on infectious diseases. *Polish Journal of Environmental Studies* 21 (3).

Morens, D.M., Folkers, G.K., and Fauci, A.S. (2004). The challenge of emerging and re-emerging infectious diseases. *Nature* 430: 242–249.

Morley, N.J. and Lewis, J.W. (2014). Temperature stress and parasitism of endothermic hosts under climate change. *Trends in Parasitology* 30 (5): 221–227.

Morse, S.S. (2001). Factors in the emergence of infectious diseases. In: *Plagues and Politics* (ed. A.T. Price-Smith), 8–26. Palgrave Publishers Ltd.

Nava, A., Shimabukuro, J.S., Chmura, A.A., and Luz, S.L.B. (2017). The impact of global environmental changes on infectious disease emergence with a focus on risks for Brazil. *ILAR Journal* 58 (3): 393–400.

Patz, J.A., Campbell-Lendrum, D., Holloway, T., and Foley, J.A. (2005). Impact of regional climate change on human health. *Nature* 438 (7066): 310–317.

Plowright, R.K., Parrish, C.R., McCallum, H. et al. (2017). Pathways to zoonotic spillover. *Nature Reviews Microbiology* 15 (8): 502–510.

Pulliam, J.R., Epstein, J.H., Dushoff, J. et al. (2012). Agricultural intensification, priming for persistence and the emergence of Nipah virus: a lethal bat-borne zoonosis. *Journal of the Royal Society Interface* 9 (66): 89–101.

Rogalski, M.A., Gowler, C.D., Shaw, C.L. et al. (2017). Human drivers of ecological and evolutionary dynamics in emerging and disappearing infectious disease systems. *Philosophical Transactions of the Royal Society, B: Biological Sciences* 372 (1712): 20160043.

Rohr, J.R., Raffel, T.R., Blaustein, A.R. et al. (2013). Using physiology to understand climate-driven changes in disease and their implications for conservation. *Conservation Physiology* 1 (1): cot022.

Rulli, M.C., Santini, M., Hayman, D.T., and D'Odorico, P. (2017). The nexus between forest fragmentation in Africa and Ebola virus disease outbreaks. *Scientific Reports* 7 (1): 1–8.

Sakai, A.K., Allendorf, F.W., Holt, J.S. et al. (2001). The population biology of invasive species. *Annual Review of Ecology and Systematics* 32 (1): 305–332.

Suzán, G., Marcé, E., Giermakowski, J.T. et al. (2008). The effect of habitat fragmentation and species diversity loss on hantavirus prevalence in Panama. *Annals of the New York Academy of Sciences* 1149 (1): 80–83.

Telfer, S., Lambin, X., Birtles, R. et al. (2010). Species interactions in a parasite community drive infection risk in a wildlife population. *Science* 330 (6001): 243–246.

Tilman, D. (1999). Global environmental impacts of agricultural expansion: the need for sustainable and efficient practices. *Proceedings of the National Academy of Sciences* 96 (11): 5995–6000.

Vaz, V.C., D'Andrea, P.S., and Jansen, A.M. (2007). Effects of habitat fragmentation on wild mammal infection by *Trypanosoma cruzi*. *Parasitology* 134 (12): 1785–1793.

Vittor, A.Y., Gilman, R.H., Tielsch, J. et al. (2006). The effect of deforestation on the human-biting rate of *Anopheles darlingi*, the primary vector of falciparum malaria in the Peruvian Amazon. *The American Journal of Tropical Medicine and Hygiene* 74 (1): 3–11.

Vittor, A.Y., Pan, W., Gilman, R.H. et al. (2009). Linking deforestation to malaria in the Amazon: characterization of the breeding habitat of the principal malaria vector, *Anopheles darlingi*. *The American Journal of Tropical Medicine and Hygiene* 81 (1): 5.

Weiss, R.A. (2001). The Leeuwenhoek lecture 2001. Animal origins of human infectious disease. *Philosophical Transactions of the Royal Society of London. Series B: Biological Sciences* 356 (1410): 957–977.

Wilcox, B.A. and Gubler, D.J. (2005). Disease ecology and the global emergence of zoonotic pathogens. *Environmental Health and Preventive Medicine* 10 (5): 263–272.

Xu, Z., Shi, L., Wang, Y. et al. (2020). Pathological findings of COVID-19 associated with acute respiratory distress syndrome. *The Lancet Respiratory Medicine* 8 (4): 420–422.

Yasuoka, J. and Levins, R. (2007). Impact of deforestation and agricultural development on anopheline ecology and malaria epidemiology. *The American Journal of Tropical Medicine and Hygiene* 76 (3): 450–460.

Zhou, F., Yu, T., Du, R. et al. (2020). Clinical course and risk factors for mortality of adult inpatients with COVID-19 in Wuhan, China: a retrospective cohort study. *The Lancet* 395 (10229): 1054–1062.

3

Environmental Interfaces for One Health

Rasika Jinadasa

Department of Veterinary Pathobiology, Faculty of Veterinary Medicine & Animal Science, University of Peradeniya, Peradeniya, Sri Lanka

3.1 Environment is the Most Dynamic Component of the One Health Triad

The environment is the most dynamic component of the One Health triad. However, it is often the most neglected component, particularly in resource-limited low- and middle-income countries (Abbassi et al. 2022; Taing et al. 2022). Unprecedented demographic and climatic change has taken place in the past few decades associated with the global population growth leading to ever increasing urbanization and increasing demand for international travel (Yabsley et al. 2021; Baker et al. 2022). Since 2007, more people live in urban areas than rural areas, and the number of commercial passenger flights has doubled since 2000 (Baker et al. 2022). Urbanization and urban expansion are major threats to ecosystems leading to habitat loss, fragmentation, loss of biodiversity, and species extinction (Yabsley et al. 2021). Environmental degradation and loss of biodiversity facilitate the spread of disease vectors and pathogens to new geographic localities, allowing the transposition of pathogens between different species and creating the ideal conditions for the transmission of pathogens from wild animals to humans known as zoonotic spillover events (Ellwanger and Chies 2021; Yuen et al. 2021). Wild animals are natural reservoirs of many unknown pathogens, and it is currently estimated that 60% of the existing human infectious diseases are zoonotic, while at least 75% of emerging infectious diseases originate in wild animals (UNEP and ILRI 2020; Ellwanger and Chies 2021; Yuen et al. 2021). Many pathogens survive outside their natural hosts without losing viability and transmissibility for significantly longer periods. Therefore, the environment acts as a reservoir for the transmission of such pathogens between different species and to humans (Alegbeleye and Sant'Ana 2020; Ellwanger and Chies 2021). Therefore, the interaction between humans, environment, and wildlife plays a significant role in the emergence of new human diseases. Most of the major recent zoonotic events resulted in severe morbidity and mortality in humans. These transboundary outbreaks and pandemics caused substantial economic losses in multiple countries (Baker et al. 2022). These major events include the 2003 severe acute respiratory syndrome coronavirus (SARS-CoV) outbreak, the 2009 swine flu pandemic, the 2012 Middle East respiratory syndrome coronavirus (MERS-CoV) outbreak, the 2013–2016 Ebola virus disease epidemic in West Africa, the 2015 Zika virus disease epidemic, and the 2019 SARS-CoV-2 (COVID-19) pandemic (Rothan and Byrareddy 2020; Wu et al. 2020; Baker et al. 2022). These outbreaks and pandemics were associated with changes in the behavior of wildlife due to anthropogenic modifications of the natural environment (Amaya and Broder 2020; Jacob et al. 2020; Pillai et al. 2020).

3.2 Anthropogenic Alteration of Natural Landscapes Reduces Biodiversity and Promotes Emergence and Spread of Infectious Diseases

Anthropogenic alteration of natural landscapes, such as intensification of agriculture and transformation of forests into pasture lands, reduces the biodiversity, which is directly associated with the emergence and spread of infectious diseases, including zoonotic infections. Natural ecosystems, such as forests with high biodiversity, have a "dilution effect" on zoonotic spillover events (Gibb et al. 2020; Halsey and Miller 2020; Ellwanger and

One Health: Human, Animal, and Environment Triad, First Edition. Edited by Meththika Vithanage and Majeti Narasimha Vara Prasad.

Chies 2021). High diversity of host species reduces or "dilutes" the prevalence of infection in high competent reservoir hosts and thereby reduces the risk of spillover events (Halsey and Miller 2020). Additionally, ecosystems with high biodiversity have many species that interfere with the transmission of pathogens through multiple mechanisms, reducing the risk of human infections. For example, increased vertebrate host diversity reduces the density of tick vectors for zoonotic Lyme disease (Halsey and Miller 2020).

The reduction in the richness and abundance of species in the natural environment promotes the proliferation of generalist small species, such as rodents, that host many pathogens (Gibb et al. 2020). It also increases the pathogen load in such species and contributes to climate change, which further alters vector dynamics (Ellwanger et al. 2018; Mendoza et al. 2020; Ostfeld and Keesing 2020). Classic examples include the expansion of the geographical ranges of mosquitoes that transmit malaria and several arboviral diseases including Chikungunya virus disease, dengue fever, eastern and western equine encephalitis, Japanese encephalitis, yellow fever, and Zika virus disease (Girard et al. 2020; Ogunah et al. 2020; WHO 2020; World Health Organization 2021). Management of arboviral diseases using conventional insecticide-based mosquito control methods is becoming ineffective and not environmentally friendly at the same time due to the widespread development of insecticide resistance, environmental contamination, and effects on non-target organisms including beneficial pollinator insects (Ogunah et al. 2020). Furthermore, adaptive changes in vector behavior in response to insecticide-based mosquito control interventions make it further challenging to control these diseases. These behavioral adaptations include changes in the time of biting, proportion of indoor biting, changes in vector species composition, and increased survival of vectors in urban environments (Ogunah et al. 2020; Sinka et al. 2020; Sougoufara et al. 2020; Youssefi et al. 2022). Holistic vector control approaches incorporating entomopathogenic bacteria, insect growth regulators, sterile males, and larvivorous native fish have proven very effective (Ogunah et al. 2020).

Similarly, bats (order: Chiroptera) are important reservoir hosts for many emerging zoonotic viruses such as Nipah virus in Malaysia, Ebola virus in Africa, and Hendra virus in Australia. These recently emerged zoonotic pathogens have caused multiple human outbreaks (Yuen et al. 2021). Similar to the role played by rodents in harboring heavy zoonotic pathogen loads in anthropogenically altered sites, bats in altered landscapes have been directly attributed to several major zoonotic disease outbreaks (Yabsley et al. 2021). For example, the gray-headed flying fox *(Pteropus poliocephalus)* bat population that migrated and settled in South Australia from other parts of the country in 2010 has been exposed to the zoonotic Hendra virus (Boardman et al. 2020; Yuen et al. 2021).

Intensification of the environmental degradation, loss of biodiversity, modifications in reservoir behavior, and disturbances to wildlife could lead to the recurrence of zoonotic spillover events with the same pathogen, involving single or multiple reservoirs. The human immunodeficiency virus originated from the simian immunodeficiency virus (SIV), which is found in several species of nonhuman primates in Africa. Two of these viruses, SIVcpz from chimpanzees and SIVsm from sooty mangabeys, had been spilled over to humans causing acquired immunodeficiency syndrome (AIDS) on at least seven different occasions (Ellwanger and Chies 2021). Ebola virus disease (EVD) outbreaks in humans usually start with a single case that could be directly attributable to zoonotic transmission originating from areas with forest fragmentation or deforestation. Modifications in reservoir behavior and disturbances to wildlife, including hunting and bushmeat consumption, have been associated with most of the outbreaks (Jacob et al. 2020; Rugarabamu et al. 2020; Gupta et al. 2021).

3.3 Climate Change Modify the Behavior of Reservoir Species of Zoonotic Pathogens and the Viability of the Pathogens in the Environment

In addition to direct anthropogenic activities, extreme environmental effects arising from climate change, such as altered rainfall patterns, may also modify the behavior of reservoir species of zoonotic pathogens and the viability of the pathogens in the environment (Rees et al. 2021; Yabsley et al. 2021; Louvrier et al. 2022). As a result, climate change directly affects the occurrence of pathogens in the environment and spillover events. Many pathogens survive outside their natural hosts without losing viability and transmissibility for significantly longer periods. Therefore, the environment acts as a reservoir for the transmission of such pathogens between different species and to humans. This is particularly true for waterborne pathogens (Alegbeleye and Sant'Ana 2020; Ellwanger and Chies 2021). The inherent survivability of the pathogen in the environment determines the success of the transmission between species. For example, non-enveloped viruses and capsulated bacteria are more resistant compared to enveloped and non-capsulated bacteria in the environment (Chiarelli et al. 2020; Durso et al. 2021; Anand et al. 2022). Multiple studies have shown that concentrations of human pathogens in natural waterbodies increase in the rainy season (González-Fernández et al. 2021). However, extreme changes in rainfall patterns lead to the "concentration-dilution effect" of pathogens and other contaminants entering natural surface waterbodies. Rainfall following prolonged dry periods may flush excess pathogen loads into surface water, increasing the pathogen concentration in the water, whereas rainfall following wet periods can dilute pathogen concentrations in surface water (Kraay et al. 2020). Certain deadly zoonotic diseases, such as anthrax, only transmit via the environment and not directly between hosts. The causative bacteria, *Bacillus anthracis*, survives in the soil for decades, and the occurrence of anthrax outbreaks is directly related to rainfall patterns (Huang et al. 2021).

3.4 Urbanization Creates Novel Habitats for Adaptable Species and New Niches for Diseases

Though urbanization is a major threat to natural ecosystems, it also creates novel habitats where adaptable species can establish and thrive. Several highly mobile host species of zoonotic pathogens, including bats, and disease vectors, including mosquitoes, are readily adapting to urban ecosystems (Yabsley et al. 2021; Yuen et al. 2021). The underlying reasons for these adaptations are rather complex. For example, recent urban and per-urban settlement of the gray-headed flying-fox (*P. poliocephalus*) in Australia is thought to be either due to loss or fragmentation of its natural foraging habitats or increasing food resources in urban areas, or both (Yabsley et al. 2021; Yuen et al. 2021). Historically, these bat colonies would roost seasonally in urban areas, probably according to the availability of food resources. However, in recent years, many urban roosts are occupied year-round (Yabsley et al. 2021). Similarly, an unusual outbreak of urban malaria was reported from the capital of Djibouti in 2012, as a result of the introduction of a new mosquito vector (*Anopheles stephensi*) into the region (Sinka et al. 2020). This Asian mosquito species is well adapted to urban environments in Africa now. Increasingly, severe outbreaks have been reported annually in Djibouti, and the new vector has been identified in Ethiopia and Sudan since then (Sinka et al. 2020). The increased presence of these host species and disease vectors in urban and peri-urban areas facilitates zoonotic spillover events under completely contrasting circumstances to historic spillover events, where sociocultural factors such as hunting, trade, and consumption of bushmeat put humans in close contact with wildlife, fresh meat, offal, and blood of wild animals that can host pathogens (Jacob et al. 2020). Furthermore, certain host species of zoonotic diseases that are adapting to human-dominated landscapes are endangered or threatened protected species, making it challenging to manage and conserve them (Yabsley et al. 2021).

3.5 Antimicrobial Resistance (AMR) Is One of the Largest Threats to Global Public Health

Antimicrobial resistance (AMR) is one of the largest threats to global public health in the twenty-first century, and according to some estimates, infections by pathogenic antimicrobial resistant bacteria (ARB) may cause most human mortalities by 2050 (Fouz et al. 2020; Lee et al. 2020; Samreen et al. 2021; Abbassi et al. 2022). It is a highly complex global threat that extends beyond national and regional boundaries, much similar to the magnitude and spread of recent pandemics (Lee et al. 2020; Torres et al. 2021). Resistance against critically important or last-resort antibiotics used in human medicine, such as colistin, carbapenems, extended-spectrum β-lactams (ESBL), and vancomycin, has been reported from environmental, livestock, or wildlife associated bacteria from most parts of the world (Koutsoumanis et al. 2021; Olaitan et al. 2021; Shi et al. 2021; Valiakos and Kapna 2021; Peng et al. 2022; Ramos et al. 2022). Alarmingly, several specific ARBs of highest priority for public health have also been reported among environmental isolates. This includes carbapenem or extended-spectrum cephalosporin and/or fluoroquinolone-resistant Enterobacterales (including *Salmonella enterica*), fluoroquinolone-resistant *Campylobacter* spp., methicillin-resistant *Staphylococcus aureus* (MRSA), and glycopeptide-resistant *Enterococcus faecium* and *Enterococcus faecalis* (Koutsoumanis et al. 2021). Among the highest priority ARGs reported from environmental bacteria are $blaCTX_{M}$, bla_{VIM}, bla_{NDM}, $bla_{OXA\text{-}48\text{-}like}$, $bla_{OXA\text{-}23}$, *mcr, armA, vanA, cfr*, and *optrA* (Koutsoumanis et al. 2021).

3.6 Transmission Dynamics of AMR in the Environmental and Wildlife Are Less Understood, or Neglected

Recent trends and mechanisms of the emergence and spread of AMR in medical and veterinary settings are relatively well understood (Torres et al. 2021; Lota et al. 2022). However, the complex transmission dynamics of AMR in the environmental and wildlife compartments, including the environmental contamination from animal husbandry and aquaculture, are less understood or neglected (Torres et al. 2021; Abbassi et al. 2022; Lota et al. 2022; Taing et al. 2022). This is partially due to the comparatively low research priorities on the dynamics of AMR in the environment and wildlife in recent years (Taing et al. 2022). A recent review has clearly shown that from 1990 to 2020 topics on plant, wildlife, and environment-related AMR threats, are frequently under prioritized as compared to topics on human and food animal health. Particularly, topics on the role of water sources play in AMR development and spread are under prioritized (Taing et al. 2022). Similar to other global health challenges, low- and middle-income countries will be the most affected by the rapidly increasing AMR, both in terms of its impact on public health and its stain on their economies (Fouz et al. 2020; Hedman et al. 2020).

3.7 Major Anthropogenic Drivers of Zoonotic Disease Emergence Also Drives the Emergence and Spread of AMR in Environment

Several major anthropogenic drivers of zoonotic disease emergence that are directly linked to the global population increase play a direct role in the emergence and spread of AMR in the environment. These factors include the increasing demand for animal protein and the associated unsustainable agricultural intensification and changes in food supply chains (UNEP and ILRI 2020). In addition to population growth, the demand for quality sources of animal protein increases with the development of countries, further promoting intensive animal husbandry (Hedman et al. 2020). Despite being essential for food security, large-scale intensive animal husbandry and aquaculture operations inherently increase the risk of AMR burden in the environment (Hedman et al. 2020). Large-scale intensive poultry operations are responsible for the largest portion of global antimicrobial use (Hedman et al. 2020). Commercial dairies, intensive pig farms, and intensive aquaculture systems also use considerable amount of antibiotics (Koutsoumanis et al. 2021).

3.8 Food-Producing Environments Play a Critical Role in the Emergence and Spread of AMR

Large-scale use of antibiotics in animal production systems at sub-therapeutic doses for growth promotion provides optimal conditions for bacteria to develop AMR. Animal manure from such production systems invariably contains antibiotic residues and their metabolites, ARB, and antibiotic resistance genes (ARGs) as contaminants (Checcucci et al. 2020; Dandeniya et al. 2022). Animal manure application to soil is a main cause of the propagation and dissemination of antibiotic residues, ARB, and ARGs in the soil–water system of the environment (Checcucci et al. 2020). The ARGs are often located on mobile genetic elements (MGEs), and the horizontal transfer (HGT) of MGEs between a broad range of bacteria, including human pathogens and human commensals, has been identified as the main mode of their persistence and dissemination (Checcucci et al. 2020). Several antibiotics used in human medicine and animal husbandry are analogs of each other, which aids in the transmission of resistance between humans and animals.

Additionally, treated or untreated farm and agricultural wastewater and sewage from anthropogenic sources such as hospitals, wastewater treatment plants, and pharmaceutical industries are frequently released to the natural environmental systems (Baros Jorquera et al. 2021). These effluents could contain antibiotic residues and their metabolites, ARB, and ARGs. These contaminants are further disseminated by water, which is the main transmission medium for such contaminants (Baros Jorquera et al. 2021). Wastewater is a significant environmental reservoir of AMR and acts as an ideal environment for ARB and ARGs to persist (Fouz et al. 2020). Although wastewater treatment processes can remove or reduce the ARB load, they have limited impact on ARGs (Fouz et al. 2020). The ARGs are relatively stable under normal wastewater treatment conditions, and therefore, they can spread the AMR among microbial communities in the environment through HGT, which is the main mechanism for acquiring AMR in most Gram-negative bacteria, including pathogens (Fouz et al. 2020; Worsley-Tonks et al. 2021).

Food-producing environments play a critical role in the emergence and spread of AMR (Koutsoumanis et al. 2021). Antibiotic-resistant human pathogens and human commensals may enter the food chain through both animal and plant-based foods including fresh vegetables and leafy greens (Koutsoumanis et al. 2021; Dandeniya et al. 2022). The sources and transmission routes include manure and fertilizers of fecal origin, irrigation water, and water for aquaculture (Koutsoumanis et al. 2021). It is clearly established that foods of plant origin are sources of foodborne exposure to ARB. Accordingly, vegetables harvested from manured soils and/or irrigated using wastewater or contaminated surface water are important sources of ARBs and antimicrobial residues entering the food chain. Therefore, the prevalence and diversity of livestock-associated ARBs in a particular food-producing environment are related to antimicrobial usage, farming, husbandry, and biosecurity practices. The selection pressure for AMR emergence in the environmental bacteria depends on the concentrations of antimicrobials/residues/metabolites in the environment and the duration of exposure (Koutsoumanis et al. 2021; Dandeniya et al. 2022). Interestingly, ARB persist in agricultural soils and continue to contaminate vegetable crops long after the exposure to manure, waste water, or other inputs that contain antibiotic residues, ARB, or ARGs (Food and Agriculture Organization and World Health Organization 2019; Koutsoumanis et al. 2021; Dandeniya et al. 2022). Several ARGs have low or no fitness cost to the bacteria or may even confer a fitness benefit (Lundberg et al. 2008; Li et al. 2020; Kloos et al. 2021; Pietsch et al. 2021). Thus, ARB carrying these ARGs would not be outcompeted by non-resistant bacteria at antimicrobial residue/metabolite concentrations below the minimal selective concentrations. Therefore, ARBs may persist within soil microbial communities even in the absence of continued antimicrobial selection pressure (Li et al. 2020; Perrin-Guyomard et al. 2020; Kloos et al. 2021).

3.9 Wildlife Also Plays a Very Significant Role in the Ecology and Dissemination of AMR

In addition to the persistence in soil and dissemination by water, wildlife also plays a very significant role in the ecology and dissemination of AMR (Guyomard-Rabenirina et al. 2020; Baros Jorquera et al. 2021). Wild animals harbor and disseminate ARB into a wide range of environmental niches and ecosystems far beyond national and regional borders (Baros Jorquera et al. 2021). For example, migrating birds may disseminate ARB across continents and pristine environments that were never exposed to ARB or ARGs (Khan et al. 2020; Hwengwere et al. 2022). Migratory wild birds travel long distances annually from Europe and Siberia to warmer parts of Asia. In several studies, β-lactam-resistant *Escherichia coli* have been identified in wild migratory birds inhabiting remote areas with low human activity (Khan et al. 2020). Resistance to multiple antibiotics including β-lactams had been reported from Antarctica, which is one of the remotest and most extreme environments, relatively free from the negative impacts of human activities. Furthermore, Antarctica is considered as the last pristine continent on Earth (Hwengwere et al. 2022).

Furthermore, wildlife plays an important role in the maintenance and dispersal of AMR at the interface of humans, domestic animals, and natural ecosystems (Guyomard-Rabenirina et al. 2020; UNEP and ILRI 2020; Baros Jorquera et al. 2021; Torres et al. 2021). Anthropogenically derived ARB and ARGs have been detected frequently in wildlife. The likelihood of detecting ARB and ARGs in wildlife increases with exposure to anthropogenic sources of AMR. For example, relatively higher AMR was reported from *E. coli* isolates from a wastewater treatment plant compared to isolates not exposed to wastewater (Worsley-Tonks et al. 2021). Similarly, ARB had been isolated from free-ranging yellow-legged gull (*Larus michahellis*) chicks that are only one week old from colonies in Europe that commonly live in industrialized areas and forage in landfills (Vittecoq et al. 2022). Furthermore, it was reported that ARB in chicks increased over time and was not spatially structured within the colony (Vittecoq et al. 2022).

Resistance to multiple antibiotics has been reported from bacteria originating from a wide range of wildlife species, including mammals, birds, reptiles, fish, and marine mammals, from all parts of the world (Grilo et al. 2020; Guyomard-Rabenirina et al. 2020; Khan et al. 2020; Kimera et al. 2020; Torres et al. 2020; Chen et al. 2021; Chiaverini et al. 2022; Hwengwere et al. 2022; Marin et al. 2022; Vittecoq et al. 2022; Woo et al. 2022; Zavala-Norzagaray et al. 2022). For example, resistance against multiple antibiotics including carbapenems has been reported from bacteria isolated from Australian silver gulls (*Chroicocephalus novaehollandiae*), which is a bird species that frequently inhabits anthropogenic waste sites in urban areas (Wyrsch et al. 2022). Similarly, β-lactam-resistant *E. coli* has been isolated from wild boar (*Sus scrofa*) in several European countries. Wild boar populations have dramatically increased in Europe over the last decades, and therefore, it could be considered as a perfect model species to study the emergence, spread, and persistence of AMR at the human–livestock–wildlife interface (Torres et al. 2020).

Other than their role in disseminating ARB, harboring ARB by wildlife is inherently dangerous as it may predispose endangered wild animals in natural habitats to infection with pathogenic ARB, which may be a threat for their conservation (Guyomard-Rabenirina et al. 2020; Baros Jorquera et al. 2021; Wang et al. 2022). For example, *E. coli* isolates that are resistant to multiple antibiotics including β-lactams have been isolated from giant pandas, which are endangered species, classified as vulnerable by the world wildlife foundation (Wang et al. 2022).

3.10 AMR is Not Monitored Regularly Using Standard Methods

Most of the currently available data on AMR in food production environments are originating from routine veterinary or food surveillance, or from standalone research projects. Therefore, most of these surveys are focused on specific zoonotic pathogens and/or indicator organisms in animal feces or food (Koutsoumanis et al. 2021; Torres et al. 2021). Therefore, a wide range of non-standardized methods and analysis techniques are used to characterize AMR, making it difficult to envisage the full picture of AMR in the environment. Furthermore, except in a few jurisdictions, such as the European Union, the monitoring of AMR is not undertaken at regular intervals, making it ever harder to gauge the true burden of environmental AMR (Koutsoumanis et al. 2021; Torres et al. 2021; Peng et al. 2022). *Escherichia coli* is preferred as an indicator organism for environmental AMR surveys including surveys on wildlife (Guyomard-Rabenirina et al. 2020; Torres et al. 2020; Anjum et al. 2021; Worsley-Tonks et al. 2021). For the survey of aquatic environments, *Aeromonas* spp. is frequently used as an indicator organism (Grilo et al. 2020; Chen et al. 2021; Woo et al. 2022). These organisms are ubiquitous in the environment, easily uptake and disseminate ARGs through HGT, and are easy and economical to grow in the laboratory. Additionally, some strains of *E. coli* and *Aeromonas* are human and animal pathogens (Grilo et al. 2020; Anjum et al. 2021; Chen et al. 2021; Woo et al. 2022).

Despite the non-standardized collection and analysis methods, available data suggest that environmental AMR is already a major global challenge, including high prevalence of multidrug resistance (MDR) and resistance to essential/critical antibiotics used in human medicine. Bacteria with resistance to $\geq$3 antibiotics that belongs to different structurally unrelated classes are considered as multidrug resistant isolates (Mukherjee et al. 2020). For example, a recent surveillance study using *E. coli* representing pig farms in all provinces in mainland China detected MDR in 91% of the isolates. Resistance was also reported against last-resort drugs used in human medicine including colistin, carbapenems, and tigecycline (Peng et al. 2022). Similarly, very high prevalence of colistin, extended-spectrum β-lactamase (ESBL), and carbapenemase resistance genes were detected in poultry farms in China (Shi et al. 2021). Several studies have clearly shown the widespread dispersion of plasmid borne *mcr* genes that confer colistin resistance among many bacterial species originating from livestock environments throughout the world, and colistin-resistant bacteria were detected in asymptomatic individuals and patients without known previous colistin exposure (Olaitan et al. 2021; Valiakos and Kapna 2021). In a classic positive response to curb the spread of AMR, colistin usage in livestock was banned in several countries, while some countries voluntarily withdrew it from the market in the recent past. This had an immediate effect on reducing colistin resistance in certain countries, for example in China and Portugal (Wang et al. 2020; Olaitan et al. 2021; Ribeiro et al. 2021). China is the largest producer and user of antibiotics in the world, of which more than 50% are used for animal husbandry (Xu et al. 2020). Only a few jurisdictions, such as the EU, have requirements to monitor surface water for the contamination of commonly used antibiotics, including amoxicillin, ciprofloxacin, sulfamethoxazole, and trimethoprim (Koutsoumanis et al. 2021)

3.11 Global and National Action Plans on AMR

Reducing the occurrence of fecal microbial contamination of fertilizers, water, feed, and the production environment is a major requirement to reduce the AMR burden in the environment. It is also necessary to minimize the persistence or recycling of ARB within animal production facilities (Koutsoumanis et al. 2021; Dandeniya et al. 2022). Many governments and national and international organizations have strongly suggested to adopt a holistic and multidisciplinary approach to address the emergence and spread of AMR, and accordingly, the global action plan (GAP) on AMR was launched in 2015 (WHO 2015; Lota et al. 2022; Pinto Ferreira et al. 2022). The GAP advocates the development and implementation of national action plans (NAPs) on AMR aimed at preventing, mitigating, and monitoring AMR (Pinto Ferreira et al. 2022). The NAPs and the prudent use of antimicrobials strategies of the World Organization for Animal Health (WOAH) are aligned with the GAP and recognize the importance of a One Health approach to combat AMR (Pinto Ferreira et al. 2022). However, the development and implementation of NAPs are often complicated due to the multifaceted nature of AMR and socioeconomic aspects favoring widespread availability of antimicrobials without prescription and irrational use across sectors in many developing countries (Hoque et al. 2020; Lota et al. 2022).

References

Abbassi, M.S., Badi, S., Lengliz, S. et al. (2022). Hiding in plain sight – wildlife as a neglected reservoir and pathway for the spread of antimicrobial resistance: a narrative review. *FEMS Microbiology Ecology* 98 (6): https://doi.org/10.1093/femsec/fiac045.

Alegbeleye, O.O. and Sant'Ana, A.S. (2020). Manure-borne pathogens as an important source of water contamination: an update on the dynamics of pathogen survival/transport as well as practical risk mitigation strategies. *International Journal of Hygiene and Environmental Health* https://doi.org/10.1016/j.ijheh.2020.113524.

Amaya, M. and Broder, C.C. (2020). Vaccines to emerging viruses: Nipah and Hendra. *Annual Review of Virology* https://doi.org/10.1146/annurev-virology-021920-113833.

Anand, U., Li, X., Sunita, K. et al. (2022). SARS-CoV-2 and other pathogens in municipal wastewater, landfill leachate, and solid waste: a review about virus surveillance, infectivity, and inactivation. *Environmental Research* https://doi.org/10.1016/j.envres.2021.111839.

Anjum, M.F., Schmitt, H., Börjesson, S. et al. (2021). The potential of using E. coli as an indicator for the surveillance of antimicrobial resistance (AMR) in the environment. *Current Opinion in Microbiology* https://doi.org/10.1016/j.mib.2021.09.011.

Baker, R.E., Mahmud, A.S., Miller, I.F. et al. (2022). Infectious disease in an era of global change. *Nature Reviews Microbiology* https://doi.org/10.1038/s41579-021-00639-z.

Baros Jorquera, C., Moreno-Switt, A.I., Sallaberry-Pincheira, N. et al. (2021). Antimicrobial resistance in wildlife and in the built environment in a wildlife rehabilitation center. *One Health* https://doi.org/10.1016/j.onehlt.2021.100298.

Boardman, W.S.J., Baker, M.L., Boyd, V. et al. (2020). Seroprevalence of three paramyxoviruses; Hendra virus, Tioman virus, Cedar virus and a Rhabdovirus, Australian bat lyssavirus, in a range expanding fruit bat, the grey-headed flying fox (*Pteropus poliocephalus*). *PLoS One* https://doi.org/10.1371/journal.pone.0232339.

Checcucci, A., Trevisi, P., Luise, D. et al. (2020). Exploring the animal waste resistome: the spread of antimicrobial resistance genes through the use of livestock manure. *Frontiers in Microbiology* https://doi.org/10.3389/fmicb.2020.01416.

Chen, J.S., Hsu, G.J., Hsu, B.M. et al. (2021). Prevalence, virulence-gene profiles, antimicrobial resistance, and genetic diversity of human pathogenic *Aeromonas* spp. from shellfish and aquatic environments. *Environmental Pollution* https://doi.org/10.1016/j.envpol.2021.117361.

Chiarelli, A., Cabanel, N., Rosinski-Chupin, I. et al. (2020). Diversity of mucoid to non-mucoid switch among carbapenemase-producing *Klebsiella pneumoniae*. *BMC Microbiology* https://doi.org/10.1186/s12866-020-02007-y.

Chiaverini, A., Cornacchia, A., Centorotola, G. et al. (2022). Phenotypic and genetic characterization of *Klebsiella pneumoniae* isolates from wild animals in Central Italy. *Animals* 12 (1347): https://doi.org/10.3390/ani12111347.

Dandeniya, W.S., Herath, E.M., Lowe, A.M. et al. (2022). Antibiotic use in commercial broiler chicken farming and its consequential resistance development in root colonizing bacteria of carrot grown in manure-applied soils in a middle-income country. *Canadian Journal of Soil Science* https://doi.org/10.1139/cjss-2021-0001.

Durso, L.M., Gilley, J.E., and Miller, D.N. (2021). Differential survival of non-O157 Shiga toxigenic *Escherichia coli* in simulated cattle feedlot runoff. *Foodborne Pathogens and Disease* https://doi.org/10.1089/fpd.2021.0024.

Ellwanger, J.H. and Chies, J.A.B. (2021). Zoonotic spillover: understanding basic aspects for better prevention. *Genetics and Molecular Biology* https://doi.org/10.1590/1678-4685-GMB-2020-0355.

Ellwanger, J.H., Zambra, F.M.B., Guimarães, R.L. et al. (2018). MicroRNA-related polymorphisms in infectious diseases-tiny changes with a huge impact on viral infections and potential clinical applications. *Frontiers in Immunology* https://doi.org/10.3389/fimmu.2018.01316.

Food and Agriculture Organization and World Health Organization (2019). *Joint FAO/WHO Expert Meeting in Collaboration with OIE on Foodborne Antimicrobial Resistance: Role of the Environment, Crops and Biocides – Meeting Report, Microbiological Risk Assessment Series*, vol. 34. Food and Agriculture Organization.

Fouz, N., Pangesti, K.N.A., Yasir, M. et al. (2020). The contribution of wastewater to the transmission of antimicrobial resistance in the environment: implications of mass gathering settings. *Tropical Medicine and Infectious Disease* https://doi.org/10.3390/tropicalmed5010033.

Gibb, R., Redding, D.W., Chin, K.Q. et al. (2020). Zoonotic host diversity increases in human-dominated ecosystems. *Nature* https://doi.org/10.1038/s41586-020-2562-8.

Girard, M., Nelson, C.B., Picot, V. et al. (2020). Arboviruses: a global public health threat. *Vaccine* https://doi.org/10.1016/j.vaccine.2020.04.011.

González-Fernández, A., Symonds, E.M., Gallard-Gongora, J.F. et al. (2021). Relationships among microbial indicators of fecal pollution, microbial source tracking markers, and pathogens in Costa Rican coastal waters. *Water Research* https://doi.org/10.1016/j.watres.2020.116507.

Grilo, M.L., Sousa-Santos, C., Robalo, J. et al. (2020). The potential of *Aeromonas* spp. from wildlife as antimicrobial resistance indicators in aquatic environments. *Ecological Indicators* https://doi.org/10.1016/j.ecolind.2020.106396.

Gupta, S., Gupta, N., Yadav, P. et al. (2021). Ebola virus outbreak preparedness plan for developing nations: lessons learnt from affected countries. *Journal of Infection and Public Health* https://doi.org/10.1016/j.jiph.2020.12.030.

Guyomard-Rabenirina, S., Reynaud, Y., Pot, M. et al. (2020). Antimicrobial resistance in wildlife in Guadeloupe (French West Indies): distribution of a single blaCTX–M–1/IncI1/ST3 plasmid among humans and wild animals. *Frontiers in Microbiology* https://doi.org/10.3389/fmicb.2020.01524.

Halsey, S.J. and Miller, J.R. (2020). Maintenance of *Borrelia burgdorferi* among vertebrate hosts: a test of dilution effect mechanisms. *Ecosphere* https://doi.org/10.1002/ecs2.3048.

Hedman, H.D., Vasco, K.A., and Zhang, L. (2020). A review of antimicrobial resistance in poultry farming within low-resource settings. *Animals* https://doi.org/10.3390/ani10081264.

Hoque, R., Ahmed, S.M., Naher, N. et al. (2020). Tackling antimicrobial resistance in Bangladesh: a scoping review of policy and practice in human, animal and environment sectors. *PLoS One* https://doi.org/10.1371/journal.pone.0227947.

Huang, Y.H., Joel, H., Küsters, M. et al. (2021). Disease or drought: environmental fluctuations release zebra from a potential pathogen-triggered ecological trap. *Proceedings of the Royal Society B: Biological Sciences* https://doi.org/10.1098/rspb.2021.0582.

Hwengwere, K., Paramel Nair, H., Hughes, K.A. et al. (2022). Antimicrobial resistance in Antarctica: is it still a pristine environment? *Microbiome* 10: https://doi.org/10.1186/s40168-022-01250-x.

Jacob, S.T., Crozier, I., Fischer, W.A. et al. (2020). Ebola virus disease. *Nature Reviews. Disease Primers* https://doi.org/10.1038/s41572-020-0147-3.

Khan, S.A., Imtiaz, M.A., Sayeed, M.A. et al. (2020). Antimicrobial resistance pattern in domestic animal – wildlife – environmental niche via the food chain to humans with a Bangladesh perspective; a systematic review. *BMC Veterinary Research* https://doi.org/10.1186/s12917-020-02519-9.

Kimera, Z.I., Mshana, S.E., Rweyemamu, M.M. et al. (2020). Antimicrobial use and resistance in food-producing animals and the environment: an African perspective. *Antimicrobial Resistance and Infection Control* https://doi.org/10.1186/s13756-020-0697-x.

Kloos, J., Gama, J.A., Hegstad, J. et al. (2021). Piggybacking on niche adaptation improves the maintenance of multidrug-resistance plasmids. *Molecular Biology and Evolution* https://doi.org/10.1093/molbev/msab091.

Koutsoumanis, K., Allende, A., Álvarez-Ordóñez, A. et al. (2021). Role played by the environment in the emergence and spread of antimicrobial resistance (AMR) through the food chain. *EFSA Journal* https://doi.org/10.2903/j.efsa.2021.6651.

Kraay, A.N.M., Man, O., Levy, M.C. et al. (2020). Understanding the impact of rainfall on diarrhea: testing the concentration-dilution hypothesis using a systematic review and meta-analysis. *Environmental Health Perspectives* https://doi.org/10.1289/EHP6181.

Lee, S., Mir, R.A., Park, S.H. et al. (2020). Prevalence of extended-spectrum β-lactamases in the local farm environment and livestock: challenges to mitigate antimicrobial resistance. *Critical Reviews in Microbiology* https://doi.org/10.1080/1040841X.2020.1715339.

Li, L., Dechesne, A., Madsen, J.S. et al. (2020). Plasmids persist in a microbial community by providing fitness benefit to multiple phylotypes. *The ISME Journal* https://doi.org/10.1038/s41396-020-0596-4.

Lota, M.M.M., Chua, A.Q., Azupardo, K. et al. (2022). A qualitative study on the design and implementation of the national action plan on antimicrobial resistance in the Philippines. *Antibiotics* 11 (820): https://doi.org/10.3390/antibiotics11060820.

Louvrier, J.L.P., Planillo, A., Stillfried, M. et al. (2022). Spatiotemporal interactions of a novel mesocarnivore community in an urban environment before and during SARS-CoV-2 lockdown. *The Journal of Animal Ecology* https://doi.org/10.1111/1365-2656.13635.

Lundberg, J.O., Weitzberg, E., and Gladwin, M.T. (2008). The nitrate-nitrite-nitric oxide pathway in physiology and therapeutics. *Nature Reviews Drug Discovery* 7 (2): 156–167. https://doi.org/10.1038/nrd2466.

Marin, C., Martín-Maldonado, B., Cerdà-Cuéllar, M. et al. (2022). Antimicrobial resistant Salmonella in chelonians: assessing its potential risk in zoological institutions in Spain. *Veterinary Sciences* 9 (6): 264. https://doi.org/10.3390/vetsci9060264.

Mendoza, H., Rubio, A.V., García-Peña, G.E. et al. (2020). Does land-use change increase the abundance of zoonotic reservoirs? Rodents say yes. *European Journal of Wildlife Research* https://doi.org/10.1007/s10344-019-1344-9.

Mukherjee, M., Gentry, T., Mjelde, H. et al. (2020). Escherichia coli antimicrobial resistance variability in water runoff and soil from a remnant native prairie, an improved pasture, and a cultivated agricultural watershed. *Water (Switzerland)* https://doi.org/10.3390/W12051251.

Ogunah, J.A., Lalah, J.O., and Schramm, K.W. (2020). Malaria vector control strategies. What is appropriate towards sustainable global eradication? *Sustainable Chemistry and Pharmacy* https://doi.org/10.1016/j.scp.2020.100339.

Olaitan, A.O., Dandachi, I., Baron, S.A. et al. (2021). Banning colistin in feed additives: a small step in the right direction. *The Lancet Infectious Diseases* https://doi.org/10.1016/S1473-3099(20)30915-4.

Ostfeld, R.S. and Keesing, F. (2020). Species that can make us ill thrive in human habitats. *Nature* https://doi.org/10.1038/d41586-020-02189-5.

Peng, Z., Hu, Z., Li, Z. et al. (2022). Antimicrobial resistance and population genomics of multidrug-resistant *Escherichia coli* in pig farms in mainland China. *Nature Communications* https://doi.org/10.1038/s41467-022-28750-6.

Perrin-Guyomard, A., Jouy, E., Urban, D. et al. (2020). Decrease in fluoroquinolone use in French poultry and pig production and changes in resistance among *E. coli* and *Campylobacter*. *Veterinary Microbiology* https://doi.org/10.1016/j.vetmic.2020.108637.

Pietsch, M., Pfeifer, Y., Fuchs, S. et al. (2021). Genome-based analyses of fitness effects and compensatory changes associated with acquisition of blacmy-, blactx-m-, and blaoxa-48/vim-1-containing plasmids in *Escherichia coli*. *Antibiotics* https://doi.org/10.3390/antibiotics10010090.

Pillai, V.S., Krishna, G., and Veettil, M.V. (2020). Nipah virus: past outbreaks and future containment. *Viruses* https://doi.org/10.3390/v12040465.

Pinto Ferreira, J., Gochez, D., Jeannin, M. et al. (2022). From OIE standards to responsible and prudent use of antimicrobials: supporting stewardship for the use of antimicrobial agents in animals. *JAC-Antimicrobial Resistance* https://doi.org/10.1093/jacamr/dlac017.

Ramos, B., Rosalino, L.M., Palmeira, J.D. et al. (2022). Antimicrobial resistance in commensal *Staphylococcus aureus* from wild ungulates is driven by agricultural land cover and livestock farming. *Environmental Pollution* https://doi.org/10.1016/j.envpol.2022.119116.

Rees, E.M., Minter, A., Edmunds, W.J. et al. (2021). Transmission modelling of environmentally persistent zoonotic diseases: a systematic review. *The Lancet Planetary Health* https://doi.org/10.1016/S2542-5196(21)00137-6.

Ribeiro, S., Mourão, J., Novais, Â. et al. (2021). From farm to fork: colistin voluntary withdrawal in Portuguese farms reflected in decreasing occurrence of mcr-1-carrying *Enterobacteriaceae* from chicken meat. *Environmental Microbiology* https://doi.org/10.1111/1462-2920.15689.

Rothan, H.A. and Byrareddy, S.N. (2020). The epidemiology and pathogenesis of coronavirus disease (COVID-19) outbreak. *Journal of Autoimmunity* https://doi.org/10.1016/j.jaut.2020.102433.

Rugarabamu, S., Mboera, L., Rweyemamu, M. et al. (2020). Forty-two years of responding to Ebola virus outbreaks in sub-Saharan Africa: a review. *BMJ Global Health* https://doi.org/10.1136/bmjgh-2019-001955.

Samreen, Ahmad, I., Malak, H.A. et al. (2021). Environmental antimicrobial resistance and its drivers: a potential threat to public health. *Journal of Global Antimicrobial Resistance* https://doi.org/10.1016/j.jgar.2021.08.001.

Shi, X., Li, Y., Yang, Y. et al. (2021). High prevalence and persistence of carbapenem and colistin resistance in livestock farm environments in China. *Journal of Hazardous Materials* https://doi.org/10.1016/j.jhazmat.2020.124298.

Sinka, M.E., Pironon, S., Massey, N.C. et al. (2020). A new malaria vector in Africa: predicting the expansion range of *Anopheles stephensi* and identifying the urban populations at risk. *Proceedings of the National Academy of Sciences of the United States of America* https://doi.org/10.1073/pnas.2003976117.

Sougoufara, S., Ottih, E.C., and Tripet, F. (2020). The need for new vector control approaches targeting outdoor biting *Anopheline* malaria vector communities. *Parasites & Vectors* https://doi.org/10.1186/s13071-020-04170-7.

Taing, L., Bhatia, H., Kaiser, R.A. et al. (2022). A rapid review of environmental health gaps in antimicrobial resistance and water-related research from 1990–2020. *International Journal of Environmental Research and Public Health* 19 (6549): https://doi.org/10.3390/ijerph19116549.

Torres, R.T., Fernandes, J., Carvalho, J. et al. (2020). Wild boar as a reservoir of antimicrobial resistance. *The Science of the Total Environment* https://doi.org/10.1016/j.scitotenv.2019.135001.

Torres, R.T., Carvalho, J., Cunha, M.V. et al. (2021). Temporal and geographical research trends of antimicrobial resistance in wildlife – a bibliometric analysis. *One Health* https://doi.org/10.1016/j.onehlt.2020.100198.

UNEP and ILRI (2020). *Preventing the Next Pandemic: Zoonotic Diseases and How to Break the Chain of Transmission*. United Nations Environment Programme.

Valiakos, G. and Kapna, I. (2021). Colistin resistant mcr genes prevalence in livestock animals (swine, bovine, poultry) from a multinational perspective. A systematic review. *Veterinary Sciences* https://doi.org/10.3390/vetsci8110265.

Vittecoq, M., Brazier, L., Elguero, E. et al. (2022). Multiresistant *Enterobacteriaceae* in yellow-legged gull chicks in their first weeks of life. *Ecology and Evolution* 12 (e8974): https://doi.org/10.1002/ece3.8974.

Wang, Y., Xu, C., Zhang, R. et al. (2020). Changes in colistin resistance and mcr-1 abundance in *Escherichia coli* of animal and human origins following the ban of colistin-positive additives in China: an epidemiological comparative study. *The Lancet Infectious Diseases* https://doi.org/10.1016/S1473-3099(20)30149-3.

Wang, X., Zhang, Y., Li, C. et al. (2022). Antimicrobial resistance of *Escherichia coli*, Enterobacter spp., *Klebsiella pneumoniae* and *Enterococcus* spp. isolated from the feces of giant panda. *BMC Microbiology* 22 (102): https://doi.org/10.1186/s12866-022-02514-0.

WHO (2015). *Organization World Health. Global Action Plan on Antimicrobial Resistance*. World Health Organization.

WHO (2020). WHO World Malaria Report 2020. Malaria Report.

Woo, S.J., Kim, M.S., Jeong, M.G. et al. (2022). Establishment of epidemiological cut-off values and the distribution of resistance genes in *Aeromonas hydrophila* and *Aeromonas veronii* isolated from aquatic animals. *Antibiotics* https://doi.org/10.3390/antibiotics11030343.

World Health Organization (2021). Word Malaria Report 2021, Word Malaria Report Geneva: World Health Organization. (2021). Licence: CC.

Worsley-Tonks, K.E.L., Miller, E.A., Anchor, C.L. et al. (2021). Importance of anthropogenic sources at shaping the antimicrobial resistance profile of a peri-urban mesocarnivore. *The Science of the Total Environment* https://doi.org/10.1016/j.scitotenv.2020.144166.

Wu, Y.C., Chen, C.S., and Chan, Y.J. (2020). The outbreak of COVID-19: an overview. *Journal of the Chinese Medical Association* https://doi.org/10.1097/JCMA.0000000000000270.

Wyrsch, E.R., Nesporova, K., Tarabai, H. et al. (2022). Urban wildlife crisis: Australian silver Gull is a bystander host to widespread clinical antibiotic resistance. *ASM Journals* https://doi.org/10.1128/msystems.00158-22%0A.

Xu, J., Sangthong, R., McNeil, E. et al. (2020). Antibiotic use in chicken farms in Northwestern China. *Antimicrobial Resistance and Infection Control* https://doi.org/10.1186/s13756-019-0672-6.

Yabsley, S.H., Meade, J., Martin, J.M. et al. (2021). Human-modified landscapes provide key foraging areas for a threatened flying mammal: the grey-headed flying-fox. *PLoS One* https://doi.org/10.1371/journal.pone.0259395.

Youssefi, F., Zoej, M.J.V., Hanafi-Bojd, A.A. et al. (2022). Temporal monitoring and predicting of the abundance of malaria vectors using time series analysis of remote sensing data through google earth engine. *Sensors (Basel, Switzerland)* https://doi.org/10.3390/s22051942.

Yuen, K.Y., Fraser, N.S., Henning, J. et al. (2021). Hendra virus: epidemiology dynamics in relation to climate change, diagnostic tests and control measures. *One Health* https://doi.org/10.1016/j.onehlt.2020.100207.

Zavala-Norzagaray, A.A., Alonso Aguirre, A.A., Angulo-Zamudio, U.A. et al. (2022). Isolation, characterization, and antimicrobial susceptibility of bacteria isolated from sea lion (Zalophus californianus) pups in Northwestern Mexico. *Journal of Willife Diseases* (In Press). https://doi.org/10.7589/JWD-D-21-00183.

4

Zoonoses

The Rising Threat to Human Health

B.G.D.N.K. de Silva[1,2], *H. Harischandra*[2], *and S.U. Nimalratna*[1]

[1] *Centre for Biotechnology, Faculty of Applied Sciences, University of Sri Jayewardenepura, Nugegoda, Sri Lanka*
[2] *Genetics and Molecular Biology Unit, Faculty of Applied Sciences, University of Sri Jayewardenepura, Nugegoda, Sri Lanka*

Zoonotic diseases is a hotly discussed topic owing to the global COVID-19 pandemic, a prime example of the chaos caused by zoonoses. COVID-19 is caused by the SARS-CoV-2 virus, a virus family found in bats, which gave rise to many concerns and speculations as to how it transmitted to humans. Many were put forth and investigated by the World Health Organization (WHO): direct transmission from bats to humans (spillover); transmitted to an intermediate host, followed by spillover; transmitted through the (cold) food chain; and transmitted via a laboratory incident. After much investigation, the most likely yet unconfirmed explanation for the outbreak is thought to be that the SARS-CoV-2 virus was transmitted to humans from its natural host, bats, via pangolin as an intermediate host. Regardless of the mode of transmission, this should be considered a wake-up call to the global damage that can be caused by zoonosis.

4.1 What is a Zoonotic Disease?

WHO describes a zoonotic disease or zoonosis (zoonoses, plural) as an infectious disease naturally transmitted from a vertebrate animal to humans and vice versa. The word "zoonoses" is derived from the Greek words "Zoon," meaning an animal, and "nosos," meaning illness. It was coined and first used by Rudolf Virchow, who defined it for communicable diseases. Some zoonotic diseases originate in animals, are spread to humans, and then are spread between humans and animals interchangeably, such as the SARS-CoV-2 virus. The first human cases of COVID-19 were reported from Wuhan City, China, in December 2019 and spread fast to humans in other regions of the world (WHO 2021). Interestingly, there were a few incidents where animals around the world were reported to have been infected by the SARS-CoV-2 virus after being in contact with infected humans. These animals include companion animals or pets such as cats, dogs, and ferrets, animals in zoos and sanctuaries around the world such as several types of big cats, otters, non-human primates, a binturong, a coatimundi, a fishing cat, and hyenas, as well as wild white-tailed deer in several states of the USA (Gollakner and Capua 2020). Mink on mink farms in multiple countries, including the Netherlands, Denmark, and the United States, have been reported to be infected as well. Interestingly, investigations have revealed that mink and a few of the people infected with SARS-CoV-2 from these farms shared unique mink-related mutations in the virus, suggesting that mink to human transmission of the virus might have occurred.

Some zoonotic diseases originate in animals but, once transmitted to humans, spread only between humans. Human immunodeficiency virus (HIV) infection and acquired immunodeficiency syndrome (AIDS), which is the last stage of an HIV infection is a global epidemic that has claimed at least 36 million lives since the first reported case in 1981. It is caused by the human immunodeficiency virus 1 (HIV-1), which originated from the simian immunodeficiency virus (SIV) of chimpanzees and HIV-2 from the SIV of the sooty mangabey monkey, and is now spread directly from human to human. The mode of transmission from the primates to humans is not known but is speculated to have happened during hunting and processing these primates for food by the indigenous people of these areas in Central and Western Africa, where these primate species live. It is likely that after the initial transmission of these SIVs to humans, these infected humans transmitted the human form of the viruses (HIV-1, HIV-2) to other people in their

One Health: Human, Animal, and Environment Triad, First Edition. Edited by Meththika Vithanage and Majeti Narasimha Vara Prasad.

communities, from where it spread, worldwide and remains an incurable, deadly disease to date. Measles is another zoonotic disease which originated in animals, namely cattle, and then diverged to spread between humans.

The impact of zoonotic diseases is graver than we think. Not only does it impede the physical and mental health of affected individuals, but it also affects the family in many ways. Zoonotic diseases, like other diseases, tend to spread among and have the biggest impact on populations at the lower end of the monetary scale in developing countries due to many reasons such as scarcity of resources, poor management, and lack of flow of information. Having a diseased individual in such a household affects the economy of the entire family, especially if the affected individual is the breadwinner and can no longer engage in his or her occupation. Additional expenses for medicine and disease management aggravate the burden. If the disease burden of a country is high, it, in turn, affects the economy of the country due to the loss of workforce and increased investments in medical expenses and disease management efforts. Lymphatic filariasis (LF) is a prime example of a disease with such consequences. LF, characterized by the gross swelling of extremities, is the second leading cause of permanent disability and has resulted in over US$100.5 billion economic burden for treatment, cost of healthcare and potential income loss in developing countries. Recent studies have implicated zoonosis of the disease, exacerbating the risk of spread and making control or mitigation a challenging task.

Interactions between humans, animals, and the environment are increasing in unhealthy proportions in the face of development, creating an unhealthy imbalance between the triad. This in turn is triggering zoonoses at an unprecedented rate, presenting a significant threat to both human and animal health, reflecting the complexities of the ecosystems in which humans and animals coexist. Human invasion of wilderness and forest areas to acquire land for agriculture, habitation, and infrastructure development degrades the natural barriers of disease transmission and increases the area of human–animal borders, increasing the risk of contracting zoonotic diseases. It also brings wild animals that were once well isolated from humans closer to them. Moreover, reduced feeding grounds provoke wild animals such as bears, racoons, deer, elephants and bats to wander into human habitation in search of food, yet again increasing the risk of incidence. Other human activities, such as animal domestication, intensive agriculture, excessive hunting, illegal wildlife trade, among others, increase the chances of contact between infected animals and humans, increasing the risk of zoonosis. Moreover, heightened global mobilization through travel and trade rapidly increases the global spread of pathogens, leading to pandemics of various magnitudes.

4.2 Classification of Zoonotic Diseases

Zoonotic diseases can be classified based on three main criteria. They are

1) Etiological agents
2) Mode of transmission
3) Direction of transmission

Zoonoses classified based on the direction of transmission are specified by a collection of terms such as anthropozoonoses, zooanthroponoses, and amphixenoses. Anthropozoonoses are diseases that cross the species barrier and are transmitted to humans from vertebrate animals, a phenomenon known as "spillover." Rabies, leptospirosis, plague, brucellosis, and Q fever are examples of anthropozoonoses that resulted from spillover events. Zooanthroponoses refer to diseases transmitted from humans to vertebrate animals, a phenomenon described as a spillback event or reverse zoonosis because transmission occurs from human to animal. Tuberculosis and other bacterial diseases causing streptococci in cattle, cats, and monkeys are examples of zooanthroponoses. Diseases such as salmonellosis and staphylococcus infections that can be transmitted bidirectionally to and from both humans and animals are termed amphixenoses (Figure 4.1).

Zoonoses can be caused by a wide range of pathogens such as viruses, bacteria, fungi, protozoans, helminths, and prions. The following table lists the major zoonotic diseases classified based on the characterization of the etiological agents (Rahman et al. 2020).

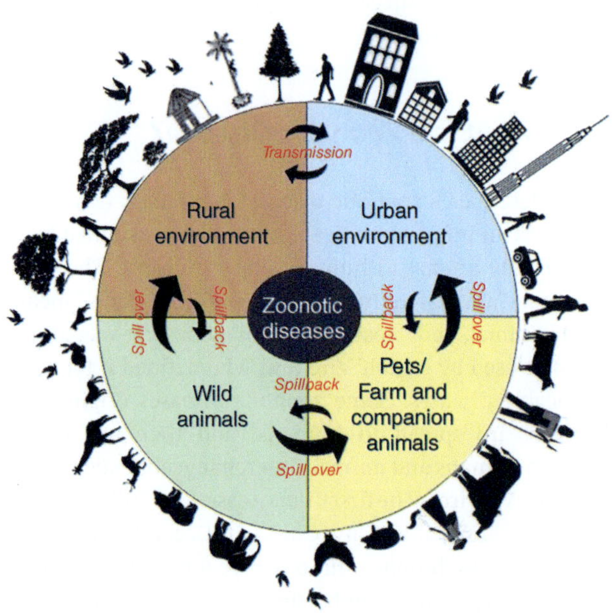

Figure 4.1 The zoonotic interrelationship between humans in rural and urban environments and animals in domestic, farm, and forest environments.

Type of zoonoses	Disease	Etiological agent	Mode of transmission	Reservoir vertebrate host
Bacterial zoonoses	Anthrax	*Bacillus anthracis*	Direct contact, contaminated food, water and biological products, air	Cattle, horses, sheep, pigs, dogs, bison, elks, white-tailed deer, goats, and mink
	Bubonic plague	*Yersinia pestis*	Vectors: infected fleas	Rock squirrels, wood rats, ground squirrels, prairie dogs, mice, voles, chipmunks, and rabbits
	Leprosy	*Mycobacterium leprae*	Air	Monkeys, rats, mice, and cats
	Lyme disease	*Borrelia burgdorferi*	Vectors: infected ticks	Cats, dogs, and horses
	Tuberculosis	*Mycobacterium bovis*, *Mycobacterium caprae*, *Mycobacterium microti*	Air	Cattle, sheep, swine, deer, wild boars, camels, and bison
	Brucellosis	*Brucella abortus*, *Brucella melitensis*, *Brucella suis*, *Brucella canis*	Direct contact, placenta, contaminated food, and biological products	Cattle, goats, sheep, pigs, and dogs
	Leptospirosis	*Leptospira interrogans*	Urine of infected animals	Wild and domestic animals including pet dogs
	Helicobacter infection	*Helicobacter pullorum*, *Helicobacter suis*	Direct contact with biological products of infected animals and contaminated food or water	Poultry and pigs
	Vibriosis	*Vibrio parahaemolyticus*	Contaminated food or water	Farm animals
	Salmonellosis	*Salmonella enterica*, *Salmonella bongor*	Contaminated food or water	Domestic animals, birds, and dogs
Rickettsial zoonoses	Q-fever epidemic	*Coxiella burnetti*	Air	Cattle, sheep, goats, dogs, cats, chickens, and wild animals
	Rocky mountain spotted fever	*Rickettsia rickettsii*	Vector borne: infected ticks	Rodents and dogs
	Scrub typhus	*Orientia tsutsugamushi*	Vector borne: chigger mites	Rodents
	Epidemic typhus	*Rickettsia prowazekii*	Vector borne: infected lice	Dogs, lambs, goat kids, calves, donkeys, and young camels
Chlamydial zoonoses	Enzootic abortion	*Chlamydia abortus*	Contaminated aerosols, ingestion of organisms shed in vaginal fluids and placental membranes at the time of abortion	Cattle, horses, sheep, pigs, cats, and rabbits
	Chlamydiosis	*Chlamydia felis*, *Chlamydia trachomatis*	Vaginal, anal, or oral sex with infected person	Cats and mice
	Psittacosis	*Chlamydia psittaci*	Direct contact of infected animals, inhalation of infectious agent	Parrots, parakeets, lories, cockatoos, cattle, sheep, and goats
Viral zoonoses	Rabies	*Rabies virus*	Direct contact with saliva or brain/nervous system tissue from an infected animal	Cattle, horses, cats, dogs, bats, monkeys, wolves, skunks, rabbits, and coyotes
	Avian influenza	*Influenza A virus*	Direct contact with infected animals biological secretions, air, and contaminated food or water	Ducks, chickens, turkeys, dogs, cats, pigs, whales, horses, seals, and wild birds

(*Continued*)

Type of zoonoses	Disease	Etiological agent	Mode of transmission	Reservoir vertebrate host
	Rift valley fever	*Rift Valley fever virus*	Direct contact of infected blood, body fluids, and tissues	Buffaloes, camels, cattle, goats, and sheep
	Ebola virus disease (Ebola hemorrhagic fever)	*Ebola virus*	Direct contact of infected blood and body fluids	Monkeys, gorillas, chimpanzees, apes, and wild antelopes
	AIDS	*HIV*	Exchange of body fluids, transplacental transmission	Monkeys and chimpanzees
	Severe acute respiratory syndrome (SARS)	*SARS coronavirus (SARS-CoV)*	Respiratory droplets and aerosols	Bats, dogs, cats, ferrets, minks, tigers, and lions
	Monkey pox	*Monkeypox virus*	Direct contact of infected animals or material contaminated with the virus	Squirrels, Gambian poached rats, dormice, different species of monkeys, and others
	Dengue fever	*Dengue virus*	Vector borne: infected mosquitoes	Monkeys and dogs
	Zika fever	*Zika virus*	Vector borne: infected mosquitoes	Apes and monkeys
	West Nile fever	*West Nile virus*	Vector borne: infected mosquitoes	Horses, birds, and reptiles
	Chikungunya fever	*Chikungunya virus*	Vector borne: infected mosquitoes	Monkeys, birds, and rodents
Parasitic zoonoses	Trichinellosis	*Trichinella* spp.	Consumption of uncooked meat of infected animals	Pigs, dogs, cats, rats, and other wild species
	Cutaneous larval migrans	*Ancylostoma braziliense*	Direct contact with infected animal feces	Dogs and cats
	Cryptococcosis	*Cryptococcus neoformans*	Direct contact, food and pigeon droppings	Dogs, cattle, horses, sheep, goats, birds, and wild animals
	Cryptosporidiosis	*Cryptosporidium parvum*	Contaminated food or water	Cattle, sheep, pigs, goats, horses, and deer
	Fascioliasis	*Fasciola hepatica, Fasciola gigantica*	Consumption of water plants contaminated with immature parasite larvae	Cattle, sheep, goats, and other ruminants mycotic/ fungal
	Hydatidosis	*Echinococcus granulosus*	Accidental consumption of contaminated food, water, or soil	Buffaloes, sheep, goats, and adult stray or shepherd dogs
Mycotic/ fungal zoonoses	Tinea/ringworm infection	*Microsporum* spp., *Trichophyton* spp.	Direct skin to skin contact with infected animal	All animals like cattle, sheep, goats, cats, and dogs
	Aspergillosis	*Aspergillus* spp.	Air	All domestic animals and birds
	Histoplasmosis	*Histoplasma capsulatum var. capsulatum*	Air	Cats, dogs, rabbits, and rats
	Cryptococcosis	*Cryptococcus neoformis*	Direct contact with infected pigeon droppings and contaminated food	Cats, dogs, cattle, horses, sheep, goats, birds, and wild animals
	Coccidioidomycosis	*Coccidioides immitis, Coccidioides posadasii*	Air	Dogs, horses, pigs, and ruminants

Type of zoonoses	Disease	Etiological agent	Mode of transmission	Reservoir vertebrate host
Protozoal zoonoses	Trypanosomiasis	*Trypanosoma brucei*	Bite of an infected tsetse fly	Antelopes, cattle, camels, and horses
	African sleeping sickness	*Trypanosoma brucei*	Bite of an infected tsetse fly	Antelopes, cattle, cats, camels, and horses
	Leishmaniasis	*Leishmania infantum*	Bite of an infected female phlebotomine sand flies	Cats, dogs, horses, and bats
	Giardiasis	*Giardia lamblia*	Contaminated water, food, surfaces, or objects	Dogs, cats, ruminants, and pigs
	Balantidiasis	*Balantidium coli*	Contaminated food, water	Ruminants, pigs, guinea pigs and rats
	Toxocariasis	*Toxocara canis, Toxocara cati*	Accidental swallowing dog or cat feces that contain infectious toxocara eggs	Dogs and cats
	Toxoplasmosis	*Toxoplasma gondii*	Ingestion of oocytes from contaminated food, soil, fecal matter and trans-placental transmission	Pigs, sheep, goats, poultry, and rabbits
	Chagas disease	*Trypanosoma cruzi*	Vector: infected kissing bugs	Domestic pigs and cats, wildlife reservoirs, include opossums, armadillos, raccoons, and woodrats
Disease caused by acellular nonviral pathogenic agents	Variant Creutzfeldt–Jakob disease (vCJD), caused by Mad Cow Disease also known as Bovine Spongiform Encephalopathy (BSE) is the only zoonotic animal prion disease	Prion protein	Consumption of beef from an infected cow	Cattle, sheep, goats, mink, deer, and elks

Zoonotic diseases can also be classified according to the mode of transmission. Zoonotic pathogens can be transmitted to humans through direct contact with an infected animal or indirectly via air, food, water, contaminated surfaces, or arthropod vectors. Direct transmission occurs when humans come in contact with saliva, mucous, blood, urine, faeces, and other body fluids of an infected animal when handling infected pets, farm animals and wild animals. Indirect transmission occurs when humans come into contact with surfaces contaminated with the disease-causing agent. Zoonotic diseases transmitted through contaminated food, water, and air are known as foodborne, waterborne, and airborne zoonotic diseases, respectively. Zoonotic diseases transmitted through the bite of infected arthropods such as mosquitoes, sandflies, ticks, and fleas are known as vector-borne zoonotic diseases. The most efficient way of controlling the spread of zoonotic diseases is by hindering transmission, and therefore, we will focus mainly on the modes of transmission of zoonotic diseases, causes and preventive measures in this chapter.

4.3 Direct Contact

Zoonotic diseases can be contracted via viruses and bacteria transmitted from saliva or body fluids of infected animals. Rabies, caused by the rabies virus, is a disease that is transmitted from saliva of an infected animal. It is a disease of the nervous system and is almost always lethal. The risk of contracting rabies from domesticated dogs is quite low due to the availability of the anti-rabies vaccine. Humans are at a higher risk of contracting the disease from stray cats and dogs and wild animals such as bats, raccoons, foxes, and skunks. Bacteria of *Pasteurella* species can be transmitted to humans by dog or cat bites, licks, or scratches, causing soft tissue infection, meningitis, arthritis, and respiratory infections. *Capnocytophaga canimorsus*, transmitted to humans by dog bites, can cause sepsis, especially in the elderly, the immunocompromised and people lacking normal spleen function. It can also lead to other fatal infections including osteomyelitis, lung abscess, and endocarditis.

4.4 Indirect Contact

4.4.1 Vector-Borne Zoonotic Diseases

4.4.1.1 Definition and Transmission

Vector-borne zoonotic diseases are those caused by viruses, bacteria, protozoans, fungi, and helminths transmitted by arthropods including mosquitoes, ticks, and fleas. Almost all vector-borne diseases originated from the sylvatic (forest) transmission cycle and then shifted to an urban transmission cycle where human and urban arthropod vectors have established a relationship with pathogens. The sylvatic cycle occurs in non-human primates (NHPs) living in forest habitats where arboreal mosquitoes transmit arboviruses from infected to naïve NHPs (NHP-mosquito-NHP-mosquito). When people invading these forest habitats for deforestation, hunting, lodging, and agriculture are bitten by infected mosquitoes, or these mosquitoes disperse to human habitation to feed, the sylvatic transmission cycle "spills over" into the urban transmission cycle. In some such cases, the sylvatic cycles will continuously be maintained with NHPs. This helps to maintain the virus in reservoirs until becoming viremic in the event of a spillover to humans, or the viral genome is changed in the event of a spillback to NHPs. However, some arboviruses fully adapt to the urban transmission cycle, eliminating the need to maintain the sylvatic cycle (Figure 4.2).

4.4.1.2 Common Examples

Malaria is a devastating parasitic and vector-borne disease that has been in the tropical world for centuries and is the disease causing the highest morbidity and mortality even today. Anopheline mosquitoes are the only genus of mosquitoes that transmit the malaria parasite. Out of the five *Plasmodium* species that carry human malaria, *Plasmodium falciparum* and *Plasmodium vivax* are the most important species and are both strict anthroponoses with no significant animal reservoir. *Plasmodium ovale* and *Plasmodium malariae* are responsible for a small percentage of infections. *P. knowlesi* causes malaria in humans and old-world monkeys (Simian malaria) connecting with sylvatic cycles.

Dengue, caused by the dengue virus (DENV), is the fastest-spreading, mosquito-borne viral infectious disease prevalent in urban and semi-urban areas of tropical and subtropical regions in the world (WHO 2022a). In forest habitats of Africa and Asia, the zoonotic or sylvatic dengue cycle is common. *Aedes* species, including *Aedes africanus*, *Aedes luteocephalus*, and *Aedes furcifer*, and monkeys maintain the zoonotic cycle, whereas the urban cycle or epidemic cycle involves transmission among humans by *Aedes aegypti* and *Aedes albopictus* found in urban cities. DENV is responsible for an estimated 390 million infections, resulting in up to 36,000 deaths annually.

Chikungunya is a mosquito-borne viral disease transmitted to humans through the bites of *Aedes* species mosquitoes infected with the chikungunya virus (CHIKV). CHIKV was first isolated in Tanzania in 1952. This is a reemerging virus. Sylvatic CHIKV has been isolated from African green monkeys (*Chlorocebus sabaeus*), patas monkeys (*Erythrocebus patas*), Guinea baboons (*Papio papio*), guenons (*Cercopithecus aethiops*), and a bushbaby (*Galago senegalensis*) in Senegal. The mosquitoes that contribute to

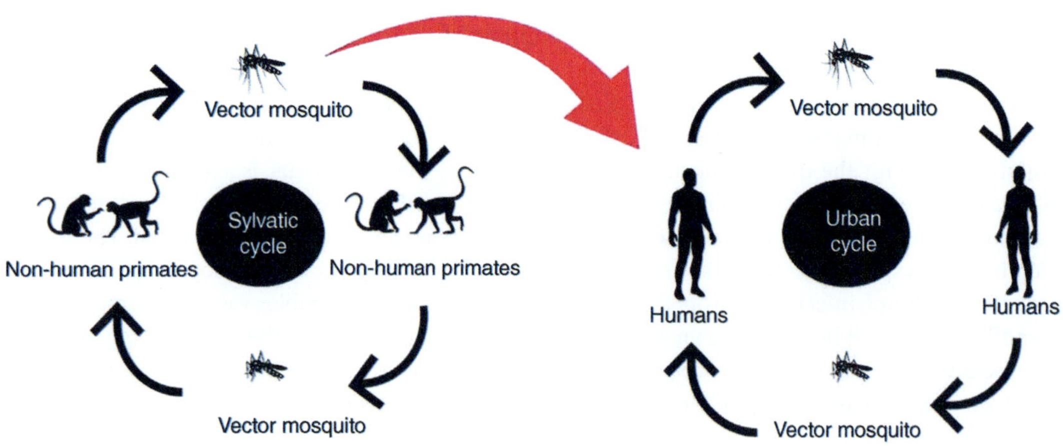

Figure 4.2 Sylvatic and urban cycles of zoonotic vector-borne diseases

the sylvatic transmission cycle are mainly *Ae. furcifer*, *Aedes taylori*, *Ae. africanus*, *Ae. Luteocephalus*, and *Aedes neoafricanus*, whereas *Ae. aegypti* and *Ae. albopictus* ensure the urban (epidemic) transmission cycle. Due to the challenges in making an accurate diagnosis, the real estimate of the number of people affected by this disease globally on an annual basis is uncertain.

West Nile virus (WNV) is one of the best-known zoonotic mosquito-borne viruses, first isolated in 1937 in Uganda and recently endemic to America and Canada. The WNV cycle occurs between mosquitoes (especially *Culex* species) and birds. Some infected birds develop a high titer of the virus in their bloodstream. Mosquitoes become infected by ingesting the virus while feeding on infected birds. The virus is ready to be transmitted to birds after about a week. The danger in infecting birds lies in that the virus can spread long distances via migratory birds. Mosquitoes with the WNV also bite and infect people, horses, and other mammals. However, they are "dead end hosts" because their viral titer in the bloodstream is quite low and therefore cannot be transmitted to mosquitoes.

Rift Valley fever (RVF) is a deadly mosquito-borne disease that affects both humans and valuable livestock in Africa. RVF can be transmitted through direct contact with blood, body fluids, or tissues of infected animals, or through bites of infected mosquitoes. Local enzootic transmission of RVF occurs at a low level during periods of average rainfall. The virus is maintained through transovarial transmission from the eggs of *Aedes* mosquitoes and occasional amplification cycles in susceptible livestock. The epizootic-epidemic cycle is triggered during unusually heavy rainfall, which provides an ideal environment for naturally infected mosquito eggs to hatch.

The best-known zoonotic disease caused by bacteria is the plague from the fourteenth century. It was caused by a bacterium called *Yersinia pestis*. The classic vector of the plague is the oriental rat flea, *Xenopsylla cheopis*. Many types of animals, such as rock squirrels, wood rats, ground squirrels, prairie dogs, chipmunks, mice, voles, and rabbits, can be affected by the plague. Wild carnivores can become infected by eating other infected animals. The epizootic-epidemic cycle occurs in the southwestern United States, more likely during cooler summers that follow wet winters. In addition to the transmission by vectors, the plague can be transmitted through contact with contaminated fluid or tissues and infectious droplets as well.

Lyme disease is a vector-borne disease caused by the bacterium *Borrelia burgdorferi* and, rarely, *Borrelia mayonii*. It is transmitted to humans through the bite of infected black-legged ticks in the genus *Ixodes*. Lyme disease is the most common disease spread by ticks in the northern hemisphere. Although the white-footed mouse (*Peromyscus leucopus*) acts as the principal reservoir of *Borrelia burgdorferi*, chipmunks (*Tamias striatus*), short-tailed and masked shrews (*Blarina brevicauda* and *Sorex cinereus*), and eastern gray squirrels (*Sciurus carolinensis*) also serve as infectious hosts.

Leishmaniasis is a zoonotic disease caused by nearly 20 species of obligate intercellular protozoa of the genus *Leishmania* and transmitted by 30 species of female phlebotomine sandflies including two main genera, *Phlebotomus* (old-world sandflies) and *Lutzomia* (new-world sandflies). The disease manifests in three clinical forms in humans; cutaneous leishmaniasis (CL), mucocutaneous leishmaniasis (MCL), and visceral leishmaniasis (VL). The most common is CL, which is classified as African Cutaneous Leishmaniasis caused by *Leishmania tropica* (human strain), *Leishmania major* (animal strain), *Leishmania aethiopica* (human strain), and South American CL caused by *Leishmania mexicana* and *Leishmania braziliensis*. VL is the most serious form caused by *Leishmania donovani* (African) and *Leishmania chagasi* (South American). Mucocutaneous leishmaniasis is the most disabling form of leishmaniasis.

Many forms of zoonotic filariasis are spread by vectors worldwide. Zoonotic lymphatic filariasis, zoonotic onchocerciasis, dirofilariasis, and Bung-eye disease are a few examples of zoonotic filariasis. Infective larvae that fall onto the skin of animals or humans during a blood meal enter the human through the puncture wound left behind by a bloodsucking arthropod. These larvae develop into adults within the animal or human host, causing lesions in the eye, the lungs, the glands, or subcutaneous tissues in humans. The adults mate and produce millions of microfilariae. These microfilariae are then ingested again by a vector, where they develop into the infective stage and so the cycle continues. The three main parasitic worm species that cause lymphatic filariasis are *Wuchereria bancrofti*, *Brugia malayi*, and *Brugia timori*. Even though the vector of these worms is mosquitoes, when it comes to *W. bancrofti* so far, no evidence has been found to show the existence of adult worms in wild species. Therefore, *W. bancrofti* is mainly described as a parasitic worm that has one definitive host, humans, and an intermediate host, mosquitoes. Mostly *Culex* species act as the vector and the intermediate host of these worms. Unlike the genus *Wuchereria*, the genus *Brugia* can be commonly seen in other vertebrate animals. *Brugia malayi* has been found in a variety of animal species and humans. Mainly four species of monkeys: *Macaca irus*, *Presbytis obscurus*, *Presbytis melalophus*, and *Presbytis cristatus*; the civet cat, *Paradoxttrus hermaphroditus*; the pangolin, *Manis javanicus*; and the domestic cats act as the reservoir hosts to *B. malayi*. Other *Brugia* species can also be found in domestic cats, dogs, panthers, gorillas, and monkeys.

4.4.1.3 Prevention and Control

Many factors contribute to successful zoonosis of diseases such as the adaptability of the pathogen in the vector, vector competency, adaptability of the pathogen in the final host, be it human or animal. The rate of transmission is dependent on many factors including the density of parasites, abundance of vectors, and rate of human–vector–animal contact. Using protective clothing, nets, or insect repellents to reduce the chance of being bitten by an infected arthropod are inexpensive yet effective preventive measures for vector-borne zoonotic diseases. Identifying and destroying breeding grounds of the vector is also imperative in controlling the vector population. The use of insecticides can also curb the disease-bearing vector population. Continuous entomological surveys in endemic areas are a must to identify emerging potential vectors of these diseases, enabling authorities to implement control measures early on.

4.4.2 Foodborne Zoonoses

4.4.2.1 Definition and Transmission

A foodborne disease (FBD) is classified by the WHO as the infectious or toxic nature caused by the consumption of food or water. Foodborne zoonotic diseases are a huge concern in the European Union, as they cause over 350,000 human infections per year. Bacteria are the causative agents of two-thirds of human food-borne diseases worldwide with a high burden in developing countries. Foodborne microorganisms are a major class of pathogens affecting food safety and causing human illnesses worldwide via contaminated food, mainly animal products contaminated with vegetative pathogens or their toxins (European Food Safety Authority 2022). Most of these microbes have zoonotic importance resulting in a significant impact on both public health and economic sectors. Food sources can get contaminated either at the farm level such as infected food-producing animals and milk contaminated with zoonotic pathogens, or during slaughter, food processing, and food preparation.

4.4.2.2 Common Examples

Bacteria are the most common of all infectious agents causing foodborne illnesses. *Campylobacter*, *Salmonella*, *Yersinia*, *Escherichia coli*, and *Listeria* are some of the most common bacteria causing foodborne diseases. Most of these pathogens are commonly found in the intestines of domestic livestock, including poultry, which can act as a reservoir for bacteria, causing foodborne illnesses (Alam et al. 2020).

More than 90% of bacterial infections are caused by *Salmonella* and *Campylobacter*. Salmonellosis is one of the most prevalent foodborne infections in industrialized countries. However, *Salmonella* has a broad range of animal hosts and has been isolated from several animal species such as birds, rodents, hedgehogs, poultry, farm animals, and insects. *Salmonella* bacteria typically live in animal and human intestines and are shed through feces. Humans can get infected with *Salmonella* through many sources, contaminated food and water being the most common ones. People can also get a *Salmonella* infection if they do not wash their hands after being in contact with animals carrying *Salmonella* or their environments, such as their bedding, food, or tank water. Humans also get salmonellosis on occasion during birth if the mother is infected.

Edible insects, beetles, caterpillars, ants, bees, wasps, grasshoppers, locusts, true bugs, dragonflies, termites, flies, cockroaches, and spiders also can harbor different pathogens like *Campylobacter spp., Staphylococcus spp., and Lactobacillus spp.* Consumption of raw or improperly cooked aquatic animals such as shellfish may also cause several foodborne diseases, where *Aeromonas hydrophila, E. coli, Yersinia spp., Brucella spp., Shigella spp., Salmonella spp., Streptococcus iniae, Clostridium botulinum, Klebsiella spp.*, and *Edwardsiella tarda* play an important role.

The most common zoonotic foodborne viral infection, acute viral hepatitis, is caused by the hepatitis E virus (HEV), an enteric nonenveloped single-stranded RNA responsible for over 20 million cases worldwide (WHO 2022b). Although acute viral hepatitis resolves by itself over a few weeks, some infections can lead to chronic infections, liver failure, and infections in other organs and can be fatal. Once thought to be contained within Asia and Africa, hepatitis E infections are now increasingly being detected in economically developed countries as well. Eight genotypes of the hepatitis E virus have been identified, of which five are capable of infecting humans. HEV is thought to spread primarily through contaminated pork. Consumption of contaminated water and aquatic animals such as shellfish are also postulated as possible transmission routes. HEV infections can cause liver damage. Some genotypes of HEV are especially dangerous to pregnant women, resulting in a high lethality ratio.

Norovirus (NoV) is responsible for nonbacterial gastroenteritis. There are several forms of noroviruses, some specific to humans and some to other animals such as swine and cattle. Noroviral gastroenteritis is mainly spread from human to human. However, studies have revealed that the NoVs in porcine are similar to the human NoV strain and that the human NoV strain is capable of eliciting an immune response in swine. These findings suggest that swine can serve as reservoirs for human NoVs. Moreover, human GII.4-like noroviruses were found in animal fecal samples and retail raw pork, suggesting that although undocumented, there might be a route of zoonotic transmission of NoVs from infected pigs and cows as well. It is, therefore, imperative to closely monitor the NoV genomes for the first signs of a change favoring zoonosis to prevent an outbreak of it.

Toxoplasmosis is a fatal foodborne zoonotic disease caused by protozoa *Toxoplasma gondii. T. gondii* is present in cats and can be passed through their fecal matter. Food contaminated with the feces of infected cats can cause toxoplasmosis in humans. There are also reports of toxoplasmosis being contracted via consumption of undercooked meat from venison, lamb, and pork. Toxoplasmosis is usually asymptomatic. However, it can cause severe conditions in pregnant women and immunocompromised individuals. It can also lead to birth defects in the unborn child if the mother contracts toxoplasmosis during pregnancy.

Taeniasis and Trichinosis are caused by several species of tapeworm of the genus *Taenia* and roundworms of the genus *Trichinella* respectively. Humans get infected by *Taenia* worms by consuming raw or undercooked beef (*Taenia saginata*) or pork (*Taenia solium* and *Taenia asiatica*). Humans act as the natural definitive host, while pigs are the intermediate hosts of larval stage parasites. People can also become infected after ingestion of microscopic viable eggs via the fecal-oral route from *T. solium* tapeworm carriers, in which case, humans act as an intermediate host (Liu et al. 2021). Symptoms of taeniasis are usually mild or nonexistent. Ingesting food contaminated with *T. solium* ova excreted by an infected human can cause cysticercosis, a foodborne zoonotic infection caused by *T. solium* larvae. Cysticercosis too is usually asymptomatic and is most prevalent in Latin America, Asia, and Africa. If larvae invade the brain and central nervous system, it can cause seizures and other neurological damage, a condition known as neurocysticercosis responsible for over 50,000 deaths per year worldwide. *Trichinella* roundworm infections are common in bears, cougars, pigs, and wild boar, and Trichinosis can be contracted by consuming the meat of infected animals.

In addition to the foodborne pathogens, different types of toxins produced by different pathogenic organisms can also cause foodborne zoonoses. The verodoxin produced by Shiga toxin-producing *Escherichia coli* (STEC) is responsible for a serious illness in humans, by posing a risk of developing haemolytic uremic syndrome (HUS) (Ievy et al. 2020; Yara et al. 2020). Ruminants are considered the main source of STEC of human infections. Food sources can be contaminated during milking and slaughter. Moreover, STEC in fecal matter can remain stable for long periods of time and, when used as fertilizer, can contaminate fresh produce. STEC in the environment can also be transmitted to humans via contaminated waterways.

In addition to various classes of organisms, prions, which are misfolded proteins that trigger normal proteins of the same variant to misfold as well, have also been reported to cause foodborne zoonosis. Variant Creutzfeldt-Jakob disease (vCJD), first reported in 1996, is one such disease that causes fatal brain damage. vCJD has been connected to the bovine spongiform encephalopathy (BSE) epidemic in cattle, and there is strong evidence suggesting that it was contracted by consuming meat from cows with BSE.

4.4.2.3 Prevention and Control

Farmers and workers in food production chains should be made aware of good sanitary practices such as washing hands, wearing gloves and masks when handling produce, livestock and animal products. Authorities should take measures to ensure slaughterhouses and food processing plants have the facilities to provide their workers with protective gear and sanitary products, including access to clean water and disinfectants. They should also make sure that the right conditions imperative for incapacitating transmission, such as maintaining the cold food chain, are in place through routine inspections. Safe food manufacturing practices such as cooking thoroughly, reheating of food, pasteurization (boiling) of milk, adequate refrigeration to prevent bacterial multiplication and toxin formation, preventing contamination and exclusion of pets and other animals from food-handling areas can prevent foodborne diseases. Restaurants and other food preparation plants should also be closely monitored to ensure that food safety procedures are in place and strictly adhered to.

Awareness programs associated with risk factors of foodborne zoonotic bacterial pathogens and control programs, including improvement in personal hygiene practices among food handlers, can be carried out. It is compulsory to educate food handlers regarding decontamination of equipment, surfaces and clothing; judicious use of antibiotics; and proper cooking and storage of food. Food safety guidelines such as Hazard Analysis and Critical Control Points (HACCP) and Good Manufacturing Practice (GMP) developed by the WHO should be implemented strictly (Tumbarski 2020).

Individuals more prone to contracting diseases than others, like pregnant women, the elderly, and the immune-suppressed, are advised to avoid consuming undercooked meat, poultry, raw milk, eggs, and food that contain raw eggs. Some countries are adopting standards for the pasteurization of ice cream and frozen desserts to reduce listeriosis. Also, in the case of Salmonellosis, attenuated DNA recombinant live *Salmonella* vaccines are used in combination with a comprehensive control strategy in animals, feed, and animal foodstuff to reduce disease incidence.

4.4.3 Waterborne Zoonoses

4.4.3.1 Definition and Transmission

Waterborne zoonotic diseases are diseases caused by zoonotic pathogens transmitted between animals and humans through contaminated water. Waterborne diseases are transmitted in different ways, such as consumption of contaminated drinking water, fecal droplet inhalation, and exposure through contact (e.g. recreational and occupational). Of the modes of transmission, consumption of contaminated drinking water is the leading cause of waterborne diseases, where transmission is directly via the fecal-oral route. Also, these diseases are interconnected with the consumption of shellfish and indirect exposure to water in foodstuffs when the water is used in irrigation, in food processing, or as an ingredient.

4.4.3.2 Common Examples

Most bacteria and viruses causing foodborne zoonoses are also transmitted via contaminated water. Bacteria like *Salmonella enterica, Campylobacter, E. coli*, and *Leptospira interrogans*; protozoa like *Giardia, Cryptosporidium*; and viruses like rotavirus, hepatitis E, and adenovirus are the most common examples of zoonotic diseases transmitted by water. Waterborne zoonotic pathogens cause both gastrointestinal diseases such as diarrhea and other illnesses such as leptospirosis and hepatitis. Diarrhea is the central symptom, where it has become the second leading cause of death for children under the age of five. Several waterborne zoonotic diseases, such as cryptosporidiosis and giardiasis, occur regularly in a range of countries; others, such as leptospirosis, occur more frequently in tropical countries.

Schistosomiasis is a neglected tropical disease caused by various trematode species of the genus Schistosoma such as *Schistosoma haematobium, Schistosoma intercalatum, Schistosoma japonicum, Schistosoma mansoni*, and *Schistosoma mekongi*. Schistosomiasis is prevalent in tropical and subtropical areas, especially in poor communities without access to clean water and sanitation. People become infected when larval forms of the parasite released by freshwater snails penetrate the skin during contact with infested water. Once inside a human host, the larvae develop into adult schistosomes. Adult worms live in the blood vessels where the females release eggs. Some of the eggs are passed out of the body through feces or urine, which in turn infect snails, the intermediate hosts.

Cryptosporidiosis and giardiasis are waterborne zoonoses caused by protozoans of the genus Cryptosporidium and Giardia, respectively. Ingestion of cysts of these parasites can lead to gut infections.

4.4.3.3 Control and Prevention

Control of waterborne zoonoses can be done at three levels: control of zoonotic waterborne pathogens in animal reservoirs, animal waste, and drinking water.

Of these, control of the zoonotic pathogens within animal reservoirs is the most challenging. Both domestic and wild animal populations need to be taken into consideration when devising control measures. Extra precautions can be taken when entering wilderness areas to avoid contacting water sources that are potentially contaminated with zoonotic pathogens from wild animals. Continuous surveillance of diseases within domestic and farm animals, immediate isolation of infected animals, provision of clean water, feed and housing facilities can limit zoonoses in domestic and farm animals. Selective disease-resistant animal breeding, competitive exclusion, bacteriophage therapy, use of antimicrobials, and active and passive immunization are also measures that can be taken to reduce the risk of creating animal reservoirs of zoonotic pathogens. Proper disposal of animal waste is crucial since the zoonotic pathogens in animal waste can persist in the soil for long periods, contaminating waterways, leading to waterborne zoonosis.

Survival, infectivity, and virulence of pathogens in water depend on a wide array of factors such as pH, salinity, light exposure, temperature, UV light (duration, intensity), rainfall, runoff, dispersal, suspended solids, turbidity, nutrients, organic content, organic foams, water quality, biological community in the water column, water depth, stratification, mixing (e.g. wind and waves), presence of aquatic plants, biofilms, and predation. Chlorination helps curb waterborne pathogens to some extent. However, other measures, such as ultraviolet light treatment, must be considered to eliminate chlorine-resistant forms of zoonotic pathogens.

4.4.4 Airborne Zoonoses

4.4.4.1 Definition and Transmission

Zoonotic diseases that are transmitted by pathogenic organisms expelled into the air by an infected person are known as airborne zoonotic diseases. Pathogens can be released into the environment via coughing, sneezing, laughing, and close personal contact with an infected organism or aerosolization. Direct inhalation of pathogenic organisms or, in some cases, the infective agents like spores and toxins cause disease spread. Additionally, these pathogens can be transmitted indirectly through food and water contaminated with aerosol particles (e.g. anthrax) and aerosols generated from biological waste products that accumulate in garbage cans, caves, and dry arid containers. Airborne particles are considered as the most infectious mode of transmission in comparison to the other modes of zoonotic disease transmission since the pathogenic agents remain suspended in the air and travel by air to different places where there is a higher potential of them being inhaled by others. It is more likely that those transmitted via aerosols will cause a pandemic over those transmitted via vectors, the reason being that vector-borne pathogens have to go through two sequential hosts to maintain their life cycle. This limits the spread of vector-borne pathogens both spatially and temporally to the geographic spread of the vector and climates favorable for the vector.

4.4.4.2 Common Examples

The commonly known airborne pathogens include bacteria like *Mycobacterium tuberculosis*, *M. bovis*, *Streptococcus pneumoniae*, and *Bordetella pertussis* and viruses like variola virus, measles virus, influenza A, and SARS-CoV-2 virus.

A well-known example of airborne zoonotic disease is anthrax, an acute zoonotic disease of livestock and humans caused by *Bacillus anthracis*. This pathogen affects wild and domestic animals such as sheep, cattle, and goats, as well as humans. *B. anthracis* spores can spread in many ways, with airborne being the deadliest since the respiratory form of the disease is highly lethal. Being highly resistant to sunlight, temperature, and disinfectants, *B. anthracis* spore poses a threat as a bioweapon. *Bordetella bronchiseptica* is a bacterium present in dogs and can cause pneumonia and upper respiratory tract infections in humans if spread through the aerosols of infected dogs, although the incidence is very rare.

The newest zoonotic coronavirus, SARS-CoV-2, which has caused an outbreak in humans, is a zoonotic airborne virus. This virus is known to infect humans and other animals, including birds and mammals. Since the epithelial cells in the respiratory tract are the primary target cells of this virus, transmission can occur through airborne particles.

Mycobacterium tuberculosis and *M. bovis* have been implicated in zoonotic airborne transmission of tuberculosis in different instances, with the former being transmitted to humans from elephants and the latter from rhinoceros. *M. bovis* is generally considered as a strain prevalent in animals, and zoonotic transmission is generally associated with contaminated milk. However, the report of airborne transmission of the *M. bovis* strain opens the possibility of nonconventional routes of transmission of pathogens between animals and humans, emphasizing the need for routine monitoring to prevent outbreaks.

4.4.4.3 Control and Prevention

Since airborne disease transmission is the most infectious mode of transmission, it is impossible to completely avoid airborne pathogens. However, steps can be taken to avoid disease propagation and transmission by taking precautionary measures such as wearing protective gear when in close contact with infected animals or housing facilities of infected animals and thorough sanitization afterward. Vaccination against several airborne diseases can greatly reduce the risk of getting and transmitting the diseases, like chickenpox, diphtheria, influenza, measles, mumps, and TB.

4.4.5 Zoonoses Contracted via Contaminated Soil and Surfaces

Some forms of the life cycle of many pathogens causing foodborne and waterborne zoonotic diseases can persist in soil and surfaces for prolonged periods, exacerbating the risk of disease spread.

4.5 Who Is at Risk of Zoonoses?

Those in close contact with animals or animal habitats, be it domestic, farm, or wild, are at a higher risk of zoonoses than others. People working in agricultural areas with high use of antibiotics for farm animals are at increased risk of zoonosis because these pathogens may be resistant to current antimicrobial drugs. People living near forests, wilderness areas, or semi-urban areas are at risk of zoonosis from wild animals such as non-human primates, rodents, foxes, or racoons either through direct transmission by being bitten or indirect transmission via surfaces contaminated with zoonotic pathogens. Wild animals that lose their natural habitats due to deforestation and urbanization encroach on human habitats frequently for food. People who visit or work in forest or wilderness areas and hunt, handle, and transport wild animals (including carcasses) are at greater risk of infection. Zoonotic diseases span a wide severity spectrum, and the impact is highly unpredictable, as seen by pandemics such as the plague, Spanish flu, and currently, COVID-19. Although anyone can get infected with a zoonotic disease, some people are at a higher risk of contracting a zoonotic disease, developing serious consequences, or even dying from these zoonotic diseases than others. Children younger than 5 years, adults older than 65 years, pregnant women, and people with weakened immune systems and other pre-existing conditions or complications are at higher risk of serious implications from zoonotic diseases than the rest of the population.

4.6 Factors Contributing to the Emergence and Reemergence of Zoonotic Diseases

During the last 70 years, at least 250 zoonoses were listed as emerging and reemerging zoonotic diseases. Anthropozoonoses, zooanthroponoses, and amphixenoses all share one factor in common: the exchange of pathogens between animals and humans, as a result of either spillover or spillback events. Spillover events are when a pathogen adapted to one species for a long time successfully infects another species (Ellwanger and Chies 2021), whereas spillback events are those that result in the transmission of pathogens from humans to animals. For successful zoonosis, there should be a considerable density of pathogens and reservoir hosts in each area, and the rate of release of the pathogen either by shedding, via a vector, or during slaughter must be high. Once released, the ability of the pathogen to survive and develop in the new environment, be it in a water body, on food, in the air, on a surface, or within a vector, and the efficacy of the mode of transmission are also major determining factors of the rate of zoonosis. The occurrence and rate of zoonosis are also dependent on the frequency of human–pathogen interactions and the adaptability of the pathogens to new intermediate and definitive hosts, vectors, and environments. Many environmental, societal, and genetic factors contribute to successful zoonosis and must be explored and well understood for effective prevention and control of zoonoses.

Changes in ecosystems due to human activities increase the risk and incidence of zoonoses. Deforestation and acquiring land for agriculture, habitation, and infrastructure lead to the loss of natural habitats, loss of natural barriers of disease transmission, and increased proximity of wild animals to humans and other domestic and farm animals, thus increasing the risk of spillover events. Moreover, hunting, handling, and transporting wildlife (including carcasses) with limited precautions, consumption of wild meat (such as bush meat), and increased usage of wildlife products also increases the risk of contracting a zoonotic disease. Increased vector movement and increased vector–human encounters due to the increased area of wilderness–human borders due to deforestation and urbanization also contribute greatly to the spread of zoonoses. The accelerating human population growth and decreasing numbers of stable ecosystems lead to a deficit of clean water and air, resulting in a higher risk of zoonosis.

The societal impact on the spread of zoonoses is also phenomenal. Those at the higher end of the monetary hierarchy self-increase the risk of zoonosis by entering forests for recreational activities such as fishing, gaming wild animals, trophy hunting, and camping, while those at the lower end of the monetary hierarchy are stricken with poverty that even something as simple as accessing clean water is nearly impossible, resulting in poor hygiene and increased susceptibility to zoonosis. They are also forced to encroach on forests to secure their livelihood and therefore are at a higher risk of zoonoses. Furthermore, this encroachment could result in damaged ecosystems, which otherwise would provide clean water and food, endangering them yet again to zoonosis. Furthermore, intensified agriculture and livestock production could lead to malpractices during handling, harvesting and slaughter; food-processing leading to foodborne zoonoses; and contamination of waterways leading to waterborne zoonoses. Transport of contaminated meat and animal products to other regions increases the mobility of the parasite and the spread of the disease. Moreover, high and improper use of veterinarian antibiotics leads to antibiotic resistance, creating favorable conditions for zoonosis. Another societal factor that increases the spread of zoonoses is the mistrust of governments. For example, lockdowns imposed by governments to break the transmission chain were disregarded by civilians at times in attempts to rally resources for survival for those in need. Improper planning by governments and degraded trust that their decisions consider the best interests of all citizens are reasons for this. High globalized movement of humans is also a major contributing factor to the fast global spread of zoonoses, resulting in pandemics of large scale, as we are currently experiencing.

Changes in the genetic makeup of the pathogens, adaptability of pathogens and vectors to new environments, intermediate and definitive hosts also play a big role in enabling transmission of pathogens between animals and humans. Mutations in the genomes of the pathogens can cause a break in the natural cycle within non-human hosts, favoring other intermediate and definitive hosts including humans. Pathogens also have their own mechanisms for evading and manipulating the immune responses of hosts to favor parasitism. Prolonged use of insecticides results in resistant vector populations, deeming it difficult to eliminate them. Spillover events could either lead to the spread of the pathogen within the human population by human-to-human transmission or via vectors or could be a dead-end event, where although infected, the disease is not transmitted to other humans. Intermediate hosts can serve as mixing vessels for pathogens, especially viruses, creating new more infectious strains that are pathogenic to humans. An intermediate host can be infected by two sources carrying two strains or can be infected by a new strain while already carrying one strain. NoVs are a prime example of this. Regardless of how these strains are introduced, genetic material of the new and existing strains can exchange and recombine within the intermediate host, creating a strain permissive to human infection. Phylogenetic distance between source and recipient hosts is also an important factor that influences zoonosis, with the incidence being high within phylogenetically closer species.

4.7 Prevention of Zoonotic Diseases

Zoonotic diseases do not get their due attention and can result in pandemics; COVID-19 being the most recent global zoonotic pandemic and the plague from the fourteenth century being the deadliest zoonotic pandemic in history. There are many challenges to mounting effective preventive and control measures against zoonosis. Genetic variations in the genomes of pathogens favoring adaptation, survival, and evolution of the pathogens within vectors, intermediate hosts, and humans make diagnosis and treatment of these diseases challenging. Moreover, most diseases show varying clinical manifestations within humans and heightened severity, deeming it difficult for early diagnosis.

Although prevention measures differ from pathogen to pathogen due to the many variables between the myriad of zoonotic diseases, such as fitness of pathogens, vectors and hosts, mode and rate of transmission, and disease severity, some overarching measures can be taken to control the spread of zoonotic diseases. First and foremost, at-risk populations must be identified. Sensitive warning systems to identify early warning signs must be designed and implemented for early detection of zoonotic threats. Continuous surveys on wild animals that are frequently in contact with humans, existing zoonotic diseases in terms of changes of the pathogens' genomes, and modes of transmission are a must. Early diagnostics must be developed to monitor the spread of zoonotic diseases. It is imperative to have a thorough reporting system and that data be shared between all responsible organizations for successful detection of early warning signs. Once detected, at-risk populations must be notified immediately and made aware of the risk and impact of these zoonotic diseases and potential preventive measures tailored to each disease.

Proactive preventive measures can ease the burden of zoonotic diseases. Limiting human–animal contact and exposure to contaminated surfaces and vectors is key to hindering zoonosis. Good sanitary practices and temporary immobilization are essential for limiting the spread of zoonoses during pandemics. The guidelines set forth by the health authorities for workers in agriculture and livestock farming must be followed strictly and closely monitored. Early diagnosis and prompt actions for containing the spreading of the disease are important aspects for health authorities and governments. Infected humans and animals must be quarantined or isolated to contain the spread of the diseases.

Protecting and restoring damaged ecosystems can also reduce the risk of zoonosis (Everard et al. 2020). However, restoration must be done with great care; for if not properly executed, it could exacerbate the problem by creating favorable conditions for zoonosis. For example, the creation of unmonitored open waterways could turn into breeding grounds for vectors of zoonotic pathogens such as mosquitoes.

4.8 One Health Initiative

The One Health approach recognizes the delicate balance between the human–animal–environment triad which if broken, leads to dire consequences, and the necessity of considering all three elements in preventing further outbreaks disrupting human and animal health and the economy (Aggarwal and Ramachandran 2020). The WHO plays a major role in designating emerging diseases and has given a directive to control the spreading of zoonotic diseases. WHO collaborates with the Food and Agriculture Organization of the United Nations (FAO) and the World Organization for Animal Health (OIE) on the Global Early Warning System for Major Animal Diseases (GLEWS), an initiative that helps share information quickly and take prompt actions on emerging animal diseases or zoonoses. The UN One Health initiative identifies the importance of uniting medical, veterinary, and environmental expertise to seek solutions for zoonotic diseases. The Center for Disease Control (CDC) leads One Health Zoonotic Disease Prioritization (OHZDP) workshops in regions where prioritizing zoonotic diseases is of high importance and develops action plans to address these concerns in collaboration with One Health partners.

In addition to these global organizations, several countries have also recognized the importance of a One Health approach and have launched their national organizations. One Health and Development Initiative (OHDI) is one such nonprofit organization launched in Nigeria. Their mission is to promote education, advocacy, and solutions to correlated issues of human, animal, and environmental health using the integrated "One Health" approach through community-based projects, media, research, advocacy, and policy influencing. One Health is in its infancy in India, but many policies and regulatory measures are coming into place with the OH approach, as they recognize the importance of the integrated well-being of all three elements. Preventing Zoonotic Diseases Emergence (PREZODE) is an initiative taken by France, where they are also teaming up with many organizations in agriculture, food, environment, and occupational health from many countries, including the Netherlands and Germany. PREZODE was also welcomed by the European Commission.

The combined efforts of these groups help civil societies, health authorities, and governments implement preventive measures as well as ensure sustainable use of the environment for the betterment of human and animal life.

References

Aggarwal, D. and Ramachandran, A. (2020). One health approach to address zoonotic diseases. *Indian Journal of Community Medicine* 45: S6–S8.

Alam, S.B., Mahmud, M., Akter, R. et al. (2020). Molecular detection of multidrug resistant salmonella species isolated from broiler farm in Bangladesh. *Pathogens* 2020 (9): 1–12.

Ellwanger, J.H. and Chies, J.A.B. (2021). Zoonotic spillover: understanding basic aspects for better prevention. *Genetics and Molecular Biology* 44: e20200355.

European Food Safety Authority (2022). Food borne zoonotic diseases. https://www.efsa.europa.eu/en/topics/topic/foodborne-zoonotic-diseases#:~:text=Foodborne%20zoonotic%20diseases%20are%20a,safety%20from%20farm%20to%20fork (accessed 7 March 2022).

Everard, M., Johnston, P., Santillo, D., and Staddon, C. (2020). The role of ecosystems in mitigation and management of COVID-19 and other zoonoses. *Environmental Science and Policy-Elsevier* 111 (2020): 7–17.

Gollakner, R. and Capua, I. (2020). Is COVID-19 the first pandemic that evolves into a panzootic? *Veterinaria Italiana* 56 (1): 7–8.

Ievy, S., Islam, S., Sobur, A. et al. (2020). Molecular detection of avian pathogenic *Escherichia coli (APEC)* for the first time in layer farms in Bangladesh and their antibiotic resistance patterns. *Microorganisms* 8: 1021.

Liu, Y., Dong, Z., Pang, J. et al. (2021). Prevalence of meat-transmitted Taenia and *Trichinella* parasites in the Far East countries. *Parasitology Research* 12: 4145–4151.

Rahman, T., Sobur, A., Islam, S. et al. (2020). Zoonotic diseases: etiology, impact, and control. *Microorganisms* 2020: 8.

Tumbarski, Y.D. (2020). Foodborne zoonotic agents and their food bioterrorism potential: a review. *Bulgarian Journal of Veterinary Medicine* 23 (2): 147–159.

World Health Organization (WHO) (2021). WHO-spiepr DHYPconvened global study of origins of SARS-spiepr DHYPCoV-spiepr DHYP2: China part. Joint Report, pp. spiepr NONBREAK61–120.

World Health Organization (WHO) (2022a). Dengue. https://www.worldmosquitoprogram.org/en/learn/mosquito-borne-diseases/dengue (accessed 7 March 2022).

World Health Organization (WHO) (2022b). Hepatitis E. https://www.who.int/news-room/fact-sheets/detail/hepatitis-e#:~:text=Hepatitis%20E%20is%20an%20inflammation,symptomatic%20cases%20of%20hepatitis%20E (accessed 7 March 2022).

WHO (2021). WHO-convened global study of origins of SARS-CoV-2: China part. Joint Report, pp. 61–120.

Yara, D.A., Greig, D.R., Gally, D.L. et al. (2020). Comparison of Shiga toxin-encoding bacteriophages in highly pathogenic strains of Shiga toxin-producing *Escherichia coli* O157:H7 in the UK. *Microbial Genomics* 2020: 6.

5

Microplastics in Soil and Water

Vector Behavior

Ewa Wiśniowska

Department of Sanitary Networks and Installations, Częstochowa University of Technology, Częstochowa, Poland

5.1 Introduction

Many researchers have well documented the presence of microplastics in surface water and soil. They are tiny particles of plastics with sizes not larger than 5 mm. The lower limit is considered, depending on the source, to be 1–1000 nm (Kim and Lee 2021; Menéndez-Pedriza and Jaumot 2020). Microplastics can be divided into primary ones, which can be found, e.g. in personal care products, cosmetics, medicines, or textiles (Menéndez-Pedriza and Jaumot 2020), and secondary ones. Secondary microplastics derive from the fragmentation of the larger plastic materials under UV degradation, mechanical crushing, biological decomposition, thermo-oxidative and thermal degradation, hydrolysis, and other factors (Menéndez-Pedriza and Jaumot 2020; Park and Park 2021). Essential sources of plastics in the environment are land flow (plastic wastes such as fragments of plastic bags, foam, fibers, coastal tourism, ship transportation, and fishing activities) and wastewater treatment plants (Li et al. 2021; Wiśniowska et al. 2018).

Plastic use has soared worldwide since the 1960s (Kim and Lee 2021). The first information on the pollution of the environment by microplastics was given by Carpenter and Smith in the early 1970s of the twentieth century (Carpenter and Smith 1972). Since then, many studies focused on the concentration of these pollutants in various environmental elements have been performed. Plastics can be divided into two categories: thermoplastics and thermosets. Thermoplastics are the ones that are reversible and can be altered by altering temperatures. In this group, such plastics as polypropylene (PP), polystyrene (PS), polyethylene terephthalate (PET), polyvinyl chloride (PCV), and polyamides (PA) can be classified. Thermosets are plastics that cannot be reversed after heating. Among the most popular plastics in this group, e.g. polyurethane (PUR) can be included (Verla et al. 2019).

The presence of microplastics in surface water, seawater, drinking water, wastewater, sludge, sediments, soil, air, and biota (fish and other aquatic organisms, birds, mammals) has been confirmed. The global value of primary microplastic release to the marine environment in 2017 was estimated to be 0.8/2.5 Mtons. It consisted of about 15/31% of the total microplastic load released to this receiver (Boucher and Friot 2017, cited in Menéndez-Pedriza and Jaumot 2020). The total release of plastics into the ocean is estimated at 8 Mtons (Li et al. 2021).

Microplastic distribution in the environment, including biota, depends on their shapes, sizes, and densities; complex interactions between these micropollutants and physical, chemical, and biological processes also affect the environmental fates of microplastic particles (Menéndez-Pedriza and Jaumot 2020). For example, in oceans, it has a toxic effect on fish and other biotas via reducing food intake, affecting body weight, delaying growth, or causing abnormal behavior. Because fish are an essential group in the marine ecosystem, changes and damage in their population affect the stability and structure of them (Li et al. 2021). It was stated that microplastics had been detected, among others, in 17% of the species on the International Union for Conservation of Nature (IUCN) Red List (Hardesty et al. 2015). The data given by Kühn et al. (2015) indicate that the risk for marine organisms caused by microplastics is mainly a result of ingestion. The data on the number of species with documented records of marine debris ingestion are presented in Table 5.1.

The data on microplastics in a food chain is limited to marine organisms (van Raamsdonk et al. 2020). However, these micropollutants can also pose a severe risk for terrestrial ecosystems. First of all, nowadays, it is estimated that agricultural soils might store more microplastics than ocean basins. Microplastics in a surface layer of soil might persist for more than 100 years. They may, among others,

One Health: Human, Animal, and Environment Triad, First Edition. Edited by Meththika Vithanage and Majeti Narasimha Vara Prasad.

Table 5.1 Number of marine species with documented plastic litter ingestion.

Type of organism	Number of species with documented ingestion	Percentage of species with documented ingestion in total number of species
Toothed whales	40	61.5
Whales	7	53.8
Dugongs and sea cows	3	60
Eared seals	8	61.5
True seals	4	21.1
Fish	92	0.28
Turtles	7	100
Penguins	5	27.8
Invertebrates	6	>0.001
Pelicans, gannets and boobies, tropicbirds	16	23.9
Gulls, skuas, terms, and auks	55	39.6
Albatross and other procellariforms	84	59.6

Source: Adapted from Kühn et al. (2015).

be transported by some organisms such as earthworms or springtails both in horizontal and vertical directions. The presence of microplastics in the soil causes structural changes in their burrows and, as a result, causes changes in soil aggregation and function. Even if soil microorganisms do not ingest microplastics, this pollutant can affect their growth and reproduction (de Sousa Machado et al. 2018). The smaller the microplastics, the more chemically active they are. Larger plastic particles in terrestrial systems cause mainly physical effects by changing soil physico-chemistry (de Sousa Machado et al. 2018). Microplastic is present at many stages of the food chain, including humans; however, the effect of microplastics on the human body is poorly understood. It was confirmed that microplastics could cause tissue damage and oxidative stress and affect immune-related gene expression in fish.

Fish exposed to microplastics suffered from growth retardation, behavioral abnormalities, and neurotoxic problems. Similar effects can also be expected in humans. Humans may experience neurotoxicity, oxidative stress, and cytotoxicity (Bhuyan 2022). The mechanism of toxic interactions between microplastics and living organisms is not clear, but toxic micropollutants adsorbed on the surface of microplastic particles are likely to have a significant impact on this phenomenon.

The fact that microplastic particles can adsorb other micropollutants, both organic and inorganic, was recently confirmed by many researchers. Because of this fact, the presence of microplastics in the environment also increases the risk of exposure to other pollutants (Kim and Lee 2021). Detailed studies on organic and inorganic pollutants' concentrations and sorption behavior on microplastics are relatively late. A good illustration of the varied affinity of different microplastics for inorganic and organic micropollutants was well presented by Tan et al. (2021) (Figure 5.1).

Microplastics are frequently considered sorbents for organic hydrophobic pollutants. However, research indicates that these types of plastic debris can also adsorb inorganic micropollutants, such as heavy metals and hydrophilic organic ones. Microplastics themselves tend to be more hydrophobic because they exhibit low polarity on their surface. It promotes hydrophobic adsorption of

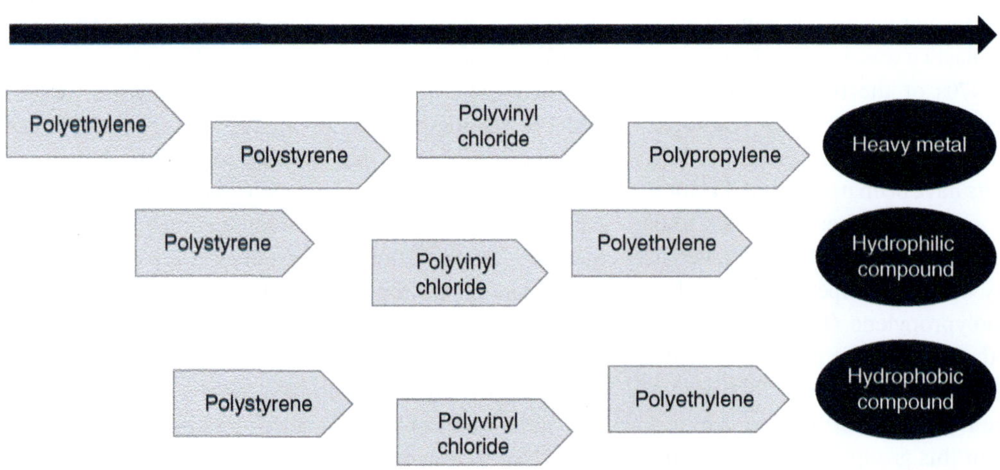

Figure 5.1 The affinity of different microplastics to different environmental pollutants. *Source:* Adapted from Tan et al. (2021).

chemicals onto their surfaces, and as a result, they act as hydrophobic adsorbents. It is expected that lipid-loving micropollutants will adsorb and cumulate on hydrophobic plastic structures, forming micelle shape-like structures (Verla et al. 2019). The tendency for adsorption of micropollutants can be indicatively evaluated based on adsorption partition coefficients (Kpw) calculated as the ratio of pollutant concentration adhered to microplastics to the environmental medium in equilibrium. Microplastic particles also show low polarity on their surface due to pH and electrostatic interactions. This low polarity is, among others, responsible for the adsorption of metal ions from the solution (Verla et al. 2019).

Some researchers indicate six main mechanisms of pollutants' adsorption onto the surface of plastics (Torres et al. 2021):

- Hydrophobic interaction – interactions between two nonpolar substances, causing them to aggregate or cluster; as a result, hydrophobic pollutants are adsorbed onto the surface of hydrophobic sorbent.
- Electrostatic interaction – the attraction between pollutant and sorbent occurs as a result of oppositely charged particles, and repulsion occurs between particles with the same charge.
- Pore-filling – contaminants enter nanoscale pores on the surface of microplastics and stay trapped there.
- Van der Waals forces – based on distance-dependent interactions between molecules, they are comparatively weak.
- Hydrogen bonding – occurs when proton donors and acceptors play a role in sorption processes.
- π–π interaction – a special dispersion force established between unsaturated (poly)cyclic molecules.

Concerning the sorption of individual groups of micropollutants on microplastics, various aforementioned mechanisms may play the most important role.

5.2 Concentrations of Inorganic Pollutants Adsorbed on Microplastics

Heavy metals have a density higher than 4.5 g/ml. Part of them are toxic to living organisms only at high concentrations, but low concentrations are necessary. These types of heavy metals are copper, zinc, and iron. The second type of heavy metal is toxic for living organisms even at low concentrations. These heavy metals are cadmium, lead, and mercury (Fan et al. 2021). Permissible levels of heavy metals for humans compared to those in food and drinking water are listed in Table 5.2. The first report on the presence of heavy metals on the surface of microplastics occurred in 2010 (Ashton et al. 2010). Until now, it has

Table 5.2 Permissible levels of heavy metals in food and drinking water, as well as safe values for human.

Heavy metal	Permissible level for human, mg/l	Permissible level in food according to EU legislation, mg/kg	Permissible levels in drinking water according to EU legislation proposal, mg/l
Cadmium	0.06	0.05–1.0	0.005
Lead	0.1	0.02–1.5	0.005
Mercury	0.01	0.1–1.0	0.001
Zinc	15	No limit	No limit
Chromium	0.05	No limit	0.025
Copper	0.1	No limit	2.0

Source: Adapted from Singh et al. (2011); Commission Regulation (EC) 1881/2006; Commission Regulation (EU) 2015/1006; Proposal for the EU Directive COM2017/753, 2018.

been shown that adsorption of heavy metals on the surface of microplastics is possible because the plastic debris have a high specific surface area, small sizes, and hydrophobicity, as well as because of the formation of biofilm on the surface of microplastics (Fan et al. 2021).

Concentrations of heavy metals on the surface of heavy metal particles are presented in Table 5.3. Concentrations of individual heavy metals on microplastics can reach even several milligrams per gram. As can be seen from the data collected in Table 5.3, extreme concentrations of individual metals can reach even several hundred milligrams per gram. Recent studies have confirmed that in the marine environment, microplastics can both adsorb and desorb heavy metals (Weber et al. 2022). Because heavy metal concentration in the environment, including sea and fresh water, is relatively high due to, e.g. industrial wastewater discharge or fuel combustion, these metals adsorption on the surface of the plastic is relatively common (Oz et al. 2019).

Moreover, because of their non-degradable nature, heavy metals are recycled and enriched in the environment, especially the water environment (Liu et al. 2021). Research work made by Oz et al. (2019) has indicated that the adsorption capacities of metals onto microplastics depend not only on the type of plastics and heavy metals but also on environmental conditions, e.g. pH.

Other factors that should be considered important in heavy metal adsorption on microplastics are aging of the microplastics, temperature, contact time, and ionic strength (Liu et al. 2021).

The mechanism of heavy metal adsorption on microplastic particles can be described by electrostatic interactions, π–π interactions, and van der Waals forces (Liu et al. 2021).

Table 5.3 Concentrations of selected heavy metals on the microplastics found in various elements of the environment.

Heavy metal (sorbate)	Type of microplastics (sorbent)	Concentration, µg/g	Type of environment in which microplastic was found	Source
Lead	Red and yellow pellets or fragments	$>10^3$	Beaches in south-west England	Massos and Turner (2017)
Cadmium		$>10^3$		
Zinc	Polymers such as PVC, LDPE, PS, PE, PP, nylon, HDPE, PC, PET, PUR, POM	Up to 6,667	Plastic debris collected from intertidal regions in Burrard Inlet, Vancouver, Canada	Munier and Bendell (2018)
Copper		Up to 188		
Lead		Up to 698,000		
Cadmium		Up to 930		
Nickel	No data available	40–131	South-west England	Holmes et al. (2012)
Nickel	No data available	0.01–1	San Diego, Bay	Rochman et al. (2014)
Zinc	No data available	0–0.121	Maidao, Huangdao, and Baian (China)	Gao et al. (2019)
Zinc	No data available	2,414.8–11,284.9	Beijiang River, China	Wang et al. (2017)
Cobalt	No data available	17.7–107	South-west, England	Holmes et al. (2012)

As an important factor for metal sorption on plastic surfaces, aging is considered. Two main processes affecting plastic aging are indicated: physicochemical deterioration and microbial colonization (Binda et al. 2021). Physicochemical process is among other UV irradiation but also UV-based oxidation. Aging by UV irradiation can increase the sorption capacity of microplastics toward heavy metals, mainly by increasing their specific surface area. Photodegradation can also break the bonds on the surface of microplastics and, as a result, change, e.g. hydrophobicity or reactivity (Liu et al. 2021). Results obtained by Seyfi et al. have shown that aging of microplastics with UV radiation can increase microplastics' power to adsorb such metals as Cr, Zn, Cu, Cd, and Zn by 20–60% (Seyfi et al. 2021).

Simultaneously, pH affects many processes, including heavy metal adsorption, because it affects heavy metal solubility in water. Under alkaline conditions, heavy metals can precipitate, which affects the adsorption process. However, it also depends on the form of heavy metal in the environment, e.g. it was stated that under acidic conditions, negatively charged ions such as CrO_4^{2-} were effectively attracted to positively charged polyethylene particles. On the other hand, polyethylene particles become negatively charged under higher pH, which decreases CrO_4^{2-} adsorption (Liu et al. 2021). However, the results of the studies on the pH effect on heavy metal adsorption gave different results. Guo et al. (2020) have observed that the sorption capacity of selected microplastics toward Cd^{2+} increased as pH increased. The results obtained by Tang et al. (2020) have indicated that Pb^{2+} was not effectively adsorbed under strongly acidic conditions (pH = 2.5), but at pH = 6, sorption efficiency was over 90%. Also, Oz et al. have observed the high adsorption efficiency of microplastics (PET, PA, and EVA) toward Pb^{2+} at pH = 5.5 (Oz et al. 2019). Research done by Wang et al. (2020) has confirmed that in the range of pH 3–7, adsorption capacity toward Zn^{2+} and Cu^{2+} increased as pH increased.

Metal adsorption on plastic microparticles is also affected by the salinity of the solution. The increased ionic strength of the solution can enhance the competition of heavy metals with other ions present in the solution for binding sides. Adsorption of positively charged ions is expected to be inversely related to salinity. As salinity increases, such metal ions as Pb, Cd, Zn, and Cu compete for the adsorption on plastics with Na^+ (Binda et al. 2021). At the same time, the presence of chloride ions may promote the formation of Cl^- transition metals homoleptic complexes and hydrates (Binda et al. 2021). Salinity can also affect the electric double layer on the surface of plastics if it has been formed. This layer is expected to form over the surface of weathered and partially charged surfaces. If the salinity of the solution varies, the thickness of the double layer also can vary, which influences the rate of diffusion and adsorption of ions (Binda et al. 2021). Also, redox potential can affect the adsorption of heavy metals by affecting the surface charge of plastics. A potential factor affecting metal adsorption on plastics' surfaces is also a concentration of suspended solids because the solids significantly affect the speciation and mobility of metals (Binda et al. 2021). It was also confirmed that higher temperature benefits heavy metal adsorption process, what was explained by Liu et al., as a result of the fact that adsorption is an endothermic reaction (Liu et al. 2021).

Biofilm formation also can affect heavy metal adsorption on the surface of microplastics. Tu et al. (2020) have stated that the formation of biofilm on the surface of microplastics reduces the hydrophobicity of polyethylene microparticle surface, as well as it increases the number of such chemical groups as carboxyl and ketone. Research by Qiongjie et al. (2022) has indicated that biofilm on polystyrene had a larger adsorption capacity for Cu^{2+} and Pb^{2+} than this microplastic aged by UV and was not affected by any factors. The authors have also confirmed that adsorption mechanisms included physical sorption, chemical sorption, and biosorption. What was important after the adsorption of the metals was that changes in the microbial community on the polyethylene surface occurred. The results obtained by the authors confirmed that the formation of biofilm strongly affects not only the adsorption behavior of the investigated metals but also a microbial community.

Heavy metals adsorbed onto microplastics can be transferred to a variety of organisms, especially the aquatic ones, because it is stated that heavy metal microplastics have bioaccumulation potential throughout the food chain (Oz et al. 2019).

5.3 Concentrations of Organic Micropollutants Adsorbed on Microplastics

Microplastic particles can adsorb on the surface of persistent organic pollutants such as polycyclic aromatic hydrocarbons (PAHs), polychlorinated biphenyls (PCBs), organochlorine pesticides, or pharmaceuticals (e.g. ciproflaxin, trimethoprim, amoxicillin, tetracycline, sulfamethoxazole, carbamazepine) (Ugwu et al. 2021; Wang et al. 2020a; Wiśniowska and Włodarczyk-Makuła 2021).

The adsorption mechanisms vary depending on the type of pollutant and other factors (e.g. presence of other pollutants, pH, salinity). An important part of them are hydrophobic partitioning interactions, van der Waals forces, π–π interaction, hydrogen bonding reactions, electrostatic interactions, and pore filling (Wang et al. 2020a). As mentioned by Guo et al. (2020), significant factor is also a type of microplastic polymer of which microplastic particle is made, e.g. PE is aliphatic, has only C—H bonds, and has no functional groups. As a result, mainly van der Waals forces can bound hydrophobic pollutants to their surface. Different plastics have different functional groups.

The pollutants' sorption behavior on microplastics depends on sorbent and sorbate properties. More detailed studies have shown that the sorption of organic micropollutants on plastics surface is affected by polymer type (Sørensen et al. 2020). Among other polymers, polyethylene (PE) and polystyrene (PS) have been identified as the ones with the highest sorption capacity for organic, hydrophobic pollutants (Sørensen et al. 2020). Of course, an important factor affecting micropollutants' adsorption onto microplastic surface is the size of polymer particles. The sorption rate of microplastics is lower than the ones reported for nanoplastics (Arienzo et al. 2021).

The sorption behavior of micropollutants on the microplastic surface is also affected by the chemistry of the solution, including pH, ionic strength, and concentration of dissolved organic matter (Wang et al. 2020a).

The lower the molecular weight of the contaminant and the lower its hydrophobicity, the lower its mass diffusion (Arienzo et al. 2021). The presence of other pollutants in the solution is also essential, and the pollutants can interact with the surface of MPs or other compounds.

Ingestion of microplastics with adsorbed organic pollutants on their surface influences the bioavailability of organic contaminants to living organisms because of the desorption of these micropollutants from the plastic microdebris. This can result in increased exposure levels of organisms to carcinogenic and mutagenic toxicants (Sørensen et al. 2020). Adsorption and desorption mechanisms of organic micropollutants are complex and, until now, not well investigated by researchers. There are some similarities and differences between the sorption behavior of various organic micropollutants such as polycyclic aromatic hydrocarbons, polychlorinated biphenyls, organochlorine pesticides, and pharmaceuticals.

Polycyclic aromatic hydrocarbons (PAHs) are a group of chemicals that consists of two or more condensed aromatic rings. They are widely detected in many parts of the environment, including water, soil, air, and living organisms. They are also common pollutants of the wastewater. They also were found on the microplastic particles; PAHs adsorption on microplastic particles is well documented. Oil spill accidents are indicated among the most concerning exposure events of microplastics to the PAHs (Honda and Suzuki 2020). Table 5.4 presents concentrations of selected PAHs on the microplastics in various environmental elements. It should be emphasized that not always the results are comparable because of the variances in sampling, handling, cleaning, separation, and analysis of microplastics and PAHs.

More detailed studies on the sorption behavior of PAHs have indicated that it was affected by the type of microplastics, e.g. the results obtained by Teuten et al. (2007) had indicated that in seawater, PE showed the higher Kd values when phenanthrene was adsorbed than PVC and PP. The results obtained for the

Table 5.4 Concentrations of selected PAH compounds on the microplastics found in various elements of the environment.

PAH compound (sorbate)	Type of microplastics (sorbent)	Concentration, μg/g	Type of environment in which microplastic was found	Source
Total PAHs	No detailed data available	0.071–1.509	Sedimentary microplastic (0.2–5 mm), beach sediments, Hong Kong	Lo et al. (2019)
Benzo(a)pirene	No detailed data available	0.250	Beaches from three island of the Pacific Ocean (Easter Island, Guam, and Hawaii)	Pannetier et al. (2019)
Total 16 PAHs	Polystyrene foams, polyethylene films and lines, other plastic pellets	3.4–119	Surface of Bohai and Huanghai Seas, China	Mai et al. (2018)
Total 15 PAHs	PE PET	Average 0.552 (mainly naphthalene)	Indonesian Cilacap coast	Bouhroum et al. (2019)
Total PAHs	No detailed data available	$2\cdot10^{-5}$–0.016 (with dominant concentrations of pyrene, phenanthrene, chrysene, and fluoranthene)	Pellets collected from Portuguese coastline	Frias et al. (2010)
Total PAHs	No detailed data available	0.018–0.21	North to South of San Diego County, California, USA	Van et al. (2012)
Total PAHs	No detailed data available	0–9.297	Kugenuma, Kanagawa	Hirai et al. (2011)

phenanthrene in freshwater (Wang and Wang 2018) showed that the order of sorption capabilities was PE > PS > PVC. The sorption capacity of PAHs to microplastics is 0.08 to even 0.4 mg/g (Wang et al. 2020a).

The results obtained by Teuten et al. (2007) have simultaneously shown that the adsorption of polycyclic hydrocarbons on microplastics is rather rapid, about 20 minutes. This phenomenon was also confirmed by Wiśniowska and Włodarczyk-Makuła (2021). Osorio Prado has stated that in the case of phenanthrene sorption on PS and PE, sorption equilibrium was reached after five minutes of contact time (Osorio Prado 2020). Sorption capacity was generally stated to be more effective at higher temperatures. For example, Sørensen et al. (2020) have confirmed that in most cases, sorption of fluoranthene and phenanthrene on the surface of PS was higher at 20 °C than at 10 °C. The authors have explained that when sorption of selected PAHs on microplastics is an endothermic process, sorption is more effective at higher temperatures. When the process is exothermic (e.g. in the case of tiny microplastics), this phenomenon is not observed.

Adsorption of PAHs on microplastic surface is also affected by salinity. For example, Osorio Prado has stated that as salinity increased, sorption capabilities of PE and PS toward phenanthrene increased as well, which was explained by the salting-out effect (Osorio Prado 2020).

Fisner et al. (2017) observed an interesting phenomenon connected with PAHs adsorption onto MPs particles. The authors have observed that the color of pellets had an essential effect on PAHs sorption behavior; both PE and PP pellets demonstrated predictable increases in total PAHs adsorbed across a spectrum of darkening color tones. Lighter colored pellets comprised lower molecular weight PAHs.

It has been confirmed that the sorption of PAHs on the microplastic surface is governed by partitioning interaction, π–π interaction, and van der Waals forces (Wang et al. 2020a).

Polychlorinated biphenyls are organochlorine compounds that were and partially are used as dielectrics and cooling liquids in electrical equipment (Torres et al. 2021). First records of the presence of PCBs on microplastic particles were published in 1972, and it was 5 μg/g (Verla et al. 2019).

Since then, determined PCB concentrations adsorbed on the microplastic particles usually did not exceed 0.1 μg/g (Table 5.5). However, some research indicated extremely high PCB concentrations, reaching even 14 μg/g.

PCBs are common in water environment, including both marine and other types of surface water. Their toxic effect on the environment due to sorption into microplastics has been well documented. Good adsorption of PCBs on microplastics is connected with the fact that microplastics offer a high amorphous to crystalline ratio. Hydrophobic PCBs readily diffuse into polymer's amorphous regions (Syberg et al. 2020). Mato et al. (2001) PE contains more

Table 5.5 Concentrations of PCBs adsorbed onto microplastic particles in the environment.

PCB compound (sorbate)	Type of microplastics (sorbent)	Concentration, μg/g	Type of environment in which microplastic was found	Source
Total PCBs	No detailed data available	0.013–1.083	Sedimentary microplastic (0.2–5 mm), beach sediments, Hong Kong	Lo et al. (2019)
Total of 13 PCBs	No detailed data available	$4 \cdot 10^{-5}$–0.124	27 locations in the Pacific Ocean and around the coast of Japan	Yeo et al. (2020)
Total 7 PCBs	No detailed data available	0.003–0.06	Pellets with the diameter of 4.0 ± 0.6 cm; Lenga Beach (San Vicente Bay)	Pozo et al. (2020)
Total 61 PCBs	PE PET	At average 14	Indonesian Cilacap coast	Bouhroum et al. (2019)
Total PCBs	No detailed data available	0.015–0.399	Los Angeles, USA	Hirai et al. (2011)

areas of amorphous structure than PS and adsorbs PCBs more rapidly. Microplastics are also suitable for PCBs because they have nonpolar surfaces (Syberg et al. 2020).

PCBs are rapidly adsorbed onto the surface of microplastics. However, the adsorption process can be continued for a longer time; for example, Mato et al. have observed that the concentration of PCBs on the surface of PP increased during six-day experiment, which means that the concentration of these pollutants on a plastic surface can vary significantly during more extended periods (Mato et al. 2001). The field studies observed that PCB concentrations on PVC and PET are relatively low, with significantly higher ones adsorbed to LDPE, HDPE, and PP (Agboola and Benson 2021).

PCB accumulation on microplastic particles poses a severe risk to the environment because most of them are known carcinogens and endocrine disruptors. Exposure of humans to PCBs can result in low birth weight, eye secretion, and facial enema.

Organochlorine pesticides are the biocides belonging to the group of chlorinated hydrocarbon derivatives. The most frequently analyzed organochlorine derivatives are dichlorodiphenyltrichloroethane (DDT), dicholordiphenyldichloroethylene (DDE), dichlorodiphenyldichloroethane (DDD), and hexachlorocycloxexane (HCH) (Verla et al. 2019). Concentrations of selected organochlorine pesticides on microplastic particles are presented in Table 5.6.

The data on pollution of the environment by organochlorine pesticides are strongly limited to DDT. Some data on HCHs and chlordane are also available. It was confirmed that organochlorine pesticides have a higher affinity to microplastics than e.g. phenanthrene. DDT and its derivatives are present in the environment in relatively low concentrations compared to other hydrophobic micropollutants. As can be seen from Table 5.6, the concentration does not usually exceed 0.1 μg/g. DDT seems to have a stronger affinity to microplastics than selected PAHs and heptachlor pesticides, endosulfan class, and endrin class ones. DDT is also better adsorbable than HCHs isomer class (Scutariu et al. 2019). Rocha-Santos and Duarte showed that DDT is the most sorbed onto PET (Rocha-Santos and Duarte 2017).

Contamination of the environment by pharmaceuticals and the sorption behavior of these pollutants is of high importance because this class of pollutants is classified as emerging for the water environment. As factors controlling adsorption of pharmaceuticals onto a microplastic surface, biofouling and formation of biofilms are considered (Agboola and Benson 2021). On the other hand, adsorbed pharmaceuticals can reduce bacterial biofilm formation if they act as biocides (Magadini et al. 2020). McDougal et al. (2021) showed that an essential factor for pharmaceutical desorption was pH because it affects pharmaceutical speciation and microplastic surface change.

5.4 Microplastics as Source of Plastic Additives and Decomposition Products

Microplastics are also a source of environmental pollution by various plastic additives, e.g. phthalates and bisphenol A (BPA). These compounds can affect, e.g. the reproduction of living organisms, produce various genetic malformations, and affect hormonal systems (Ugwu et al. 2021). BPA is known for its estrogenic activity both in vertebrates and in some invertebrate species (De Sousa

Table 5.6 Concentrations of selected organochlorine pesticides adsorbed onto microplastic particles in the environment.

Organochlorine pesticide compound (sorbate)	Type of microplastics (sorbent)	Concentration, μg/g	Type of environment in which microplastic was found	Source
DDT	No detailed data available	0.002–0.626	Sedimentary microplastic (0.2–5 mm), beach sediments, Hong Kong	Lo et al. (2019)
DDT	No detailed data available	0.0001–0.007	Pellets with the diameter of 4.0 ± 0.6 cm; Lenga Beach (San Vicente Bay)	Pozo et al. (2020)
DDT	No detailed data available	$1.6 \cdot 10^{-4}$–$4.05 \cdot 10^{-3}$	Pellets collected from Portuguese coastline	Frias et al. (2010)
HCHs	No detailed data available	$2 \cdot 10^{-4}$–0.019	Remote islands in the Pacific, Atlantic, Indian Oceans and the Caribbean Sea	Heskett et al. (2012)
Chlordane	No detailed data available	0.004–0.0144	(From seabird) Southern Brazil	Colabuono et al. (2010)

Machado et al. 2018). Plastic additives are of high molecular weight and are used in concentrations of 10–80% w/w or more of total plastic composition (Nerland et al. 2014).

The risk connected with endocrine-disrupting plastics released to the environment increases as larger particles are crushed into smaller ones because of the exponential increase in the surface/volume ratio (De Sousa Machado et al. 2018). As a result of degradation processes, microplastic particles can crush into smaller nanoplastic particles. This particles can be toxic to living organisms directly, e.g. due to physical damage in microalgae cells, but this is not a rule (Sheela et al. 2022).

The property that is key in how fast the additives migrate through and out of the plastic is molecular size. The smaller the additive's molecular size, the faster it can migrate (Nerland et al. 2014). Concentrations of Bisphenol A in plastic particles can be in the wide range from 2.10–4 to 0.73 μg/g (Nerland et al. 2014).

The problem connected with microplastics' presence in the environment could also be other additives and decomposition products of microplastics, including some UV stabilizers (e.g. UV-328, UV-236, UV-237), which contain functional groups altering endocrine systems. Also, some flame retardants, such as hexabromocyclododecane (HBCDD) and decabromodiphenylether (deca-BDE), can be a real problem for the environment. Moreover, microplastics also contain UV filters such as benzophenone 3 (BP-3), 4-methyl benzylidene camphor (4-MBC), octocrylene (OC), octyl-methoxycinnamate (OMC), or ethylhexyl dimethyl p-aminobenzoic acid (OD-PABA) (Ugwu et al. 2021).

5.5 Microplastics as a Base for Microorganisms Growth

Microplastic particles can be covered by diverse communities of bacteria and other microorganisms, such as protozoans, algae, and fungi (Menéndez-Pedriza and Jaumot 2020). The type of biofilm and its composition can be affected by the plastics' roughness, topography, surface charge or wettability, and the amount and composition of additives in the polymer. Also, environmental conditions such as temperature, pH, ionic strength, and trophic status affect biofilm formation. It was observed that colonization of the microplastic surface by the biofilm of microorganisms is rapid – it takes place within hours. Because of the variety of factors influencing biofilm formation on the surface of the microplastics, various microbial communities can colonize them (Rummel et al. 2017). Microorganisms settling on the polymer surface can also be affected by degradation processes that modify its surface, e.g. photooxidation, propagation, and termination (Rummel et al. 2017).

The presence of the biofilm on the surface of microplastics can affect the environmental fates of these pollutants. First of all, the formation of the biofilm can lead to an increase in the density of the particles and, as a result, decrease its buoyancy and sedimentation behavior (Rummel et al. 2017). Biofilm can also increase the immiscibility of the surface of microplastics in water (Verla et al. 2019). The presence of the biofilm on the surface of microplastics can also promote the formation of heteroaggregates that show better sedimentation properties than individual microplastic particles (Rummel et al. 2017).

Microbial biofilm also increases the surface area available for sorption processes (Verla et al. 2019). The composition of bacterial biofilms is very diversified and can change over time (Binda et al. 2021).

Biofilm, which covers the surface of the microplastics, also affects the fates of other micropollutants present in water, especially the hydrophobic ones. It is connected both to the fact that these pollutants can adsorb on their surface or can be degraded by biofilm microorganisms (Rummel et al. 2017). However, in the experiments regarding the sorption of hydrophobic micropollutants to the surface of microplastics, the role of biofilm is usually disregarded (Rummel et al. 2017). In contrast, they should be taken into consideration because of their ability to degrade most of the organic micropollutants adsorbed on the surface of the biofilm (Rummel et al. 2017).

It was also confirmed that the biofilm is a sorbent for metals. It is because of the fact that microorganisms form the biofilm through a process called quorum sensing, which is known to control gene expression in which microbial cells form a matrix of extracellular polymeric substance (EPS) by adhering to each other on living and nonliving surfaces. EPS can act as a ligand and, by chelation, bind or release metals (Verla et al. 2019).

It is also important to note that such microorganisms as *Bacillus cereus*, *Micrococcus* sp., *Pseudomonas* sp., and *Corynebacterium* sp. are capable of degrading plastics. Mineralization of the microplastic polymers results in the formation of various compounds, salts, and minerals that can promote or inhibit the growth of biofilm microorganisms (Sheela et al. 2022).

The effect of contaminants adsorbed onto the surface of microplastics on living organisms is difficult to predict. Both degradation and bioaccumulation of them in living organisms are not well understood.

5.6 Conclusions

Based on the data presented earlier, it can be stated that:

1) Microplastic particles effectively adsorb both inorganic and organic pollutants. As a result, they may act as vectors that transport other contaminants through all environment elements.
2) The sorption process of pollutants onto the surface of microplastics is influenced by multiple factors, including microplastic parameters such as type and crystallinity of polymer, polarity, functional groups, size, and aging. Also, other factors, such as being connected with the environment: pH, ionic strength, temperature, and presence of other contaminants, are essential. Important factors affecting sorption onto microplastics connected with the characteristics of sorbates are their hydrophobicity, concentration, and type (organic and inorganic).
3) The fates of pollutants sorbed onto plastic surface depends not only on physical and chemical properties but also on biofilm formation that plays an essential role in such phenomena as biofilm formation. Biofilm microorganisms can partially degrade plastics and change the density of the particle, immiscibility of the surface, and increase the surface area.
4) Data on the toxicity of microplastics to living organisms are still insufficient. It was confirmed that it could be caused by the release of plasticizers from microplastics, the accumulation of carcinogenic hydrophobic compounds such as PAHs, and physical damage in cells of living organisms.

References

Agboola, O.D. and Benson, N.U. (2021). Physisorption and chemisorption mechanisms influencing micro(nano) plastics-organic chemical contaminants: a review. *Front. Environ. Sci.* https://doi.org/10.3389/fenvs.2021.678574.

Arienzo, M., Ferrara, L., and Trifuoggi, M. (2021). The dual role of microplastics in marine environment: sink and vectors of pollutants. *Mar. Sci. Eng.* 9 (6): 642. https://doi.org/10.3390/jmse9060642.

Ashton, K., Holmes, L., and Turner, A. (2010). Association of metals with plastics production pellets in the marine environment. *Mar. Pollut. Bull.* 60 (11): 2050–2055, cited after: Fan et al. (2021).

Bhuyan, S. (2022). Effects of microplastics on fish and in human health. *Front. Environ. Sci.* https://doi.org/10.3389/fenvs.2022.827289.

Binda, G., Spanu, D., Monticelli, D. et al. (2021). Unfolding interaction the between microplastics and (trace) elements in water: a critical review. *Water Res.* 204: 117637.

Boucher, J. and Friot, D. (2017). *Primary Microplastics in the Oceans: A Global Evaluation of Sources*. Gland: IUCN. ISBN: 9782831718279.

Bouhroum, R., Boulkamh, A., Asia, L. et al. (2019). Concentrations and fingerprints of PAHs and PCBs adsorbed onto marine plastic debris from the Indonesian

Cilacapcoast and the North Atlantic gyre. *Regional Studies in Marine Science* 29: 100611. https://doi.org/10.1016/j.rsma.2019.100611-02194342.

Carpenter, E.J. and Smith, K.L. (1972). Plastics on the sargasso sea surface. *Science* 175: 1240–1241.

Colabuono, F.I., Taniguchi, S., and Montone, R.C. (2010). Polychlorinated biphenyls and organochlorine pesticides in plastics ingested by seabirds. *Mar. Pollut. Bull.* 60 (4): 630–634. https://doi.org/10.1016/j.marpolbul.2010.01.018.

Commission Regulation (EC) No 1881/2006 of 19 December 2006 setting maximum levels for certain contaminants in foodstuffs, OJL 20.12.2006, L 364/5.

De Sousa Machado, A., Kloas, W., Zarfi, C. et al. (2018). Miroplastics as an emerging threat to terrestrial ecosystems. *Glob. Chang. Biol.* 24 (4): 1405–1416. https://doi.org/10.1111/gcb.14020.

European Commission (2018). Proposal for a Directive of the European Parliament and of the Council on the Quality of Water Intended for Human Consumption (COM/2017/753). Brussels: European Commission.

Fan, T., Zhao, J., Chen, Y. et al. (2021). Coexistence and adsorption properties of heavy metals by polypropylene microplastics. *Adsorpt. Sci. Technol.* 2021: 4938749.

Fisner, M., Taniguchi, S., Moreira, F. et al. (2017). Colour spectrum and resin-type determine the concentration and composition of polycyclic aromatic hydrocarbons (PAHs) in plastic pellets. *Mar. Pollut. Bull.* 122: 323–330.

Frias, J.P.G.L., Sobral, P., and Ferreira, A.M. (2010). Organic pollutants in microplastics from two beaches of the Portuguese coast. *Mar. Pollut. Bull.* 60 (11): 1988–1992.

Gao, F., Li, J., Sun, C. et al. (2019). Study on the capability and characteristics of heavy metals enriched on microplastics in marine environment. *Mar. Pollut. Bull.* 144: 61–67. https://doi.org/10.1016/j.marpolbul.2019.04.039.

Guo, X., Hu, G., Fan, X., and Jia, H. (2020). Sorption properties of cadmium on microplastics: the common practice experiment and a two-dimensional correlation spectroscopic study. *Ecotoxicol. Environ. Saf.* 190: 110118. https://doi.org/10.1016/j.ecoenv.2019.110118.

Hardesty, B.D., Good, T.P., and Wilcox, C. (2015). Novel methods, new results and science-based solutions to tackle marine debris impacts on wildlife. *Ocean Coast. Mang.* 115: 4–9, cited after: Ugwu et al. (2021).

Heskett, M., Takada, H., Yamashita, R. et al. (2012). Measurement of persistent organic pollutants (POPs) in plastic resin pellets from remote islands: toward establishment of background concentrations for International Pellet Watch. *Mar. Pollut. Bull.* 64: 445–448.

Hirai, H., Takada, H., Ogata, Y. et al. (2011). Organic micropollutants in marine plastics debris from the open ocean and remote and urban beaches. *Mar. Pollut. Bull.* 62: 1683–1692.

Holmes, L.A., Turner, A., and Thompson, R.C. (2012). Adsorption of trace metals to plastic resin pellets in the marine environment. *Environ. Pollut.* 160 (1): 42–48.

Honda, M. and Suzuki, N. (2020). Toxicities of polycyclic aromatic hydrocarbons for aquatic animals. *Int. J. Environ. Res. Public Health* 17: 1363.

Kim, H. and Lee, J. (2021). Emerging concerns about microplastic pollution on groundwater in South Korea. *Sustainability* 12 (13): https://doi.org/10.3390/su12135275.

Kühn, S., Bravo Rebolledo, E.L., and van Franeker, J.A. (2015). Deleterious effect of litter on marine life. In: *Marine Anthropogenic Litter* (ed. M. Bergmann, L. Gutow and M. Klages). Cham: Springer. https://doi.org/10.1007/978-3-319-16510-3_4.

Li Y., Sun Y., Li J. et al. (2021). Research on the influence of microplastics on marine life. *3rd International Conference on Air Pollution and Environmental Engineering. IOP Conf. Series: Earth and Environmental Science*, Vol. 631, 012006. IOP Publishing. https://doi.org/10.1088/1755-1315/631/1/012006.

Liu, S., hi, J., Wang, J. et al. (2021). Interactions between microplastics and heavy metals in aquatic environments: a review. *Front. Microbiol.* https://doi.org/10.3389/fmicb.2021.652520.

Lo, H.S., Wong, C.Y., Tam, N.F.Y., and Cheung, S.G. (2019). Spatial distribution and source identification of hydrophobic organic compounds (HOCs) on sedimentary microplastic in Hong Kong. *Chemosphere* 219: 418–426. https://doi.org/10.1016/j.chemosphere.2018.12.032.

Magadini, D.L., Goes, J.I., Ortiz, S. et al. (2020). Assesing the sorption of pharmaceuticals to microplastics through in-situ experiments in New York City waterways. *Sci. Total Environ.* 729: 138766. https://doi.org/10.1016/j.scitotenv.2020.138766.

Mai, L., Bao, L., Shi, L. et al. (2018). Polycyclic aromatic hydrocarbons affiliated with microplastics in surface waters of Bohai and Huanghai Seas, China. *Environ. Pollut.* 241: 834–840. https://doi.org/10.1016/j.envpol.2018.06.012.

Massos, A. and Turner, A. (2017). *Cadmium, Lead and Bromine in Beached Microplastics.* University of Plymouth. https://pearl.plymouth.ac.uk/bitstream/handle/10026.1/9235/Massos%20and%20TurnTu%202017%20Env%20Poll%202017.pdf?sequence=1.

Mato, Y., Isobe, T., Takada, H. et al. (2001). Plastic resin pellets as a transport medium for toxic chemicals in the marine environment. *Environ. Sci. Technol.* 35: 318–324. https://doi.org/10.1021/es0010498, cited after: Syberg et al. (2020).

McDougal, L., Thomson, L., Brand, S. et al. (2021). Adsorption of a diverse range of pharmaceuticals to polyethylene microplastics in wastewater and their desorption in environmental matrices. *Sci. Total Environ.* 152071: https://doi.org/10.1016/j.scitotenv.2021.152071.

Menéndez-Pedriza, A. and Jaumot, J. (2020). Interaction of environmental pollutants with microplastic: a critical rewiev of sorption factors, bioacummulation and ecotoxicological effects. *Toxics* 8 (2): 40. https://doi.org/10.3390/toxics8020040.

Munier, B. and Bendell, L. (2018). Macro and microplasics sorb and desorb metals and act as a point source of trace metals to coastal ecosystems. *PLoS One* https://doi.org/10.1371/journal.pone.0191759.

Nerland, I.L., Halsband, C., Allan, I., and Thomas, K.V. (2014). Microplastics in Marine Environments: Occurrence, Distribution and Effects, Report NIVA, Norway.

Osorio Prado, N. (2020). Sorption of polycyclic aromatic hydrocarbons (PAHs) on microplastics in the freshwater, brackish, and saline environments. MSc thesis. University of Tokyo.

Oz, N., Kadizade, G., and YurtSever, M. (2019). Investigation of heavy metal adsorption on microplastics. *Appl. Ecol. Environ. Res.* 17 (4): 7301–7310.

Pannetier, P., Cachot, J., Clérandeau, C. et al. (2019). Toxicity assessment of pollutants sorbed on environmental sample microplastics collected on beaches: part I – adverse effects on fish cell line. *Environ. Pollut.* 248: 1088–1097. https://doi.org/10.1016/j.envpol.2018.12.091.

Park, H. and Park, B. (2021). Review of microplastics distribution, toxicity, analysis methods, and removal technologies. *Water* 13 (19): 2736. https://doi.org/10.3390/w13192736.

Pozo, K., Urbina, W., Gómez, V. et al. (2020). Persistent organic pollutants sorbedin plastic resin pellet – "Nurdles" from coastal areas of Central Chile. *Mar. Pollut. Bull.* 151: 110786. https://doi.org/10.1016/j.marpolbul.2019.110786.

Qiongjie, W., Yong, Z., Yangyang, Z. et al. (2022). Effects of biofilm on metal adsorption behavior and microbial community of microplastics. *J. Hazard. Mater.* 424, part A: 127340.

Rocha-Santos, T.A. and Duarte, A.C. (2017). *Characterization and Analysis of Microplastics*. Elsevier, cited after: Agboola and Benson (2021).

Rochman, C., Hentschel, B.T., and Teh, S.J. (2014). Long-term sorption of metals is similar among plastic types: implications for plastic debris in aquatic environments. *PLoS One* https://doi.org/10.1371/journal.pone.0085433.

Rummel, C.D., Jahnke, A., Gorokhova, E., and Kühnel, D. (2017). *Environ. Sci. Technol. Lett.* 4: 258–267.

Scutariu, R.E., Puiu, D., Nechifor, G. et al. (2019). *in vitro* sorption study of some organochlorine pesticides on polyethylene terephthalate microplastics. *Revis. Chim.* 70 (12): 4620–4626. https://doi.org/10.37358/RC.19.12.7803, cited after: Agboola and Benson (2021).

Seyfi, S., Katibeh, H., and Heshami, M. (2021). Investigation of the process of adsorption of heavy metals in coastal sands containing micro-plastics, with special attention to the effect of aging process and bacterial spread in micro-plastics. *Arch. Environ. Prot.* 47 (3): 50–59.

Sheela, A., Manimekalai, B., and Dhinagaran, G. (2022). Review on the distribution of microplastics in oceans and its impacts: need for modeling-base approach to investigate the transport and risk of microplastic pollution. *Environ. Eng. Res.* 27 (4): 210243.

Singh, R., Gautam, N., Mishra, A., and Gupta, R. (2011). Heavy metals and living systems: an overview. *Indian J. Pharm.* 43 (3): 246–253.

Sørensen, L., Rogers, E., Altin, D. et al. (2020). Sorption of PAHs to microplastic and their bioavailability and toxicity to marine copepodus under co-exposure conditions. *Environ. Pollut.* 258: 113844.

Syberg, K., Knudsen, K., Tairova, Z. et al. (2020). Sorption of PCBs to environmental plastic pollution in the North Atlantic Ocean: importance of size and polymer type. *Environ. Eng.* 2: 100062.

Tan, S.A., Khalik, W., Ong, M. et al. (2021). Marine microplastics as vectors of major ocean pollutants and its hazards to the marine ecosystem and humans. *Prog. Earth Planet. Sci.* 8: 12.

Tang, S., Lin, L., Wang, X. et al. (2020). Pb(II) uptake onto nylon microplastics: interaction mechanism and adsorption performance. *J. Hazard. Mater.* 386: 121960. https://doi.org/10.1016/j.jhazmat.2019.121960.

Teuten, E.L., Rwoland, S.J., Galloway, T.S., and Thompson, R.C. (2007). Potential for plastics to transport hydrophobic contaminants. *Environ. Sci. Technol.* 2007 (41): 7759–7764. https://doi.org/10.1021/ES071737S, cited after: Osorio Prado (2020).

Torres, F., Dioses-Salinas, D., Pizarro-Ortega, C., and De-la-Torre, G. (2021). Sorption of chemical contaminants on degradable and non-degradable microplastics: recent progress and research trends. *Sci. Total Environ.* 757: 143875.

Tu, C., Chen, T., Zhou, Q. et al. (2020). Biofilm formation and its influences on the properties of microplastics as affected by exposure time and depth in the seawater. *Sci. Total Environ.* 734: 139237. https://doi.org/10.1016/j.scitotenv.2020.139237, cited after: Liu et al. (2021).

Ugwu, K., Herrera, A., and Gómez, M. (2021). Microplastics in marine biota: a review. *Mar. Pollut. Bull.* 169: 112540.

Van Raamsdonk, L.W., van der Zande, M., Koelmans, A.A. et al. (2020). Current insights into monitoring, bioaccumulation, and potential health effects of microplastics present in the food chain. *Foods* 9 (1): 72. https://doi.org/10.3390/foods9010072.

Van, A., Rochman, C.M., Flores, E.M. et al. (2012). Persistent organic pollutants in plastic marine debris found on beaches in San Diego, California. *Chemosphere* 86: 258–263.

Verla, A.W., Enyoh, C.E., Verla, E.N. et al. (2019). Microplastic–toxic chemical interaction: a review study on quantified levels, mechanism and implication. *SN Appl. Sci.* 1: 1400. https://doi.org/10.1007/s42452-019-1352-0.

Wang, W. and Wang, J. (2018). Different partition of polycyclic aromatic hydrocarbon on environmental particulates in freshwater: microplastics in comparison to natural sediment. *Ecotoxicol. Environ. Saf.* 147: 648–655, cited after: Osorio Prado (2020).

Wang, J., Jinping, P., Zhi, T. et al. (2017). Microplastics in the surface sediments from the Beijiang River littoral zone: composition, abundance, surface textures and interaction with heavy metals. *Chemosphere* 171: 248–258.

Wang, Q., Zhang, Y., Wangjin, X. et al. (2020). The adsorption behavior of metals in aqueous solution by microplastics effected by UV radiation. *J. Environ. Sci.* 87: 272–280. https://doi.org/10.1016/j.jes.2019.07.006.

Wang F., Zhang M., Sha W., Wang Y., Hao H., Dou Y., Li Y., Sorption behavior and mechanisms of organic contaminants to nano and microplastics, Molecules, 2020a, 25: 1827, https://doi.org/10.3390/molecules25081827.

Weber, C.J., Hahn, J., and Opp, C. (2022). Spatial connections between microplastics and heavy metal pollution within floodplain soils. *Appl. Sci.* 12: 595. https://doi.org/10.3390/app12020595.

Wiśniowska, E. and Włodarczyk-Makuła, M. (2021). Adsorption of selected 3-ring and 4-ring polycyclic aromatic hydrocarbons on polyester microfibers – preliminary studies. *Desalin. Water Treat.* 232: 414–420.

Wiśniowska, E., Moraczewska-Majkut, K., and Nocoń, W. (2018). Efficiency of microplastics removal in selected wastewater treatment plants – preliminary studies. *Desalin. Water Treat.* 134: 316–323.

Yeo, B.G., Takada, H., Yamashita, R. et al. (2020). PCBs and PBDEs in microplastic particles and zooplankton in open water in the Pacific Ocean and around the coast of Japan. *Mar. Pollut. Bull.* 151: 110806. https://doi.org/10.1016/j.marpolbul.2019.110806.

Section II

Environmental Domains for One Health

6

Cyanotoxin in Hydrosphere and Human Interface

Dhammika N. Magana-Arachchi[1] *and Rasika P. Wanigatunge*[2]

[1] *Molecular Microbiology and Human Diseases Unit, National Institute of Fundamental Studies, Kandy, Sri Lanka*
[2] *Department of Plant and Molecular Biology, Faculty of Science, University of Kelaniya, Kelaniya, Sri Lanka*

6.1 Introduction

Cyanobacteria are ubiquitous, prokaryotic, and the only bacteria capable of photosynthesis. The phylum Cyanobacteria comprises about 150 genera and nearly 2000 species, among which 46 are identified as toxigenic (Magana Arachchi and Wanigatunge 2020). Cyanotoxins, a secondary metabolite produced by cyanobacteria, threaten humans, animals, and the environment. The hydrosphere or the aqua sphere is the total water on the earth in any form, as vapor, liquid, and solid with its dissolved constituents. One Health is a trio that brings humans, animals, and the environment they share as one unit (Figure 6.1). The chapter will outline how cyanotoxins in hydrosphere cause health complications within the "One Health Triad" practice.

6.2 Cyanobacteria and Cyanotoxins

6.2.1 Cyanobacteria and Cyanotoxins

Cyanobacteria are an ancient group of prokaryotic organisms that are more than 3500 million years old and prokaryotic. They are rich in natural products and produce many chemical compounds with different chemical structures as secondary metabolites. Cyanobacteria are microscopic and exhibit high variability in their morphology. They can exist as single cells, in groups, as colonies, or in filamentous forms. They possess specific characteristics of algae, such as cell wall structure and pigments. Hence earlier, they were called blue-green algae. Cyanobacteria are capable of growing in diverse environments, including terrestrial or aquatic habitats. These bacteria can survive under low-light conditions with the help of their accessory pigments, specially phycocyanin, phycobilins, and phycoerythrin.

The favorable environmental conditions and nutrient availability enhance cyanobacteria's proliferation, leading to cyanobacterial blooms (Weralupitiya et al. 2022). They occur naturally in most surface waters in low to moderate numbers. Most of these bloom formers can produce cyanotoxins (Table 6.1). Whether these toxins cause adverse health issues will depend on their genetic composition and the cyanobacterial biomass (Ibelings et al. 2021).

Cyanotoxin production is not limited to freshwater systems, but the highest cyanotoxin levels have been reported from algal blooms and scums in freshwater ecosystems (Benayache et al. 2019; Weralupitiya et al. 2022). Most of the time, the cyanotoxins are kept within the live cells (intracellular). However, both live and dead cyanobacterial cells could release the toxins into the aquatic environments. Certain cyanobacteria, such as *Cylindrospermopsis*, naturally excrete the toxin cylindrospermopsin, into waters. In contrast, others release the toxins when their cell walls rupture, or encounter any stress, or when the cell dies.

These cyanotoxins are hazardous to humans, animals, and the environment. Major cyanotoxins, including microcystins (MCs), cylindrospermopsin (CYN), anatoxins, saxitoxins, lyngbyatoxins, nodularins (NODs), aplysiatoxin, lipopolysaccharides, can be grouped according to their chemical structure (Table 6.1). Different genera of cyanobacteria can produce one single cyanotoxin. Microcystins are produced by multiple cyanobacteria genera, including *Microcystis*, *Dolichospermum* (previously *Anabaena*), *Planktothrix*, *Nostoc*, *Oscillatoria*, and *Anabaenopsis* (Figure 6.2) (Filatova et al. 2021). Microcystins are seven amino acid peptide molecules that contain a characteristic Adda moiety [(2*S*,3*S*,4*E*,6*E*,8*S*,9*S*)-3-amino-9-methoxy-2,6,8-trimethyl-10-phenyldeca 4,6-dienoic acid] or its derivatives. By 2019, around 279 different microcystin isoforms had been identified (Bouaïcha et al. 2019). But the number reached 300 by

One Health: Human, Animal, and Environment Triad, First Edition. Edited by Meththika Vithanage and Majeti Narasimha Vara Prasad.

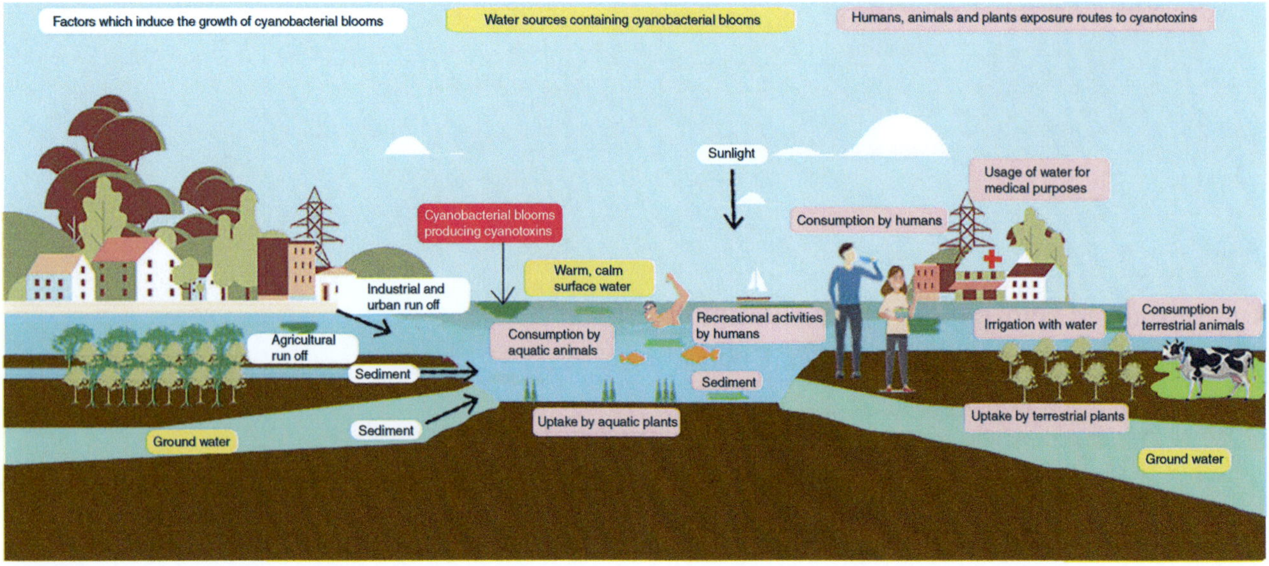

Figure 6.1 A schematic representation of the fate of cyanotoxin in the environment: a growing threat to human and animal health.

Table 6.1 Summary of common cyanotoxins, chemical structures, affecting organs, and producing genera.

Name of cyanotoxin	Structure	Affecting organs	Producing genera	References
Microcystins	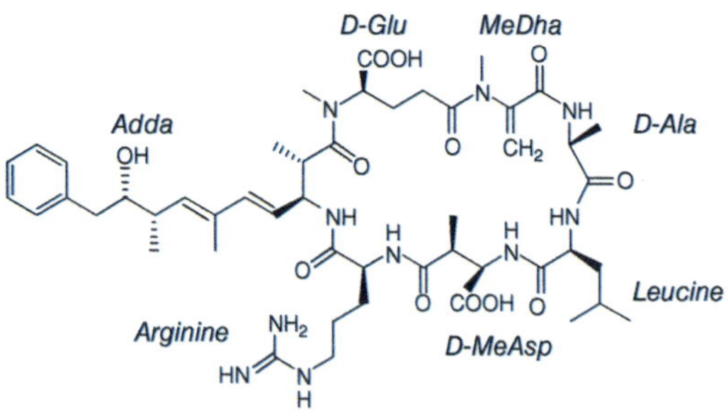	Lungs, liver, immune system, gastrointestinal tract, cardiovascular system	*Dolichospermum*, *Anabaenopsis*, *Aphanocapsa*, *Arthrospira*, *Hapalosiphon*, *Microcystis*, *Nostoc*, *Oscillatoria*, *Planktothrix*, *Snowella*, *Woronichinia*, *Aphanizomenon*, *Limnothrix*, *Phormidium*	Kubickova et al. (2019), Cao et al. (2019), Abdallah et al. (2021)
Nodularins	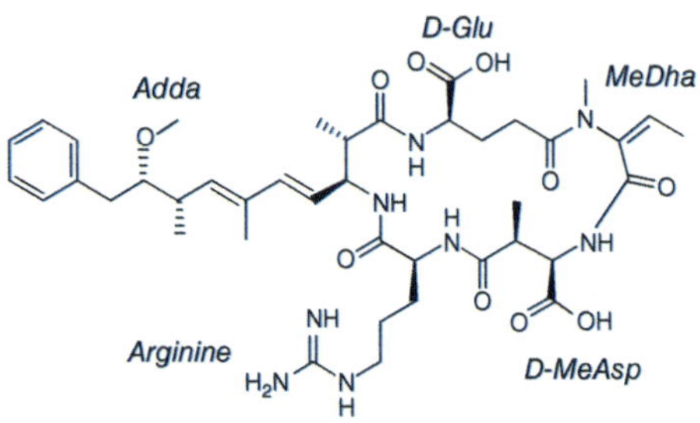	Lungs, liver	*Nodularia*	Kubickova et al. (2019)
Cylindrospermopsin	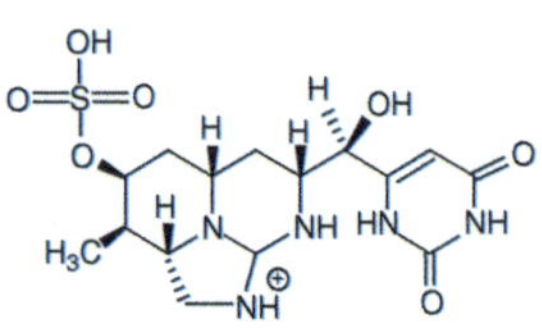	Lungs, liver, kidney, immune system, gastrointestinal tract	*Dolichospermum*, *Aphanizomenon*, *Cylindrospermopsis*, *Raphidiopsis*, *Umezakia, Lyngbya*, *Planktothrix*	Kubickova et al. (2019), Abdallah et al. (2021)
Anatoxin-a	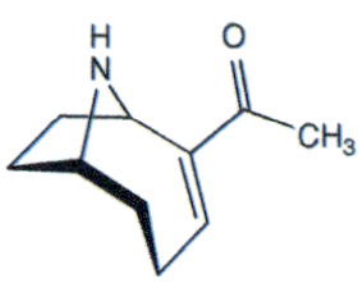	Nervous tissue, brain	*Dolichospermum*, *Oscillatoria*, *Cylindrospermum*, *Aphanizomenon*	Kubickova et al. (2019), Abdallah et al. (2021)

Table 6.1 (Continued)

Name of cyanotoxin	Structure	Affecting organs	Producing genera	References
Homoanatoxin-a	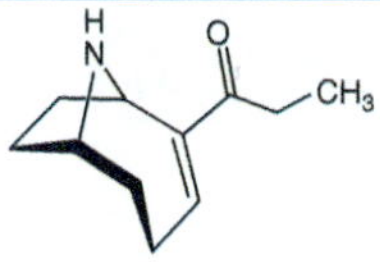	Nervous tissue, brain	*Phormidium, Raphidiopsis*	Kubickova et al. (2019)
Anatoxin-a(s)	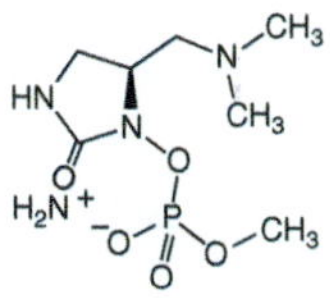	Nervous tissue, brain	*Dolichospermum*	Kubickova et al. (2019)
Saxitoxin	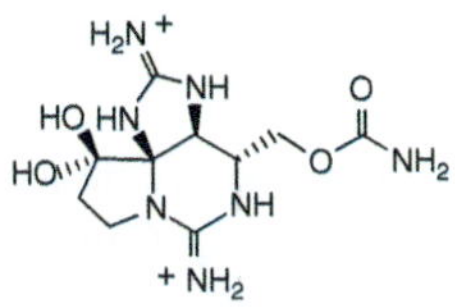	Nervous tissue, brain	*Dolichospermum, Aphanizomenon, Cylindrospermopsis, Lyngbya, Planktothrix, Raphidiopsis, Fischerella, Geitlerinema, Scytonema*	Meriluoto et al. (2017), Abdallah et al. (2021)
β-*N*-methylamino-l-alanine	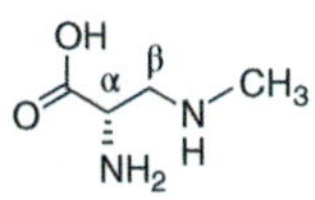	Nervous tissue	*Nostoc, Trichodesmium, Synechococcus, Fischerella*	Meriluoto et al. (2017)

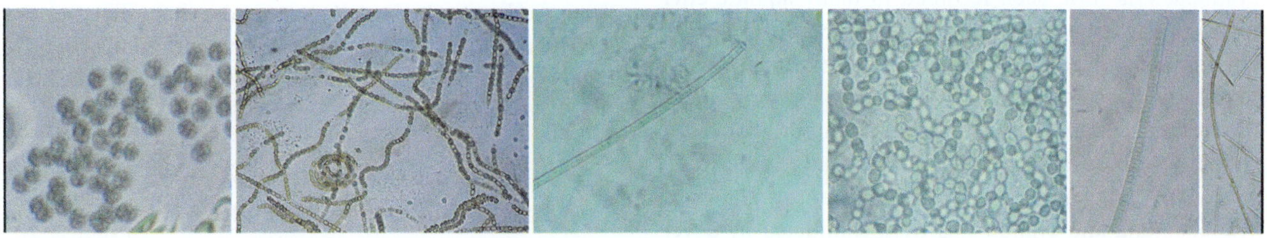

Figure 6.2 Micrographs showing microcystin producing cyanobacteria: (a) *Microcystis* sp., *Dolichospermum* sp. (previously *Anabaena*), *Planktothrix* sp., *Nostoc* sp., *Oscillatoria* sp., and *Anabaenopsis* sp.

2021 (Jones et al. 2021). Cylindrospermopsin is a cyclic guanidine alkaloid mainly produced by freshwater cyanobacteria; *Cylindrospermopsis*, *Anabaena*, *Aphanizomenon flos-aquae*, and many other genera. In addition, the other genera *Lyngbya*, *Oscillatoria*, and *Phormidium* can also produce toxins. Mostly, as these are benthic cyanobacteria, they can release toxins when rising to the surface, being attached to the bottom, or while dispersed in the water. *Nodularia*, which is mainly present in marine systems, produces nodularin. This cyclic non-ribosomal pentapeptide cyanotoxin has been identified as a potent toxin affecting the health of humans, wild animals, and the environment. A variety of cyanobacterial species can produce more than one cyanotoxin; *Anabaena* species, for example, produce microcystin, cylindrospermopsin and anatoxins.

Certain cyanobacteria, during optimum conditions, regulate their buoyancy to stay in surface waters or pursue the bottom of the water bodies. The ability to passage through the water column is a plus point for cyanobacteria over other microorganisms that contest for nutrients and light. In addition, their floatation capacities (due to gas vesicles) allow scum-forming cyanobacteria (e.g. *Microcystis* spp.) to occupy the first centimeters of the water column. Floating cyanobacteria, such as *Anabaena* and *Microcystis*, may drift upward when mixing is weak and accumulate in dense surface blooms (Figure 6.3). Benthic cyanobacteria, such as *Lyngbya*, *Oscillatoria*, and *Phormidium*, also produce cyanotoxins and, therefore, may be hazardous if they detach and rise to the surface or disperse in the water.

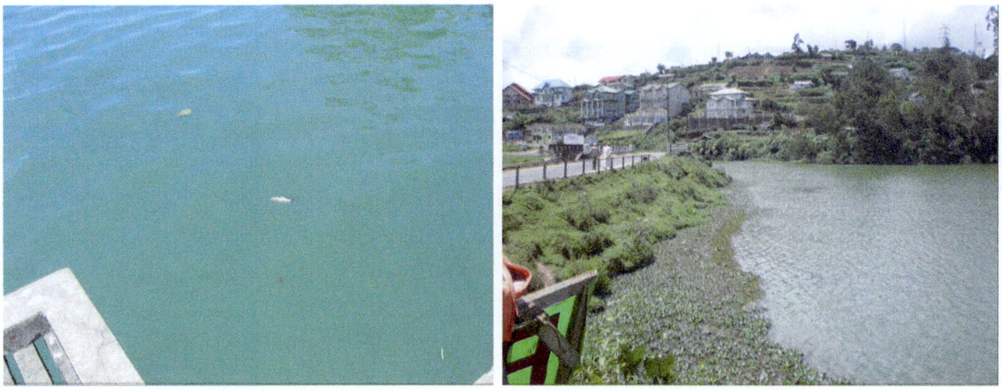

Figure 6.3 Photographs showing dense cyanobacterial blooms in surface waters of Lake Beria and Gregory Lake, Sri Lanka.

6.2.2 Occurrence of Cyanobacteria in the Hydrosphere

Scientific studies on the ecology and fate of cyanotoxins in temperate freshwater environments are abundant, whereas limited studies have been reported from humid tropics. A review article by Svirčev et al. (2019) reported 1118 documentations of major cyanotoxins in 869 freshwater ecosystems from 66 countries worldwide, with microcystin being the most commonly detected. They reported ~183 recorded cyanotoxin poisonings in humans and animals. Globally, cyanobacteria have been recorded in many aquatic environments, whether fresh, marine, or brackish. In aquatic environments, cyanobacteria occur in diverse habitats: suspended in dispersed form or as aggregates in the water, on the water surface, on the bottom sediment, or attached to shoreline rocks, sediments, and plants (Meriluoto et al. 2017). According to the literature, most studies on cyanobacteria and cyanotoxins were conducted by developed countries, while certain countries did not possess any data on the said issue (Svirčev et al. 2019).

During seasonal studies, microcystins and anatoxin-a have been frequently reported from the countries in Europe, spanning from the United Kingdom, Poland, Italy, Poland, Czech Republic, Germany, Russia, France, and the Netherlands (Filatova et al. 2020; Hartnell et al. 2020).

There are many reports about substantial hazards triggered by the moving cyanobacterial blooms from streams to rivers, estuaries, and beaches (Camacho-Munoz et al. 2021). The shellfish and other animals accumulate the cyanotoxins released by these blooms and potentially transfer those toxins into the food web. A study by Camacho-Munoz et al. (2021) mimicking the coastal environment within the laboratory has shown the uptake of the two cyanotoxins, microcystins and nodularins, getting into mussels.

Officially launched in 2016 by the United States and its federal partners, the One Health Harmful Algal Bloom System (OHHABS) is a surveillance system. The system collects information to help Centers for Disease Control and Prevention (CDC) and their partners understand Harmful Algal Blooms (HABs) and prevent humans and animals from getting ill. OHHABS of the United States (18 States of the US) in their report presented 421 harmful cyanobacterial bloom occurrings. Human illnesses included 389 cases, while animal diseases records counted 413 cases. The reporting period was from 2016 to 2018. According to the report, the majority happened from May to October, numbering 413. Among the recorded, 90% were from freshwater bodies. Human and animal illnesses primarily occurred from June to September, numbering 378 (98%), and from May to September, it was 410, which is 100% (Roberts et al. 2020).

6.2.3 Impacts of Climate Changes on Cyanobacterial Occurrence in the Hydrosphere

The prevalence of cyanobacteria is increasing in freshwaters due to climate change. The direct sunlight, rise in water temperatures, pH changes due to biological activities, heavy rainfalls, and flooding are some of the physical parameters that influence the cyanobacterial bloom formation. According to a recent review (Moreira et al. 2022), the effects of climatic changes have been more studied in marine systems. Still, they discussed the factors such as an increase in temperature or global warming and gales accompanying substantial rainfalls that facilitated the cyanobacterial distribution worldwide. In temperate regions, certain cyanotoxin-producing species could be observed in the lakes in the early summer. In contrast, certain others occurred in late summer, when temperatures rose above 20 °C. However, there are records of some cyanobacteria's ability to bloom even in winter by withstanding the cold weather.

A study conducted in Fehérvárcsurgó reservoir in Hungary describes the presence of *Aphanizomenon flos-aquae, Microcystis flos-aquae, Microcystis wesenbergii, Cuspidothrix issatschenkoi, Dolichospermum fos-aquae*, and *Snowella litoralis* in the reservoir. They observed histopathological changes in the gills and kidney tissues of the fish. They witnessed more damage in the summer months, correlating that to increased cyanobacterial biomass and the adverse impact on the ecosystem (Drobac Backović et al. 2021).

According to published data, environmental pressures exerted on ecosystems are the decisive factor in population dynamics and the toxicity of cyanobacterial blooms. Temperature stratifications influence cyanobacterial bloom formation and its accumulation as a surface scum. However, some other lake characteristics, including turbidity of the water, water mixing due to winds, water stagnation, and the nature of the water column, might influence the bloom development or get dissolved (Ibelings et al. 2021).

6.2.4 Impacts of Anthropogenic Activities on Cyanobacterial Occurrence in the Hydrosphere

According to a recent WHO document, primary anthropogenic sources that release nutrients such as nitrogen (N) and phosphorus (P) into water bodies are agricultural runoffs, sewage, and municipal wastewaters (WHO 2020a). These wastes are generated by people while engaged in their daily activities, domestically or during their occupations. Fertilizers, pesticides, and the excretory releases of farming animals contribute to the waste generated due to agricultural activities. The population growth and urbanization have also led to a rapid rise in human activities, releasing a large amount of waste and polluting the environment. All these wastes could be directly dumped or transported via different routes to water bodies, making the aquatic systems rich with nutrients and facilitating the global occurrence and spreading of cyanobacteria.

Cyanobacteria thrive in eutrophic lakes and ponds with phosphorus concentrations >50 μg/l. Theoretically, any nutrient could be limiting, but practically, the two macronutrients P in soluble form or as total, and, in some cases, N is decisive for the amount of cyanobacterial biomass that can occur in a particular water body (Chorus and Zessner 2021). Considerable cyanobacterial biomasses can often be found in mesotrophic ecosystems when the total phosphorus concentrations are between 20 and 50 μg/l. The *Planktothrix rubescens* growing in deep sub-alpine lakes is one such example (Humbert and Fastner 2017).

In general, many physicochemical and biotic factors and processes are recognized as influencing the population dynamics of cyanobacteria and their vertical and horizontal distribution in water bodies (Humbert and Fastner 2017).

6.3 Modes of Human Exposure to Cyanotoxins and Illnesses Associated with Cyanotoxins

6.3.1 Modes of Human Exposure to Cyanotoxins

Eutrophication paves the way for harmful cyanobacterial blooms, enhancing the risk of surface freshwater contamination. It causes significant health issues in humans and animals.

Recently WHO-updated guideline values have been finalized for the four cyanotoxins: microcystins, cylindrospermopsins, anatoxin-a, and saxitoxins. The previous WHO guideline value for total microcystins-LR (MC-LR) in drinking water is 1 μg/l. However, the MC-LR value and the total microcystins' content are also considered in the new update. The value for a lifetime is 1 μg/l and for short-term events, 12 μg/l in drinking water (WHO 2020a). Additionally, threshold values for cylindrospermopsin, anatoxin-a, and saxitoxins are now also taken into account, with values of 3, 30, and 3 μg/l in drinking water, respectively (WHO 2020b–d).

The US Environmental Protection Agency (USEPA) has set up a 10-day health guideline for drinking water for microcystin-LR at 1.6 μg/l. For cylindrospermopsin, the limit is 3.0 μg/l for school-age children and adults. In infants, the values are set at 0.3 and 0.7 μg/l (USEPA 2015).

The most common way for humans to become exposed to cyanotoxins is through unintentionally drinking cyanotoxin-contaminated water. Other ingestion routes involve consuming food prepared from toxin-contaminated water, cyanotoxin-accumulated seafood or aquatic fish, mollusks, etc., or cyanotoxin-contaminated edible plant parts (Abdallah et al. 2021; Weralupitiya et al. 2022). It is unclear whether cooking affects cyanotoxins, as most are heat stable and nonvolatile (Abdallah et al. 2021). In addition to ingestion, the other exposure routes are dermal contact via participating in recreational activities such as swimming and fishing or even while undergoing medical treatments such as dialysis.

Interestingly, there are records regarding potential cyanotoxin inhalation via dust particles (Abdallah et al. 2021). As cyanotoxins are non-volatile, inhalation can happen during a spray if the liquid is contaminated with cyanotoxins or cells. There is a possibility of inhalation while engaging in certain recreational activities such as water skiing or even swimming (WHO 2020a).

Exposure to cyanotoxins via drinking water differs from country to country and even within a country. Because most people in the developed world drink treated drinking water, and as such, exposure to drinking raw water is minimal. For them, exposure to cyanotoxins is mainly through recreational activities. But around 152 nations are still developing, and people living in some of these countries lack access to clean water. Hence, the water they primarily consume is raw, taken from dug wells, and there is a potential risk of cyanotoxin ingestion via drinking the untreated water.

The accumulation of cyanotoxins in plants is a result of several factors. Cyanotoxin accumulation produces severe toxic effects such as reduced plant growth, seed germination, and enhanced oxidative stress. Additionally, a lowered rate of mineral uptake, a decrease in photosynthetic efficiency, and a loss in chlorophyll content are possible (Weralupitiya et al. 2022). The persistence of cyanotoxins in water used to irrigate plants will lead to bioaccumulation of these cyanotoxins in plants and phytotoxicity, as well as the potential risk of pollution in groundwater (Weralupitiya et al. 2022). Compared to agricultural plants, bioaccumulation of microcystin is three times higher in edible parts of leafy vegetables (Zhang et al. 2021).

Most developed and some developing countries perform quantitative analysis on their food and dietary supplements for cyanotoxin detection as it is a major route for acute food poisoning. A study from Brazil has shown how fish accumulate MCs, and these toxins caused oxidative stress, neurotoxicity, and molecular damage (Calado et al. 2019). The study demonstrated how persistent MCs are within these fish tissues. For more data on cyanotoxins and seafood contamination by cyanotoxins, readers are advised to refer to an up-to-date overview of the contamination of cyanotoxins in food from all the developing nations in Africa, Asia, and Latin America (Abdallah et al. 2021).

6.3.2 Illnesses Associated with Cyanotoxins

6.3.2.1 Human Illnesses

Currently, cyanobacteria are considered a microbial contaminant. In 1998, the cyanotoxins were included in the USEPA drinking water candidate contaminating list (CCL), considering how they transmit through drinking waters (Magana-Arachchi and Wanigatunge 2020).

Cyanotoxins are causative agents for many chronic and acute diseases in humans. Depending on the source, route, and duration of cyanotoxin exposure, the toxicity exerted on the human body could be different and decide whether the illness is acute or chronic.

Acute exposure to cyanobacterial blooms and their toxins can cause various symptoms in humans. Depending on the exposure site, it could be a headache, body aches with muscle and joint pains, allergic reactions, eye irritation, etc. Gastrointestinal discomforts such as vomiting, diarrhea, abdominal pain, and cramps are also possible if ingested. Further, it will cause fever and ulcers in the mouth. According to published reports, there is a possibility of getting acute pneumonia or dermatitis. In severe cases, seizures, damage to the liver, cardiac or respiratory arrest, and death might happen (US EPA 2019). Chronic exposure to cyanotoxin may cause liver and kidney damage and also neurotoxicity (Figure 6.4).

According to a recent publication, a total of 389 human cases of illness due to cyano exposure were reported by the US OHHABS, with 341, ~88% being classified as probable. Among the reported, 51% of the cases were in July, when a single freshwater harmful algal bloom caused the incident. Starting in a large lake, the cyanobacterial bloom spread to connected waterways, such as rivers, canals, and reservoirs, and lasted more than three months (Roberts et al. 2020).

All reported illnesses (~98%) occurred from June to September. The 380 cases displayed various signs and symptoms; among them, gastrointestinal problems were frequent (67%). Further, ~43% had symptoms such as headache, fever, or lethargy; 27% had skin-related issues; and 16% displayed ear, nose, or throat-related symptoms. There were no deaths. Time to the onset of initial signs or symptoms was available for 124 people with a one-time exposure ranging from one minute to eight days (Roberts et al. 2020).

The documented and scientifically proven human deaths due to cyanotoxins are limited. Though guidelines could be imposed for the protection of public water supply systems, rules and regulations cannot be applied to privately owned wells. Most developing countries use well water for their drinking, and it is the same in most parts of Sri Lanka. Chronic Kidney Disease of unknown etiology (CKDu) has been a major health problem in Sri Lanka for the last three decades, and more than 2500 patients have died due to the disease. Most patients are from the dry zone of Sri Lanka, where people consume well water to satisfy their thirst. Research from Sri Lanka has shown the presence of cyanobacteria with toxin-generating ability in well waters in the dry zone of the country and an increased risk for chronic renal disease for people living in the dry zone of Sri Lanka (Liyanage et al. 2016).

MCs employ diverse cellular mechanisms in inducing severe organ impairments. These include enhanced oxidative stress, cytoskeletal disruption, endoplasmic reticulum dysfunction, mitochondrial dysfunction, DNA damage, and apoptosis (Cao et al. 2019; Xu et al. 2020). The kidney is another target of MC toxicity in humans. Severe cytotoxic effects are induced in the renal tissues due to MC toxicity in humans. In a reported case study from Montevideo, Uruguay, a 20-month-old infant was hospitalized following repeated recreational exposure to *Microcystis* blooms containing MCs at up to 8200 μg/l (Vidal et al. 2017). The infant's liver was excised and subjected to histopathological examination. It was revealed that heavy bleeding was involved with severe damage to the liver and nodular degeneration without inflammation. A liver sample was

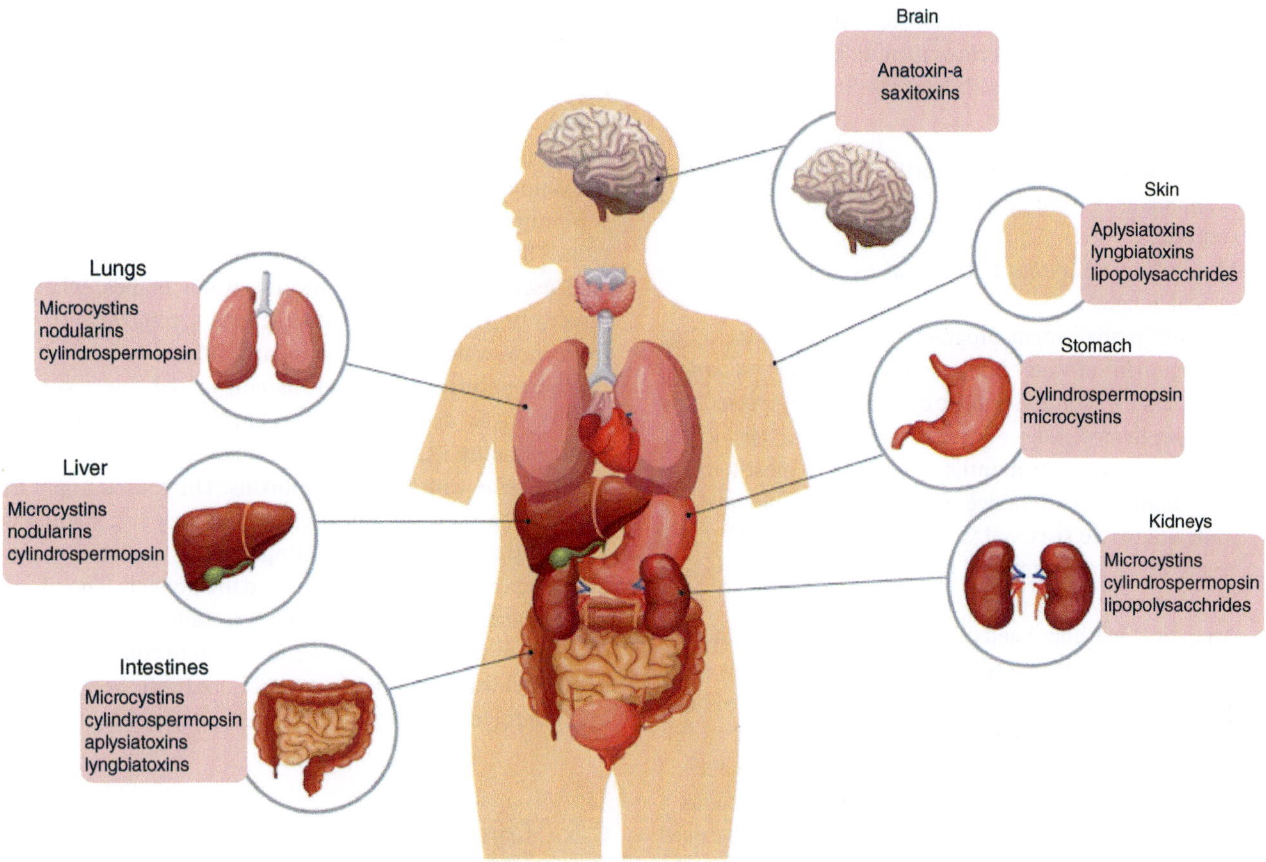

Figure 6.4 Possible target organs affected by different cyanotoxins.

extracted with methanol, and the presence of MC-LR and [D-Leu1] MC-LR in substantial amounts confirmed the toxicity experienced by the infant (Vidal et al. 2017).

Certain Chinese studies have shown a relationship between the frequency of cyanobacterial blooms and cancers in the digestive tract and prostate gland. Still, more concrete evidence is needed for a conclusion. Though there are records of cyanobacterial presence in the human gut, it has not yet been proven that cyanobacteria multiply within the human body. As such, there is no release of cyanotoxins within the human body.

When published data are considered, the human data are inadequate due to a lack of quantitative exposure information and potential coexposure to other microorganisms and contaminants. There are no long-term studies of MC carcinogenicity (WHO 2020a).

6.3.2.2 Animal Intoxications

There are many records of animal intoxications due to cyanotoxins. A recent review discusses an incident where Portugal had encountered the death of farmed cows, and when investigating the deaths, it was recorded that cows had microcystins in their kidneys. Interestingly, the adjacent water bodies that these animals used for drinking had cyanobacterial blooms (Moreira et al. 2022). The decay of cyanobacterial blooms consumes the oxygen in the water, creating hypoxic conditions in water bodies leading to animal and plant deaths.

Based on OHHABS 64 animal case reports, at least 413 animals became ill, and around 89% perished. Most (81%) animal cases of illness were classified as suspected. About 89% of the animals were exposed while being in fresh waters. Even one giant bird died. Around 73% of cases happened in May 2018. Around 99% of illnesses occurred from May to September. Domestic pets accounted for 52 cases. Livestock affected was 42, while wildlife accounted for 319. Among them, 96% were dogs, 86% cattle, and 97% birds. (Roberts et al. 2020).

6.4 The Future Directions for Effective Risk Management of Toxic Cyanobacteria

Many countries around the globe have taken steps to protect their people from cyanotoxin exposure, mainly when used as drinking water, whether the source is groundwater wells, lakes, reservoirs, rivers, or any other means. Implementing and adhering to guidelines minimizes cyanotoxins' risks and health hazards. Some of the factors that need attention are

- Need for continuous monitoring programs to detect cyanotoxins in the reservoirs used as drinking water sources.
- Monitoring reservoirs is essential to maintain the ecological balance.
- Efficient management programs are required, including management of water bodies, correct toxicity assessment by accurately identifying toxic cyanobacterial species, and whether the reservoirs adhere to the recommended levels.
- During the summer months, reservoirs in most temperate countries experience cyanobacterial blooms. To understand the seasonal variation of cyanotoxins in the reservoirs, a more-detailed temporal resolution needs to be practiced, with a weekly frequency.
- Analytical methods used for the detection of cyanotoxins should have easy accessibility. Standard protocols must also be used; tests should be rapid, convenient to handle, and low-cost. For example, multiplex PCR could simultaneously identify the presence of genes in potential MCs, CYNs, and NODs, releasing cyanobacteria as a rapid and economical test. However, these can be used only for monitoring, and quantifications are essential for confirming cyanotoxins.
- Studies on other cyanotoxins, such as neurotoxins, dermatotoxins, produced by cyanobacteria to address more health impairments.
- Most developing countries do not practice the correct usage of fertilizers and the amount to be used. As such, farmers could be effectively educated on proper agricultural practices to minimize the excessive use of pesticides and inorganic fertilizers in farming and how these have to be used without polluting aquatic water bodies.

People need to be concerned about the water used in irrigating grown plants. The plants will take these up if the waters are contaminated with cyanotoxins. Therefore, monitoring of waters that are used in agriculture is vital. It is crucial to refrain from growing leafy vegetables on agricultural lands. However, even if this is done, it is critical to monitor the cultivations for cyanotoxins to prevent the risk of cyanotoxin contamination (Zhang et al. 2021).

Monitoring the aquaculture plants and fish ponds is vital. The effluents are rich in nutrients. When the generated excreta are released into the water bodies, whether directly or treated, the procedures used to remove nutrients from wastewaters must be standardized.

When published literature is considered, most studies are on MCs, describing the occurrence and effects on humans, animals, and the environment. However, it was not the same with other cyanotoxins. The reason might be that a wide range of analytical techniques and standards are easily assessable in detecting MCs. Still, there is adequate data on other cyanotoxins and their effects. Therefore, when managing the risks from cyanobacterial blooms and implementing safety measures, it is vital to consider all the potential cyanotoxin producers and not limit them only to MC-producing taxa (Codd et al. 2020).

6.5 Conclusion

Why do cyanobacteria produce cyanotoxins? This is a global problem for which the answer is not yet known. Hence the topic "Cyanotoxin in hydrosphere and human interface" within the One Health Triad is an important area of research to be involved.

Acknowledgment

We are expressing our sincere appreciation to Ms. Sanduni Bandara and Ms. Sammani De Silva for technical support in the preparation of Figures 6.1 and 6.4 and Table 6.1.

References

Abdallah, M.F., Van Hassel, W.H., Andjelkovic, M. et al. (2021). Cyanotoxins and food contamination in developing countries: review of their types, toxicity, analysis, occurrence and mitigation strategies. *Toxins* 13 (11): 786.

Benayache, N.Y., Nguyen-Quang, T., Hushchyna, K. et al. (2019). An overview of cyanobacteria harmful algal bloom (CyanoHAB) issues in freshwater ecosystems. In: *Limnology-Some New Aspects of Inland Water Ecology* (ed. D. Gökçe), 1–25. https://doi.org/10.5772/intechopen.84155.

Bouaïcha, N., Miles, C.O., Beach, D.G. et al. (2019). Structural diversity, characterization and toxicology of microcystins. *Toxins* 11 (12): 714.

Calado, S.L.M., Santos, G.S., Wojciechowski, J. et al. (2019). The accumulation dynamics, elimination and risk assessment of paralytic shellfish toxins in fish from a water supply reservoir. *Science of the Total Environment* 651: 3222–3229.

Camacho-Muñoz, D., Waack, J., Turner, A.D. et al. (2021). Rapid uptake and slow depuration: health risks following cyanotoxin accumulation in mussels? *Environmental Pollution* 271: 116400.

Cao, L., Massey, I.Y., Feng, H., and Yang, F. (2019). A review of cardiovascular toxicity of microcystins. *Toxins* 11 (9): 507.

Chorus, I. and Zessner, M. (2021). Assessing and controlling the risk of cyanobacterial blooms: nutrient loads from the catchment. In: *Toxic Cyanobacteria in Water* (ed. I. Chorus and M. Welker), 433–503. CRC Press.

Codd, G.A., Testai, E., Funari, E., and Svirčev, Z. (2020). Cyanobacteria, cyanotoxins, and human health. In: *Water treatment for purification from cyanobacteria and cyanotoxins* (ed. A.E. Hiskia, T.M. Triantis, M.G. Antoniou, et al.), 37–68. Wiley.

Drobac Backović, D., Tokodi, N., Marinović, Z. et al. (2021). Cyanobacteria, cyanotoxins, and their histopathological effects on fish tissues in Fehérvárcsurgó reservoir, Hungary. *Environmental Monitoring and Assessment* 193 (9): 1–14.

Filatova, D., Picardo, M., Núñez, O., and Farré, M. (2020). Analysis, levels and seasonal variation of cyanotoxins in freshwater ecosystems. *Trends in Environmental Analytical Chemistry* 26: e00091.

Filatova, D., Jones, M.R., Haley, J.A. et al. (2021). Cyanobacteria and their secondary metabolites in three freshwater reservoirs in the United Kingdom. *Environmental Sciences Europe* 33 (1): 1–11.

Hartnell, D.M., Chapman, I.J., Taylor, N.G. et al. (2020). Cyanobacterial abundance and microcystin profiles in two Southern British Lakes: the importance of abiotic and biotic interactions. *Toxins* 12 (8): 503.

Humbert, J.F. and Fastner, J. (2017). *Ecology of Cyanobacteria*, 11–18. Chichester: Wiley.

Ibelings, B.W., Kurmayer, R., Azevedo, S.M. et al. (2021). Understanding the occurrence of cyanobacteria and cyanotoxins. In: *Toxic Cyanobacteria in Water* (ed. I. Chorus and M. Welker), 213–294. CRC Press.

Jones, M.R., Pinto, E., Torres, M.A. et al. (2021). CyanoMetDB, a comprehensive public database of secondary metabolites from cyanobacteria. *Water Research* 196: 117017.

Kubickova, B., Babica, P., Hilscherová, K., and Šindlerová, L. (2019). Effects of cyanobacterial toxins on the human gastrointestinal tract and the mucosal innate immune system. *Environmental Sciences Europe* 31 (1): 1–27.

Liyanage, H.M., Arachchi, D.M., Abeysekara, T., and Guneratne, L. (2016). Toxicology of freshwater cyanobacteria. *Journal of Environmental Science and Health, Part C* 34 (3): 137–168.

Magana-Arachchi, D.N. and Wanigatunge, R.P. (2020). Ubiquitous waterborne pathogens. In: *Waterborne Pathogens* (ed. M.N.V. Prasad and A. Grobelak), 15–42. Butterworth-Heinemann.

Meriluoto, J., Spoof, L., and Codd, G.A. (ed.) (2017). *Handbook of Cyanobacterial Monitoring and Cyanotoxin Analysis*. Wiley.

Moreira, C., Vasconcelos, V., and Antunes, A. (2022). Cyanobacterial blooms: current knowledge and new perspectives. *Earth* 3 (1): 127–135.

Roberts, V.A., Vigar, M., Backer, L. et al. (2020). Surveillance for harmful algal bloom events and associated human and animal illnesses – one health harmful algal bloom system, United States, 2016–2018. *Morbidity and Mortality Weekly Report* 69 (50): 1889.

Svirčev, Z., Lalić, D., Bojadžija Savić, G. et al. (2019). Global geographical and historical overview of cyanotoxin distribution and cyanobacterial poisonings. *Archives of Toxicology* 93 (9): 2429–2481.

USEPA (2015). *Drinking Water Health Advisory for the Cyanobacterial Microcystin Toxins* (EPA Document Number: 820R15100). United States Environment Protection Agency.

USEPA (2019). *Cyanobacteria and Cyanotoxins: Information for Drinking Water Systems* (EPA-810F11001). United States Environmental Protection Agency.

Vidal, F., Sedan, D., D'Agostino, D. et al. (2017). Recreational exposure during algal bloom in Carrasco Beach, Uruguay: a liver failure case report. *Toxins* 9 (9): 267.

Weralupitiya, C., Wanigatunge, R.P., Gunawardana, D. et al. (2022). Cyanotoxins uptake and accumulation in crops: phytotoxicity and implications on human health. *Toxicon* 211: 21–35.

World Health Organization (2020a). Cyanobacterial toxins: microcystins. Background document for development of WHO guidelines for drinking-water quality and guidelines for safe recreational water environments. In: *World Health Organization*, 1–55. Geneva: (WHO/HEP/ECH/WSH/2020.6). Licence: CC BY-NCSA 3.0 IGO.

World Health Organization (2020b). *Cyanobacterial Toxins: Cylindrospermopsins* (No. WHO/HEP/ECH/WSH/2020.4). World Health Organization.

World Health Organization (2020c). *Cyanobacterial Toxins: Anatoxin-a and Analogues* (No. WHO/HEP/ECH/WSH/2020.1). World Health Organization.

World Health Organization (2020d). *Cyanobacterial Toxins: Saxitoxins* (No. WHO/HEP/ECH/WSH/2020.8). World Health Organization.

Xu, S., Yi, X., Liu, W. et al. (2020). A review of nephrotoxicity of microcystins. *Toxins* 12 (11): 693.

Zhang, Y., Whalen, J.K., and Sauvé, S. (2021). Phytotoxicity and bioconcentration of microcystins in agricultural plants: Meta-analysis and risk assessment. *Environmental Pollution* 272: 115966.

7

Contributions to One Health Approach to Solve Geogenic Health Issues

Rohana Chandrajith[1,2] *and Johannes A.C. Barth*[2]

[1] *Department of Geology, Faculty of Science, University of Peradeniya, Peradeniya, Sri Lanka*
[2] *GeoZentrum Nordbayern, Friedrich-Alexander University Erlangen-Nürnberg (FAU), Erlangen, Germany*

7.1 Introduction

In recent years, the need for multidisciplinary approaches to solve more complex problems related to human, animal, and environmental health at local, regional, and global levels has been well recognized. With these approaches, the concept of "One Health" was introduced to tackle more complex health issues in which expert knowledge of different disciplines such as physicians, veterinarians, environmentalists, anthropologists, economists, and sociologists, among many others, is involved (Gibbs 2014; Lebov et al. 2017). "One Health" is a holistic approach that recognizes the importance of investigating the interactions between the environment and the health of humans and animals. Although One Health (OH) is not a new concept, it has become widely discussed in the recent past. These discussions address an ever-changing system due to the unconditional interactions between people, animals, plants, agriculture, and our living environment.

One Health approaches are complex due to many interactions between different disciplines, and they must be seen as a multidisciplinary subject. For instance, in human health-related investigations physicians, nurses, public health practitioners, and epidemiologists are required, while in animal health and agro-environment studies, veterinarians and agricultural experts need to become involved. In order to solve problems in the OH approach, collaborating and coordinating activities among all disciplines are necessary, and no individual persons, organizations, or sectors can address issues related to the interface of animal-human-environment health. In other words, OH is the incorporation of elements from all three domains – that is human, animal and environmental health (Figure 7.1).

Humans and animals can be considered an integral part of our natural environment and part of the large geochemical cycles (Dissanayake and Chandrajith 2009). Although geoscience seems far from health, rocks and minerals are the fundamental building blocks of the earth and supply important chemical elements to the natural environment. Therefore, earth materials serve as the preliminary sources of major and trace elements that are essential for the survival of organisms but, in excessive amounts, may also become harmful. Living organisms obtain the chemical elements that are required for their physiological functions directly or indirectly from the surrounding environment, mainly through the soil, water, or air (Dissanayake 2005). Geosciences can therefore be involved in investigating the distribution of elements in different geological and environmental materials, their mobilities, and behaviors such as speciations that are necessary to explain specific health issues.

Geoscientific disciplines that study chemical constituents of geological material and their relationships with human, animal, and plant health are now termed "Medical Geology." They have become an emerging branch of geosciences (Dissanayake and Chandrajith 1999; Finkelman et al. 2018, 2001; Selinus 2002). Geoscientists can understand and investigate irregularities and regional distributions of elements that influence animal and ecosystem health. In many cases, they are related to water. In addition, emissions from volcanic eruptions, effects of dust, natural radioactivity, and organic contaminants in water and soil can act as contributors to the concept of medical geology. Therefore, medical geology pertains to OH principles with its interdisciplinary approaches that involve different professionals and experts. In this chapter, the

One Health: Human, Animal, and Environment Triad, First Edition. Edited by Meththika Vithanage and Majeti Narasimha Vara Prasad.

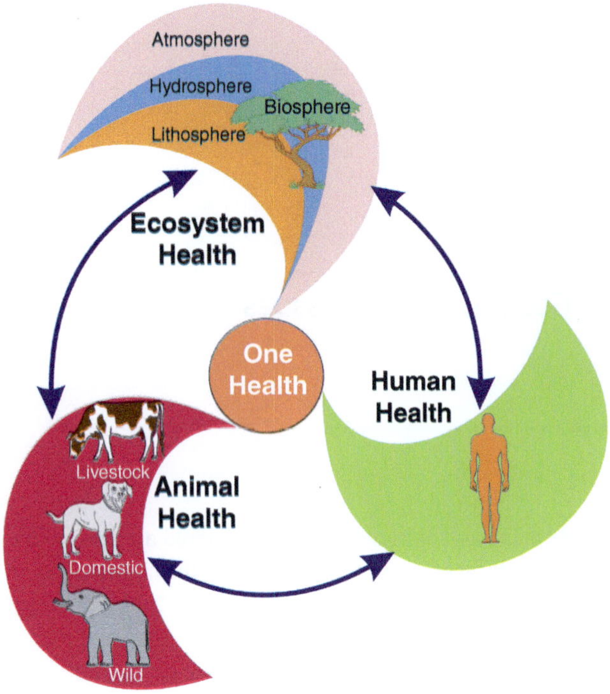

Figure 7.1 Environmental interactions, including the geosphere, with the health issues for humans and animals.

importance of geology on the health of humans and animals will be discussed with a few important examples.

7.2 Medical Geology – Historical Perspective

As mentioned earlier, OH is not a new concept. Hippocrates (460–370 BCE), who is considered the father of modern medicine, wrote that "*If you want to learn about the health of a population, look at the air they breathe, the water they drink, and the places where they live.*" This clearly indicates the importance of the natural environment on health. Hippocrates also noted that geothermal water coming through toxic metal-containing soils was unsuitable for drinking (Orem et al. 2019). A Swiss toxicologist Paracelsus (1493–1541) expressed that "*All substances are poisons; there is none which is not a poison, only the dose differentiates a poison and a remedy.*" These two approaches can be considered as the most important early concepts of OH. It is also well-known that in the ancient medical systems of Ayurveda and Chinese traditional medicine, mineral-based treatment systems were widely used for healing many ailments (Chen et al. 2020; Prajapati et al. 2006). For instance, mica-based preparations are used in treating skin disorders and respiratory problems in traditional and alternative medical systems in South Asian countries (Wijenayake

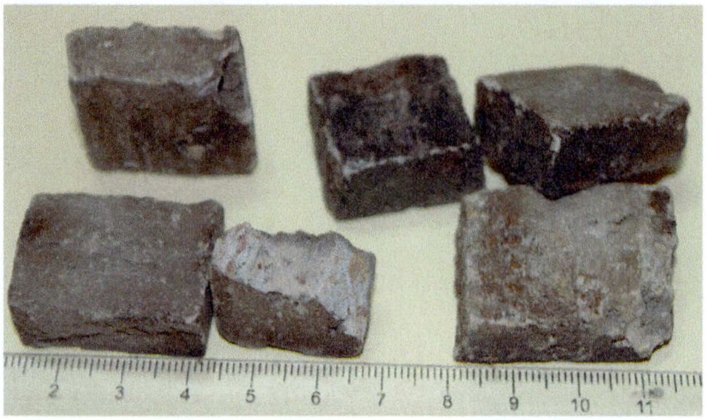

Figure 7.2 Sikor tablets (baked clay biscuit) which are commonly consumed by rural Bangladesh pregnant women. Eating earthy materials is common among rural and tribal communities in Asia, Africa, and Latin America.

et al. 2022). In addition, the habit of biting earth materials (geophagy) such as clay, soil, or minerals is common among animals as well as in rural communities in Asia, Africa, and Latin America (Dissanayake and Chandrajith 2009; Woywodt and Kiss 2002) (Figure 7.2). Also, Alexander von Humboldt (1769–1859), the great German philosopher, during one of his expeditions in the Orinoco in Venezuela (1799–1804), noticed that the Ottomac people deliberately consumed earthy materials without suffering from any illness as a result (Wilson 2003).

In the twentieth century, with the development of more reliable analytical instruments, wider attention was given to the study of the geochemistry of environmental materials including water, soil, rocks, and plants. Such studies contributed to the investigation of the geographic distributions of health issues that are related to geological environments. Terms such as Geomedicine, Medical Geochemistry, and Medical Geology are used to describe these studies. In general, medical geology is the term that is now most widely accepted. It can best be described as the science dealing with the chemistry of the elements in geological materials in relation to health in humans and animals (Davies et al. 2013). In 1996, the International Union of Geological Sciences (IUGS) under the purview of the United Nations Educational, Scientific, and Cultural Organization (UNESCO) approved "Medical Geology" as a subdiscipline of geology (Selinus et al. 2005).

7.3 Pathways of Elements in the Geoenvironment

Elements of geological origin can have a profound impact on health and the geographic distributions of diseases, such as fluorosis or skin cancer, that occur due to the intake of excess fluoride and arsenic, respectively (Dissanayake 2005).

Medical Geology attempts to understand the bioavailability, pathways, speciation, and toxicities of elements. Factors such as genetics, lifestyle, sex, age, and food habits also need to be taken into account as they interconnect with deficiencies, excesses, or imbalances of inorganic elements that could markedly influence the health of a population. The field of medical geology has become more popular since the beginning of the twenty-first century with parallel investigations of the spatial distribution of health problems that may associate with geogenic processes. Medical geology is an interdisciplinary field of science and geoscientists need to work with chemists, physicians, epidemiologists, and other allied health professionals to investigate geographic distributions of health issues caused by exposure to elements through geogenic and anthropogenic pathways (Bundschuh et al. 2017; Finkelman et al. 2018).

Most elements enter the human body from the air, via food, and via water (Figure 7.3). Geoscientists try to understand and investigate irregularities in regional distributions of elements and relate them to their geological and geochemical characteristics. They also provide an understanding of the influence on human, animal, and ecosystem health due to excess or deficiency of elements in the geoenvironment. Rocks and minerals are the preliminary geological materials that are broken down by weathering processes, forming soils on which crops and animals are raised. Therefore, the composition of rocks largely determines the availability of elements in the living environment.

From a medical geology perspective, elements can be classified as essential and toxic. Essential elements that are important for the physiological functions of an organism can further be subdivided as major (O, C, H, N), minor (Ca, Mg, Na, Cl, K, P, S), and trace (e.g. Fe, F, Se, Mo, I, Co) elements. Elements such as As, Cd, Pb, Hg are not involved in any known metabolic activities in organisms or have no recognized biological role and are therefore considered toxic elements or nonessential elements (Selinus 2004). Even the deficiency or excess intake of minor and essential trace elements may pose health implications in organisms (Figure 7.4).

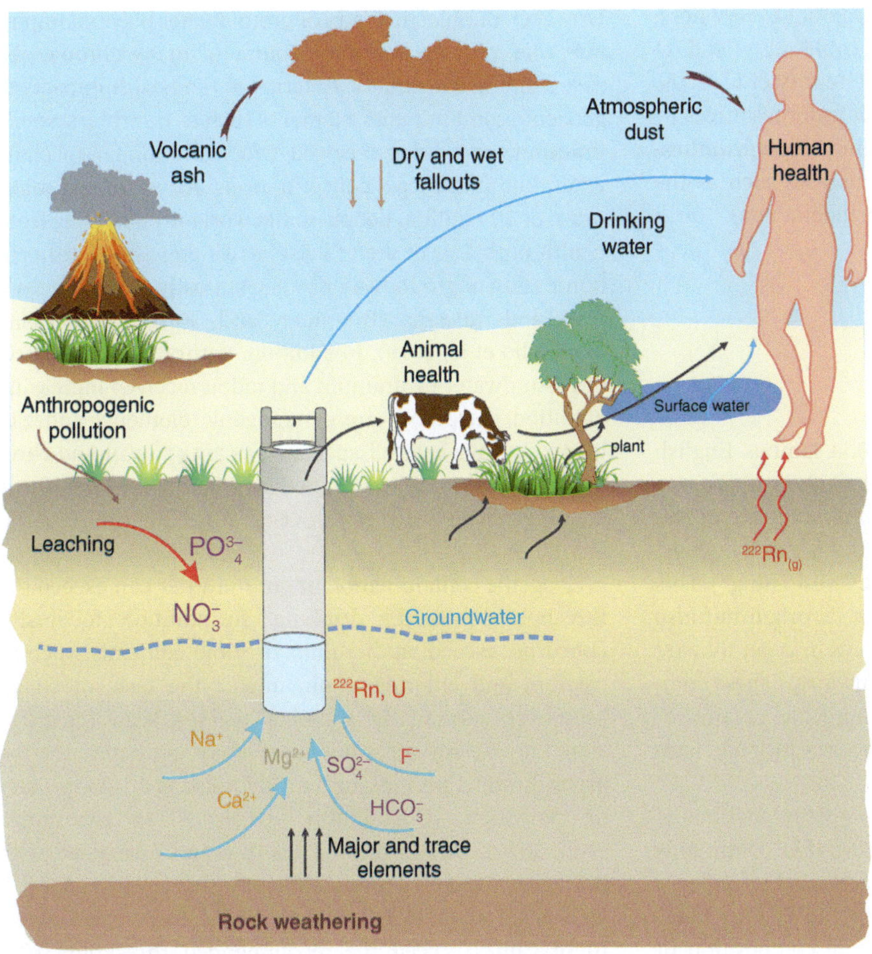

Figure 7.3 Integration of animals and humans in the geogenic environment.

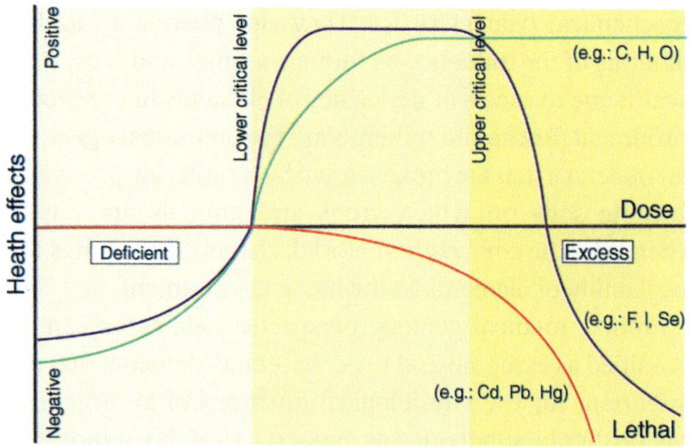

Figure 7.4 Dose–response curve indicating the relationship between the dose and health effects of major essential (green line), minor essential (blue line), and nonessential (red line) elements.

Among many geoenvironment-related health issues, excess fluoride in drinking water and dental and skeletal fluorosis, arsenic in drinking water and food and incidences of cancer are among the best-known relationships. Although low levels of radiation originating from the terrestrial environment are usually common everywhere, high natural background radiation could also lead to chronic health issues for inhabitants (Hendry et al. 2009; Nugraha et al. 2021). Contamination of water resources by nitrogenous compounds that occur mainly through anthropogenic activities can cause serious diseases such as the blue baby syndrome (or methemoglobinemia), birth defects, and cancer (Brender 2020).

7.4 The Hydrologic Cycle and One Health

David Herbert Lawrence (1885–1930), a famous English writer and poet, wrote that "*Water is H_2O, hydrogen two parts, oxygen one, but there is also a third thing, that makes it water and nobody knows what it is and where it is from*" (D.H. Lawrence; "Birds, Beasts and the Third Thing"). This statement indicates the uncertainty of its origin but also the importance of additional components in water that are usually dissolved or occur in particulate form. These components may be naturally dissolving inorganic, organic, or biological contaminants from tiny bacteria to long-chain organic molecules.

The hydrologic cycle describes the perpetual motions of water in the terrestrial system. During this continuous movement of water in the terrestrial system, chemical and microbiological compositions of water can change naturally or by anthropogenic activities. The composition of groundwater is also modified due to interactions with soil and aquifer material during the infiltration. The long resident time in aquifers usually increases dissolved ionic constituents in groundwater (Appelo and Postma 2004). However, evapotranspiration translates water back into its pure form and leaves behind dissolved components. In some cases, this increases the contaminant concentrations even further in the residual water. Apart from natural contamination, water quality can be changed chemically or microbiologically through various anthropogenic activities such as mining, ore smelting, agriculture-related activities, and other industrial and domestic activities, contributing organic and inorganic contaminants to water. Water becomes a potential source of diseases and death when contamination exceeds its natural purification ability. In addition, water can also provide a breeding ground for disease-causing vectors. Water insect-borne diseases such as malaria and dengue fever kill millions of lives every year (Boutayeb 2006). Biologically contaminated water also transmits diseases such as cholera, diarrhea typhoid, amebiasis, and hepatitis through pathogens.

The majority of the world's population depends on groundwater as the main accessible reservoir of freshwater. However, the geochemistry of groundwater plays an important role and can become a source of many chronic diseases among consumers. In terms of the health impacts of geogenic contaminants, elements such as fluoride, arsenic, uranium, and radon received wider attention, especially when found in excess concentrations. An estimated minimum of 300 million people in the world are suffering from health problems or are at least at risk due to natural contamination of groundwater by geogenically occurring fluoride and arsenic (Brammer and Ravenscroft 2009; Kimambo et al. 2019). In addition, natural contamination of groundwater by uranium and radon received increasing attention since both are carcinogenic elements and can lead to various health issues such as lung cancer and chromosomal aberrations in blood lymphocytes (Bersimbaev and Bulgakova 2015; Nayak et al. 2022; Rani et al. 2021; Stalder et al. 2012).

Geogenic contamination of groundwater can exceed the threshold limits for drinking. In addition to health concerns, exceeding the limits of some elements, such as calcium and chloride, could impact the taste of water. Moreover, particularly in coastal regions, seawater intrusion into freshwater aquifers severely contaminates the groundwater, thus making it unfit for use as drinking water or irrigation (Chandrajith et al. 2014; Jayathunga et al. 2020). Due to serious health issues associated with drinking water contaminations, the World Health Organization (WHO) set guideline values especially if these values exceed the recommended thresholds after water treatment (WHO 2011).

7.5 Geology and Health – Some Examples

The interrelationship between the health of a population and the geogenic environment is considered here in tropical terrains where weathering rates are usually intense and many inhabitants interact with the immediate surrounding environment via farming and direct drinking water supply (Dissanayake and Chandrajith 1999). Among many chronic diseases, the link between fluoride and arsenic in drinking water and human health is well established in medical geology.

7.5.1 Fluoride

Fluorine is a common element in the geogenic environment and is ranked as the 13th abundant constituent in the earth's crust (Edmunds and Smedley 2013). Due to its high reactivity, fluorine is found in water, soil, air, and plants mostly in its ionic form. Fluoride is considered an essential minor element for dental health, while excessive intake causes detrimental effects such as dental and skeletal fluorosis (Figure 7.5) (Chandrajith et al. 2020; Dissanayake 2005). These diseases are common in populations that preliminary depend on groundwater as their source of drinking water. In addition, drinking brick tea and inhaling coal smoke are other key sources of fluoride intake in humans (Choubisa and Choubisa 2016; Liu et al. 2007; Zhang and Cao 1996). As recommended by the WHO, fluoride is an essential constituent for dental health; however, higher concentrations than 1.5 mg/l in drinking water are suspected to cause detrimental effects on teeth. People who consume fluoride concentrations over 4.0 mg/l may suffer from skeletal or crippling fluorosis (WHO 2011).

Besides, health impacts on Ca-phosphate-based hard tissues, negative impacts of fluoride were also reported on soft tissues of the body such as the liver, kidney, heart, lungs, brain, and nervous and reproductive systems (Balasooriya et al. 2019; Dissanayake and Chandrajith 2019; Gulegoda et al. 2022; Nakamoto and Rawls 2018; Ozsvath 2009; Zhu et al. 2007). It is also noted that fluoride together with calcium can accumulate in the pineal gland in the brain, which produces the hormone melatonin. Subsequent calcification of the gland may result in melatonin deficiency (Chlubek and Sikora 2020). Several early studies also reported that regular consumption of high fluoride water may lower the Intelligence Quotient (IQ) levels among children (Kundu et al. 2015; Xiang et al. 2003). In addition, excessive intake of fluoride can lead to other chronic diseases including neurological complications (Choubisa 2014) and chronic kidney disease (Balasooriya et al. 2019; Liyanage et al. 2022).

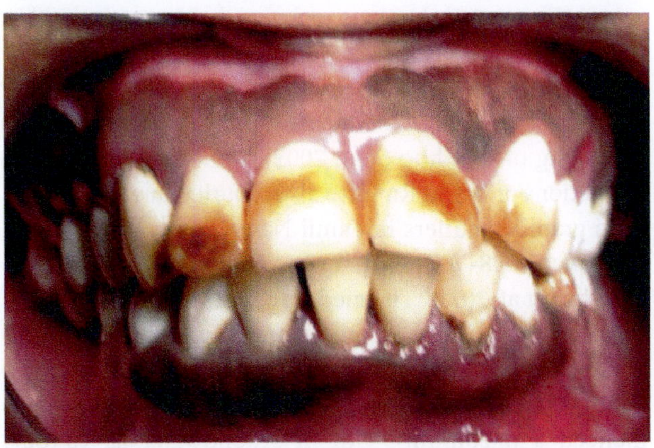

Figure 7.5 A typical case of dental fluorosis in Sri Lanka, caused by regular consumption of high-fluoride groundwater.

In addition, plants grown on fluoride-rich soils or crops irrigated with fluoride-rich groundwater can suffer from impaired growth parameters (Banerjee and Roychoudhury 2019). On the other hand, some plants, such as tea (*Camellia sinensis*), can accumulate fluoride and then release it into the infusion, thus leading to further fluoride intake in addition to regular consumption of fluoride-rich drinking water (Chandrajith et al. 2007, 2022). Rice (*Oryza sativa* L.) also showed higher fluoride accumulation when irrigated with fluoride-contaminated water (Mondal 2017). Excessive intake of fluoride, either through feed or water, can be harmful to animals. Among animals, fluoride toxicities were noted mainly among cattle and buffaloes. Chronic fluoride intoxications including dental and skeletal fluorosis were noted in bovine calves due to excessive ingestion through drinking water or feeding grasses that grown on soils contaminated with fluoride (Choubisa 2021).

Although contamination of environmental media by fluoride is primarily geogenic, anthropogenic activities also make a considerable contribution. In addition to weathering and consequent leaching from fluoride-bearing minerals, volcanic eruptions are another geogenic source of fluoride. Coal-burning, fertilizer application, glass, ceramic, steel manufacturing industries and phosphate ore processing are considered anthropogenic sources of fluoride (Brindha and Elango 2011; Prasad and Mondal 2007; Vithanage and Bhattacharya 2015).

Note that due to the importance of dental health, fluoride is added to drinking water supplies as well as toothpaste and salts (Marthaler 2013; Mullane et al. 2016). Despite these actions, the essentiality and toxicity of fluoride in drinking water are much debated in the scientific community. For many tropical countries, the WHO guideline limit (1.5 mg/l) is not applicable since health manifestations of fluoride also can be observed even at much lower levels than the recommended limits (Chandrajith et al. 2020).

7.5.2 Arsenic

One of the most interesting medical geological problems that required an OH approach is arsenic poisoning due to the consumption of naturally contaminated water. During the last few decades, a large number of studies were carried out by various disciplines to investigate the As contamination-related health issues. Millions of people in Bangladesh and West Bengal and communities in other countries such as Vietnam, Taiwan, China, Mexico, Chile, Nepal, Myanmar, Cambodia, and Argentina suffer from As-related health issues due to the consumption of As-rich natural water (Fendorf et al. 2010; Herath et al. 2016; Smedley and Kinniburgh 2002).

The prevalence of skin disorders, cancer, and cardiovascular diseases, among many others, is caused mainly by the ingestion of As via drinking water and also by food grown in arsenic-rich soils. It was also reported that contaminated groundwater was used extensively in Bangladesh for rice cultivation and thus caused higher accumulations of arsenic, possibly causing additional health impacts on consumers (Bhattacharya et al. 2010; Meharg and Rahman 2003). Due to the magnitude of the problem, particularly in Bangladesh, the WHO lowered the provisional guideline value for arsenic in drinking water from 50 to 10 μg/l (Smedley 2005). In most cases, the occurrence of As in the environment is geogenic. In particular, groundwater extracted from sedimentary aquifers that are rich with organic matter and metal oxy-hydroxides can contain high levels of As (Mukherjee and Bhattacharya 2001). For instance, groundwater extracted from Quaternary and alluvial deltaic sediments in the Bengal Basin of Bangladesh and West Bengal is typical for having high As contents (Mahanta et al. 2015). In addition, As also showed bioaccumulation in wild animals, particularly birds. Arsenic can cause biochemical impacts including oxidative stresses, detrimental effects on reproductive systems, and behavioral changes in birds (Sánchez-Virosta et al. 2015).

7.5.3 Uranium and Radon

Natural radiation is common in geogenic environments with about 60 naturally occurring radionuclides in the air, water, soil, rocks, minerals, and food (Dissanayake and Chandrajith 2009). Natural background radiation is usually the largest human exposure with an average annual effective dose per capita of 2.4 mSv (UNSCEAR 2011). Radionuclides, such as ^{238}U, ^{232}Th, and ^{40}K, are the most important radionuclides present in geological materials in detectable quantities (Chandrajith et al. 2010). Besides that, anomalously high background radiations are also noted in some areas such as Ramsar (Iran), Guarapari (Brazil), Yangjiang (China), and Kerala (India), where the geology and geochemistry of the source rocks and minerals play a major role in providing high natural radiation (UNSCEAR 2011).

Among the known radionuclides, uranium (U) and radon (Rn) are naturally occurring radiogenic elements that can pose both chemical and radiological toxicity. Radon (^{222}Rn) is a short-lived radiogenic daughter nuclide of the ^{238}U decay series and can cause health risks. In addition, particularly groundwater may contain elevated contents of Rn. Since Rn is a gaseous element, it can be released into the indoor atmosphere when using groundwater for domestic purposes (Adithya et al. 2021). Drinking water with excessively high levels of ^{222}Rn may cause a risk of cancer mostly in the gastrointestinal system, while continuous inhalation may pose elevated risks of cancer in the respiratory system (Kendall et al. 2016; Moon and Yoo 2021; Zhuo et al. 2001).

Uranium naturally occurs in some groundwater systems, and its concentration is mostly controlled by the geology of the aquifer. Regular human consumption of groundwater contaminated with uranium causes health effects, and hence the assessment of radiological and chemical toxicity on humans is essential (Ramesh et al. 2021). Uranium loadings also could be made worse through foodstuffs. Here, approximate daily intakes of U through food between 1 and 2 μg and of 1.5 μg through drinking water have been considered safe (Keith et al. 2013). Any excess intake could cause damage to the kidneys and DNA, as well as bone degeneration and reproductive disorder, brain and nerve disorders, and cancer (Brugge et al. 2005; Daniel et al. 2022).

As in the case of fluoride and arsenic, both uranium and radon can also occur above their threshold concentrations in water resources depending on the geological conditions and mineralogy of aquifers. Heavy minerals such as zircon, monazite, baddeleyite, allanite and apatite are examples of minerals that contain higher amounts of radioactive elements (Figure 7.6). Igneous rocks, such as granite, contain these minerals in reasonable quantities and groundwater obtained from granitic aquifers for instance in Fujian, China, contains high Rn levels up to 147.8 kBq/m^3 and 0.54 μg/kg of U (Zhuo et al. 2001). Abnormally high concentrations of U and Rn were also reported in groundwater from granitic aquifers in Tamil Nadu, South India, which contained 258–7072 Bq/m^3 Rn and 0.28–84.65 μg/l U (Adithya et al. 2021). The median concentrations of 1.8 μg/l and 78 Bq/l of U and Rn, respectively, were also found in groundwater obtained from granitic aquifers in Changwon, South Korea (Hwang and Kim 2021). The WHO recommended a maximum ^{222}Rn in groundwater as 100 Bq/l (WHO 2011), while UNSCEAR suggested a range of 4–40 Bq/l (UNSCER 2011).

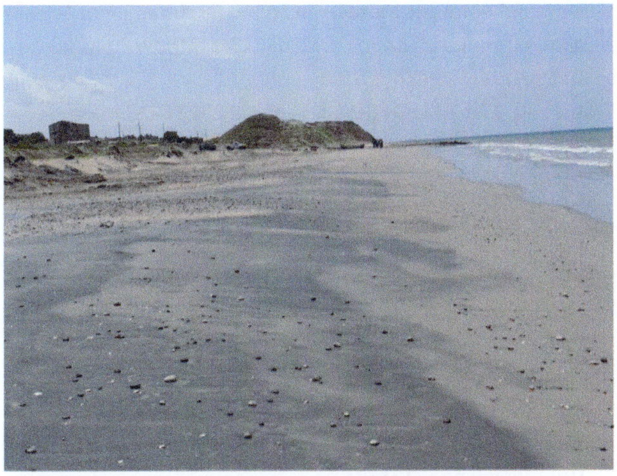

Figure 7.6 A beach rich with heavy minerals: Some of the heavy minerals can produce high background radiation, causing health effects, as in the case of Kerala Beach in India.

7.6 Conclusions

The health problems caused by geochemical anomalies are preliminary local or regional issues. Geoscientists can identify anomalies in major and trace elements in the natural environment. In this case, geochemical mapping is an important part that provides invaluable information on anomalies of elements or their species in the geogenic environment. Groundwater, soil, rock, or stream sediments can be used as media to demarcate elevated levels of toxic elements or depletion of essential elements in geological terrains. These anomalies can easily help identify local or regional distributions of health issues. In addition, as a contribution to the concept of OH, providing baseline geochemical data becomes an increasingly demanded tool in epidemiology and medical geology. With the help of geographic information systems (GIS) integrated with statistical analyses, vulnerable areas for chronic diseases can much better be outlined in recent decades (Dissanayake and Chandrajith 2009). In the framework of One Health, related professionals such as epidemiologists, veterinarians, and agriculturists then can identify possible influences of geochemical anomalies on human, animal, agricultural, or environmental health. However, collaboration across different disciplines needs to further develop within the One Health concept to assure the health and well-being of humans and animals.

References

Adithya, V.S.P., Chidambaram, S., Prasanna, M.V. et al. (2021). Health risk implication and spatial distribution of radon in groundwater along the lithological contact in South India. *Archives of Environmental Contamination and Toxicology* 80: 308–318. https://doi.org/10.1007/s00244-020-00798-9.

Appelo, C.A.J. and Postma, D. (2004). *Geochemistry, Groundwater and Pollution*. CRC Press.

Balasooriya, S., Munasinghe, H., Herath, A.T. et al. (2019). Possible links between groundwater geochemistry and chronic kidney disease of unknown etiology (CKDu): an investigation from the Ginnoruwa region in Sri Lanka. *Exposure and Health* https://doi.org/10.1007/s12403-019-00340-w.

Banerjee, A. and Roychoudhury, A. (2019). Fluorine: a biohazardous agent for plants and phytoremediation strategies for its removal from the environment. *Biologia Plantarum* 63: 104–112. https://doi.org/10.32615/bp.2019.013.

Bersimbaev, R.I. and Bulgakova, O. (2015). The health effects of radon and uranium on the population of Kazakhstan. *Genes and Environment* 37: 18. https://doi.org/10.1186/s41021-015-0019-3.

Bhattacharya, P., Samal, A.C., Majumdar, J., and Santra, S.C. (2010). Arsenic contamination in Rice, wheat, pulses, and vegetables: a study in an arsenic affected area of West Bengal, India. *Water, Air, & Soil Pollution* 213: 3–13. https://doi.org/10.1007/s11270-010-0361-9.

Boutayeb, A. (2006). The double burden of communicable and non-communicable diseases in developing countries. *Transactions of the Royal Society of Tropical Medicine and Hygiene* 100: 191–199. https://doi.org/10.1016/j.trstmh.2005.07.021.

Brammer, H. and Ravenscroft, P. (2009). Arsenic in groundwater: a threat to sustainable agriculture in South and South-East Asia. *Environment International* 35: 647–654. https://doi.org/10.1016/j.envint.2008.10.004.

Brender, J.D. (2020). Human health effects of exposure to nitrate, nitrite, and nitrogen dioxide. In: *Just Enough Nitrogen: Perspectives on How to Get There for Regions with Too Much and Too Little Nitrogen* (ed. M.A. Sutton, K.E. Mason, A. Bleeker, et al.), 283–294. Cham: Springer International Publishing.

Brindha, K. and Elango, L. (2011). Fluoride in groundwater: causes, implications and mitigation measures. In: *Fluoride Properties, Applications and Environmental Management* (ed. S.D. Monroy), 111–136. New York: Nova Science Publisher.

Brugge, D., DeLemos, J.L., and Oldmixon, B. (2005). Exposure pathways and health effects associated with chemical and radiological toxicity of natural uranium: a review. *Reviews on Environmental Health* 20: 177–194. https://doi.org/10.1515/REVEH.2005.20.3.177.

Bundschuh, J., Maity, J.P., Mushtaq, S. et al. (2017). Medical geology in the framework of the sustainable development goals. *Science of the Total Environment* 581–582: 87–104. https://doi.org/10.1016/j.scitotenv.2016.11.208.

Chandrajith, R., Abeypala, U., Dissanayake, C.B., and Tobschall, H.J. (2007). Fluoride in Ceylon tea and its implications to dental health. *Environmental Geochemistry and Health* 29: 429–434. https://doi.org/10.1007/s10653-007-9087-z.

Chandrajith, R., Seneviratna, S., Wickramaarachchi, K. et al. (2010). Natural radionuclides and trace elements in rice field soils in relation to fertilizer application: study of a chronic kidney disease area in Sri Lanka. *Environmental Earth Sciences* 60: 193–201. https://doi.org/10.1007/s12665-009-0179-1.

Chandrajith, R., Chaturangani, D., Abeykoon, S. et al. (2014). Quantification of groundwater–seawater interaction in a coastal sandy aquifer system: a study from Panama, Sri Lanka. *Environmental Earth Sciences* 72: 867–877. https://doi.org/10.1007/s12665-013-3010-y.

Chandrajith, R., Diyabalanage, S., and Dissanayake, C.B. (2020). Geogenic fluoride and arsenic in groundwater of Sri Lanka and its implications to community health. *Groundwater for Sustainable Development* 10: 100359. https://doi.org/10.1016/j.gsd.2020.100359.

Chandrajith, R., Bhagya, S., Diyabalanage, S. et al. (2022). Exposure sssessment of fluoride intake through commercially available black tea (*Camellia sinensis* L.) from areas with high incidences of chronic kidney disease with undetermined origin (CKDu) in Sri Lanka. *Biological Trace Element Research* 200: 526–534. https://doi.org/10.1007/s12011-021-02694-2.

Chen, X.-J., Jia, L.-Q., Hao, Z.-G., and Jia, T. (2020). The introduction of traditional Chinese mineral medicine. *China Geology* 2: 355–356. https://doi.org/10.31035/cg2020044.

Chlubek, D. and Sikora, M. (2020). Fluoride and pineal gland. *Applied Sciences* 10: 2885. https://doi.org/10.3390/app10082885.

Choubisa, S.L. (2014). Bovine calves as ideal bio-indicators for fluoridated drinking water and endemic osteo-dental fluorosis. *Environmental Monitoring and Assessment* 186: 4493–4498. https://doi.org/10.1007/s10661-014-3713-x.

Choubisa, S. (2021). Chronic fluoride exposure and its diverse adverse health effects in bovine calves in India: an epitomised review. *Global Journal of Biology, Agriculture and Health Sciences* 10: 1–6.

Choubisa, S.L. and Choubisa, D. (2016). Status of industrial fluoride pollution and its diverse adverse health effects in man and domestic animals in India. *Environmental Science and Pollution Research* 23: 7244–7254. https://doi.org/10.1007/s11356-016-6319-8.

Daniel, R., Tripathi, D., Singh, S. et al. (2022). Uranium: occurrence, distribution across India and its potential health effects. *Journal of Radioanalytical and Nuclear Chemistry* 331: 2805–2815. https://doi.org/10.1007/s10967-022-08373-3.

Davies, B.E., Bowman, C., Davies, T.C., and Selinus, O. (2013). Medical geology: perspectives and prospects. In: *Essentials of Medical Geology*: Revised Edition (ed. O. Selinus), 1–13. Dordrecht: Springer.

Dissanayake, C. (2005). Of stones and health: medical geology in Sri Lanka. *Science* 309: 883–885. https://doi.org/10.1126/science.1115174.

Dissanayake, C.B. and Chandrajith, R. (1999). Medical geochemistry of tropical environments. *Earth-Science Reviews* 47: 219–258. https://doi.org/10.1016/S0012-8252(99)00033-1.

Dissanayake, C.B. and Chandrajith, R. (2009). *Introduction to Medical Geology: Focus on Tropical Environment.* Heidelberg: Springer Science & business media.

Dissanayake, C.B. and Chandrajith, R. (2019). Fluoride and hardness in groundwater of tropical regions-review of recent evidence indicating tissue calcification and calcium phosphate nanoparticle formation in kidney tubules. *Ceylon Journal of Science* 48: 197–207. https://doi.org/10.4038/cjs.v48i3.7643.

Edmunds, W.M. and Smedley, P.L. (2013). Fluoride in natural waters. In: *Essentials of Medical Geology* (ed. O. Selinus), 311–336. Springer.

Fendorf, S., Michael, H.A., and Geen, A.V. (2010). Spatial and temporal variations of groundwater arsenic in South and Southeast Asia. *Science* 328: 1123–1127. https://doi.org/10.1126/science.1172974.

Finkelman, R.B., Skinner, H.C.H., Plumlee, G.S., and Bunnell, J.E. (2001). Medical geology. *Geotimes* 46: 20–23.

Finkelman, R.B., Orem, W.H., Plumlee, G.S., and Selinus, O. (2018). Applications of geochemistry to medical geology. In: *Environmental Geochemistry*, 2ee (ed. B. De Vivo, H.E. Belkin and A. Lima), 435–465. Elsevier. 10.1016/B978-0-444-63763-5.00018-5.

Gibbs, E.P.J. (2014). The evolution of one health: a decade of progress and challenges for the future. *Veterinary Record* 174: 85–91. https://doi.org/10.1136/vr.g143.

Gulegoda, C.R., Dissanayake, C.B., Amarasekara, D.S. et al. (2022). Impact of fluoride exposure on male reproductive parameters: a pilot case-control study in Sri Lanka. *Exposure and Health* https://doi.org/10.1007/s12403-022-00465-5.

Hendry, J.H., Simon, S.L., Wojcik, A. et al. (2009). Human exposure to high natural background radiation: what can it teach us about radiation risks? *Journal of Radiological Protection* 29: A29–A42. https://doi.org/10.1088/0952-4746/29/2a/s03.

Herath, I., Vithanage, M., Bundschuh, J. et al. (2016). Natural arsenic in global groundwaters: distribution and geochemical triggers for mobilization. *Current Pollution Reports* 2: 68–89. https://doi.org/10.1007/s40726-016-0028-2.

Hwang, J. and Kim, S.W. (2021). Occurrence of uranopolycrase in pegmatite related to a Jurassic granite pluton in Cheongwon, South Korea: mineral chemistry and texture of a potential source of uranium and radon in a granite aquifer. *Environmental Earth Sciences* 80: 473. https://doi.org/10.1007/s12665-021-09766-5.

Jayathunga, K., Diyabalanage, S., Frank, A.H. et al. (2020). Influences of seawater intrusion and anthropogenic activities on shallow coastal aquifers in Sri Lanka: evidence from hydrogeochemical and stable isotope data. *Environmental Science and Pollution Research* 27: 23002–23014. https://doi.org/10.1007/s11356-020-08759-4.

Keith, S., Faroon, O., Roney, N. et al. (2013). *Toxicological Profile for Uranium*. Atlanta, GA: Agency for Toxic Substances and Disease Registry (US).

Kendall, G.M., Miles, J.C.H., Rees, D. et al. (2016). Variation with socioeconomic status of indoor radon levels in Great Britain: the less affluent have less radon. *Journal of Environmental Radioactivity* 164: 84–90. https://doi.org/10.1016/j.jenvrad.2016.07.001.

Kimambo, V., Bhattacharya, P., Mtalo, F. et al. (2019). Fluoride occurrence in groundwater systems at global scale and status of defluoridation – state of the art. *Groundwater for Sustainable Development* 9: 100223. https://doi.org/10.1016/j.gsd.2019.100223.

Kundu, H., Basavaraj, P., Singla, A. et al. (2015). Effect of fluoride in drinking water on children's intelligence in high and low fluoride areas of Delhi. *Journal of Indian Association of Public Health Dentistry* 13: 116–121. https://doi.org/10.4103/2319-5932.159043.

Lebov, J., Grieger, K., Womack, D. et al. (2017). A framework for one health research. *One Health* 3: 44–50. https://doi.org/10.1016/j.onehlt.2017.03.004.

Liu, G., Zheng, L., Qi, C., and Zhang, Y. (2007). Environmental geochemistry and health of fluorine in Chinese coals. *Environmental Geology* 52: 1307–1313. https://doi.org/10.1007/s00254-006-0569-6.

Liyanage, D.N.D., Diyabalanage, S., Dunuweera, S.P. et al. (2022). Significance of Mg-hardness and fluoride in drinking water on chronic kidney disease of unknown etiology in Monaragala, Sri Lanka. *Environmental Research* 203: 111779. https://doi.org/10.1016/j.envres.2021.111779.

Mahanta, C., Enmark, G., Nordborg, D. et al. (2015). Hydrogeochemical controls on mobilization of arsenic in groundwater of a part of Brahmaputra river floodplain, India. *Journal of Hydrology: Regional Studies* 4: 154–171. https://doi.org/10.1016/j.ejrh.2015.03.002.

Marthaler, T.M. (2013). Salt fluoridation and oral health. *Acta Medica Academica* 42: 140–155. https://doi.org/10.5644/ama2006-124.82.

Mondal, N.K. (2017). Effect of fluoride on photosynthesis, growth and accumulation of four widely cultivated rice (*Oryza sativa* L.) varieties in India. *Ecotoxicology and Environmental Safety* 144: 36–44. https://doi.org/10.1016/j.ecoenv.2017.06.009.

Moon, J. and Yoo, H. (2021). Residential radon exposure and leukemia: a meta-analysis and dose-response meta-analyses for ecological, case-control, and cohort studies. *Environmental Research* 202: 111714. https://doi.org/10.1016/j.envres.2021.111714.

Mukherjee, A.B. and Bhattacharya, P. (2001). Arsenic in groundwater in the Bengal Delta plain: slow poisoning in Bangladesh. *Environmental Reviews* 9: 189–220. https://doi.org/10.1139/er-9-3-189.

Mullane, D.M.O., Baez, R.J., Jones, S. et al. (2016). Fluoride and oral health. *Community Dental Health* 33 (2): 69–99. https://doi.org/10.1922/CDH_3707O'Mullane31.

Meharg, A.A. and Rahman, M.M. (2003). Arsenic contamination of Bangladesh Paddy field soils: implications for rice contribution to arsenic consumption. *Environmental Science & Technology* 37: 229–234. https://doi.org/10.1021/es0259842.

Nakamoto, T. and Rawls, H.R. (2018). Fluoride exposure in early life as the possible root cause of disease in later life. *Journal of Clinical Pediatric Dentistry* 42: 325–330. https://doi.org/10.17796/1053-4625-42.5.1.

Nayak, T., Basak, S., Deb, A., and Dhal, P.K. (2022). A systematic review on groundwater radon distribution with human health consequences and probable mitigation strategy. *Journal of Environmental Radioactivity* 247: 106852. https://doi.org/10.1016/j.jenvrad.2022.106852.

Nugraha, E.D., Hosoda, M., Kusdiana, U. et al. (2021). Comprehensive exposure assessments from the viewpoint of health in a unique high natural background radiation area, Mamuju, Indonesia. *Scientific Reports* 11: 14578. https://doi.org/10.1038/s41598-021-93983-2.

Orem, W.H., Bunnell, J.E., Tatu, C.A., and Pavlovic, N.M. (2019). Toxicological pathways of relevance to medical geology. In: *Encyclopedia of Environmental Health*, 2e (ed. J. Nriagu), 88–98. The Netherlands: Elsevier Science.

Ozsvath, D.L. (2009). Fluoride and environmental health: a review. *Reviews in Environmental Science and Bio/Technology* 8: 59–79. https://doi.org/10.1007/s11157-008-9136-9.

Prajapati, P., Sarkar, P.K., Nayak, S.V. et al. (2006). Safety and toxicity profile of some metallic preparations of ayurveda. *Ancient Science of Life* 25: 57.

Prasad, B. and Mondal, K. (2007). Leaching characteristics of fluoride from coal ash. *Asian Journal of Water, Environment and Pollution* 4: 17–21.

Ramesh, R., Subramanian, M., Lakshmanan, E. et al. (2021). Human health risk assessment using Monte Carlo simulations for groundwater with uranium in southern India. *Ecotoxicology and Environmental Safety* 226: 112781. https://doi.org/10.1016/j.ecoenv.2021.112781.

Rani, S., Kansal, S., Singla, A.K., and Mehra, R. (2021). Radiological risk assessment to the public due to the presence of radon in water of Barnala district, Punjab, India. *Environmental Geochemistry and Health* 43: 5011–5024. https://doi.org/10.1007/s10653-021-01012-y.

Sánchez-Virosta, P., Espín, S., García-Fernández, A.J., and Eeva, T. (2015). A review on exposure and effects of arsenic in passerine birds. *Science of the Total Environment* 512–513: 506–525. https://doi.org/10.1016/j.scitotenv.2015.01.069.

Selinus, O. (2002). Medical geology: method, theory and practice. In: *Geoenvironmental Mapping: Methods, Theory and Practice* (ed. P.T. Bobrowsky), 473–496. Leiden, The Netherlands: Taylor and Francis/Balkema.

Selinus, O. (2004). Medical geology: an emerging speciality. *Terrae* 1: A1–A8.

Selinus, O., Alloway, B., Centeno, J.A. et al. (2005). *Essentials of Medical Geology*. Springer.

Smedley, P. (2005). Arsenic occurrence in groundwater in South and East Asia. In: *Towards a More Effective Operational Response. Arsenic Contamination of Groundwater in South and East Asian Countries* (ed. K. Kemper), 20–97. New Delhi, India: World Bank.

Smedley, P.L. and Kinniburgh, D.G. (2002). A review of the source, behaviour and distribution of arsenic in natural waters. *Applied Geochemistry* 17: 517–568. https://doi.org/10.1016/S0883-2927(02)00018-5.

Stalder, E., Blanc, A., Haldimann, M., and Dudler, V. (2012). Occurrence of uranium in Swiss drinking water. *Chemosphere* 86: 672–679. https://doi.org/10.1016/j.chemosphere.2011.11.022.

UNSCEAR (United Nations Scientific Committee on the Effects of Atomic Radiation) (2011). Sources and effects of ionizing radiation. UNSCEAR 2008 report to the General Assembly, Vol. II with scientific annexe. United Nations, New York, p. 179.

Vithanage, M. and Bhattacharya, P. (2015). Fluoride in the environment: sources, distribution and defluoridation. *Environmental Chemistry Letters* 13: 131–147. https://doi.org/10.1007/s10311-015-0496-4.

WHO (2011). *Guidelines for Drinking-Water Quality*, 4e. Geneva: World Health Organization.

Wijenayake, A., Abayasekara, C., Pitawala, A., and Bandara, B.M.R. (2022). Antimicrobial potential of four mica drugs and their chemical and mineralogical properties. *BMC Complementary Medicine and Therapies* 22: https://doi.org/10.1186/s12906-022-03545-w.

Wilson, M.J. (2003). Clay mineralogical and related characteristics of geophagic materials. *Journal of Chemical Ecology* 29: 1525–1547. https://doi.org/10.1023/A:1024262411676.

Woywodt, A. and Kiss, A. (2002). Geophagia: the history of earth-eating. *Journal of the Royal Society of Medicine* 95: 143–146. https://doi.org/10.1258/jrsm.95.3.143.

Xiang, Q., Liang, Y., Chen, L. et al. (2003). Effect of fluoride in drinking water on children's intelligence. *Fluoride* 36: 84–94.

Zhang, Y. and Cao, S.R. (1996). Coal burning induced endemic fluorosis in China. *Fluoride* 29: 207–211.

Zhu, L., Zhang, H.H., Xia, B., and Xu, D.R. (2007). Total fluoride in Guangdong soil profiles, China: spatial distribution and vertical variation. *Environment International* 33: 302–308. https://doi.org/10.1016/j.envint.2006.10.010.

Zhuo, W., Iida, T., and Yang, X. (2001). Occurrence of 222Rn, 226Ra, 228Ra and U in groundwater in Fujian Province, China. *Journal of Environmental Radioactivity* 53: 111–120. https://doi.org/10.1016/S0265-931X(00)00108-9.

8

Disasters

Health and Environment Interphase

Novil Wijeskara

Humphrey Fellowship Program, Department of Global Health, Rollins School of Public Health, Emory University, Atlanta, GA, USA
Disaster Preparedness and Response Division, Ministry of Health, Colombo, Sri Lanka

8.1 Key Terminology on Disasters

Disasters have been experienced by humanity since the beginning of human civilization (Leroy 2020). The origin of the word disaster is based on the belief that the unfavorable positioning of stars would bring bad luck in destructive events such as earthquakes or floods (Merriam-Webster Dictionary 2022). Even these ancient beliefs support the notion of the close interaction between disasters, human health, and the environment.

Disasters have become a reality in today's world. Extreme weather events are increasing due to climate change (IPCC 2022). Rapid population growth and unplanned urbanization are pushing communities to settle in areas with a higher risk for disasters (Patel and Burke 2009; Yahmed 1994). Environmental degradation, industrialization, and urbanization are progressively disrupting natural systems and the social safety net (Whitmee et al. 2015). As a result, disasters will continue to be a challenge that affects humanity at present and will in the future.

Many terms have been used in the discipline and practice of disaster management. Ironing out the discrepancies in terminologies, the United Nations Office for Disaster Risk Reduction (DRR) has developed a glossary of terminology on DRR (United Nations Office for Disaster Risk Reduction (UNDRR) 2017). At the onset of this chapter, let us review some key terminology concerning natural disasters. The definitions in Text Box 8.1 have been obtained from the United Nations Office for Disaster Risk Reduction.

When examining the definition of disaster closely, several essential elements within it could be found.

Functional disruption to humans: Negative effects on the institution of humanity, such as community or society, prove to be a characteristic feature of a disaster. The unit at which this disruption could be decided is based on its requirements. For example, the unit of the human organization affected by drought could be a district, country, or region.

Interaction of the hazardous events with conditions of exposure, vulnerability, and capacity: A disaster demands the interaction of the hazardous event with three other elements, indicating the multifactorial nature of factors contributing to the disaster's occurrence. This relationship will be discussed later in the chapter.

Losses and impacts: The hallmark of disasters is their negative consequences in human, material, economic, and environmental losses and impacts. The losses and impacts could lead to deaths, injuries, damage to private and public property, infrastructure, disruption of agriculture or commercial activity, and environmental pollution.

The size of the hazardous event does not matter for an event to be categorized as a disaster. Instead, the ability of the system that the disaster impacts on coping is the determining factor for defining a disaster. For example, the EMDAT, one of the largest databases that provide information on disasters, uses the following criteria to define an event as a disaster (Center for Research on the Epidemiology of Disasters 2009):

Ten or more people dead
Hundred or more people affected
The declaration of a state of emergency
A call for international assistance.

Hazard is another important concept that is used in disaster narrative. Hazard is a disaster waiting to happen. When a hazard becomes a hazardous event, it could become an emergency that could escalate into a disaster. An emergency could be managed within the capacity of the community or society. When the emergency exceeds the capacity of the community or society to manage

One Health: Human, Animal, and Environment Triad, First Edition. Edited by Meththika Vithanage and Majeti Narasimha Vara Prasad.

Text Box 8.1 Key Definitions of Disasters

Disaster: A serious disruption of the functioning of a community or a society at any scale due to hazardous events interacting with conditions of exposure, vulnerability, and capacity, leading to one or more of the following: human, material, economic and environmental losses, and impacts.
Hazard: A process, phenomenon, or human activity that may cause loss of life, injury or other health impacts, property damage, social and economic disruption, or environmental degradation.
Vulnerability: The conditions determined by physical, social, economic, and environmental factors or processes which increase the susceptibility of an individual, a community, assets, or systems to the impacts of hazards.
Exposure: The situation of people, infrastructure, housing, production capacities, and other tangible human assets located in hazard-prone areas.
Capacity: The combination of all the strengths, attributes, and resources available within an organization, community, or society to manage and reduce disaster risks and strengthen resilience.
Disaster Risk: The potential loss of life, injury, or destroyed or damaged assets which could occur to a system, society, or community in a specific period of time, determined probabilistically as a function of hazard, exposure, vulnerability, and capacity.
Disaster Risk Management: The application of DRR policies and strategies to prevent new disaster risk, reduce existing disaster risk, and manage residual risk, contributing to the strengthening of resilience and reduction of disaster losses.
Disaster Management Assessment/Disaster Risk Assessment: A qualitative or quantitative approach to determine the nature and extent of disaster risk by analyzing potential hazards and evaluating existing conditions of exposure and vulnerability that together could harm people, property, services, livelihoods, and the environment on which they depend.
Resilience: The ability of a system, community, or society exposed to hazards to resist, absorb, accommodate, adapt to, transform, and recover from the effects of a hazard in a timely and efficient manner, including through the preservation and restoration of its essential basic structures and functions through risk management.

Source: UNDRR (2017).

on its own, it becomes a disaster (Walker 2012). The relationship between hazard, emergency, and disaster is shown in Eq. (8.1):

$$\text{Hazard} \rightarrow \text{Emergency} \rightarrow \text{Disasters} \tag{8.1}$$

One crucial concept embedded in this equation is that there is an opportunity for human beings to intervene in the progression of a hazard to a disaster. Thus, disasters are not events humans have no control over.

Disaster risk is a concept used to quantify the potential for damage due to a hazard in each area within a given time. One of the commonly used disaster risk equations is shown in Eq. (8.2) (UNICEF 2014).

$$\text{Risk} = \text{Hazard} \times \text{Vulnerability} \times \text{Exposure} / \text{Capacity} \tag{8.2}$$

Risk is a combined result of several factors: hazard, vulnerability, exposure, and capacity. Hazard encompasses the event that releases the negative factors that initiate the disaster. Vulnerability is a collection of all negative attributes that increase the disaster risk, while capacity encompasses the positive attributes that reduce the disaster risk. Finally, the exposure measures the number of elements at risk. Table 8.1 provides some examples of the hazard, vulnerability exposure, and capacity concerning an earthquake disaster in a city.

Table 8.1 Examples of hazard, vulnerability, exposure, and capacity concerning an earthquake disaster in a city.

Factor	Example
Hazard	Magnitude of the earthquake (measured on Richter scale 1–9)
	Frequency of earthquakes in the area
	Closeness of the city to the epicenter of the earthquake
Vulnerability	Poorly engineered or non-engineered buildings
	Poor awareness on responses to when an earthquake is felt
Exposure	Number of buildings located in the impact zone of the earthquake
Capacity	Reinforced and adequately engineered buildings with the ability to withstand earthquakes
	Ability to do search and rescue, patient evacuation, first aid, and pre-hospital care, mass casualty management

A complex interaction between the hazard, vulnerability, exposure, and capacity produces disaster risk. Hazard, vulnerability, and exposure contribute to the increased disaster risk, whereas capacity contributes to DRR.

Hazards could be natural or man-made. The magnitude and the frequency characterize the hazard. Magnitude is a function of the energy released by the hazardous event. For example, the magnitude of earthquakes is measured using the Richter scale ranging from 0 to 9 or the Modified Mercalli intensity (I–XII) scale (California Eathquake Authority 2020). Cyclone magnitude is measured using the Saffir-Simpson scale ranging from 1 to 5 (NOAA 2022). The magnitude of Tornados is measured using Enhanced Fujita scale, ranging from 0 to 5 (NOAA US Department of Commerce 2022). Thus, with increasing magnitude, the potential for damage following a hazardous event is rising. Hazardous events are cyclical events. The frequency indicates how soon a hazardous event would return. For example, a yearly flood is more frequent than a 10-yearly flood. Similarly, the magnitude of yearly floods would often be low, while a 10-yearly flood would cause more damage.

Classification of hazards has been a challenging and evolving task globally. UNDRR and the International Society of Science have organized 302 hazard information profiles under eight hazard types (Murray et al. 2022). Further, each hazard type has clusters and hazards listed (Figure 8.1).

The eight hazard types include meteorological and hydrological, extraterrestrial, geohazards, environmental, chemical, biological, technological, and societal. In addition, different disaster databases use different types of hazard classification. Therefore, coherent definitions, nomenclature, and hazard classification are needed to better coordinate disaster risk management (DRM) efforts globally.

Even though the hazards could be natural, it has been argued that disasters may not be natural: Human involvement is essential for a hazard to become a disaster. Hence, it has been argued that all disasters are man-made, not natural. By calling all disasters to be man-made, more responsibility is called upon humanity to reduce disaster risk, rather than blaming the environment for the damages caused by disasters (Liopetriti n.d.). For the rest of this chapter, we will only focus on disasters that arise out of natural hazards. However, this chapter will use the terms natural hazards and natural disasters interchangeably.

EMDAT classified disasters into two groups, natural and technological. Another third category of complex disasters includes some major famine situations for which the drought was not the primary causal factor (Center for Research on the Epidemiology of Disasters 2009). Figure 8.2 shows the number of records on EMDAT based on the above three groups from 1900 to 2021.

Most disasters during the reporting period had been natural disasters ($n = 16{,}123$, 64%). Figure 8.3 shows the same period's trend of natural and man-made disasters.

Natural and technological disasters have shown a rising trend over the years. In 2021, 437 natural and 151 technological disasters have been reported worldwide.

The breakdown of natural disasters is shown in Figure 8.4.

When considering the same period, the most hazards were hydrological (39%), followed by meteorological (31%). Geophysical hazards accounted for 12% of the hazards, while biological hazards were responsible for 10% of the hazards. Finally, climatological hazards accounted for 8% of the events.

Figure 8.5 shows the breakdown of the technological hazard subtypes for the same period.

Road, water, and air transport accidents contribute to the most significant technological hazards, followed by explosion and fire. Rail accidents take sixth place when considering the number of reports on EMDAT.

8.1.1 Vulnerability

Another critical element of the disaster risk equation is vulnerability. Vulnerability is a multidimensional phenomenon. Some dimensions of vulnerability include physical, physiological, political, economic, and social aspects. Physical vulnerability expresses the proximity of an individual or a property to a hazard. For example, the location of a community in a river basin may determine how often it will be affected by floods. Further, the proximity of a community to a fault line may increase the vulnerability to earthquakes.

Physiological vulnerability to disasters is determined by the characteristics of an individual, such as age, gender, and health status. For example, children and the elderly are more vulnerable to most disasters. Women and pregnant mothers too are affected disproportionately. In addition, chronic medical conditions such as heart disease, lung diseases, diabetes mellitus, kidney disease, and mental health issues increase the vulnerability of individuals during or in the aftermath of disasters.

The political vulnerability could come into play in the aftermath of disasters. The local and contextual dynamics will heavily influence political vulnerability, especially in the aftermath of complex humanitarian emergencies.

Economic vulnerability is a crucial factor in the aftermath of disasters. The poor individuals, families, and communities are often clustered in areas with high physical vulnerability to disasters and are disproportionately affected by disasters. While all segments of society could be affected by disasters, the impacts and efforts needed to recover by poor

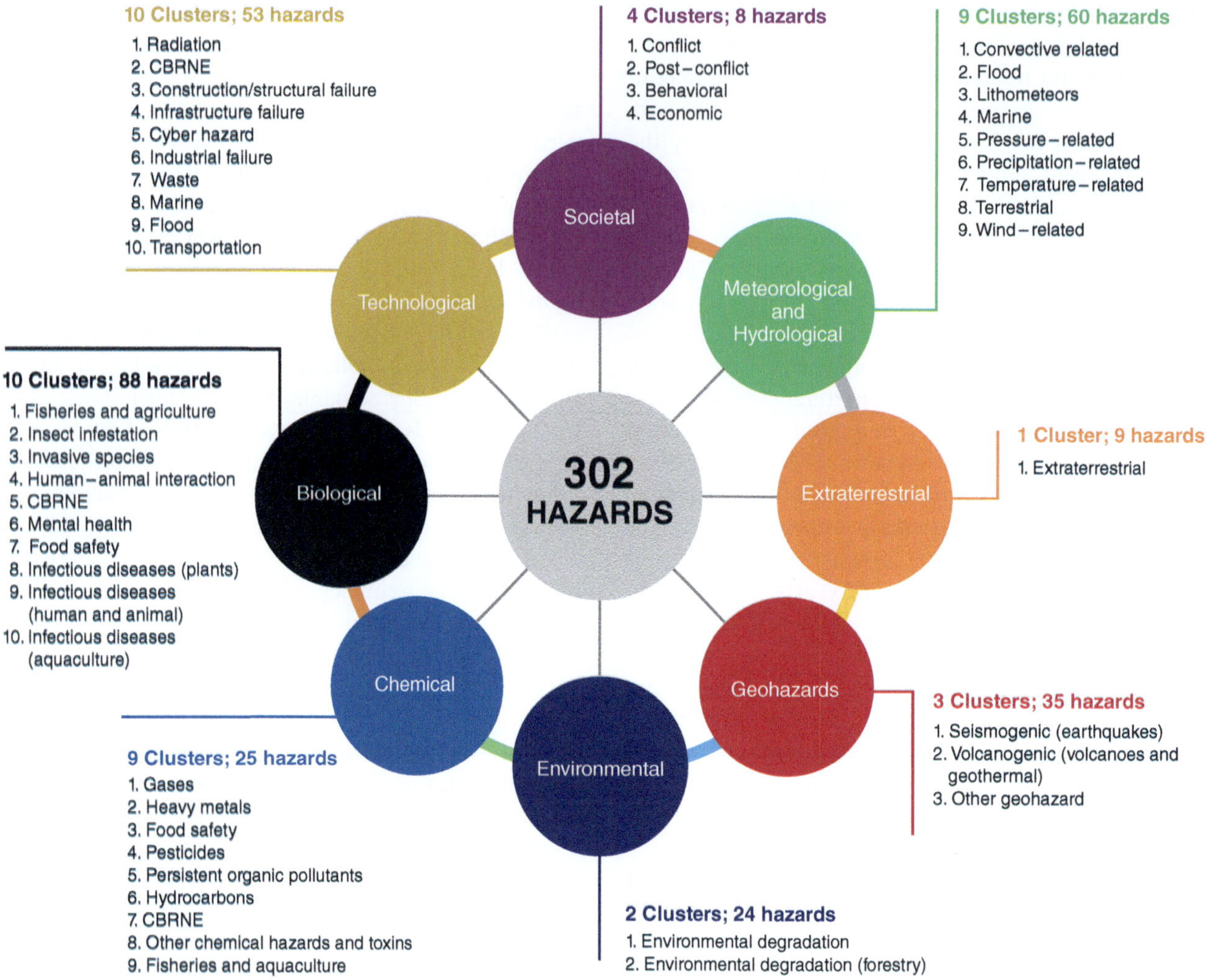

10 Clusters; 53 hazards
1. Radiation
2. CBRNE
3. Construction/structural failure
4. Infrastructure failure
5. Cyber hazard
6. Industrial failure
7. Waste
8. Marine
9. Flood
10. Transportation
4 Clusters; 8 hazards
1. Conflict
2. Post–conflict
3. Behavioral
4. Economic
9 Clusters; 60 hazards
1. Convective related
2. Flood
3. Lithometeors
4. Marine
5. Pressure–related
6. Precipitation–related
7. Temperature–related
8. Terrestrial
9. Wind–related
Societal
Technological
Meteorological and Hydrological
10 Clusters; 88 hazards
1. Fisheries and agriculture
2. Insect infestation
3. Invasive species
4. Human–animal interaction
5. CBRNE
6. Mental health
7. Food safety
8. Infectious diseases (plants)
9. Infectious diseases (human and animal)
10. Infectious diseases (aquaculture)
Biological
302 HAZARDS
Extraterrestrial
1 Cluster; 9 hazards
1. Extraterrestrial
Chemical
Geohazards
Environmental
3 Clusters; 35 hazards
1. Seismogenic (earthquakes)
2. Volcanogenic (volcanoes and geothermal)
3. Other geohazard
9 Clusters; 25 hazards
1. Gases
2. Heavy metals
3. Food safety
4. Pesticides
5. Persistent organic pollutants
6. Hydrocarbons
7. CBRNE
8. Other chemical hazards and toxins
9. Fisheries and aquaculture
2 Clusters; 24 hazards
1. Environmental degradation
2. Environmental degradation (forestry)

Figure 8.1 United Nations Office for Disaster Risk Reduction (UNDRR)/International Science Council (ISC) hazard information profiles according to 8 hazard types note: CBRNE = chemical, biological, radiological, nuclear, and high-yield explosives. *Source:* Reproduced from Fahad S Malik and Anna Schwappach, UK Health Security Agency.

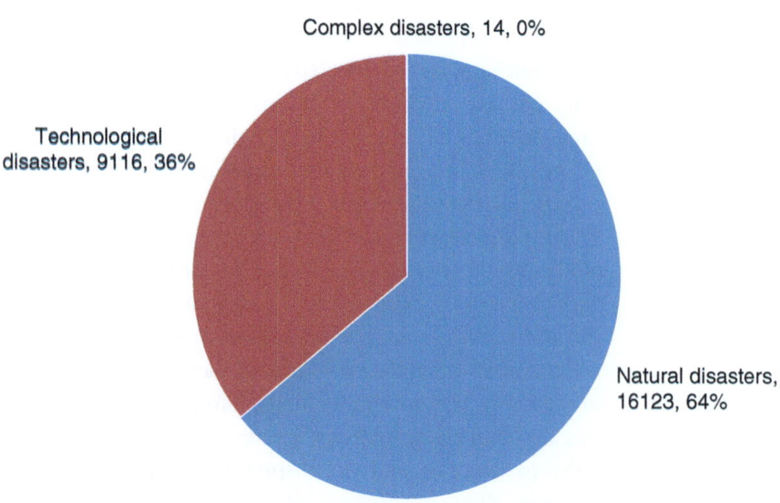

Figure 8.2 Disaster categories reported on EMDAT from 1900 to 2021.

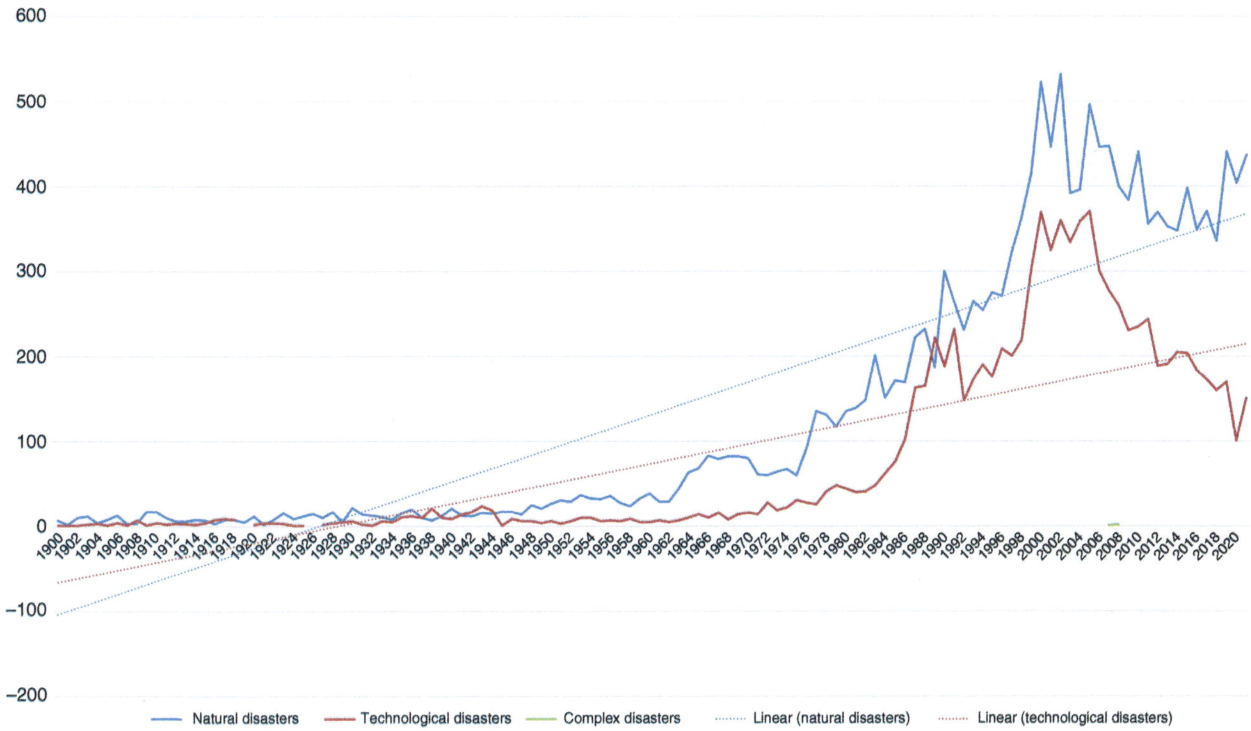

Figure 8.3 Trend of natural disasters and technological disasters from 1900 to 2021.

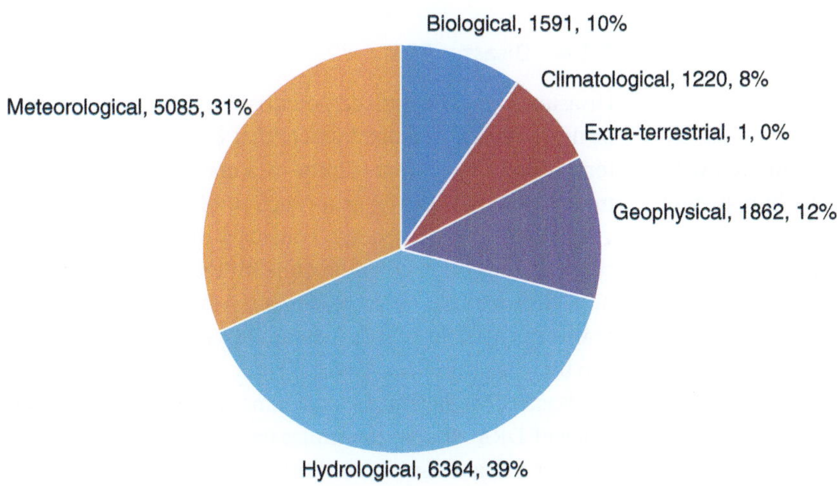

Figure 8.4 Distribution of natural disasters by subtypes on EMDAT from 1900 to 2021.

communities are much higher. Lack of savings, poor access to financial capital for recovery, and lack of new skills that are relevant in the aftermath of disasters could further aggravate economic vulnerability. Developmental approaches to reducing poverty will have additional benefits in reducing disaster vulnerability. Furthermore, risk sharing and risk transfer tools such as microinsurance benefitting needy communities could further reduce economic vulnerability.

Social vulnerability encompasses all negative aspects that restrict an individual, family, or community benefit from the safety nets available. Existing divisions and polarities within a community could increase social vulnerability. Unhealthy majority–minority relationships based on forms of social stratification such as race, ethnicity, religion, or sexual orientation could aggravate social vulnerability. The lack of solid and well-resourced community-based organizations contributes to social vulnerability. In addition, poor participation of community members and lack of fair representation could further increase social vulnerability.

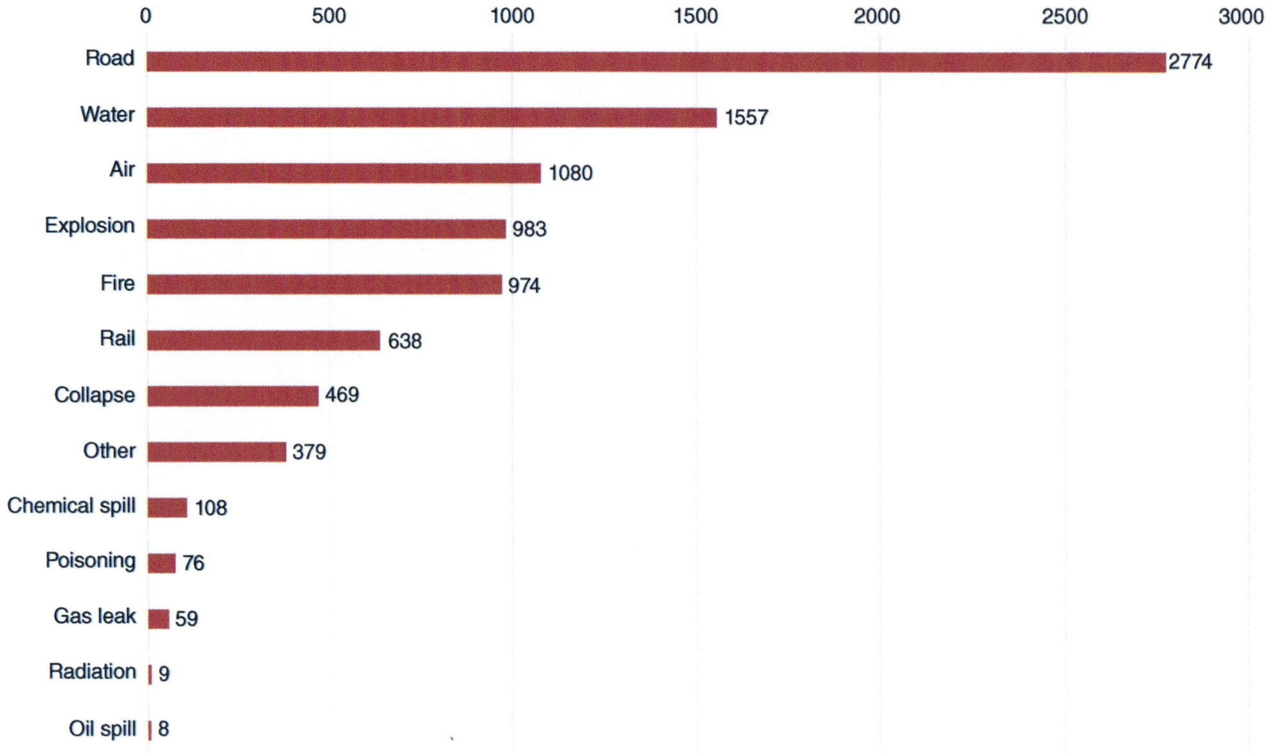

Figure 8.5 Distribution of technological disasters by subtypes on EMDAT from 1900 to 2021.

8.1.2 Exposure

Exposure is used to quantify the situation of people, infrastructure, housing, production capacities, and other tangible human assets. For example, a flood in an urban area with more houses and people would cause more human and property damage than in a rural area with fewer houses and people. On the other hand, a flood in a rural area with much agricultural land would cause more agricultural livelihood damage, while it would cause lesser property and human damage in an urban area where agricultural lands are scarce.

8.1.3 Capacity

Capacity indicates the combination of all the strengths, abilities, and resources available within an organization, community, or society to manage and reduce disaster risks and strengthen resilience. In other words, it involves all positive aspects that contribute to DRR. The building of capacity, in turn, contributes to the reduction of disaster risk and could be done at the individual, family, and community levels. Capacity building includes awareness-raising, development of preparedness and response plans, establishing early-warning systems, stockpiling of disaster relief items, and testing and improvement plans. Capacity building at all levels is a core strategy that could be used to reduce disaster risk.

8.1.4 Disaster Risk

Disaster risk indicates the potential for loss of life, injury, or destroyed or damaged assets that could occur to a system, society, or a community in a specific period, determined probabilistically as a function of hazard, exposure, vulnerability, and capacity. Perceived disaster risk by the communities often could be quite different from the measured disaster risk by professionals. Many awareness programs in the field of disasters are targeted at bridging the gap between these two types of risks.

Disaster Management Assessment forms the cornerstone of DRM and is sometimes called disaster risk assessment or risk assessment in short. It involves a qualitative or quantitative approach to determine the nature and extent of disaster risk by analyzing potential hazards and evaluating existing conditions of exposure and vulnerability that together could harm people, property, services, livelihoods, and the environment on which they depend.

A similar concept in the environmental sciences include the environmental impact assessments (EIAs), which are aimed at assessing the significant effects of a project or development proposal on the environment. (Morgan 2012) EIAs make sure that project decision-makers think about the likely effects on the environment at the earliest possible time and aim to avoid, reduce, or offset those effects. The focus in EIA is the project and the effects of a project on the environment. In contrast, disaster management assessment attempts to assess the risk of one or more hazards in a given community under the prevailing vulnerability, exposure, and capacity scenarios.

Damage indicates the replacement value of totally or partially destroyed physical assets. On the other hand, losses describe flows of the economy that arise from the temporary absence of the damaged assets. Damage and Loss Assessment (DALA) attempts to approximate the effects of a disaster on an economy from a macroeconomic perspective (Jovel and Mudahar 2010). Further, disaster recovery should not be limited only to the replacement of the damaged assets and the losses incurred by the disaster but also include recovery needs that should incorporate DRR and build back better principles. The Post Disaster Needs Assessment (PDNA) is a form of disaster management assessment carried out in the aftermath of disasters to assess the response needs caused by disasters (European Commission, The United Nations Development Group, and The World Bank 2013).

8.2 Effects of Disasters on Environment and Health

Natural disasters could affect the environment negatively in their aftermath. For example, the surface water could be contaminated after a flood. In addition, natural disasters could also damage the built environment, especially in the aftermath of disasters such as earthquakes and floods. The soil also could be affected by natural disasters, for example, due to hazards such as landslides and coastal erosion.

Some environmental changes that could occur in the aftermath of natural disasters with health implications are summarized in Figure 8.6.

In summary, changes in the environment due to components of the environment such as geosphere, hydrosphere, atmosphere, and biosphere could lead to changes in the earth/soil, water, air, plants, and animals. Some pathways that these changes could compromise human health directly and indirectly. For example, disruption of the built environment, such as the houses, roads, and public places, could lead to deaths, injuries, and diseases. Similarly, exposure to infectious agents in the water, soil, and air could also negatively impact human health. Contamination of air, water, and soil with toxic chemicals could harm humans. Plant and animal damage could lead to a food supply disruption, malnutrition, and associated adverse health consequences. In addition to the pathways shown in Figure 8.6, there could be many other ways and pathways that natural disasters could impact human health directly and indirectly.

Figure 8.7 shows the deaths and injuries resulting from natural and technological disasters from 1900 to 2022.

The number of deaths due to natural disasters has been showing a decreasing trend over the years. Peaks in deaths from 1900 to 1965 have been well above 1.5 million. However, technological disasters show an increasing trend over the years for the same period. The decreasing number of deaths due to natural disasters could be due to the DRM measures implemented over time. In addition, improving the trauma care systems to avert deaths following disasters would also have contributed to the reduction of deaths. However, the number of deaths due to technological disasters shows an increasing trend. Furthermore, industrialization and development have exposed more human lives to risks resulting in deaths. The need to address all hazards during DRM approaches, including technological disasters, is a policy recommendation that could be reached based on these findings.

Figures 8.8 and 8.9 show the trends of injured, affected, and made homeless from 1900 to 2021.

The total number of injured and displaced is increasing over time for natural and technological disasters. The same is true for the number affected by natural disasters. However, the same for technological disasters seems to be stagnating. On the other hand, the number injured and displaced due to technological disasters is also increasing, while the number affected remains almost static. These findings suggest that natural and technological disasters

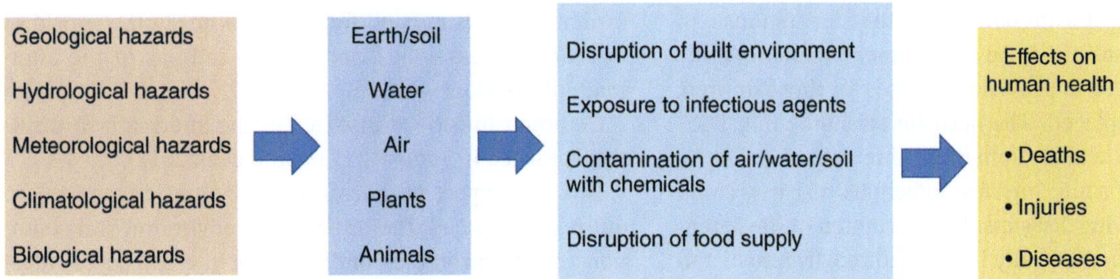

Figure 8.6 Hazards, environmental effects, and health impacts.

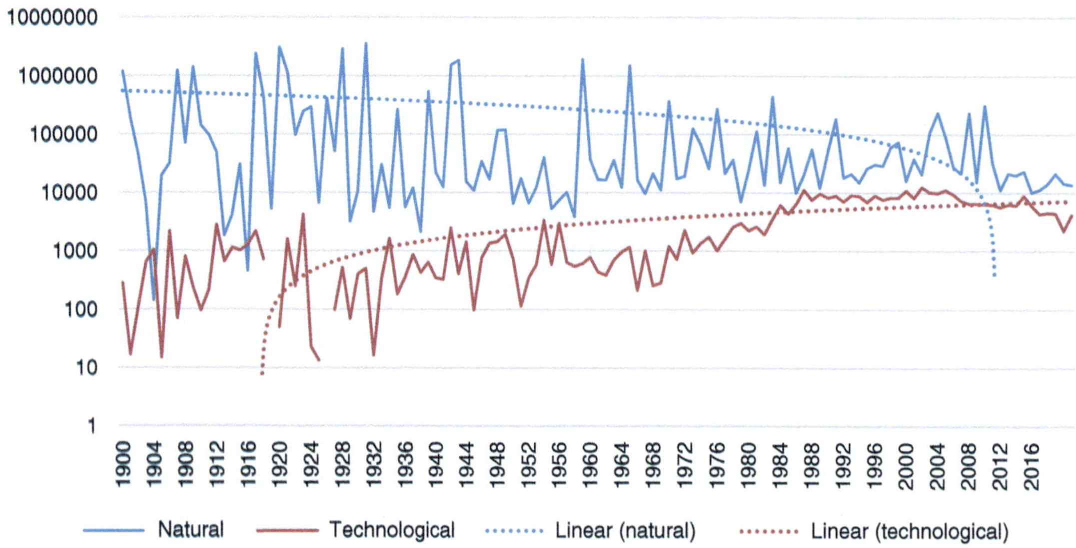

Figure 8.7 Deaths and injuries from natural and technological disasters from 1900 to 2021.

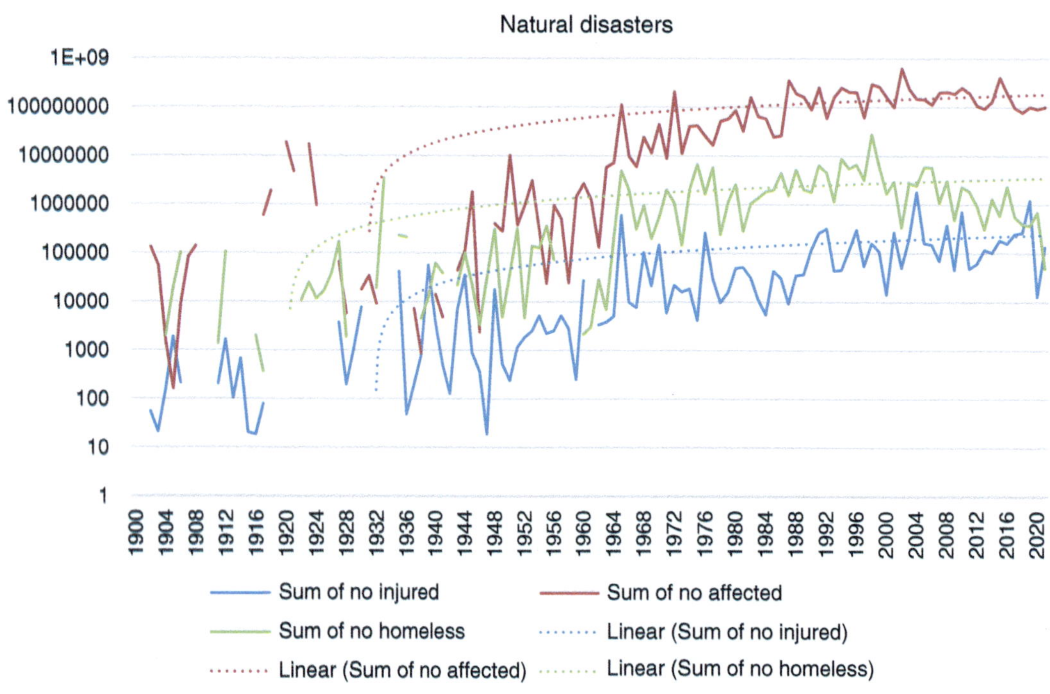

Figure 8.8 Distribution of number injured, affected, and homeless due to natural disasters on EMDAT from 1900 to 2021.

continue to be significant burdens for disaster response. In addition, they continue to be development challenges due to the cost involved in providing services for those injured, affected, and displaced. The need for strengthening DRR activities is quite evident from these observations.

In addition to acute injuries, infectious diseases could also thrive following disasters. The disruption of the defensive mechanisms, especially in the built environment following disasters, could also contribute to this increased infectious disease risk. For example, lack of safe water, sanitation, housing, and food contributes to the spread of infectious diseases in displacement settings in the aftermath of disasters.

Common infectious diseases in the aftermath of disasters are listed in Table 8.2 (Kouadio et al. 2012).

One key aspect is that disasters do not create disease outbreaks. Instead, the unfavorable environmental conditions create favorable conditions for the spread of infectious diseases. Therefore, by effective interventions to manipulate the environmental conditions using public

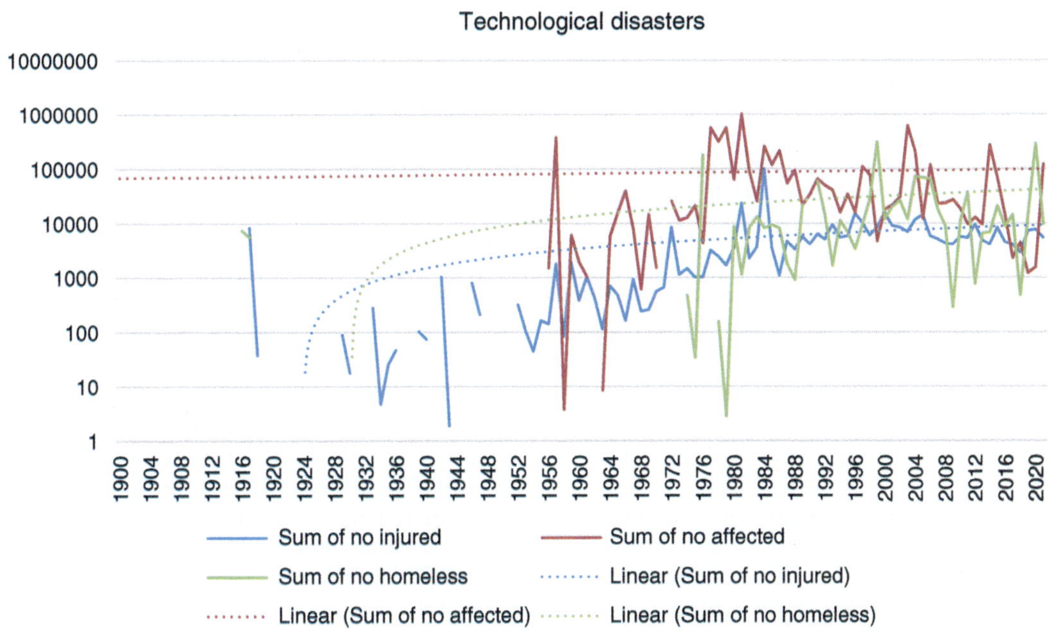

Figure 8.9 Distribution of number injured, affected, and homeless due to technological disasters on EMDAT from 1900 to 2021.

Table 8.2 Common infectious disease outbreaks in disasters.

Disease category	Diseases
Water-borne diseases	Diarrhea, dysentery, typhoid, hepatitis A
Air-borne diseases	Acute respiratory tract infections, measles, Meningococcal meningitis, tuberculosis
Vector-borne diseases	Dengue, leptospirosis
Skin diseases and infection of wound	Tetanus, cutaneous mucomycosis

health interventions, the risk of the spread of infectious diseases could be removed or reduced. Risk factors for the spread of infectious diseases and possible public health interventions to address them are given in Table 8.3 (Kouadio et al. 2012).

Several risk factors work together to increase the risk of infectious diseases in the aftermath of disasters. Even though disasters do not cause infectious disease outbreaks, the confluence of several risk factors could create situations for such diseases to spread at high speed. These risk factors could be in the affected community, the new environment they go to, and the health system that is available to serve them in the new setting (Wisner et al. 2002).

In the aftermath of disasters, communities move from non-endemic areas to endemic areas of diseases, with poor immunity to the diseases in the new area. As a result, they could get easily infected with new diseases. Furthermore, poor nutrition, primarily because of long-term disasters, could increase the risk of infectious diseases. In addition, the affected community will have poor awareness of hygiene habits and health-seeking behaviors. For example, nonadherence to healthy habits such as handwashing and using toilets for defecation may increase the risk of water-borne diseases. In addition, the affected communities will not be aware of the existing health services in the newly settled area, such as hospitals and clinics. Therefore, public health interventions such as prophylaxis for diseases, improving the quantity and quality of food, conducting nutrition rehabilitation programs, and conducting health education and hygiene promotion activities could be carried out to minimize the risk of population-related factors.

Changes in the natural and the built environment in the aftermath of disasters, such as overcrowding of shelters with poor ventilation and lighting, could create favorable conditions for spreading infectious diseases. In addition, insufficient water quantity and quality, especially for drinking purposes, could increase the risk of water-borne diseases. Furthermore, a lack of safe, sanitary facilities and waste disposal mechanisms could further increase the spread of infectious diseases. It should be noted that poor shelter, water supply, and sanitation also increase the risk of sexual and gender-based violence in displacement settings. Vector breeding could also increase in the new environmental conditions in which the displaced communities live. Further, the new settlements could increase the

Table 8.3 Risk factors for the spread of infectious diseases and possible public health interventions to address them.

Domain	Risk factors for spread of infectious diseases	Possible public health interventions to address them
Population-related factors	Movement of population from non-endemic to endemic areas	Prophylaxis (malaria, leptospirosis)
	Malnutrition	Improve quantity and quality of food, conduct nutrition rehabilitation programs
	Poor health awareness, hygiene habits, and health-seeking behavior	Health education, hygiene promotion
Environmental factors	Crowded shelters with poor ventilation and lighting	Plan shelters according to the standards. for example 3.5 m^2 per person Decongestion of overcrowded shelters
	Poor quantity and quality of water	Provide at least 20 l per person per day, ensure at 0.2 mg/l of free residual chlorine levels
	Poor sanitary facilities and waste disposal	Ensure availability of at least 1 toilet per 20 persons, mainstream camp cleaning and disposal of solid, and liquid waste disposal
	Increased breeding of vectors	Removal of vector breeding sites, use of impregnated bed nets, spraying of insecticides
Health-system factors	Disrupted vaccination	Restore vaccination program, conduct supplementary immunization programs
	Destruction or weakening of preventive and curative health services	Strengthen preventive and curative health services

population's exposure to new vectors they have not previously been exposed.

Such environmental risks could be minimized through effective shelter management. The Sphere Humanitarian Standards provide detailed guidelines and technical standards for effectively managing displaced persons' shelters (Sphere Project 2018). For example, at least 3.5 m^2 per person of indoor space is needed when establishing temporary shelters. In addition, decommissioning overcrowded camps to shelters with improved conditions could help reduce the risk of spreading infectious diseases.

Safe drinking water is a crucial requirement to ensure the health of communities. At least 20 l of water per person per day is recommended while ensuring 0.2 mg/l of free residual chlorine levels could reduce the risk of water-borne diseases. The availability of adequate toilets for disaster-affected communities is a key factor in ensuring communities' health. It is recommended to have at least one toilet per 20 persons. Further, establishing and strengthening solid and liquid waste management in a camp setting are essential to reduce the risk of water-borne disease. Removing breeding sites in a displaced camp setting is necessary to reduce vector-borne disease risk.

Due to natural disasters, health systems could be affected. For example, childhood vaccination campaigns could be disrupted, increasing the risk of infectious diseases. Further, the detection and treatment of infectious diseases could be affected in the aftermath of disasters due to the damaged health centers, reduced health human resources, and poor availability of essential medicines and supplies. On the other hand, restoration of existing vaccination programs and the launching of supplementary immunization programs based on the epidemiological patterns of the areas could contribute to reducing infectious diseases due to health-system factors. Further, strengthening preventive and curative health services can also strengthen the health system.

8.3 Managing Natural Disasters to Minimize Effects on Human Health

Minimizing the effects on human health in the form of deaths, injuries, and disasters due to disasters has been a key focus of natural disaster management. This has been done through the disaster management cycle (Figure 8.10).

The disaster management cycle shown in Figure 8.10 has three phases: response, recovery, and preparedness. The response phase starts with the occurrence of a disaster.

Response phase: The response phase commences with the onset of the disaster soon after that. Response activities aim to ensure the safety and security of the affected populations,

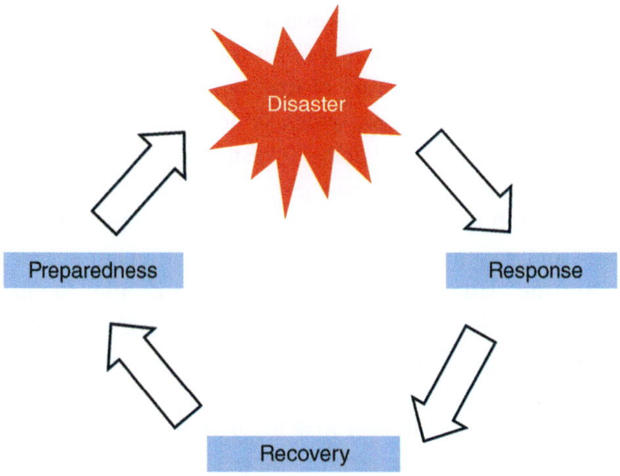

Figure 8.10 Disaster management cycle.

evacuation of at-risk populations, search and rescue, first aid and emergency health services, food, water, sanitation, and other non-food relief items. In addition, it is essential to provide treatment for common illnesses that the affected communities may face and mental health and psychosocial services.

Recovery phase: There is no clear demarcation between response and recovery phases. However, recovery indicates the commencement of the normalization of life back, shifting from the aid-dependent response phase. Therefore, two substages of recovery could be identified: rehabilitation and reconstruction. Rehabilitation includes makeshift and temporary arrangements to return life to normalcy. In comparison, the reconstruction involves more long-term measures to build back better. In addition, measures aimed at reducing the disaster risk are also carried out in the reconstruction phase.

Preparedness phase: A critical characteristic of natural disasters is that they occur cyclically. Thus, following each disaster, a time of relative peace is often observed where measures could be taken to improve the preparation for the subsequent disasters. Preparedness activities include public awareness, development of individual and institutional preparedness plans, testing of plans, stockpiling, and capacity building. These areas are often done in preparation for natural disasters (Figure 8.11).

8.4 Shifting the Focus: Response to Disaster Risk Management

The Asian Disaster Preparedness Center uses the following diagram to explain the relationship between development, DRR, and DRM (ADPC 2018).

The outermost rectangle indicates development in the above diagram. Disasters impact development, the overarching aim of human civilization. Because of disasters, the developmental trajectory could either be slowed or, in worst-case scenarios, reversed. DRR and DRM are approaches aimed at minimizing the effects of disasters on the development trajectory. Hence, disaster management is a discipline and a practice of development.

Two broad approaches could be used to deal with disaster risk generated at the interphase of hazard, vulnerability, exposure, and capacity. These are DRR and DRM, depicted as two overlapping large circles in the above diagram. DRR

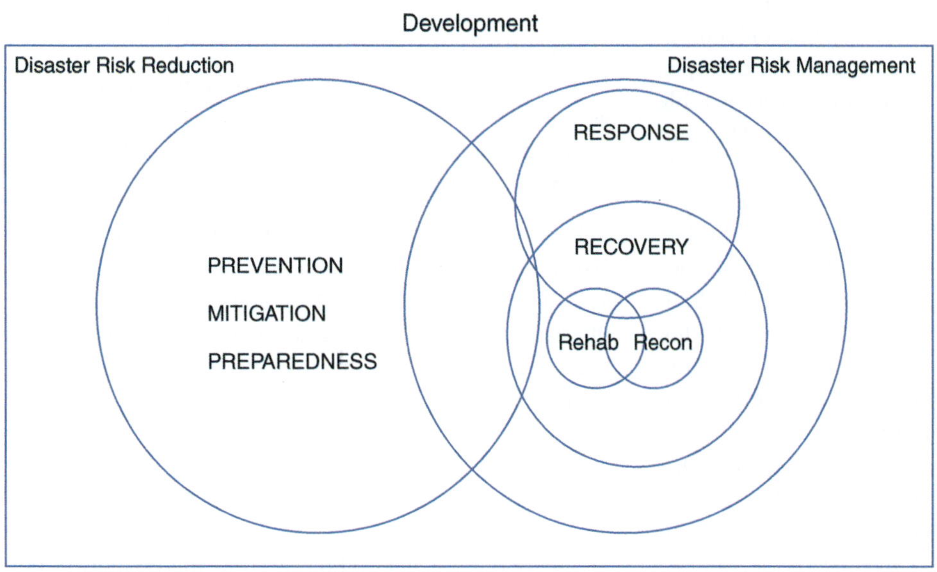

Figure 8.11 Relationship between Development, Disaster Risk Management, and Disaster Risk Reduction. Source: Asian Disaster Preparedness Center.

is aimed at reducing the disaster risk, whereas DRM is aimed at managing the residual risk. Since it is impossible to reduce the disaster risk to zero using risk reduction strategies, DRM is essential and complementary to managing the residual risk.

Under DRR, three strategies could be identified: prevention, mitigation, and preparedness. Prevention is aimed at averting the disaster risk by totally removing it. It is often not possible to bring down the disaster risk to zero, but some efforts could minimize it considerably. For example, permanently relocating a coastal community at risk to the higher ground could be an example of prevention. Mitigation is aimed at reducing the disaster risk considerably. For example, building Tsunami resilient public infrastructure in high-risk areas could be an example of mitigation.

On the other hand, preparedness assumes that disaster risk is considerably high. Hence it is worth preparing for a disaster. By preparedness measures, it is possible to reduce deaths, injuries, and property damage when a disaster is impending or happening. For example, with a functioning Tsunami early-warning system, it is possible to minimize deaths and injuries by safely evacuating people and taking ships off the sea from the harbors. Activities carried out in the preparedness phase of the disaster management cycle have been discussed earlier under the disaster management cycle.

DRM activities typically occur before or after a disaster. The response is aimed at providing life-saving services to the affected communities. These have been discussed under response in the disaster management cycle. Recovery is depicted as overlapping with the response stage. Response marked the shift from the emergency phase to the normalizing phase. Two overlapping stages again could be identified within recovery: rehabilitation and reconstruction. Rehabilitation means the immediate and temporary measures to bring life back to normalcy. For example, damaged bridges need to be repaired as quickly as possible to reestablish the supply chains in a disaster-affected community. Rehabilitation could be done with the available resources and as fast as possible.

On the other hand, it is essential to rebuild a new bridge, probably one that the next disaster will not damage. Hence it would be better than the bridge that used to be. The hallmark of such rehabilitation efforts is building back better, which could provide an opportunity to catch up with the growth trajectory and reduce future disaster risk through more resilient infrastructure and systems.

Different stages in this framework do overlap. In reality, disaster management progresses fluidly and flawlessly across different stages of the above disaster management framework. However, frameworks like the above could be beneficial for us to conceptualize different stages of disasters and their relationship to development.

The global disaster management system has traditionally been focused on responding to disasters when they occur. Due to the cyclical nature of disasters, repeated expenses on response are needed, which is not sustainable. It has been proven that every dollar invested in DRR could save eight dollars in disaster response (Abramovitz, 2001). The need to shift the focus from disaster response to DRM has been an issue that has been discussed over the last decade.

As the culmination of these efforts, the Sendai Framework for Disaster Risk Reduction 2015–2030 was adopted at the Third UN World Conference on Disaster Risk Reduction in Sendai, Japan, on 18 March 2015 (United Nations Office for Disaster Risk Reduction 2015). It was the first significant agreement of the post-2015 development agenda and called for concrete actions to protect development gains from the disaster risk. The Sendai Framework is in line with the Paris Agreement on Climate Change, the Addis Ababa Action Agenda on Financing for Development, the New Urban Agenda, and ultimately the Sustainable Development Goals. The Sendai Framework calls for "the substantial reduction of disaster risk and losses in lives, livelihoods, and health and in the economic, physical, social, cultural and environmental assets of persons, businesses, communities, and countries."

The Framework recognizes that the State has the primary role in reducing disaster risk. However, it should be collaboratively shared with the local government, the private sector, and other stakeholders.

Sendai Framework highlights seven clear targets and four priorities for action to prevent new and reduce existing disaster risks. These four priorities are

1) understanding disaster risk,
2) strengthening disaster risk governance to manage disaster risk,
3) investing in disaster reduction for resilience, and
4) enhancing disaster preparedness for effective response and to "Build Back Better" in recovery, rehabilitation, and reconstruction.

This Framework aims to substantially reduce disaster risk and losses in lives, livelihoods, and health and in persons, businesses, communities, and countries' economic, physical, social, cultural, and environmental assets over the next 15 years. Thus, the link between DRR and the protection of human health is evident.

8.5 Resilience: A New Paradigm

Resilience is a concept that has become increasingly important at the intersection of natural disasters and health. Resilience is the ability of a system, community or society exposed to hazards to resist, absorb, accommodate, adapt to, transform and recover from the effects of a hazard in a timely and efficient manner, including through the preservation and restoration of its essential basic structures and functions through risk management (UNDRR, 2017). Traditional external disaster response activities often wane off with time. However, resilience depends on the internal resources of the community to address challenges.

The concept of resilience has been applied to a different setting. Two such applications include health systems and community resilience.

8.5.1 Health Systems Resilience

When natural disasters occur, their effects could be felt not only by the community but also by the health system, which is expected to respond to the health care needs of the affected community. However, if the health system is compromised, it becomes challenging to cater to the needs of the disaster survivors. Hence, the health system needs to be resilient in the wake of such disasters.

Health systems resilience is the ability of health systems not only to plan for shocks, such as pandemics, economic crises, or the effects of climate change, but also to minimize the negative consequences of such disruptions, recover as quickly as possible, and adapt by learning lessons from the experience to become even better performing and more prepared (OECD 2020).

Some tools used for making the health systems resilient include the Safe Hospitals Initiative (WHO 2013), development of preparedness and response plans for health institutions, training of health staff, and testing of the plans through simulation exercises and drills. In addition, it is essential to mobilize emergency lifesaving assistance to provide health services in the aftermath of disasters. Further, stockpiling essential medicines also contributes to health systems' resilience. Finally, human resources become a critical element of health systems' resilience; hence, rapid mobilization mechanisms are essential.

The COVID-19 pandemic has raised the importance of focusing on health systems resilience more than ever. Therefore, WHO has made the following policy recommendations on building resilient health systems based on primary health care (WHO 2021).

1) Leverage the current response to strengthen both pandemic preparedness and health systems
2) Invest in essential public health functions, including those needed for all-hazards emergency risk management
3) Build a strong primary health care foundation
4) Invest in institutionalized mechanisms for whole-of-society engagement
5) Create and promote enabling environments for research, innovation, and learning
6) Increase domestic and global investment in health system foundations and all-hazards emergency risk management
7) Address preexisting inequities and the disproportionate impact of COVID-19 on marginalized and vulnerable populations

8.5.2 Community Resilience

The concept of resilience could also be applied to a community. A resilient community, in turn, could prepare, face, and recover from natural disasters and environmental shocks using their resources. Community resilience has been a much-researched topic in recent years. Many conceptual and operational frameworks have been developed in this regard (Figure 8.12). We will discuss the Sri Lankan Community Resilience Framework as an example of being used as a tool to promote resilience at the intersection of disasters, health, and the environment (Disaster Management Center 2015).

The Community Resilience Framework is a conceptual representation of how the community will interact with risk knowledge, subsystems, and aspects of government.

The community is at the center of the above framework. This centrality implies that promoting resilience should be started and expanded with and by communities. The engagement of communities in promoting community resilience depends mainly on their risk knowledge. Risk knowledge is a cross-cutting requirement within each resilience element. Enhancing resilience in all of these

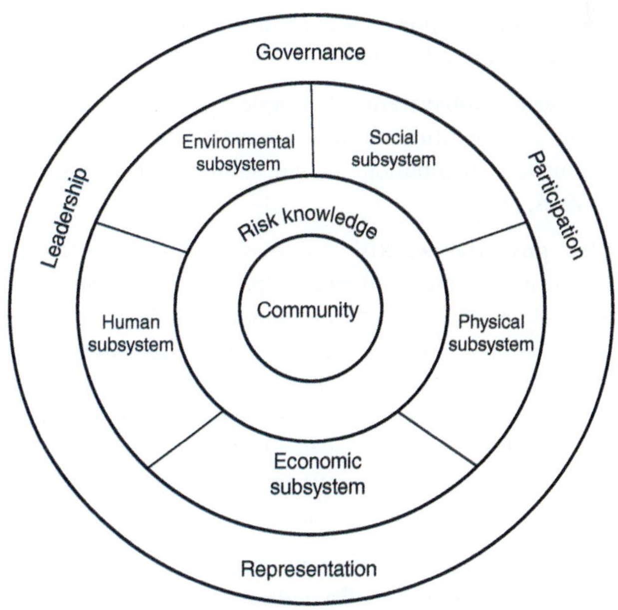

Figure 8.12 The Community Resilience Framework of Sri Lanka. Source: Disaster Management Center.

elements is essential to reduce risk from hazards, accelerate recovery from disaster events, and adapt to changing conditions in a manner consistent with community goals. The risks that are not perceived as real and relevant are unlikely to mount effective, resilient behaviors by communities.

Communities do not operate in a vacuum in promoting their resilience. Instead, a complex ecosystem comprising multiple subsystems influences the resilience-building process. Five of the above subsystems are discussed in the following text:

Physical subsystem: Physical infrastructure refers to the substructure or underlying foundation or network used for providing goods and services; especially the basic installations and facilities on which the continuance and growth of a community or state are dependent, such as the roads, water systems, communications facilities, sewers, sidewalks, cable, wiring, schools, power plants, and transportation and communication systems.

Environmental subsystem: Environmental subsystem refers to all aspects of the surrounding in which the community lives and survives. This chapter focused on the environmental subsystem's functions concerning disasters generating health problems or diseases.

Human subsystem: Human subsystem outlines the risk coping capacities of individuals in a community. Health comprises a vital component of the human subsystem. Curative, preventive, promotive, and rehabilitative health services contribute to resilience under the human subsystem.

Social subsystem: Under the social subsystem, a community is expected to have adequate risk coping strategies and positive interrelationships to endure disasters and bounce back following a disaster.

Economic subsystem: Economic systems are people, firms, and institutions that interact to accomplish the production, distribution, and consumption of goods and services.

Risk governance: Risk governance is another crosscutting issue comprising leadership, participation, and representation. Systems of governance include the public organizations (political, administrative, legislative, and judicial institutions) that contribute to the administration of government functions of the community. Governance includes the processes through which government institutions, or any group of people with a mandate or with a common purpose, make decisions.

Community Resilience is a concept that could be used to promote health in the wake of disasters. For example, the framework mentioned earlier has been used to build the capacity of religious and community leaders to assist disaster-affected communities in Sri Lanka. In addition, the Community Resilience Framework has been used to assess the pandemic preparedness in Sri Lanka. Further, the same framework has been used to explore how community-level stakeholders could assist communities during the economic crisis in Sri Lanka.

8.6 Areas for Future Research and Practice

The research on natural disasters at the interphase of health and environment is becoming increasingly important with the increasing complexity of such relationships. Some areas of further research and practice could be recommended.

Practical and successful efforts to have common terminology for disasters have been undertaken in the recent past. However, more work must be done to incorporate these definitions into national and subnational disaster management systems.

Similarly, disaster classification has been an area that has seen considerable developments in the recent past. Nevertheless, different disaster data bases maintained for different purposes still use non-uniform classification systems. In addition, different disaster management and development agencies have yet to incorporate a uniform classification system in their practice areas.

The cornerstone of both DRR and DRM activities is risk assessment. Even though the theoretical background and the methodologies for conducting disaster risk assessments are available, more support is needed for evidence-based risk assessments to be carried out in practice. The need to have readily available geo-referenced data layers on hazards, vulnerability, exposure and capacity, and geographic information-based technologies to carry out risk assessments cannot be overemphasized. In addition, quantitative–qualitative mixed-method approaches can also be used to carry out disaster risk assessments.

Environmental impact and disaster risk assessments provide a rich niche for future research and practice. Integrated approaches for combined environmental impact and disaster risk assessments could save resources and support risk-based decisions averting damages and losses in the long run.

Predictive modeling is yet another vital area for research and practice. Different environmental and disaster scenarios and conditions could be factored in to predict the health, environmental and socioeconomic impacts, and different risk reduction strategies to address them. Such exercises should support solving real-life problems that disaster management, environment, and health practitioners are trying to solve.

Chemical, Biological, Radiological, Nuclear, and Explosive (CBRNE) emergencies are gaining importance daily. Such emergencies could be accidental or intentional. Inventorying of CBRNE hazards, risk assessment, preparedness planning, capacity building, and testing of plans all need further research and improvement of practice.

Health impacts of disasters are another critical area of research gap. Global Burden of Diseases assessments needs to factor in disaster morbidity and mortality. In addition, research comparing different intervention approaches for addressing disaster morbidity, and mortality needs to be carried out.

Climate change is calling for more action against disasters at the environment-health interphase. Health impacts of climate change, especially at the national, subnational, and local levels, and strategies to mitigate them, need detailed interdisciplinary research and practice.

The COVID-19 pandemic has provided the importance of global health security. Disasters could have transboundary environmental and health impacts. Hence, it is essential to look at the disaster-environment-health interphase as a global health security issue. Cross-border collaboration and cooperation are needed in this regard.

One Health approach can be used for further research at the disaster-environment-health interphase, especially on biological hazards. The shared assessment methodologies and surveillance, preparedness, and response strategies are used in the human, animal, and environmental health fields in anticipation of biological hazards.

Planetary health and disasters are also closely linked. How different environmental disasters could arise due to the disruption of the equilibrium of the component of the planetary ecosystem as well as multidisciplinary research and practice to codesign effective solutions to address them could be affluent areas for the future.

Last but not least, more research and practice on resilience regarding the health systems, communities, and environment need to be done. Furthermore, different subsystems under each of the areas mentioned earlier could enhance resilience at the interphase of disaster, environment, and health.

Acknowledgement

The support extended by Banura Nadathilake in preparation of the manuscript is acknowledged with thanks.

References

Abramovitz, J.N. (2001). Averting Unnatural Disasters. State of the World 2001. *The Wold Watch Institute report on Progress Towards a Sustainable Society.* W.W. Norton and Company. New York, USA. pp. 123–131. https://www.preventionweb.net/files/1849_VL102116.pdf.

ADPC. 2018."Introduction to Disaster Management," Thailand Asian Disaster Preparedness Center (ADPC).

California Eathquake Authority (2020). Earthquake measurements: magnitude vs intensity. https://www.earthquakeauthority.com/Blog/2020/Earthquake-Measurements-Magnitude-vs-Intensity (accessed 11 July 2022).

Center for Research on the Epidemiology of Disasters (2009). EM-DAT. https://www.emdat.be/about (accessed 11 July 2022).

Disaster Management Center (2015). *Community Resilience Framework Sri Lanka.* Colombo Disaster Management Center.

European Commission, The United Nations Development Group, and The World Bank (2013). Post-disaster needs assessment|United Nations Development Programme. *UNDP.* https://www.undp.org/publications/post-disaster-needs-assessment (accessed 11 July 2022).

IPCC (2022). Sixth assessment report. https://www.ipcc.ch/assessment-report/ar6 (accessed 11 July 2022).

Jovel, R.J. and Mudahar, M. (2010). *Damage, Loss, and Needs Assessment Guidance Notes: Volume 1.* Design and Execution of a Damage, Loss, and Needs Assessment. Washington, DC: World Bank.

Kouadio, I.K., Aljunid, S., Kamigaki, T. et al. (2012). Infectious diseases following natural disasters: prevention and control measures. *Expert Review of Anti-Infective Therapy* 10 (1): 95–104. https://doi.org/10.1586/eri.11.155.

Leroy, S.A.G. (2020). Natural hazards, landscapes and civilizations. *Reference Module in Earth Systems and Environmental Sciences* https://doi.org/10.1016/B978-0-12-818234-5.00003-1.

Liopetriti, Yiota. (n.d.). Why disasters are not natural. *ShelterBox.* https://www.shelterbox.org/climate-change-hub/why-disasters-are-not-natural (accessed 11 July 2022).

Marriam-Webster Dictionary (2022). Disaster definition & meaning – Merriam-Webster. https://www.merriam-webster.com/dictionary/disaster (accessed 11 July 2022).

Morgan, R.K. (2012). Environmental impact assessment: the state of the art. *Impact Assessment and Project Appraisal* 30 (1): 5–14. https://doi.org/10.1080/14615517.2012.661557.

Murray, V., Abrahams, J., Ahmed, K. et al. (2022). *Policy Brief: Using UNDRR/ISC Hazard Information Profiles To Manage Risk And Implement The Sendai Framework For Disaster Risk Reduction*." 2022 Global Platform for Disaster Risk Reduction (GP2022) in Bali, Indonesia, 8. International Science Council https://council.science/publications/policy-brief-hazards-informations-profiles-drr/ and https://council.science/publications/.

NOAA (2022). Saffir-Simpson hurricane wind scale. https://www.nhc.noaa.gov/aboutsshws.php (accessed 11 July 2022).

NOAA US Department of Commerce (2022). The enhanced fujita scale (EF Scale). https://www.weather.gov/oun/efscale (accessed 11 July 2022).

OECD (2020). Health systems resilience - OECD. https://www.oecd.org/health/health-systems-resilience.htm (accessed 11 July 2022).

Patel, R.B. and Burke, T.F. (2009). Urbanization – an emerging humanitarian disaster. *New England Journal of Medicine* 361 (8): 741–743. https://doi.org/10.1056/NEJMp0810878.

Sphere Project (2018). The sphere handbook – humanitarain charter and minimum standards in humanitarian response. https://spherestandards.org/handbook-2018 (accessed 11 July 2022).

UNICEF (2014). *Child-Centered Risk Assessnebt – Regional Synthesis of UNICEF Assessment in Asia*. Kathmandu UNICEF Regional Office for South Asia (ROSA).

United Nations Office for Disaster Risk Reduction (2015). Sendai framework for disaster risk reduction 2015–2030. In: *UN World Conference on Disaster Risk Reduction, 2015 March 14–18*. Sendai, Japan. Geneva: United Nations Office for Disaster Risk Reduction http://www.wcdrr.org/uploads/Sendai_Framework_for_Disaster_Risk_Reduction_2015-2030.pdf (accessed 30 July 2022).

United Nations Office for Disaster Risk Reduction (UNDRR) (2017). Terminology. https://www.undrr.org/terminology (accessed 11 July 2022).

Walker, Bryan. (2012). Better ways to prepare for emergencies by bryan walker. https://www.obooko.com/free-social-science-books/prepare-for-emergencies-walker (accessed 11 July 2022).

Whitmee, S., Haines, A., Beyrer, C. et al. (2015). Safeguarding human health in the Anthropocene epoch: report of the Rockefeller Foundation–lancet commission on planetary health. *The Lancet* 386 (10007): 1973–2028. https://doi.org/10.1016/S0140-6736(15)60901-1.

WHO (2013). Safe hospitals in emergencies and disasters: structural, non-structural and functional indicators. https://www.who.int/publications/i/item/9789290614784 (accessed 11 July 2022).

WHO (2021). WHO's 7 policy recommendations on building resilient health systems. https://www.who.int/news/item/19-10-2021-who-s-7-policy-recommendations-on-building-resilient-health-systems (accessed 11 July 2022).

Wisner, B., Adams, J., and World Health Organization (2002). *Environmental Health in Emergencies and Disasters: A Practical Guide*. World Health Organization.

Yahmed, S.B. (1994). *Population Growth and Disasters*, vol. 47. World Health (3).

9

Role of Microorganisms in Bioavailability of Soil Pollutants

H.M.S.P. Madawala

Department of Botany, Faculty of Science, University of Peradeniya, Peradeniya, Sri Lanka

9.1 Introduction

Soil environment acts as a sink for many pollutants of either natural or synthetic in origin. Over the years, soil pollution has become a major concern due to the unwarranted release of pollutants owing to industrialization, large-scale production of hazardous chemicals, urbanization, and intensification of agriculture (Yun et al. 2018). Direct addition, atmospheric deposition, contaminated irrigation water, rainwater, and runoff are some of the known pathways of soil contamination. Once they enter the soil environment, the pollutants can remain for lengthy periods of time due to the chemically reactive nature of soils. Some chemical, physical, and biological properties of soils assist these pollutants to transform into other chemical forms, thus altering their mobility, distribution, and availability within soils. Besides soil's three-phase system (solid, liquid, and gaseous), the living component that includes microorganisms plays a vital and active role in maintaining processes and reactions within the soil environment as well as the nature of soil pollutants.

Soil quality plays a key role in maintaining human health. Approximately, 78% of the average per capita calorie consumptions by humans come directly from crops grown in soils. Moreover, another 20% of the calorie intake comes from food sources that indirectly rely on soil (Brevick 2009). Soils can also act as a natural filter to trap contaminants from water. Therefore, soil contaminants, including heavy metals, toxic chemicals, and pathogens, have the potential to cause serious health issues in humans. Hence, it is important to determine and understand the fates of soil contaminants and their potential distribution in the soil environment in order to mitigate their health impacts on humans. Therefore, processes involved in regulating the mobility and bioavailability of soil pollutants, possible pathways, and exposure events of transferring them from soils to humans are of great importance to understand possible links between the soil quality and human well-being (Petruzzelli et al. 2020) and also to minimize associated hazards.

The "One Health" concept was introduced to focus on emerging infectious diseases in a mutual context covering three important sectors: human, animal, and the environment. As all organisms, including humans, microorganisms, and animals, live in a shared environment, focusing solely on human health while disregarding other sectors and their interfaces is understandably a futile exercise. Therefore, the collective approach in "One Health" concept encourages the policy makers, scientists, and other relevant stakeholders to formulate and implement programs, policies, legislation, and research by considering all three sectors collectively to set goals and face challenges in managing human well-being. The "One Health" approach and its significance have come to the forefront since the outbreak of the current COVID-19 pandemic. Since the COVID-19 outbreak, the scientific community has realized the importance of a holistic approach to tackle such zoonotic diseases because a segregated approach to combating such global pandemics seems unrealistic. Therefore, being one of the major sectors in the "One Health" concept, the "environment" plays a central role in maintaining human health.

The synthetic elements/compounds and their various products tend to accumulate in the soil environment causing potential toxicities to both humans and animals. Though soils have inherent abilities to filter, buffer, offset, and degrade these contaminants over time, some other properties in soils determine the fate, transport, and subsequent penalties of these contaminants. Therefore, understanding the relationships between soil contaminants and soil characteristics is crucial in accomplishing one of the United Nations Environment Programme(UNEP) goals,

One Health: Human, Animal, and Environment Triad, First Edition. Edited by Meththika Vithanage and Majeti Narasimha Vara Prasad.

which is a pollution-free planet. In addition to soil chemical and physical characteristics, microorganisms and their activities play a decisive role in transforming soil pollutants that determine their fate, bioavailability, and transport within soils (Bolan et al. 2014; Biswas et al. 2015). Soil pollutant, at its solid phase, is not readily prone to environmental processes. Once in the liquid phase, pollutants become available for plants and soil microorganisms. Soil pollutants tend to transform between these phases, facilitated by soil physical, chemical, and biological reactions. The bioavailability of soil pollutants is the final outcome of a series of complex processes, influenced by the properties of the pollutant, soil characteristics, and soil organisms.

Microorganisms are widely distributed in all spheres of the globe due to their diverse nutritional requirements and their tolerance to varying growing conditions. The ability of microorganisms to biodegrade soil and aquatic pollutants through conversion, modification, and utilization has been exploited by the researchers in the bioremediation technology (Tang et al. 2007). The degradation process depends mainly on the extent of the soil microbial population and its ability to produce enzyme/s (Abatenh et al. 2017). The enzymes' affinity to the specific pollutant plays a key role in the biodegradation process. In the biodegradation process, microorganisms transform soil pollutants into more mobile and available forms, thus inflicting toxic effects on living beings. In other situations, microorganisms change chemical characteristics in the soil environment, thus indirectly influencing the bioavailability of soil pollutants. This chapter reviews different pathways and mechanisms where microorganisms act on soil pollutants altering their bioavailability that eventually influences human and environmental health at large.

9.2 Soil Pollution: The Global Scenario

The connection between environmental pollution and human health has been widely recognized for decades (Oliver and Gregory 2015). In 2017, the United Nations Environmental Assembly (UNEA) of the UNEP, at its third session held in Nairobi, Kenya, introduced "Towards a pollution-free planet" and adopted a Ministerial Declaration and nine resolutions to address soil pollution and mitigate its impacts. Accordingly, representatives from 150 countries unanimously recognized the importance of healthy soils and the need for effective steps to combat soil pollution (UNEP 2017; Khan et al. 2021).

The primary sources of soil contaminants generally are anthropogenic in origin, *viz.*, industrial waste and emissions, urban waste, agricultural and livestock waste, agrochemicals (fertilizers, pesticides, etc.), and wastewater irrigation (Kabata-Pendias 2011; Mousavi and Khodadoost 2019). Over the past few centuries, rapid industrialization, urban development, and intensive agriculture have intensified the level of soil pollution dramatically (Kabir et al. 2012; Yun et al. 2018). Despite being recognized as a global issue, a majority of available studies are focused on local- or point-scale pollution and their related issues (Venuti et al. 2016; Kim et al. 2017), while global-scale assessment of the distribution of organic and inorganic soil contaminants is scarce or even non-existent (FAO and UNEP 2021). Soil pollution and its consequences are not confined to a place or a country, as pollutants can spread across all major boundaries (at the habitat and geographical levels) due to human-mediated activities and weather patterns (Dragović et al. 2008). Pollutants that travel long distances through the air–soil–water system cause diffuse pollution, and it is largely unknown compared to local-source pollution. Nevertheless, both types of pollution can cause significant impacts on the environment and human health (Grathwohl and Halm 2003).

Soil pollution has been identified as the third most significant threat to soil functions (FAO and ITPS 2015). In addition to causing negative impacts on human and livestock health, soil pollutants can also cause nutrient imbalances and soil acidification, eventually causing detrimental impacts on soil productivity. According to the estimates carried out in the 1990s by the International Soil Reference and Information Centre (ISRIC) and the UNEP, approximately 22 million hectares have been affected by soil contaminants (Oldeman 1992). After almost three decades, it is reasonable to predict the severity of the nature and the extent of this issue at present. Despite being recognized as a global issue, only a few developed countries have taken steps to estimate the extent of their soil pollution, while developing countries may face monetary constraints to conduct studies of that magnitude. In a survey conducted in China, 16% of all soils and 19% of agricultural soils have been categorized as polluted (CCICED 2015). Approximately three million polluted/contaminated sites have been earmarked in the European Economic Area and its West Balkan countries (EEA 2014). In Australia, about 80,000 contaminated sites were recognized in 2010 (DECA 2010). However, due to the lack of information, the true extent of global-scale soil pollution is not precisely revealed (Panagiotakis and Dermatas 2015). This lack of baseline information in regard to the scale of soil pollution can be considered a major challenge to scientists and policy makers to mitigate their potential impacts.

Despite poor global estimates of the soil pollution, the negative impacts of soil pollution have been well accepted by the scientific community. Accordingly, studies have been conducted to assess and remediate soil pollution, with more emphasis on its direct influence on the human health. These studies confirm an unswerving connection between soil pollution and emerging pests and diseases as a result of the loss of ecosystem balance due to competition among organisms and vanishing predators (Landrigan et al. 2018). Also, the steady generation of antimicrobial resistance bacteria and genes is also having detrimental effects on humans as they lose their ability to cope with pathogens (WHO 2018). Moreover, soil pollutants impose negative impacts on soil quality and productivity, eventually resulting in lower crop yields over time (Tian et al. 2015; Lu and Tian 2017).

9.3 Types of Soil Pollutants

Based on the chemical nature, soil pollutants can be broadly divided into two groups: organic and inorganic. According to the International Union of Pure and Applied Chemistry (IUPAC) system of naming soil pollutants, organic and inorganic pollutants are further subdivided into chlorinated and non-chlorinated, and metal/metalloid and nonmetal, respectively (Nič et al. 2009; Swartjes 2011). The metals/metalloids are relatively of high atomic masses and are collectively known as "heavy metals." Sometimes, even nonmetal pollutants such as arsenic (As), antimony (Sb), and selenium (Se) are categorized as "heavy metals" (Kemp and Arundel 1998). Among the inorganic soil pollutants, cadmium (Cd), chromium (Cr), mercury (Hg), lead (Pb), and arsenic (As) are the most noxious. These elements are naturally present in low levels, but once they exceed a certain threshold level, they become hazardous soil pollutants (Landrigan et al. 2018). They are nonbiodegradable, thus they can remain in soils for a long time, readily accumulating in plants and other living organisms. These elements are present in soils in different oxidation states (based on soil physicochemical properties including soil pH), thus allowing them to freely interact with other chemical compounds. These interactions sometimes will lead to transform these elements into more available forms, allowing plants and microorganisms to uptake them freely. Once inside organisms, they tend to accumulate over time as they cannot be subjected to metabolic breakdown. Despite being the most essential nutrients for plant growth, nitrogen (N) and phosphorus (P) can also become soil contaminants once they occur in excess, which is a common occurrence in agricultural soils (Torrent et al. 2007). Excessive use of synthetic fertilizers can pollute groundwater through leaching and surface water bodies through runoff, causing eutrophication and/or other health and environmental consequences (Yaron et al. 2012). In addition, some heavy metals are also known to pollute soils through contaminated fertilizers (Brevik 2009).

Organic pollutants are carbon-based compounds derived mainly from anthropogenic activities with a negligible amount coming from natural events such as volcanic eruptions and forest fires. Organic pollutants of synthetic origin originate from pesticides, industrial chemicals (polychlorinated biphenyls, PCBs), and other volatile organic compounds. In contrast to inorganic pollutants and their potential impacts, the fate of organic pollutants and their effects on human health and the environment are less known (FAO and UNEP 2021). The persistence, fate, and mobility of pesticides in soils depend on various processes, including sorption–desorption, volatilization, leaching, and biological degradation (Arias-Estévez et al. 2008).

Polycyclic aromatic hydrocarbons (PAHs) are semi-volatile organic pollutants in soils viz anthracene, fluoranthene, naphthalene, and pyrene (Lerda 2011). Use of sewage sludge, mining, and combustion of coal, gas, and oil are known sources of PAHs (Aichner et al. 2013; Keyte et al. 2013). Their low water solubility and slow transfer rates from solid to liquid phase can result in poor natural attenuation through microbial processes and long retention in soils. However, once they enter the soil environment, they can be attenuated or degraded by various physicochemical and biological processes (Okere and Semple 2012).

Persistent organic pollutants (POPs) are chemical compounds that could persist in the environment and bioaccumulate in food chains (UNEP 2001). They include both chlorinated and brominated aromatics and are mainly of industrial origin. The pesticide (dichloro-diphenyl-trichloroethane [DDT]), which is still used to control mosquitoes in some parts of the world, is also a known POP. Soil is the major sink for POPs, and they form stable bonds with organic matter particles and become non-extractable. However, some soil environmental changes can modify their partitioning rates, thus converting them to readily extractable fractions (Guzzella et al. 2011).

9.4 Emerging Pollutants

Emerging pollutants are synthetic or naturally occurring chemicals that have become known in recent times. Due to their emerging nature, any work related to their monitoring, even at a local scale, is scarce (Geissen et al. 2015). Just like other soil pollutants, they are known or at least suspected to inflict adverse environmental and health consequences (Sauvé and Desrosiers 2014). Pharmaceuticals, hormones, micro- and nanoplastics, and even bacteria and viruses are considered as emerging soil pollutants (Rodríguez-Eugenio et al. 2018). In addition, personal care products, phthalates, plasticizers, and nanomaterial are also considered as emerging soil pollutants. Despite their potentially negative consequences on human health and the environment, the information related to their fate, bioavailability, distribution, and toxicities is not well understood (Pietroiusti et al. 2018). According to the global projections, there will be an approximately 3.4% annual increase in the production of emerging pollutants till 2030 (Rodríguez-Eugenio et al. 2018).

Pharmaceuticals and personal care products were identified as soil contaminants only recently, following some new health issues. Once they enter the environment through unwarranted waste disposal mechanisms, these contaminants cannot be eliminated effectively using conventional techniques (Miege et al. 2009). The land application of municipal sludge is known to be the main route of introducing these pollutants to agricultural soils (Wu et al. 2010). Furthermore, the heavy use of antimicrobial drugs in humans and livestock eventually led to the development of resistant bacterial strains and genes, causing even more serious health issues (Sun et al. 2018).

Micro- and nanoplastics, also categorized as another emerging soil contaminant, are derived from fragmentation and weathering of plastic products, where soil considered as their prime sink (Bancone et al. 2020). They found relatively in small concentrations, but the lack of knowledge of their impacts and fate in soils brings many challenges to scientists. In recent times, relatively more studies have been conducted on microplastics and their potential impacts on human and environmental health (Han et al. 2020; Azizi et al. 2021; Bai et al. 2021; Huang et al. 2021). The formulation of standard methodologies to detect their levels in the environment is still ongoing. These miniscule particles may also be able to end up in humans and other organisms through various sources, including water and food, causing health scares (da Costa et al. 2016; Ding et al. 2019; Ragusa et al. 2021).

Plasticizers are chemical additives used to enhance the flexibility of polymer-based products. Due to their hazardous nature, the use of plasticizers has since been strictly regulated. In addition, plasticizers are also used in lubricating oils, paints, automobile parts, perfumes, food packaging, etc. (Rodríguez-Eugenio et al. 2018). Man-made nanoparticles are another emerging soil pollutant that needs further investigation. They can be present in paints, cosmetic products, textiles, paper plastics, and food (Fiorino 2010). Due to their emerging nature, the information related to their solubility, transformations, and interactions that determine their fates in soils is still limited (Liang et al. 2013).

9.5 Fates of Soil Pollutants

Soils have an inherent ability to filter, buffer, and transform soil pollutants into other forms as a part of their natural cleansing process (Blum 2005). Hence, once pollutants enter soils, they undergo various physicochemical and biochemical reactions to transform them into other forms, leading to either reduction in their toxicity or degradation. These processes are governed mainly by both soil characteristics (such as soil texture, soil organic matter, pH, moisture, and temperature) and pollutant itself (size, molecular status, solubility, charge distribution, etc.) (Gevao et al. 2000). Some processes transform soil pollutants either into more available forms, enabling plants and microorganisms to absorb, or into less available forms.

Earlier, soil pollutants had been quantified for standard guidelines and regulatory frameworks based on their total contents rather than their available fractions. However, once it was realized that the total contents can lead to overestimation of the issue and cause futile expenses to introduce costly remediation techniques (Meers et al. 2007). It is also known that organisms are influenced by the "available fraction" of soil pollutants (Lanno et al. 2004), but not the fraction considered as "unavailable." Therefore, the "available fraction" of soil contaminants has since been taken into consideration when preparing risk-based regulatory frameworks to assess soil pollutant levels and introduce mitigatory measures (Harmsen 2007; Kim et al. 2015). Nonetheless, the precise definition of "bioavailability" across different scientific disciplines is also debatable. Despite many definitions (Lanno et al. 2004), the "bioavailability" generally represents the fraction of the chemical that is readily available for the uptake by organisms. Environmental scientists define "bioavailability" as the accessibility of a solid-bound chemical for assimilation with a probable toxicity (Alexander 2000). The reliable and standard methods to measure the bioavailable fraction of soil contaminants also have their own merits and drawbacks (Kim et al. 2015).

Of many chemically, physically, and biologically driven transformations of soil pollutants that take place in the soil environment, microorganisms play a pivotal role. In the bioremediation technique, microorganisms act on soil pollutants, destroying or reducing their toxicities with the help of their catabolic processes. Therefore, the degradation of soil pollutants with the help of native and exotic microorganisms is considered as an efficient and low-cost technique for remediating soil pollutants.

9.6 Why Microbes?

Microorganisms play a vital role in biogeochemical cycles mainly with the help of their intense enzymatic capacity (Ehrlich 1998; Alexander 2000). Soil microorganisms consider organic and/or inorganic pollutants as their substrates to generate nutrients and energy for their own growth. In nature, soil microorganisms face a limited amount of utilizable carbon to generate energy for their growth and survival. Thus, when they come across new carbon sources in the form of an organic pollutant, they act on them to generate energy (Annweiler et al. 2000). In addition to act as a carbon source, soil pollutants also provide nutrients for microorganisms such as nitrogen, sulfur, phosphorus, and even metals (Stamper et al. 2002). Moreover, some organic pollutants may inflict toxic effects on microbial cells (Rodriguez et al. 2018). In such situations, microorganisms alter the properties of these organic pollutants through their enzymatic activities, transforming them into less-toxic forms (Hamme 2004). Some organic pollutants that bear a resemblance to the natural substrate of the microbial enzyme system allow microbes to act on the soil pollutant in place of their actual substrate.

Microorganisms act on pollutants mainly through extracellular/intracellular/membrane-bound enzymes, chelating agents, vesicles, and cell surface agents (Hamme 2004). Biodegradation is known as the catalytic reduction of pollutants by microbial enzymes, thus splitting bonds and converting soil pollutants into inorganic forms (Basak et al. 2021; Bhatt et al. 2021). However, when metabolic activities did not move toward mineralization, the resulting products may possess different characteristics in terms of their bioavailability (biodegradability and toxicity) and mobility within soils. As a result, once microorganisms act on soil pollutants, the toxicity of pollutants can be reduced by transforming them into less-available forms for uptake through complexation with minerals or polymerization (Bressler and Fedorak 2001). In addition to reactions catalyzed by enzymes, microbes are also known to possess genes that are responsible for metabolizing a given pollutant (Whyte et al. 2002). Some microbes have the metabolic potential to degrade more than one pollutant, while others possess more than one group of enzymes (extra- or intracellular) to metabolize a particular substrate (Van Hamme et al. 2003). Such capabilities allow soil microorganisms to act on pollutants efficiently and transform them into other forms. Recent studies confirmed that a "consortium of bacteria" or "biofilms" is more effective in acting on organic and inorganic pollutants than a single microbial strain (Li et al. 2022).

Despite all these enzymatic and metabolic capabilities, the biodegradable capacity of soil pollutants can be hindered due to various other intrinsic and extrinsic factors including insufficient substrate and cofactor and lack of appropriate metabolic machinery (van Hamme 2004). If the pollutant is naturally occurring or else closely resembles its natural substrate, microorganisms tend to biodegrade it easily. If the pollutant is a "xenobiotic," the existing mechanisms may not be able to fully accommodate the novel properties of the xenobiotic. In order to act on such pollutants, microorganisms possess catabolic enzymes that catalyze reactions and also additional mechanisms to protect from possible toxic effects. These additional mechanisms include chemotaxis, the production of biosurfactants, modifications to cell surface characteristics, and energy-consumed uptake and efflux. In instances, the appropriate microorganisms may not present in the environment in order to biodegrade the particular soil contaminant/s (Daly 2000; Fredrickson et al. 2000). The enzyme/s involved in the biodegradation process will only be expressed when the contaminant or the cofactor levels are above a certain threshold level (Van Hamme 2004). Moreover, higher the concentration of the pollutant, it is more likely that the microorganism is unable to act on it and defend its toxicity. In order to avoid these obstacles, microorganisms have developed various other mechanisms (i.e. chemotaxis, cell surface characteristics, etc.) to improve their chances of biodegrading environmental pollutants.

9.7 Organic Soil Pollutants

Microorganisms are responsible for degrading most organic matter in soils, releasing carbon dioxide, minerals, and water as end products. Similarly, microorganisms act on organic pollutants in soils through transformation, mineralization, or complexation, thus transforming pollutants into available or unavailable forms. In recent years, more emphasis has been placed on soil organic pollutants such as organochlorine pesticides, polybrominated diphenyl ethers (PBDEs), halohydrocarbons, and polycyclic aromatic hydrocarbons (PAHs), which are collectively known as POPs (Ren et al. 2018) and known for their high toxic effects at low concentrations (Tang et al. 2014, 2016).

Microbes play an important role in remediating POPs through their degradation process, but it is often limited by their low bioavailability. Microorganisms absorb POPs through cellular membranes with the help of sorption/desorption processes (Ehlers and Luthy 2003; Ren et al. 2018). When pollutants come across soil conditions that make them poorly available (such as strongly binding soil organic matter and minerals), microorganisms tend to adjust their characteristics in terms of morphology, physiology, and behaviour to fit into these environmental conditions (Fester et al. 2014).

In terms of morphological adaptations, fungal mycelia facilitate efficient mobilization and distribution of soil pollutants (Furuno et al. 2012; Fester et al. 2014), while others modify their cell surface characteristics (composition and surface charges) in order to increase their absorption power under low-soluble soil pollutants, sometimes even by

70-fold (Wick et al. 2002; de Carvalho et al. 2009). Microbes also tend to alter their cell wall composition to enhance its potential of adhesion when in contact with pollutants of low solubility. Some microbes (mostly fungi) have developed a multidimensional arrangement in order to increase the area of contact with the pollutants (Furuno et al. 2012; Otto et al. 2016).

In terms of physiological adjustments, microbes expedite the rate of transferring pollutants by decreasing the transport distance or increasing the chemical gradient that eventually speeds up the desorption process (Wick et al. 2002). Moreover, microorganisms discharge surface-active molecules, known as biosurfactants, to improve the bioavailability of soil pollutants by decreasing the interfacial tension while increasing the mobility and solubility (Adrion et al. 2016). Some microbes secrete electron shuttles (i.e. favin, mononucleotide, riboflavin, etc.), thus aiding the redox biotransformation (Yu et al. 2015). All these physiological adaptations facilitate microbes to have direct contact with pollutants, thus improving their bioavailability (Ren et al. 2018). Chemotaxis and mobility modes are some of the behavioral adaptations shown by microbes to improve their access to contaminants (Fester et al. 2014) and to increase their bioavailability (Krell et al. 2013).

Using these morphological, physiological, and behavioral adaptations, adsorbed pollutants can be made available for microorganisms through two potential means (Chen and Ding 2012). They are (i) biosurfactant-assisted release of soil-adsorbed pollutants and (ii) direct degradation of adsorbed pollutants by intracellular/extracellular enzymes. Research has shown that microbes biodegrade soil pollutants more easily when they are present in soil solution than when they are in their adsorbed state (Megharaj et al. 2011; Zhu et al. 2016). However, once the readily available fraction is exhausted, the adsorbed pollutants can also be made available for microorganisms to act on (Yang et al. 2009).

9.7.1 Chemotaxis

Research into soil organic pollutants revealed that chemotactic movement of bacteria increases their bioavailability, which facilitates the process of bioremediation (Krell et al. 2012). Chemotaxis involves both chemoattraction and chemorepellent reactions in contact with pollutants, where chemoattraction tends to increase the bioavailability of organic pollutants while chemorepellent decreases it. The chemoattraction process enhances the bioavailability of soil pollutants through various microbial-driven mechanisms (Marx and Aitken 2000; Law and Aitken 2003). Studies have revealed that bacterial species like *Rhizobium* sp., *Bradyrhizobium* sp., *Pseudomonas* sp., *Azospirillum* sp., *Ralstonia* sp., *Burkholderia* sp., and *Flavimonas oryzihabitans* show chemoattraction potential toward environmental pollutants such as toluene, naphthalene and their derivatives, explosives, aliphatic hydrocarbons, and herbicides (Leungsakul et al. 2005; Liu et al. 2009). In most instances, these bacterial species use these pollutants as a source of carbon or energy to power their own metabolic processes. Some bacterial strains show chemorepellant responses toward soil pollutants that are toxic for their growth, thus transforming them into less available forms. These repulsive responses shown by bacteria are considered as a part of their survival strategy to lessen the harmful effects of toxic pollutants (Krell et al. 2012). These highly complex chemotactic responses are mediated by a concerted action of chemoreceptors, which are plasmid- or genome-encoded signaling proteins (Beilen et al. 2001). Comparative studies have been carried out to test the ability of microorganisms to degrade soil pollutants through their chemotactic approaches (Krell et al. 2012). Studies also confirmed the close link between the biodegradation and chemotaxis as even structurally similar non-substrate compounds do not act as chemoattractants (Krell et al. 2012).

9.7.2 Cell Surface Properties

Properties of the microbial cell surfaces are important determinant of interactions between microorganisms and soil pollutants, as they are the interface (via transport and exchanges) through which microbes interact with the environment (Van Hemme et al. 2004). Organic soil pollutants are generally hydrophobic (Dewangan et al. 2021), thus microorganisms employ various mechanisms to access them. Microbes have the potential of altering their cell surface properties such as surface charge density, wettability, roughness, and topography either to increase access or to avoid pollutants (Krasowska and Sigler 2014; Zheng et al. 2021).

9.7.3 Biosurfactants

Microorganisms release biosurfactants, amphipathic molecules with a molecular weight of 500–1500 Da, to enhance the bioavailability of pollutants while serving many other physiological functions (Roane et al. 2015). Biosurfactants increase pollutant bioavailability through their involvement in reducing surface and interfacial tensions between the two immiscible phases (Nikolova and Gutierrez 2021). The surfactant-driven facilitation of solubilization or desorption was observed not only with organic pollutants but with metals as well (Christofi and Ivshina 2002). Surfactants are located on cell surfaces or secreted into the medium, thus assisting the uptake of hydrophobic pollutants through direct cellular contact or micellarization (Ward 2010). In the event that the pollutant is too toxic, biosurfactant micelles may inhibit the microbial uptake of contaminants, indicating that their action is also determined by several other factors such as environmental conditions and pollutant properties. (van Hamme 2004; Ward 2010). Soils tend to bind surfactants strongly, thus making the desorption process of pollutants more complex; thus the use of commercially available biosurfactants in the bioremediation of aquifers faces many challenges (Ji et al. 2021).

9.7.4 Pesticides

With the intensification of agriculture, the use of synthetic pesticides has been increased dramatically over time. Some fractions of pesticides tend to remain in soils as a major soil pollutant, and once exposed, they cause serious health concerns in human beings (Heard et al. 2017; Kim et al. 2017). Based on their chemical composition, synthetic pesticides are categorized into four main groups: organochlorines, organophosphates, carbamates, and pyrethrins and pyrethroids (Raffa and Chiampo 2021). During the microbial-driven degradation process, pesticides are fully mineralized or transformed into other products driven by intra- and extracellular enzymes such as hydrolases, peroxidases, and oxygenases. According to Raffa and Chiampo (2021), the trajectory of the enzyme-driven biotransformation can be divided into three phases.

1) Pesticides are transformed into less-toxic products through oxidation, reduction, or hydrolysis reactions.
2) The products of Phase I are converted into highly soluble sugars and amino acids.
3) Convert the Phase II metabolites into less-toxic secondary conjugates.

In bacterial degradation, sometimes the metabolites produced can cause additional issues than their original pesticide. The hydrolyzed product (3,5,6-trichloro-2-pyridinol) of chlorpyrifos (an organophosphate) possesses higher water solubility than that of chlorpyrifos, resulting in widespread soil and water contamination (Raffa and Chiampo 2021). Research also noted that a consortium of bacteria can be more effective in the biodegradation of pesticides in comparison to a single strain, perhaps through the reduction of the accumulation of intermediary products (Jariyal et al. 2018; Doolotkeldieva et al. 2021). In addition to bacteria, fungi also show some superior ability of degrading pesticides due to their inherent attribute of producing many enzymes (Oliveira et al. 2015) and high resistance to pollutants (Purnomo et al. 2020). The mineralization process also converts pesticides into their ultimate inorganic products including carbon dioxide, minerals, and water. Both biodegradation and mineralization processes are influenced by many factors including the type of the microbe, soil properties, microbial population, and the type of the pollutant (Nguyen et al. 2018; Raffa and Chiampo 2021). For example, low mineralization of glyphosate in acidic soils is either due to the formation of strong linkages with carboxylic or phosphonic acid groups of the pesticide (leading to reducing its bioavailability) or due to aluminum toxicity on soil microbes (Nguyen et al. 2018). When the pollutant is not supporting the growth of microbes, pesticides are transformed into other compounds with the help of microorganisms and their enzymes (hydrolytic enzymes, transferases, oxidases, and reductases) using a chain of reactions, which is known as "co-metabolism" (Ma et al. 2014).

9.7.5 Petroleum Hydrocarbons

Contamination caused by petroleum hydrocarbons is considered as a serious environmental issue as they can be harmful for many life forms. Primary soil pollution by petroleum hydrocarbons can lead to the secondary pollution of groundwater and air, causing even further detrimental actions (Hu et al. 2013; Galitskaya et al. 2021). Contamination by crude oil is common due to its widespread use, dumping, and accidental spills. Petroleum products are a mixture of a wide range of high and low molecular weight hydrocarbons and consist of saturated and branched alkenes, alkanes, and homo- and heterocyclic naphthenes. They also contain different functional groups (ethers, carboxylic acids, etc.) and aromatic molecules (asphaltenes, resins, etc.) (Srivastava and Singh 2019). Broadly, petroleum hydrocarbons can be divided into aliphatics, aromatics, asphaltenes, and resins, and the latter two groups show the lowest biodegradable ability.

Once they enter the soil environment, they undergo numerous transformations *viz*., physical (dispersion), physicochemical (evaporation, dissolution, sorption), chemical (photo-oxidation), and biological (catabolism). Just like most other pollutants, microorganisms act on these petroleum hydrocarbons as an alternative source of carbon and energy, during which the toxic effects of petroleum hydrocarbons lessened. As a result, soil microorganisms are used in bioremediation techniques to eliminate petroleum hydrocarbons from soils. However, hydrocarbons can impose both direct (causing membrane dysfunctions, cell lysis, growth inhibition) and indirect (structure and function of populations driven by changes to soil properties) consequences on soil microbial communities (Fan et al. 2014). Therefore, despite some microbes showing the ability to biodegrade petroleum hydrocarbons, a majority of them cannot survive in soils contaminated with them, thus reducing their diversity and total biomass (Sutton et al. 2013). Nevertheless, microorganisms that possess hydrocarbon-tolerant and hydrocarbon-degrading abilities could survive and even proliferate under these polluted conditions (Chikere et al. 2011). Though hydrocarbons impose immediate negative impacts on the indigenous soil microorganisms, they also possess many adaptive mechanisms (producing spores and secondary metabolites, forming biofilms, etc.) to withstand those detrimental impacts (Blagodatskaya et al. 2007; Jia et al. 2017). The microorganisms with the ability of tolerating and degrading hydrocarbons demonstrate varying abilities and mechanisms in catabolizing petroleum hydrocarbons. A majority of them are using their ability to secrete extracellular enzymes to breakdown inorganic and organic pollutants (Tang et al. 2012), while others establish symbiotic relationships to aid the enzyme-catalyzed breakdown. The main pathway of microbial breakdown of hydrocarbons is under aerobic conditions. Nevertheless, some bacteria utilize hydrocarbons anaerobically as well (van Hamme et al. 2003; Widdel et al. 2010). While bacteria prefer to decompose aliphatic and aromatic compounds using very specific metabolic pathways, fungi degrade polycyclic aromatics with the help of nonspecific enzyme complexes (Harms et al. 2011; Galitskaya et al. 2021). In addition, environmental conditions, indigenous microbial composition and abundance, and soil physicochemical properties influence sorption and desorption of hydrocarbons in soils, thus in turn affecting their toxicity and bioavailability (Sutton et al. 2013; Liu et al. 2017).

9.8 Potentially Toxic Elements (Heavy Metals)

Due to the ambiguity in definitions, the general public believes that all "heavy metals" are toxic. In fact, some heavy metals in minute quantities such as copper (Cu), iron (Fe), aluminum (Al), nickel (Ni) play a vital role in life processes of organisms (Bruins et al. 2000). Some heavy metals such as cadmium (Cd), arsenic (As), lead (Pb) are relatively toxic and have no specific biological role in organisms. To avoid this vagueness, the elements that cause harmful effects on living organisms are categorized as "potentially toxic elements" (PTEs) (Pourret and Hursthouse 2019) or "toxic trace elements" (TTEs) (Niemeyer et al. 2012; Shen et al. 2016; Polyak et al. 2018). According to estimates, the concentration of "heavy metals" in soils could range from 1 to 100,000 mg/kg and can contaminate food chains, inflicting major issues both in animal and human health (Antoniadis et al. 2017). The fate of heavy metals is governed by both biotic and abiotic processes in soils (Zhang et al. 2020). In addition to abiotic factors (complexation, adsorption–desorption, precipitation–dissolution, etc.), microorganisms play a role in dissolving minerals directly or indirectly under both aerobic and anaerobic conditions (Kurek 2002). Indirectly, microbes have the ability to dissolve minerals due to their production of organic and inorganic acids. On the other hand, heavy metals inhibit the biodegradation of organic pollutants in soils causing heavy metal toxicity to microorganisms.

As the risks of PTEs are due to their available fractions, the mobility and bioavailability of PTEs in the soil environment are of great concern. Therefore, processes leading to immobilizing and stabilizing of PTEs are crucial in order to reduce their availability for plants, microbes, and humans (Park et al. 2011; Bolan et al. 2014). Microorganisms play a vital role in biogeochemical cycles of PTEs and also in the natural remediation of the environment polluted by them (Alm et al. 2003). When PTEs (will be known as heavy metals hereafter) are present in high concentrations, they are toxic for soil microorganisms. Therefore, in order to survive in the presence of PTEs, microorganisms display various mechanisms (extracellular barriers, efflux and re-oxidation of metal ions, and extracellular and intracellular sequestration) to reduce or tolerate their toxic effects (Alm et al. 2003; Gonzalez Henao and Ghneim-Herrera 2021).

There are varying mechanisms responsible for transforming heavy metals maintaining either their retention (sorption, precipitation, and complexation) or losses (plant uptake, leaching, and volatilization) in soils. All these reversible (i.e. adsorption/desorption and precipitation/dissolution) and irreversible (i.e. leaching, volatilization) reactions together with other soil properties and environmental factors will eventually determine the available metal fraction in the soil solution. Just like organic pollutants, microorganisms are unable to biodegrade heavy metal pollutants in soils. Nevertheless, microorganisms can alter/modify soil physicochemical features, which eventually defining the bioavailability of heavy metals. Though heavy metals are nonbiodegradable, they can transform into different oxidation states and form organic complexes depending on the soil physicochemical properties. As a result, the mobility and availability of heavy metals in the soil environment are largely governed by abiotic processes such as precipitation–dissolution, adsorption–desorption, complexation, redox reactions, and leaching (El-Naggar et al. 2019). These abiotic processes are driven by soil properties such as pH, ion exchange capacity, redox potential, electrical conductivity, organic matter, clay minerals, and bulk density, thus controlling the mobility of heavy metals in soils (Beiyuan et al. 2017). In addition, biotic factors such as microbial-driven transformation and immobilization and plant uptake are also considered as decisive but indirect factors in determining the bioavailability of heavy metals.

Heavy metals are present in the environment in different fractions viz exchangeable, bound (bound to carbonates, Fe and Mg oxides, organic matter, etc.), and residual (found in primary and secondary minerals) (Rinklebe and Shaheen 2014). Soil physicochemical properties such as pH, clay, redox potential, and organic matter are considered major factors controlling the bioavailability of heavy metals (Peijnenburg et al. 2002), thus their toxicities. Some metals tend to form complexes with humus, clay minerals, and Fe and Mn hydrous oxides, while others form soluble salts such as calcium carbonate (Morgan 2013). Most sorption processes of heavy metals are pH dependent, thus the sorption is highest in alkaline soils, while acidic conditions favor the opposite process (desorption), thus increasing the bioavailability of metals.

Microorganisms, though they cannot biodegrade heavy metals readily, play an important role in remediating them in soils through various direct and ancillary mechanisms with the sole intention of tolerating their toxic effects. Unlike organic pollutants, microorganisms rely on detoxification and immobilization processes to reduce heavy metal toxicities and to impede their mobility in soils (Roane et al. 2001). Microorganisms also have the ability to sequester, precipitate, biosorb, and transform heavy metals from one oxidation state to another (Yin et al. 2019; Rizvi et al. 2020). Through various mechanisms, microorganisms are able to remove heavy metals from soils or to convert them into less-toxic forms (Saha et al. 2022). They are

1) Reduction – microorganisms reduce toxic forms of heavy metals using biological agents (i.e. conversion of Hg^{2+} to Hg^0, Cr^{6+} to Cr^{3+})
2) Precipitation – heavy metals bind with chelating agents and precipitate, thus reducing their bioavailability
3) Intracellular assimilation – microbes absorb/accumulate heavy metals in the cell to protect them from toxic effects
4) Solubility/mobilization – microorganisms produce siderophores, chelators, and organic acids to increase the solubility and mobility of heavy metals
5) Immobilization – heavy metals get immobilized by microorganisms through their extracellular sequestration to control their toxicities
6) Complexation – heavy metals bind with extra polymeric substances (EPS) forming complexes
7) Membrane biosorption – sequester by bacterial cells

Through these mechanisms, contaminants can be transformed into less toxic or immobilized forms (Smets and Pritchard 2003).

Microorganisms also can readily react on heavy metals, mediating the "speciation" process with the help of their metabolic reactions (Bolan et al. 2013). Speciation can enhance the bioavailability of heavy metals, thus facilitating the uptake process by living organisms (Olaniran et al. 2013). For example, microorganisms with arsM genes (Hg-methylating bacteria) transform HgS into methylmercury, making them available for plant uptake (Graham et al. 2012), causing toxic effects. The microbial-driven speciation is also used traditionally in bioremediation techniques to minimize the impacts of PTEs and to enhance the metal stability, and in turn reducing the bioavailability of heavy metals for uptake (Saha et al. 2022).

Microorganisms also use their oxidation and reduction reactions to facilitate the speciation and the mobility of heavy metals such as As, Cr, Hg, and Se in soils (Bolan and Duraisamy 2003; Banks et al. 2006). Metals are less available in their higher oxidation states, while the solubility of metalloids (elements possessing intermediate properties between those of metals and solid nonmetals) depends on both the oxidation state and the ionic form (Ross 1994). Arsenic (As) is a redox-active metalloid whose toxicity and mobility depend strongly on its oxidation state (Jiang et al. 2009). In soils, the bacterial-driven oxidation of As^{3+} into As^{5+} makes the heavy metal less mobile (Battaglia-Brunet et al. 2002; Bachate et al. 2012). In contrast to arsenic, the oxidation of Cr^{3+} to Cr^{6+} enhances the mobility and bioavailability of Cr, though this oxidation is mainly driven by abiotic factors including oxidizing agents (Seshadri et al. 2015).

Microorganisms tend to secrete a variety of metabolites as a result of their intense metabolic processes, and they play a critical role in facilitating their acts on soil pollutants (Coelho et al. 2015; Dixit et al. 2015; Ahemad 2019). For example, bacteria and fungi secrete siderophores, low molecular weight organic compounds with a primary function to act as a chelating agent of ferric ions that reduce metal bioavailability in contaminated soils. Recent studies noted that siderophores have the potential of binding with various other metals and metalloids (Roskova et al. 2022). In addition to their distinctive ability to solubilize and mobilize heavy metals and metalloids, siderophores also mediate the production of reactive oxygen species, thus assisting the degradation of organic contaminants (Roskova et al. 2022). Some bacterial cells tend to alter their morphology to increase the production of siderophores in order to assist the intercellular accumulation of metals (Manoj et al. 2020).

A gram-negative, sulfate-reducing bacterium, *Desulfovibrio desulfuricans* transforms sulfate to hydrogen sulfate and reacts with heavy metals like Cd and Zn to form insoluble metal sulfides (Chibuike and Obiora 2014).

Microbes also possess negatively charged functional groups (i.e. phosphate, hydroxyl, carbonyl, etc.) in their cell walls that rapidly bind with toxic metal ions (Dixit et al. 2015). Fungi too show bioremediation ability of metal ions through similar mechanisms as bacteria (accumulation, transformation, precipitation, etc.) (Ayangbenro and Babalola 2017).

Recent studies revealed that consortia of fungi and bacteria (or fungal-bacteria biofilms) have shown some superior potential in acting on heavy metal pollutants in soils over single species/strains (Hassan et al. 2020; Njoku et al. 2020). Biofilms, which are more tolerant of contaminants and abiotic stress conditions, together with their various catabolic pathways, act more efficiently on soil pollutants, breaking down complex molecules, mobilizing metal ions, and increasing their bioaccumulation (Sharma 2021).

9.8.1 Rhizosphere Microorganisms

The soil–plant interface, known as the "rhizosphere," is the region where complex interactions take place between its resident organisms and plants, leading to stimulatory effect on the growth of plants. The rhizosphere also acts as a sink for soil contaminants (Seshadri et al. 2015). The rhizospheric microorganisms seem playing a crucial role in heavy metal bioavailability in polluted soils (Mishra et al. 2017), which is known as "rhizoremediation" (Kuiper et al. 2004). Rhizosphere microorganisms either bind metal ions on to their cell surfaces or absorb them into cells, making heavy metals less available for other soil organisms (Ehrlich 1997). In soils, rhizospheric microbes are capable of modifying speciation, toxicity, mobility, dissolution, and deterioration of heavy metals (Gadd 2010). However, their ability to transform metals in the rhizosphere environment is largely controlled by physicochemical properties of soils, type and concentration of metal species, metabolic activity, and diversity of microbes (Kong and Glick 2017; Mishra et al. 2017).

Plant growth promoting bacteria (PGPB) secrete various organic acids, chelators, enzymes, hormones, and polymeric compounds that stimulate the plant growth and its survival (Ma et al. 2011; Fasani et al. 2018). In addition to their growth-promoting ability, organic acids decline the soil pH in the immediate vicinity of the root system, thus increasing the metal bioavailability. In contrast, polymeric compounds help to decrease the mobility of heavy metals (Chen et al. 2017). Chelators (siderophores) enhance metal bioavailability through their metal-binding ability, thus improving root-shoot translocation and metal uptake (Yan et al. 2020). Leguminous plants inoculated with PGPB have demonstrated a higher efficiency of metal accumulation under low-contaminated soils in comparison to their un-inoculated counterpart (Checcucci et al. 2017; Saadani et al. 2019).

Arbuscular mycorrhizal fungi (AMF) form the most exclusive symbiotic association in most terrestrial plants on earth. Studies revealed that AMF was found in highly disturbed as well as in highly polluted ecosystems (Yan et al. 2020), indicating that AMF-colonized plants seem to have the ability to tolerate heavy metal contaminants (Xu et al. 2012). The evidence also confirms that some mycorrhizal plants increase metal phytostabilization through metal sequestration by roots and hyphae (Saha et al. 2020), hence making them less available for other soil organisms to uptake. Based on these promising findings, in recent times, relatively more studies have been carried out to explore the role of AMF on heavy metal pollutants (Yan et al. 2020; Solìs-Ramos et al. 2021; Zhang and Chen 2021).

9.9 Microplastics

Plastics are organic polymers produced from nonrenewable sources with exclusive characteristics (Worm et al. 2017). Due to its many uses, plastic consumption has increased dramatically over the years, with a predicted threefold increase by 2050 from the usage of 359 million tons between 2008 and 2018 (Chia et al. 2020). Though plastics are apparently nonbiodegradable, they can degrade at a slow pace (ranging from 10 to 1000 years) depending on the environmental conditions, type of plastic, and treatments (Othman et al. 2021). Therefore, over time, plastics disintegrate into smaller particles known as "microplastics." In addition to being a soil pollutant itself, microplastics also have the potential to act as a carrier of many other types of co-contaminants such as pharmaceutical pollutants, heavy metals, and nanomaterials (Chatterjee and Sharma 2019).

Microplastics enter the environment through many human-mediated activities (He et al. 2019; Ding et al. 2020) and are known to inflict many detrimental impacts on human health and functions and other terrestrial and marine life (Liu et al. 2017; de Souza Machado et al. 2018; Panebianco et al. 2019). In particular, microplastics are known to impact plants by affecting their nutrient uptake and growth by modifying soil characteristics (Khalid et al. 2020; Othman et al. 2021; Weerasinghe and Madawala 2022). Also, plants tend to accumulate microplastics in their bodies causing oxidative damage through antioxidative enzyme activity (Yu et al. 2020). Moreover, microplastics affect animals and are known to cause ecotoxicities (Chagas et al. 2020; Cheng et al. 2020). Humans are prone to the detrimental impacts of microplastics through contaminated food chains, inflicting inflammatory responses, neurotoxic effects, and cancerous growth in humans (Hwang et al. 2019; Ju et al. 2019).

Microorganisms that tend to survive in microplastic-contaminated soils are showing many adaptations to tolerate stressful conditions incurred by the pollutant (Guan and Liu 2020; Yang et al. 2020). While they perform these stress responses to withstand microplastic pollution, enzymes and their activities play a major role in regulating cell functions in microorganisms (Cheng et al. 2021). These regulatory enzymes are involved not only in cell functions but also in degrading other pollutants in soils, including microplastics. They depolymerize the structure of microplastics to form monomers, eventually utilizing them as a carbon source for energy production (Gong et al. 2018; Kawai et al. 2019). According to studies, there are many enzyme groups that are capable of depolymerizing microplastics viz oxidases, amidases, laccases, hydrolases, and proxidases (Ashter 2016). Although deploymerization is known to take place with the help of extracellular enzymes, the complete mineralization of microplastics is still questionable and less explored.

As a solution to address microplastic pollution and its consequences, more focus is drawn lately on biodegradable plastics. Biodegradable plastics are made of petrochemicals and bio-based sources such as corn starch, lignin, and cellulose. Though its uses are limited, at the end of their life cycle, plastics biodegrade and are converted into water, carbon dioxide, and biomass with the help of microorganisms. The specific conditions needed for the biodegradation process of biodegradable microplastics are not always available under natural conditions. Therefore, if the conditions for biodegradation process are not met, then both plastics and biodegradable plastics will have similar longevities in the environment, thus causing comparable environmental impacts (Wei et al. 2021). Some suggests that biodegradable microplastics act as even stronger vectors of pollutants and microorganisms due to their persistence nature in comparison to microplastics (Zuo et al. 2019; Wang et al. 2021).

9.9.1 Nanomaterials

According to the European Commission States, nanomaterials (NM) can be defined as materials that are measured, at least one of the three dimensions, between 1 and 100 nm. Particles with all three dimensions that are in the nanoscale are known as nanoparticles (NP). These NMs can possess exclusive physical and chemical characteristics (extra reactivity, increased subcellular level transport, and interactions), thus may impose greater risks in both aquatic and terrestrial ecosystems compared to many other soil pollutants, causing serious impacts on organisms (Lead et al. 2018). These NMs can undergo several transformations and reach the environment as soil pollutants. As they are novel materials, the knowledge on their behavior in the environment is still scarce. If NMs reach soils in large amounts, they may pose a serious threat. However, due to lack of studies on NMs and NPs, their mobility can be predicted from naturally occurring NPs, which are known as colloids. Colloids are naturally occurring particles in soils possessing a spherical diameter between 1 and 1000 nm. According to many reviews, detachment and attachment of NPs are the key processes observed to define their mobility in soils (Klaine et al. 2008; Tourinho et al. 2012; Batley et al. 2013).

Their novel characteristics may not necessarily imply that they impose unusual behaviors in aquatic and terrestrial ecosystems. Loureiro et al. (2018) predict that microorganisms have the potential to initiate modifications as NP coatings such as citrate, gum Arabic, and PVP (polyvinylpyrrolidone) consist of simple organic molecules that can serve as a substrate for them. As a result, the surface coatings of NPs with these compounds may degrade rapidly in the environment. Others provide evidence to suggest that rhizosphere microorganisms may also influence the functionalization of NPs (Kirschling et al. 2011). Furthermore, studies confirm that arbuscular mycorrhizal colonization (AMF) plays no significant role in Au NP uptake from soils, indicating the zero influence on its bioavailability (Judy et al. 2012).

9.10 A Final Inference

With the growing populations and ever-increasing industrialization and agricultural activities, various soil pollutants have been introduced into the environment over the years, causing detrimental impacts on all life processes either directly or indirectly. The role of microorganisms in determining the solubility, availability, and transport of soil pollutants has gained attention from the scientists. Over time, information has been gathered to highlight the decisive role played by microorganisms in alleviating the toxic effects of soil pollutants by altering their bioavailability. The metabolic capacity of microorganisms plays a critical role in modifying the bioavailability of pollutants in soils. In addition, they also use various direct and indirect mechanisms to reduce the toxic effects of soil pollutants by reducing their bioavailability, mobility, and sometimes even transforming them into harmless forms. Further, microorganisms evolved many strategies to tolerate heavy metal toxicities, as well as other strategies to detoxify them. More studies are needed to reveal the molecular-level mechanisms behind these strategies that lead to changes in the bioavailability of heavy metals. This information can be used to design remediation interventions in the future.

Environmental factors also determine the action of microorganisms on soil pollutants. This information has long been used in introducing bioremediation operations to contaminated sites. Most studies and on-site trials have been conducted using a single microbial strain or species. However, recent studies confirm more promising outcomes with consortia of microorganisms or biofilms, as they can enhance their metabolic activities, and their collective actions on soil pollutants far better than single microbial strain/species due to their unique ability to tolerate abiotic stresses. Understanding of the role of microorganisms in emerging pollutants and in determining their mobility and fates in the soil environment is lacking, necessitating further attention from scientists.

References

Abatenh, E., Gizaw, B., Tsegaye, Z., and Wassie, M. (2017). The role of microorganisms in bioremediation: a review. *Open Journal of Environmental Biology* 2 (1): 38–46.

Adrion, A.C., Singleton, D.R., Nakamura, J. et al. (2016). Improving polycyclic aromatic hydrocarbon biodegradation in contaminated soil through low-level surfactant addition after conventional bioremediation. *Environmental Engineering Science* 33 (9): 659–670.

Ahemad, M. (2019). Remediation of metalliferous soils through the heavy metal resistant plant growth promoting bacteria: paradigms and prospects. *Arabian Journal of Chemistry* 12 (7): 1365–1377.

Aichner, B., Bussian, B., Lehnik-Habrink, P., and Hein, S. (2013). Levels and spatial distribution of persistent organic pollutants in the environment: a case study of German forest soils. *Environmental Science & Technology* 47 (22): 12703–12714.

Alexander, M. (2000). Aging, bioavailability, and overestimation of risk from environmental pollutants. *Environmental Science & Technology* 34 (20): 4259–4265.

Alm, E.W., Burke, J., and Spain, A. (2003). Fecal indicator bacteria are abundant in wet sand at freshwater beaches. *Water Research* 37 (16): 3978–3982.

Annweiler, E., Richnow, H.H., Antranikian, G. et al. (2000). Naphthalene degradation and incorporation of naphthalene-derived carbon into biomass by the thermophile *Bacillus thermoleovorans*. *Applied and Environmental Microbiology* 66 (2): 518–523.

Antoniadis, V., Levizou, E., Shaheen, S.M. et al. (2017). Trace elements in the soil–plant interface: phytoavailability, translocation, and phytoremediation: a review. *Earth-Science Reviews* 171: 621–645.

Arias-Estévez, M., López-Periago, E., Martínez-Carballo, E. et al. (2008). The mobility and degradation of pesticides in soils and the pollution of groundwater resources. *Agriculture, Ecosystems & Environment* 123 (4): 247–260.

Ashter, S.A. (2016). Types of biodegradable polymers. *Introduction to Bioplastic Engineering* 81–151.

Ayangbenro, A.S. and Babalola, O.O. (2017). A new strategy for heavy metal polluted environments: a review of microbial biosorbents. *International Journal of Environmental Research and Public Health* 14 (1): 94.

Azizi, S.M.M., Hai, F.I., Lu, W. et al. (2021). A review of mechanisms underlying the impacts of (nano) microplastics on anaerobic digestion. *Bioresource Technology* 329: 124894.

Bachate, S.P., Khapare, R.M., and Kodam, K.M. (2012). Oxidation of arsenite by two β-proteobacteria isolated from soil. *Applied Microbiology and Biotechnology* 93 (5): 2135–2145.

Bai, Z., Wang, N., and Wang, M. (2021). Effects of microplastics on marine copepods. *Ecotoxicology and Environmental Safety* 217: 112243.

Bancone, C.E., Turner, S.D., and Ivar do Sul, J. A., and Rose, N. L. (2020). The paleoecology of microplastic contamination. *Frontiers in Environmental Science* 8: 574008.

Banks, M.K., Schwab, A.P., and Henderson, C. (2006). Leaching and reduction of chromium in soil as affected by soil organic content and plants. *Chemosphere* 62 (2): 255–264.

Basak, B., Patil, S.M., Saha, S. et al. (2021). Rapid recovery of methane yield in organic overloaded-failed anaerobic digesters through bioaugmentation with acclimatized microbial consortium. *Science of the Total Environment* 764: 144219.

Batley, G.E., Kirby, J.K., and McLaughlin, M.J. (2013). Fate and risks of nanomaterials in aquatic and terrestrial environments. *Accounts of Chemical Research* 46 (3): 854–862.

Battaglia-Brunet, F., Dictor, M.C., Garrido, F. et al. (2002). An arsenic(III)-oxidizing bacterial population: selection, characterization, and performance in reactors. *Journal of Applied Microbiology* 93 (4): 656–667.

van Beilen, J.B., Panke, S., Lucchini, S. et al. (2001). Analysis of Pseudomonas putida alkane-degradation gene clusters and flanking insertion sequences: evolution and regulation of the alk genes The EMBL accession numbers for the sequences reported in this paper are AJ245436 [P. putida (oleovorans) GPo1 alk gene clusters and flanking DNA],

AJ233397 (P. putida P1 alk gene clusters and flanking DNA), AJ249793 (P. putida P1 nahKJ genes), AJ249825 [P. putida (oleovorans) GPo1 16S RNA gene] and AJ271219 (P. putida P1 16S RNA gene). *Microbiology* 147 (6): 1621–1630.

Beiyuan, J., Awad, Y.M., Beckers, F. et al. (2017). Mobility and phytoavailability of As and Pb in a contaminated soil using pine sawdust biochar under systematic change of redox conditions. *Chemosphere* 178: 110–118.

Bhatt, P., Gangola, S., Bhandari, G. et al. (2021). New insights into the degradation of synthetic pollutants in contaminated environments. *Chemosphere* 268: 128827.

Biswas, B., Sarkar, B., Rusmin, R., and Naidu, R. (2015). Bioremediation of PAHs and VOCs: advances in clay mineral–microbial interaction. *Environment International* 85: 168–181.

Blagodatskaya, E.V., Blagodatsky, S.A., Anderson, T.H., and Kuzyakov, Y. (2007). Priming effects in Chernozem induced by glucose and N in relation to microbial growth strategies. *Applied Soil Ecology* 37 (1–2): 95–105.

Blum, W.E. (2005). Functions of soil for society and the environment. *Reviews in Environmental Science and Biotechnology* 4 (3): 75–79.

Bolan, N.S. and Duraisamy, V.P. (2003). Role of inorganic and organic soil amendments on immobilisation and phytoavailability of heavy metals: a review involving specific case studies. *Soil Research* 41 (3): 533–555.

Bolan, N., Mahimairaja, S., Kunhikrishnan, A., and Choppala, G. (2013). Phosphorus–arsenic interactions in variable-charge soils in relation to arsenic mobility and bioavailability. *Science of the Total Environment* 463: 1154–1162.

Bolan, N., Kunhikrishnan, A., Thangarajan, R. et al. (2014). Remediation of heavy metal (loid) s contaminated soils – to mobilize or to immobilize? *Journal of Hazardous Materials* 266: 141–166.

Bressler, D.C. and Fedorak, P.M. (2001). Purification, stability, and mineralization of 3-hydroxy-2-formylbenzothiophene, a metabolite of dibenzothiophene. *Applied and Environmental Microbiology* 67 (2): 821–826.

Brevik, E.C. (2009). *Plant Growth and Crop Production* (ed. W. Verheye). Oxford: Encyclopedia of Life Support Systems (EOLSS) Publishers (accessed February 2022).

Bruins, M.R., Kapil, S., and Oehme, F.W. (2000). Microbial resistance to metals in the environment. *Ecotoxicology and Environmental Safety* 45 (3): 198–207.

de Carvalho, C.C.C.R., Wick, L.Y., and Heipieper, H.J. (2009). Cell wall adaptations of planktonic and biofilm *Rhodococcus erythropolis* cells to growth on C5 to C16 n-alkane hydrocarbons. *Applied Microbiology and Biotechnology* 82: 311–320.

Chagas, B.R.C., Utsunomiya, H.S.M., Fernandes, M.N., and Carvalho, C.S. (2020). Metabolic responses in bullfrog, *Lithobates catesbeianus* after exposure to zinc, copper and cadmium. *Comparative Biochemistry and Physiology Part C: Toxicology & Pharmacology* 233: 108768.

Chatterjee, S. and Sharma, S. (2019). Microplastics in our oceans and marine health. *Field actions science reports. The Journal of Field Actions*, (Special Issue) 19: 54–61.

Checcucci, A., Bazzicalupo, M., and Mengoni, A. (2017). Exploiting nitrogen-fixing rhizobial symbionts genetic resources for improving phytoremediation of contaminated soils. In: *Enhancing Cleanup of Environmental Pollutants* (ed. N.A. Anjum, S.S. Gill and N. Tuteja), 275–288. Cham: Springer.

Chen, B. and Ding, J. (2012). Biosorption and biodegradation of phenanthrene and pyrene in sterilized and unsterilized soil slurry systems stimulated by *Phanerochaete chrysosporium*. *Journal of Hazardous Materials* 229: 159–169.

Chen, Y., Yang, W., Chao, Y. et al. (2017). Metal-tolerant *Enterobacter* sp. strain EG16 enhanced phytoremediation using *Hibiscus cannabinus* via siderophore-mediated plant growth promotion under metal contamination. *Plant and Soil* 413: 203–216.

Cheng, Y., Zhu, L., Song, W. et al. (2020). Combined effects of mulch film-derived microplastics and atrazine on oxidative stress and gene expression in earthworm (*Eisenia fetida*). *Science of the Total Environment* 746: 141280.

Cheng, Y., Song, W., Tian, H. et al. (2021). The effects of high-density polyethylene and polypropylene microplastics on the soil and earthworm *Metaphire guillelmi* gut microbiota. *Chemosphere* 267: 129219.

Chia, W.Y., Tang, D.Y.Y., Khoo, K.S. et al. (2020). Nature's fight against plastic pollution: algae for plastic biodegradation and bioplastics production. *Environmental Science and Ecotechnology* 4: 100065.

Chibuike, G.U. and Obiora, S.C. (2014). Heavy metal polluted soils: effect on plants and bioremediation methods. *Applied Environment and Social Sciences* 214: 1–12.

Chikere, C.B., Okpokwasili, G.C., and Chikere, B.O. (2011). Monitoring of microbial hydrocarbon remediation in the soil. *Biotechnology* 1 (3): 117–138.

China Council for International Cooperation on Environment and Development [CCICED] (2015). Evaluation and Prospects for a Green Transition Process in China. CCICED Task Force Report. http://www.cciced.net/encciced/policyresearch/report/201504/P020150413497198320874.pdf.

Christofi, N. and Ivshina, I. (2002). Microbial surfactants and their use in soil remediation. In: *Bioremediation of Aquatic and Terrestrial Ecosystems* (ed. M. Fingerman and R. Nagabhushanam). UK: Science Publishers, Inc. 311 pp.

Coelho, L.M., Rezende, H.C., Coelho, L.M. et al. (2015). Bioremediation of polluted waters using microorganisms. In: *Advances in Bioremediation of Wastewater and Polluted Soil* (ed. N. Shiomi), 1–22. Shanghai: IntechOpen https://doi.org/10.5772/60770.

da Costa, J.P., Santos, P.S., Duarte, A.C., and Rocha-Santos, T. (2016). (Nano) plastics in the environment – sources, fates and effects. *Science of the Total Environment* 566: 15–26.

Daly, M.J. (2000). Engineering radiation-resistant bacteria for environmental biotechnology. *Current Opinion in Biotechnology* 11 (3): 280–285.

DECA (Department of Environment and Conservation, Australia) (2010). Assessment levels for soil, sediment and water. https://www.der.wa.gov.au/images/documents/your-environment/contaminated-sites/guidelines/2009641 (accessed 23 July 2022).

Dewangan, S., Bhatia, A.K., Singh, A.K., and Carabineiro, S.A. (2021). Removal of hydrophobic contaminants from the soil by adsorption onto carbon materials and microbial degradation. *C – Journal of Carbon Research* 7 (4): 83.

Ding, J., Li, J., Sun, C. et al. (2019). Detection of microplastics in local marine organisms using a multi-technology system. *Analytical Methods* 11 (1): 78–87.

Ding, L., Zhang, S., Wang, X. et al. (2020). The occurrence and distribution characteristics of microplastics in the agricultural soils of Shaanxi Province, in North-Western China. *Science of the Total Environment* 720: 137525.

Dixit, R., Malaviya, D., Pandiyan, K. et al. (2015). Bioremediation of heavy metals from soil and aquatic environment: an overview of principles and criteria of fundamental processes. *Sustainability* 7 (2): 2189–2212.

Doolotkeldieva, T., Bobusheva, S., and Konurbaeva, M. (2021). The improving conditions for the aerobic bacteria performing the degradation of obsolete pesticides in polluted soils. *Air, Soil and Water Research* 14: 1178622120982590.

Dragović, S., Mihailović, N., and Gajić, B. (2008). Heavy metals in soils: distribution, relationship with soil characteristics and radionuclides and multivariate assessment of contamination sources. *Chemosphere* 72 (3): 491–495.

Ehlers, L.J. and Luthy, R.G. (2003). Peer reviewed: contaminant bioavailability in soil and sediment. *Environmental Science & Technology* 37 (15): 295A–302A.

Ehrlich, H.L. (1997). Microbes and metals. *Applied Microbiology and Biotechnology* 48 (6): 687–692.

Ehrlich, H.L. (1998). Geomicrobiology: its significance for geology. *Earth-Science Reviews* 45 (1–2): 45–60.

El-Naggar, A., El-Naggar, A.H., Shaheen, S.M. et al. (2019). Biochar composition-dependent impacts on soil nutrient release, carbon mineralization, and potential environmental risk: a review. *Journal of Environmental Management* 241: 458–467.

European Environment Agency (EEA) (2014). Soil degradation. http://www.eea.europa.eu/publications/92-9157-202-0/page306.html (accessed March 2022).

Fan, F., Yin, C., Tang, Y. et al. (2014). Probing potential microbial coupling of carbon and nitrogen cycling during decomposition of maize residue by 13C-DNA-SIP. *Soil Biology and Biochemistry* 70: 12–21.

FAO & ITPS (2015). Status of the world's soil resources (SWSR) – main report. In: *Food and Agriculture Organization of the United Nations and Intergovernmental Technical Panel on Soils*. Rome: FAO. http://www.fao.org/3/a-i5199e.pdf.

FAO & UNEP (2021). Global Assessment of Soil Pollution: Report, Italy.

Fasani, E., Manara, A., Martini, F. et al. (2018). The potential of genetic engineering of plants for the remediation of soils contaminated with heavy metals. *Plant, Cell & Environment* 41 (5): 1201–1232.

Fester, T., Giebler, J., Wick, L.Y. et al. (2014). Plant–microbe interactions as drivers of ecosystem functions relevant for the biodegradation of organic contaminants. *Current Opinion in Biotechnology* 27: 168–175.

Fiorino, D.J. (2010). Voluntary initiatives, regulation, and nanotechnology oversight: charting a path. In: *Project on Emerging Nanotechnologies No. 19*. Washington, DC: Woodrow Wilson Center for Scholars.

Fredrickson, J.K., Zachara, J.M., Kennedy, D.W. et al. (2000). Reduction of U(VI) in goethite (α-FeOOH) suspensions by a dissimilatory metal-reducing bacterium. *Geochimica et Cosmochimica Acta* 64 (18): 3085–3098.

Furuno, S., Foss, S., Wild, E. et al. (2012). Mycelia promote active transport and spatial dispersion of polycyclic aromatic hydrocarbons. *Environmental Science & Technology* 46 (10): 5463–5470.

Gadd, G.M. (2010). Metals, minerals and microbes: geomicrobiology and bioremediation. *Microbiology* 156 (3): 609–643.

Galitskaya, P., Biktasheva, L., Blagodatsky, S., and Selivanovskaya, S. (2021). Response of bacterial and fungal communities to high petroleum pollution in different soils. *Scientific Reports* 11 (1): 1–18.

Geissen, V., Mol, H., Klumpp, E. et al. (2015). Emerging pollutants in the environment: a challenge for water resource management. *International Soil and Water Conservation Research* 3 (1): 57–65.

Gevao, B., Semple, K.T., and Jones, K.C. (2000). Bound pesticide residues in soils: a review. *Environmental Pollution* 108 (1): 3–14.

Gong, J., Kong, T., Li, Y. et al. (2018). Biodegradation of microplastic derived from poly (ethylene terephthalate) with bacterial whole-cell biocatalysts. *Polymers* 10 (12): 1326.

Gonzalez Henao, S. and Ghneim-Herrera, T. (2021). Heavy metals in soils and the remediation potential of bacteria associated with the plant microbiome. *Frontiers in Environmental Science* 15.

Graham, A.M., Bullock, A.L., Maizel, A.C. et al. (2012). Detailed assessment of the kinetics of hg-cell association, hg methylation, and methylmercury degradation in several Desulfovibrio species. *Applied and Environmental Microbiology* 78 (20): 7337–7346.

Grathwohl, P. and Halm, D., 2003. Integrated Soil and Water Protection against Diffuse Pollution (SOWA).

Guan, N. and Liu, L. (2020). Microbial response to acid stress: mechanisms and applications. *Applied Microbiology and Biotechnology* 104 (1): 51–65.

Guzzella, L., Poma, G., De Paolis, A. et al. (2011). Organic persistent toxic substances in soils, waters and sediments along an altitudinal gradient at Mt. Sagarmatha, Himalayas, Nepal. *Environmental Pollution* 159 (10): 2552–2564.

Hamme, J.D.V. (2004). Bioavailability and biodegradation of organic pollutants – a microbial perspective. In: *Biodegradation and Bioremediation*, 37–56. Berlin, Heidelberg: Springer.

Han, S., Bang, J., Choi, D. et al. (2020). Surface pattern analysis of microplastics and their impact on human-derived cells. *ACS Applied Polymer Materials* 2 (11): 4541–4550.

Harms, H., Schlosser, D., and Wick, L.Y. (2011). Untapped potential: exploiting fungi in bioremediation of hazardous chemicals. *Nature Reviews Microbiology* 9 (3): 177–192.

Harmsen, J. (2007). Measuring bioavailability: from a scientific approach to standard methods. *Journal of Environmental Quality* 36 (5): 1420–1428.

Hassan, A., Periathamby, A., Ahmed, A. et al. (2020). Effective bioremediation of heavy metal-contaminated landfill soil through bioaugmentation using consortia of fungi. *Journal of Soils and Sediments* 20 (1): 66–80.

He, P., Chen, L., Shao, L. et al. (2019). Municipal solid waste (MSW) landfill: a source of microplastics? – Evidence of microplastics in landfill leachate. *Water Research* 159: 38–45.

Heard, M.S., Baas, J., Dorne, J.L. et al. (2017). Comparative toxicity of pesticides and environmental contaminants in bees: are honey bees a useful proxy for wild bee species? *Science of the Total Environment* 578: 357–365.

Hu, Y., Liu, X., Bai, J. et al. (2013). Assessing heavy metal pollution in the surface soils of a region that had undergone three decades of intense industrialization and urbanization. *Environmental Science and Pollution Research* 20 (9): 6150–6159.

Huang, W., Song, B., Liang, J. et al. (2021). Microplastics and associated contaminants in the aquatic environment: a review on their ecotoxicological effects, trophic transfer, and potential impacts to human health. *Journal of Hazardous Materials* 405: 124187.

Hwang, J., Choi, D., Han, S. et al. (2019). An assessment of the toxicity of polypropylene microplastics in human derived cells. *Science of the Total Environment* 684: 657–669.

Jariyal, M., Jindal, V., Mandal, K. et al. (2018). Bioremediation of organophosphorus pesticide phorate in soil by microbial consortia. *Ecotoxicology and Environmental Safety* 159: 310–316.

Ji, W., Abou Khalil, C., Jayalakshmamma, M.P. et al. (2021). Behavior of surfactants and surfactant blends in soils during remediation: a review. *Environmental Challenges* 2: 100007.

Jia, J., Bi, C., Guo, X. et al. (2017). Characteristics, identification, and potential risk of polycyclic aromatic hydrocarbons in road dusts and agricultural soils from industrial sites in Shanghai, China. *Environmental Science and Pollution Research* 24 (1): 605–615.

Jiang, J., Bauer, I., Paul, A., and Kappler, A. (2009). Arsenic redox changes by microbially and chemically formed semiquinone radicals and hydroquinones in a humic substance model quinone. *Environmental Science & Technology* 43 (10): 3639–3645. https://doi.org/10.1021/es803112a. PMID: 19544866.

Ju, H., Zhu, D., and Qiao, M. (2019). Effects of polyethylene microplastics on the gut microbial community, reproduction and avoidance behaviors of the soil springtail, Folsomia candida. *Environmental Pollution* 247: 890–897.

Judy, J.D., Unrine, J.M., Rao, W. et al. (2012). Bioavailability of gold nanomaterials to plants: importance of particle size and surface coating. *Environmental Science & Technology* 46: 8467–8474.

Kabata-Pendias, A. (2011). *Trace Elements in Soils and Plants*, 4e. Boca Raton, FL: CRC Press.

Kabir, E., Ray, S., Kim, K.H. et al. (2012). Current status of trace metal pollution in soils affected by industrial activities. *The Scientific World Journal* 2012: 916705.

Kawai, F., Kawabata, T., and Oda, M. (2019). Current knowledge on enzymatic PET degradation and its possible application to waste stream management and other fields. *Applied Microbiology and Biotechnology* 103 (11): 4253–4268.

Kemp, R. and Arundel, A., 1998. Survey Indicators for Environmental Innovation. IDEA Paper Series 8/1998. Step Group, Oslo.

Keyte, I.J., Harrison, R.M., and Lammel, G. (2013). Chemical reactivity and long-range transport potential of polycyclic aromatic hydrocarbons – a review. *Chemical Society Reviews* 42 (24): 9333–9391.

Khalid, N., Aqeel, M., and Noman, A. (2020). Microplastics could be a threat to plants in terrestrial systems directly or indirectly. *Environmental Pollution* 267: 115653.

Khan, S., Naushad, M., Lima, E.C. et al. (2021). Global soil pollution by toxic elements: current status and future perspectives on the risk assessment and remediation strategies–A review. *Journal of Hazardous Materials* 417: 126039.

Kim, R.Y., Yoon, J.K., Kim, T.S. et al. (2015). Bioavailability of heavy metals in soils: definitions and practical implementation – a critical review. *Environmental Geochemistry and Health* 37 (6): 1041–1061.

Kim, K.H., Kabir, E., and Jahan, S.A. (2017). Exposure to pesticides and the associated human health effects. *Science of the Total Environment* 575: 525–535.

Kirschling, T.L., Golas, P.L., Unrine, J.M. et al. (2011). Microbial bioavailability of covalently bound polymer coatings on model engineered nanomaterials. *Environmental Science & Technology* 45 (12): 5253–5259.

Klaine, S.J., Alvarez, P.J., Batley, G.E. et al. (2008). Nanomaterials in the environment: behavior, fate, bioavailability, and effects. *Environmental Toxicology and Chemistry: An International Journal* 27 (9): 1825–1851.

Kong, Z. and Glick, B.R. (2017). The role of plant growth-promoting bacteria in metal phytoremediation. *Advances in Microbial Physiology* 71: 97–132.

Krasowska, A. and Sigler, K. (2014). How microorganisms use hydrophobicity and what does this mean for human needs? *Frontiers in Cellular and Infection Microbiology* 4: 112.

Krell, T., Lacal, J., Guazzaroni, M.E. et al. (2012). Responses of pseudomonas putida to toxic aromatic carbon sources. *Journal of Biotechnology* 160 (1–2): 25–32.

Krell, T., Lacal, J., Reyes-Darias, J.A. et al. (2013). Bioavailability of pollutants and chemotaxis. *Current Opinion in Biotechnology* 24 (3): 451–456.

Kuiper, I., Lagendijk, E.L., Bloemberg, G.V., and Lugtenberg, B.J. (2004). Rhizoremediation: a beneficial plant–microbe interaction. *Molecular Plant-Microbe Interactions* 17 (1): 6–15.

Kurek, E. (2002). 5 microbial mobilization of metals. *Interactions Between Soil Particles and Microorganisms: Impact on the Terrestrial Ecosystem* 8: 189.

Landrigan, P.J., Fuller, R., Hu, H. et al. (2018). Pollution and global health – an agenda for prevention. *Environmental Health Perspectives* 126 (8): 084501.

Lanno, R., Wells, J., Conder, J. et al. (2004). The bioavailability of chemicals in soil for earthworms. *Ecotoxicology and Environmental Safety* 57 (1): 39–47.

Law, A.M. and Aitken, M.D. (2003). Bacterial chemotaxis to naphthalene desorbing from a nonaqueous liquid. *Applied and Environmental Microbiology* 69 (10): 5968–5973.

Lead, J.R., Batley, G.E., Alvarez, P.J. et al. (2018). Nanomaterials in the environment: behavior, fate, bioavailability, and effects – an updated review. *Environmental Toxicology and Chemistry* 37 (8): 2029–2063.

Lerda, D. (2011). *Polycyclic Aromatic Hydrocarbons (PHA) Factsheet*, 4e. JCR Technical Notes EURAL, JCR 66955-2011.

Leungsakul, T., Keenan, B.G., Smets, B.F., and Wood, T.K. (2005). TNT and nitroaromatic compounds are chemoattractants for *Burkholderia cepacia* R34 and *Burkholderia* sp. strain DNT. *Applied Microbiology and Biotechnology* 69 (3): 321–325.

Li, J., Liu, Q., Sun, S. et al. (2022). Degradation characteristics of crude oil by a consortium of bacteria in the existence of chlorophenol. *Biodegradation* 1–16.

Liang, Y., Bradford, S.A., Simunek, J. et al. (2013). Sensitivity of the transport and retention of stabilized silver nanoparticles to physicochemical factors. *Water Research* 47 (7): 2572–2582.

Liu, X., Wood, P.L., Parales, J.V., and Parales, R.E. (2009). Chemotaxis to pyrimidines and identification of a cytosine chemoreceptor in *Pseudomonas putida*. *Journal of Bacteriology* 191 (9): 2909–2916.

Liu, F., Niu, L., Chen, H. et al. (2017). Seasonal changes of polycyclic aromatic hydrocarbons in response to hydrology and anthropogenic activities in the Pearl River estuary, China. *Marine Pollution Bulletin* 117 (1–2): 255–263.

Loureiro, A., Noro, J., Abreu, A.S. et al. (2018). Absence of albumin improves in vitro cellular uptake and disruption of poloxamer 407-based nanoparticles inside cancer cells. *Molecular Pharmaceutics* 15 (2): 527–535.

Lu, C. and Tian, H. (2017). Global nitrogen and phosphorus fertilizer use for agriculture production in the past half century: shifted hot spots and nutrient imbalance. *Earth System Science Data* 9 (1): 181–192.

Ma, Y., Prasad, M.N.V., Rajkumar, M., and Freitas, H.J.B.A. (2011). Plant growth promoting rhizobacteria and endophytes accelerate phytoremediation of metalliferous soils. *Biotechnology Advances* 29 (2): 248–258.

Ma, Y., Zhai, S., Mao, S.Y. et al. (2014). Co-metabolic transformation of the neonicotinoid insecticide imidacloprid by the new soil isolate Pseudoxanthomonas indica CGMCC 6648. *Journal of Environmental Science and Health, Part B* 49 (9): 661–670.

Manoj, S.R., Karthik, C., Kadirvelu, K. et al. (2020). Understanding the molecular mechanisms for the enhanced phytoremediation of heavy metals through plant growth promoting rhizobacteria: A review. *Journal of Environmental Management* 254: 109779.

Marx, R.B. and Aitken, M.D. (2000). Bacterial chemotaxis enhances naphthalene degradation in a heterogeneous aqueous system. *Environmental Science & Technology* 34 (16): 3379–3383.

Meers, E., Vandecasteele, B., Ruttens, A. et al. (2007). Potential of five willow species (*Salix* spp.) for phytoextraction of heavy metals. *Environmental and Experimental Botany* 60 (1): 57–68.

Megharaj, M., Ramakrishnan, B., Venkateswarlu, K. et al. (2011). Bioremediation approaches for organic pollutants: a critical perspective. *Environment International* 37 (8): 1362–1375.

Miege, C., Choubert, J.M., Ribeiro, L. et al. (2009). Fate of pharmaceuticals and personal care products in wastewater treatment plants – conception of a database and first results. *Environmental Pollution* 157 (5): 1721–1726.

Mishra, J., Singh, R., and Arora, N.K. (2017). Alleviation of heavy metal stress in plants and remediation of soil by rhizosphere microorganisms. *Frontiers in Microbiology* 8: 1706.

Morgan, R. (2013). Soil, heavy metals, and human health. In: *Soils and Human Health* (ed. E.C. Brevik and L.C. Burgess), 59–82. Boca Raton: CRC Press.

Mousavi, S.A. and Khodadoost, F. (2019). Effects of detergents on natural ecosystems and wastewater treatment processes: a review. *Environmental Science and Pollution Research* 26 (26): 26439–26448.

Nguyen, T.T.N., Wallace, H.M., Xu, C.Y. et al. (2018). The effects of short term, long term and reapplication of biochar on soil bacteria. *Science of the Total Environment* 636: 142–151.

Nič, M., Jirát, J., Košata, B. et al. (2009). *IUPAC Compendium of Chemical Terminology: Gold Book*, 2.1.0e. Research Triagle Park, NC: IUPAC. http://goldbook.iupac.org.

Niemeyer, J.C., Lolata, G.B., de Carvalho, G.M. et al. (2012). Microbial indicators of soil health as tools for ecological risk assessment of a metal contaminated site in Brazil. *Applied Soil Ecology* 59: 96–105.

Nikolova, C. and Gutierrez, T. (2021). Biosurfactants and their applications in the oil and gas industry: current state of knowledge and future perspectives. *Frontiers in Bioengineering and Biotechnology* 9: 626639.

Njoku, K.L., Akinyede, O.R., and Obidi, O.F. (2020). Microbial remediation of heavy metals contaminated media by *Bacillus megaterium* and *Rhizopus stolonifer*. *Scientific African* 10: e00545.

Okere, U. and Semple, K. (2012). Biodegradation of PAHs in 'pristine'soils from different climatic regions. *Journal of Bioremediation and Biodegradation S* 1 (2): 1–11.

Olaniran, A.O., Balgobind, A., and Pillay, B. (2013). Bioavailability of heavy metals in soil: impact on microbial biodegradation of organic compounds and possible improvement strategies. *International Journal of Molecular Sciences* 14 (5): 10197–10228.

Oldeman, L.R. (1992). Global extent of soil degradation. In: *Bi-Annual Report 1991–1992/ISRIC*, 19–36. ISRIC.

Oliveira, B.R., Penetra, A., Cardoso, V.V. et al. (2015). Biodegradation of pesticides using fungi species found in the aquatic environment. *Environmental Science and Pollution Research* 22 (15): 11781–11791.

Oliver, M.A. and Gregory, P.J. (2015). Soil, food security and human health: a review. *European Journal of Soil Science* 66 (2): 257–276.

Othman, A.R., Hasan, H.A., Muhamad, M.H. et al. (2021). Microbial degradation of microplastics by enzymatic processes: a review. *Environmental Chemistry Letters* 19 (4): 3057–3073.

Otto, R., Castro, S.A.Q., Mariano, E. et al. (2016). Nitrogen use efficiency for sugarcane-biofuel production: what is next? *Bioenergy Research* 9 (4): 1272–1289.

Panagiotakis, I. and Dermatas, D. (2015). Remediation of contaminated sites. *Bulletin of Environmental Contamination and Toxicology* 94 (3): 267–268.

Panebianco, A., Nalbone, L., Giarratana, F., and Ziino, G. (2019). First discoveries of microplastics in terrestrial snails. *Food Control* 106: 106722.

Park, S., Kim, K.S., Kim, J.T. et al. (2011). Effects of humic acid on phytodegradation of petroleum hydrocarbons in soil simultaneously contaminated with heavy metals. *Journal of Environmental Sciences* 23 (12): 2034–2041.

Peijnenburg, W., Sneller, E., Sijm, D. et al. (2002). Implementation of bioavailability in standard setting and risk assessment? *Journal of Soils and Sediments* 2 (4): 169–173.

Petruzzelli, G., Pedron, F., and Rosellini, I. (2020). Bioavailability and bioaccessibility in soil: a short review and a case study. *AIMS Environmental Science* 7 (2): 208–225.

Pietroiusti, A., Vecchione, L., Malvindi, M.A. et al. (2018). Relevance to investigate different stages of pregnancy to highlight toxic effects of nanoparticles: the example of silica. *Toxicology and Applied Pharmacology* 342: 60–68.

Polyak, Y.M., Bakina, L.G., Chugunova, M.V. et al. (2018). Effect of remediation strategies on biological activity of oil-contaminated soil – a field study. *International Biodeterioration & Biodegradation* 126: 57–68.

Pourret, O. and Hursthouse, A. (2019). It's time to replace the term "heavy metals" with "potentially toxic elements" when reporting environmental research. *International Journal of Environmental Research and Public Health* 16 (22): 4446.

Purnomo, A.S., Sariwati, A., and Kamei, I. (2020). Synergistic interaction of a consortium of the brown-rot fungus *Fomitopsis pinicola* and the bacterium *Ralstonia pickettii* for DDT biodegradation. *Heliyon* 6 (6): e04027.

Raffa, C.M. and Chiampo, F. (2021). Bioremediation of agricultural soils polluted with pesticides: a review. *Bioengineering* 8 (7): 92.

Ragusa, A., Svelato, A., Santacroce, C. et al. (2021). Plasticenta: first evidence of microplastics in human placenta. *Environment International* 146: 106274.

Ren, X., Zeng, G., Tang, L. et al. (2018). The potential impact on the biodegradation of organic pollutants from composting technology for soil remediation. *Waste Management* 72: 138–149.

Rinklebe, J. and Shaheen, S.M. (2014). Assessing the mobilization of cadmium, lead, and nickel using a seven-step sequential extraction technique in contaminated floodplain soil profiles along the central Elbe River, Germany. *Water, Air, & Soil Pollution* 225 (8): 1–20.

Rizvi, A., Zaidi, A., Ameen, F. et al. (2020). Heavy metal induced stress on wheat: phytotoxicity and microbiological management. *RSC Advances* 10 (63): 38379–38403.

Roane, T.M., Josephson, K.L., and Pepper, I.L. (2001). Dual-bioaugmentation strategy to enhance remediation of co-contaminated soil. *Applied and Environmental Microbiology* 67 (7): 3208–3215.

Roane, T. M., Pepper, I. L., & Gentry, T. J. (2015). Microorganisms and Metal Pollutants. Environmental Microbiology, 415–439. Editor(s): Ian L. Pepper, Charles P. Gerba, Terry J. Gentry, (3e), Academic Press. doi:https://doi.org/10.1016/b978-0-12-394626-3.00018-1

Rodríguez, J., Gallampois, C.M., Timonen, S. et al. (2018). Effects of organic pollutants on bacterial communities under future climate change scenarios. *Frontiers in Microbiology* 9: 2926.

Rodríguez-Eugenio, N., McLaughlin, M., and Pennock, D. (2018). *Soil Pollution: A Hidden Reality*. Rome: FAO 142 pp.

Roskova, Z., Skarohlid, R., and McGachy, L. (2022). Siderophores: an alternative bioremediation strategy? *Science of the Total Environment* 819: 153144.

Ross, S.M. (1994). Sources and forms of potentially toxic metals in soil–plant systems. In: *Toxic Metals in Soil–Plant Systems* (ed. S.M. Ross), 3–25. New York: Wiley.

Saadani, O., Jebara, S.H., Fatnassi, I.C. et al. (2019). Effect of *Vicia faba* L. var. *minor* and *Sulla coronaria* (L.) Medik associated with plant growth-promoting bacteria on lettuce cropping system and heavy metal phytoremediation under field conditions. *Environmental Science and Pollution Research* 26 (8): 8125–8135.

Saha, M., Sarkar, A., Roy, T. et al. (2020). Phytobiomes: role in nutrient stewardship and soil health. In: *Phytobiomes: Current Insights and Future Vistas*, 1–28. Singapore: Springer.

Saha, J., Adhikary, S., and Pal, A. (2022). Analyses of the heavy metal resistance pattern and biosorption potential of an indigenous *Bacillus tropicus* strain isolated from arable soil. *Geomicrobiology Journal* 1–15.

Sauvé, S. and Desrosiers, M. (2014). A review of what is an emerging contaminant. *Chemistry Central Journal* 8 (1): 15.

Seshadri, B., Bolan, N.S., and Naidu, R. (2015). Rhizosphere-induced heavy metal (loid) transformation in relation to bioavailability and remediation. *Journal of Soil Science and Plant Nutrition* 15 (2): 524–548.

Sharma, P. (2021). Role and significance of biofilm-forming microbes in phytoremediation – a review. *Environmental Technology and Innovation* 25: 102182.

Shen, W., Zhu, N., Cui, J. et al. (2016). Ecotoxicity monitoring and bioindicator screening of oil-contaminated soil during bioremediation. *Ecotoxicology and Environmental Safety* 124: 120–128.

Smets, B.F. and Pritchard, P.H. (2003). Elucidating the microbial component of natural attenuation. *Current Opinion in Biotechnology* 14 (3): 283–288.

Solís-Ramos, L.Y., Coto-López, C., and Andrade-Torres, A. (2021). Role of arbuscular mycorrhizal symbiosis in remediation of anthropogenic soil pollution. *Symbiosis* 84 (3): 321–336.

de Souza Machado, A.A., Lau, C.W., Till, J. et al. (2018). Impacts of microplastics on the soil biophysical environment. *Environmental Science & Technology* 52 (17): 9656–9665.

Srivastava, A.K. and Singh, V.K. (2019). Biological action of essential oils (terpenes). *International Journal of Biological and Medical Research* 10 (3): 6854–6859.

Stamper, D.M., Radosevich, M., Hallberg, K.B. et al. (2002). Ralstonia basilensis M91-3, a denitrifying soil bacterium capable of using s-triazines as nitrogen sources. *Canadian Journal of Microbiology* 48 (12): 1089–1098.

Sun, Y.Z., Zhang, D.H., Cai, S.B. et al. (2018). MDAD: a special resource for microbe-drug associations. *Frontiers in Cellular and Infection Microbiology* 8: 424.

Sutton, M.A., Bleeker, A., Howard, C.M. et al. (2013). *Our Nutrient World. The Challenge to Produce More Food & Energy with Less Pollution*. Centre for Ecology & Hydrology.

Swartjes, F.A. (2011). Introduction to contaminated site management. In: *Dealing with Contaminated Sites* (ed. F.A. Swartjes), 3–89. Dordrecht: Springer.

Tang, X., Zhu, Y., and Meng, Q. (2007). Enhanced crude oil biodegradability of *Pseudomonas aeruginosa* ZJU after preservation in crude oil-containing medium. *World Journal of Microbiology and Biotechnology* 23 (1): 7–14.

Tang, J., Lu, X., Sun, Q., and Zhu, W. (2012). Aging effect of petroleum hydrocarbons in soil under different attenuation conditions. *Agriculture, Ecosystems & Environment* 149: 109–117.

Tang, X., Zeng, B., Hashmi, M.Z. et al. (2014). PBDEs and PCDD/Fs in surface soil taken from the Taizhou e-waste recycling area, China. *Chemistry and Ecology* 30 (3): 245–251.

Tang, S., Yin, H., Chen, S. et al. (2016). Aerobic degradation of BDE-209 by *Enterococcus casseliflavus*: isolation, identification and cell changes during degradation process. *Journal of Hazardous Materials* 308: 335–342.

Tian, L.Y., Yang, J.Y., and Huang, J.H. (2015). Uptake and speciation of vanadium in the rhizosphere soils of rape (*Brassica juncea* L.). *Environmental Science and Pollution Research* 22 (12): 9215–9223.

Torrent, J., Barberis, E., and Gil-Sotres, F. (2007). Agriculture as a source of phosphorus for eutrophication in southern Europe. *Soil Use and Management 23*: 25–35.

Tourinho, P.S., Van Gestel, C.A., Lofts, S. et al. (2012). Metal-based nanoparticles in soil: fate, behavior, and effects on soil invertebrates. *Environmental Toxicology and Chemistry* 31 (8): 1679–1692.

UNEP (2001). United Nations Environment Program, Ozone Action Programme, Source Book of Technologies for Protecting the Ozone Layer: Alternatives to Methyl Bromide. http://www.uneptie.org/ozonaction.html (accessed 17 December 2014).

UNEP (2017). *The Emissions Gap Report 2017*. Nairobi: United Nations Environment Programme (UNEP).

Van Hamme, J.D., Singh, A., and Ward, O.P. (2003). Recent advances in petroleum microbiology. *Microbiology and Molecular Biology Reviews* 67 (4): 503–549.

Van Hamme, J.D., Fedorak, P.M., Foght, J.M. et al. (2004). Use of a novel fluorinated organosulfur compound to isolate bacteria capable of carbon-sulfur bond cleavage. *Applied and Environmental Microbiology* 70 (3): 1487–1493.

Venuti, A., Alfonsi, L., and Cavallo, A. (2016). Anthropogenic pollutants on top soils along a section of the Salaria state road, Central Italy. *Annals of Geophysics* 59 (5): G0544–G0544.

Wang, C., Zhao, J., and Xing, B. (2021). Environmental source, fate, and toxicity of microplastics. *Journal of Hazardous Materials* 407: 124357.

Ward, O.P. (2010). Microbial biosurfactants and biodegradation. In: *Biosurfactants. Advances in Experimental Medicine and Biology*, vol. 672 (ed. R. Sen). New York: Springer. https://doi.org/10.1007/978-1-4419-5979-9_5.

Weerasinghe, W.M.T.M. and Madawala, H.M.S.P. (2022). Potential impacts of two types of microplastics on *Solanum lycopersicum* L. and arbuscular mycorrhizal fungi. *Ceylon Journal of Science* 51 (2): 137–146.

Wei, X.F., Bohlén, M., Lindblad, C. et al. (2021). Microplastics generated from a biodegradable plastic in freshwater and seawater. *Water Research* 198: 117123.

WHO (2018). *Public Health and Climate Change Adaptation Policies (Final Report)*. WHO Press.

Whyte, L.G., Schultz, A., Van Beilen, J.B. et al. (2002). Prevalence of alkane monooxygenase genes in Arctic and Antarctic hydrocarbon-contaminated and pristine soils. *FEMS Microbiology Ecology* 41 (2): 141–150.

Wick, L., De Munain, A., Springael, D., and Harms, H. (2002). Responses of *Mycobacterium* sp. LB501T to the low bioavailability of solid anthracene. *Applied Microbiology and Biotechnology* 58 (3): 378–385.

Widdel, F., Knittel, K., and Galushko, A. (2010). Anaerobic hydrocarbon-degrading microorganisms: an overview. In: *Handbook of Hydrocarbon and Lipid Microbiology* (ed. K.N. Timmis), 1998–2022. Berlin, Heidelberg: Springer.

Worm, B., Lotze, H.K., Jubinville, I. et al. (2017). Plastic as a persistent marine pollutant. *Annual Review of Environment and Resources* 42 (1): 1–26.

Wu, C., Zhang, H., He, P., and Shao, L. (2010). Thermal stabilization of chromium slag by sewage sludge: effects of sludge quantity and temperature. *Journal of Environmental Sciences* 22 (7): 1110–1115.

Xu, Z.Y., Tang, M., Chen, H. et al. (2012). Microbial community structure in the rhizosphere of *Sophora viciifolia* grown at a lead and zinc mine of Northwest China. *Science of the Total Environment* 435: 453–464.

Yan, A., Wang, Y., Tan, S.N. et al. (2020). Phytoremediation: a promising approach for revegetation of heavy metal-polluted land. *Frontiers in Plant Science* 11: 359.

Yang, D.S., Pennisi, S.V., Son, K.C., and Kays, S.J. (2009). Screening indoor plants for volatile organic pollutant removal efficiency. *HortScience* 44 (5): 1377–1381.

Yang, Y., Liu, W., Zhang, Z. et al. (2020). Microplastics provide new microbial niches in aquatic environments. *Applied Microbiology and Biotechnology* 104 (15): 6501–6511.

Yaron, B., Dagan, G., and Goldshmid, J. (ed.) (2012). *Pollutants in Porous Media: The Unsaturated Zone between Soil Surface and Groundwater*, vol. 47. Springer Science & Business Media.

Yin, X., Jiang, Y., Tan, Y. et al. (2019). Co-transport of graphene oxide and heavy metal ions in surface-modified porous media. *Chemosphere* 218: 1–13.

Yu, Y.Y., Guo, C.X., Yong, Y.C. et al. (2015). Nitrogen doped carbon nanoparticles enhanced extracellular electron transfer for high-performance microbial fuel cells anode. *Chemosphere* 140: 26–33.

Yu, F., Yang, C., Huang, G. et al. (2020). Interfacial interaction between diverse microplastics and tetracycline by adsorption in an aqueous solution. *Science of the Total Environment* 721: 137729.

Yun, S.W., Baveye, P.C., Kim, D.H. et al. (2018). Analysis of metal (loid) s contamination and their continuous input in soils around a zinc smelter: development of methodology and a case study in South Korea. *Environmental Pollution* 238: 140–149.

Zhang, C. and Chen, Z. (2021). Advances in study on the effects of arbuscular mycorrhizal fungi on plants in remediation of arsenic-contaminated soil. *Acta Agriculturae Scandinavica, Section B – Soil & Plant Science* 71 (9): 825–834.

Zhang, H., Yuan, X., Xiong, T. et al. (2020). Bioremediation of co-contaminated soil with heavy metals and pesticides: influence factors, mechanisms and evaluation methods. *Chemical Engineering Journal* 398: 125657.

Zheng, S., Bawazir, M., Dhall, A. et al. (2021). Implication of surface properties, bacterial motility, and hydrodynamic conditions on bacterial surface sensing and their initial adhesion. *Frontiers in Bioengineering and Biotechnology* 9: 643722.

Zhu, X., Li, W., Zhan, L. et al. (2016). The large-scale process of microbial carbonate precipitation for nickel remediation from an industrial soil. *Environmental Pollution* 219: 149–155.

Zuo, L.Z., Li, H.X., Lin, L. et al. (2019). Sorption and desorption of phenanthrene on biodegradable poly (butylene adipate co-terephtalate) microplastics. *Chemosphere* 215: 25–32.

10

Per- and Polyfluoroalkyl Substances (PFAS) Migration from Water to Soil–Plant Systems, Health Risks, and Implications for Remediation

Viraj Gunarathne[1], Meththika Vithanage[2], and Jörg Rinklebe[1]

[1] *Laboratory of Soil- and Groundwater-Management, Water- and Waste-Management, Institute of Foundation Engineering, School of Architecture and Civil Engineering, University of Wuppertal, Wuppertal, Germany*
[2] *Ecosphere Resilience Research Centre, Faculty of Applied Sciences, University of Sri Jayewardenepura, Nugegoda, Sri Lanka*

10.1 Introduction

Per- and polyfluoroalkyl substances (PFAS) are a class of synthetic compounds comprised of more than 4000 fluorinated aliphatic substances (Al Amin et al. 2020; Nakayama et al. 2019). In general, PFAS have diverse chemical, physical, and biological features; however, they are consistent with the fully or partially fluorinated carbon chain (Cousins et al. 2020). The strong carbon–fluorine bonds (i.e. 536 kJ/mol C—F bonding strength) make these compounds thermodynamically stable, inert, and resistant to degradation by hydrolysis, metabolism, and photolysis (Al Amin et al. 2020; Podder et al. 2021). Ionizable and polar headgroups available in the long chains of PFAS grant it unique surface-active behavior (Sharifan et al. 2021), combined with the hydrophobic and oleophobic properties (Buck et al. 2011) make them excellent candidates for the production of consumer products such as nonstick cooking ware, protective coatings, firefighting materials (e.g. aqueous film-forming foams [AFFFs] utilized to extinguish fires that involve extremely flammable liquids), cosmetics, carpets, mining, and electronics.

There is growing concern over the life cycles and environmental impacts of PFAS due to their high stability and persistence in nature and their high potential for accidental contamination during fluoropolymer manufacture, usage, and improper disposal (Wang et al. 2014). This global level of contamination has been aided by the widespread use of PFAS, which could be evidently found in wildlife and the environment, even in human beings through continuous exposure to PFAS in water, food, and air (Fenton et al. 2021). Studies indicated that PFAS with long carbon chains, such as PFOA (perfluorooctanoic acid) and PFOS (perfluorooctanesulfonic acid), have much higher persistence in nature, more mobility, higher bioaccumulation tendency, and greater toxic effects (Wang et al. 2019).

The distribution of PFAS throughout the atmosphere as well as in the hydrosphere has been thoroughly studied. The soil, on the other hand, is a vital reservoir that experiences a frequent movement of PFAS in different forms. The release of these PFAS into soil layers occurs along varied paths, mainly above-ground activities such as atmospheric deposition and agricultural and sewage effluents (Mei et al. 2021). Therefore, PFAS primarily interact with the soil layer before seeping into groundwater or even interacting with surface waters. Studies up to date have found that the most predominant PFAS accumulation in soil takes place in the shallow soil horizon (Nickerson et al. 2020). Thereafter, PFAS might absorb on soil particles or disintegrate in soil solution. The sorption characteristics of PFAS in the soil environment are crucial because they determine the available concentration of PFAS for plants to uptake. Organic matter (SOM), minerals, and pH play a vital role among the factors that determine the sorption capacity of the soil (Oliver et al. 2020).

When PFAS in the soil are taken up by plants, they are transferred to the corresponding food chains. This uptake and accumulation of PFAS largely occur through roots (Wang et al. 2020a). As a result, it can ultimately pose human health-related concerns as well. Therefore, this chapter is written with the objectives of an interdisciplinary understanding of different processes that influence the migration of PFAS from water to soil–plant systems, human-health related issues, and implications and remediation measures that can be carried out to address the problems that occurred with environmental contamination.

One Health: Human, Animal, and Environment Triad, First Edition. Edited by Meththika Vithanage and Majeti Narasimha Vara Prasad.

10.2 Sources of PFAS Contamination

Due to their natural persistent characteristics, PFAS can be found in environments without being degraded for long periods of time. There are two major sources, namely point and nonpoint sources, involved in the environmental release of PFAS. Point sources are distinct and stationary, while nonpoint sources are dispersed sources whose origin or location are unknown. Industrial sites, firefighting training facilities, landfills, and wastewater treatment plants are considered point sources of PFAS contamination. Nonpoint sources include precipitation, atmospheric distribution of volatile PFAS, surface runoff, breakdown of consumer products, and breakdown/transformation of PFAS precursor compounds (Kurwadkar et al. 2021). Figure 10.1 indicates different routes of environmental contamination of PFAS by different sources. Among the varied routes by which both soil and water sources receive PFAS, a few important point sources are further discussed in this section.

10.2.1 Aqueous Film-Forming Foams (AFFFs)

One of the primary sources of PFAS in the environment includes AFFFs. Continuous discharges of AFFFs have been related to serious soil and groundwater contamination issues (Martin et al. 2019). PFAS from AFFFs can be released into terrestrial and aquatic habitats during the processes of storage, handling, usage, and post-use cleaning, making them an important point source (Cousins et al. 2019). Mishandling of these chemicals in production and storage can result in minute amounts of PFAS being discharged into the environment (Bolan et al. 2021), whereas larger quantities of AFFFs are discharged into the environment during real firefighting applications (Reinikainen et al. 2022).

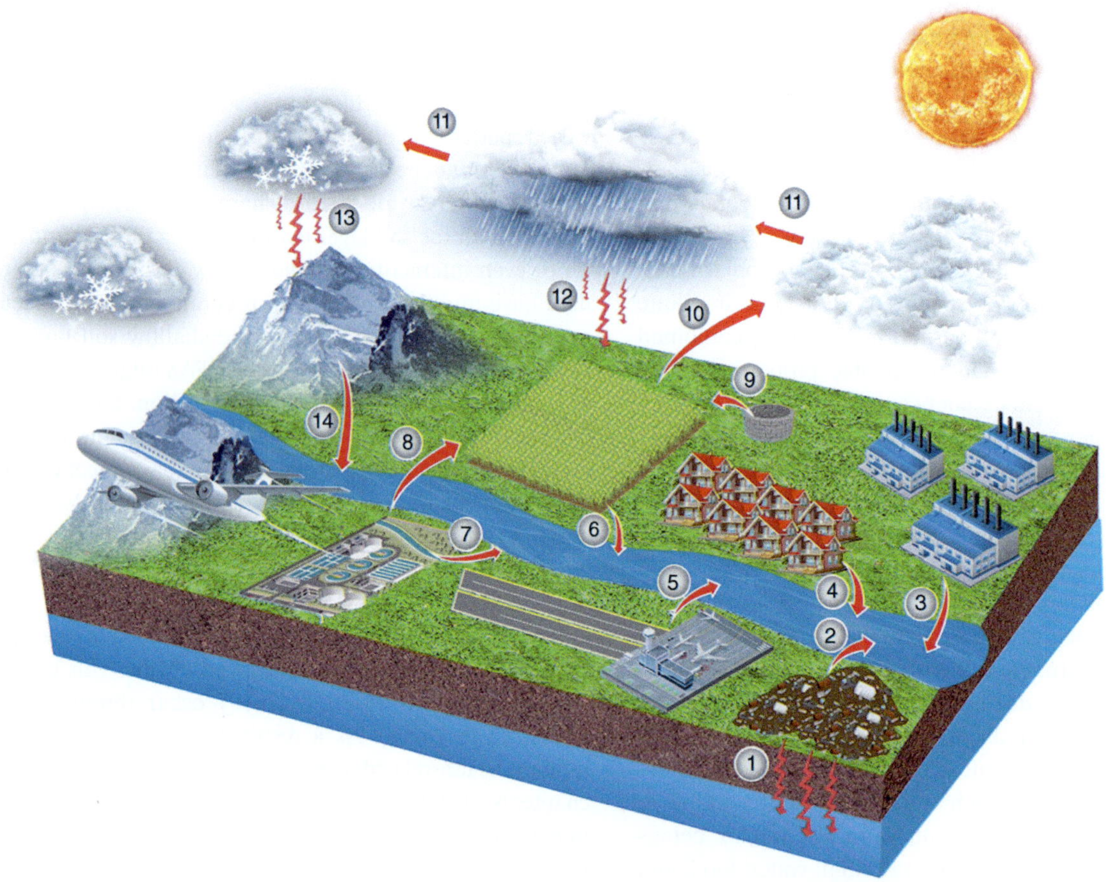

Figure 10.1 PFAS sources and environmental contamination routes (1 – direct infiltration of leachates and groundwater contamination; 2 – surface water contamination by leachates; 3 – discharge of industrial effluents; 4 – discharge of household effluents; 5 – AFFFs; 6 – pesticides; 7 – wastewater treatment plant effluents; 8 – biosolid application; 9 – contaminated groundwater application; 10 – evapotranspiration; 11 – carrying away with clouds; 12 – rainfall; 13 – snowing; 14 – icecaps and glacier melting).

Evidence found in several studies shows that AFFFs used in various places, such as firefighting drills, airports, and even defense sites such as military camps (Salice et al. 2018), collect considerably large quantities of PFAS in soil and groundwater, resulting in negative impacts on resident aquatic and terrestrial biota. Approximately 26,000 PFAS-contaminated sites are spread across the United States, and PFAS-contaminated drinking water is believed to affect six million Americans (Darlington et al. 2018).

10.2.2 Landfill Effluents

Sanitary landfilling is now the most frequent method utilized by many nations for disposing of municipal solid waste, including natural and anthropogenic organic materials such as PFAS. Thus, PFAS can become mobile in waste and seep out into pore water, resulting in contaminated leachate (Shahsavari et al. 2021). Industrial wastes, such as fabrics, construction materials, and coating materials, can be a diffuse source of PFAS and related compounds, in addition to sewage and wastewater (Janousek et al. 2019). Most modern landfill sites have proper designs to minimize the migration of leachate into groundwater, but sometimes poorly managed landfills and improper discharge of waste onto bare land can cause PFAS leakage into the environment. In such cases, PFAS will remain in landfills and will continue to accumulate over time (Gallen et al. 2018). In landfill leachates, perfluorohexane sulfonate (PFHxS) contamination was identified at relatively high concentrations (range 73–25,000 ng/l; mean 1700 ng/l), PFOA contamination was at average concentrations (range 17–7500 ng/l; mean 690 ng/l), and PFOS contamination was detected at a relatively low range of 13–2700 ng/l (mean 310 ng/l) (Shahsavari et al. 2021). Moreover, the construction and demolition waste materials were found to be key sources of PFAS at waste management sites (Hamid et al. 2018).

10.2.3 Wastewater Effluents and Biosolids

Effluents from waste disposal sites and treatment facilities and biosolids constitute the major sources of PFAS contaminants in soil and water (Ambaye et al. 2022). Many household equipment nowadays contain PFAS. Small amounts of such PFAS with low concentrations can transport through household wastewater to municipal wastewater treatment plants, where they accumulate in biosolids (Bolan et al. 2021). Short- and long-chain perfluoroalkyl acids (PFAA) were found in high concentrations in both wastewater treatment plant influents (up to 1.0 ng/l) and effluents (15 to >1500 ng/l) (Lenka et al. 2021). Generally, effluents contain higher concentrations of perfluorocarboxylic acids compared to their concentration in influents (Coggan et al. 2019). A global scale meta-analysis revealed the presence of PFOA and PFOS in wastewater at the highest measured concentrations with minimal temporal fluctuation when compared to other PFAS determined in wastewater sources (Cookson and Detwiler 2022). Another study carried out in Australia with two wastewater treatment plants determined the concentration of 11 PFAS. The PFAS concentration in influent of one treatment plant was 57 ± 3.3–94 ± 17 ng/l and the other was 31 ± 6.1–142 ± 73 ng/l. The average collective concentration of those 11 PFAS released by the nearby residents of the study area was 21 kg/year (range 15–28 kg/year), which is a substantially large amount of PFAS released to waterways (Nguyen et al. 2019). Cookson and Detwiler (2022) in their meta-analysis concluded that no conventional wastewater treatment method is effectively eliminating PFAS in wastewater influents, which consist of a significant portion of industrial components, resulting in higher PFAS concentrations in effluents. Therefore, the pollution of water resources and soil by PFAS is inevitable if the improper release of wastewater effluents and biosolids takes place into the environment or if they are used as irrigation water or fertilizers for agricultural fields.

10.3 Biotransformation of PFAS

PFAS transformation is mainly governed by abiotic and biotic degradation processes. Secondary products resulting from the transformation of precursor PFAS compounds act as indirect sources of PFAS contamination (Ruan et al. 2015). Therefore, it is essential to have a clear understanding of PFAS precursor compounds, their degradation products, biotransformation agents, and the required edaphic conditions to mitigate PFAS contamination in soil.

Microorganisms including various strains of bacteria, fungi; soil macroorganisms such as earthworms; and plants are involved in the biotransformation process of PFAS (Bolan et al. 2021). There are aerobic and anaerobic bacterial species that have capacities to degrade PFAS; however, aerobic biotransformation is the most widely investigated scenario (Zhang et al. 2022b). For instance, Zhao and Zhu (2017) reported biodegradation pathways of 10 : 2 fluorotelomer alcohol (10 : 2 FTOH) by soil microorganisms, earthworms (*Eisenia fetida*), and wheat (*Triticum aestivum* L.) roots and identified a number of perfluorocarboxylic acids as biodegradation products of 10 : 2 FTOH. The microbial degradation of 10 : 2 FTOH took place in soil, resulting in PFOA, perfluorodecanoate (PFDA), and perfluorononanate (PFNA). Perfluoroundecanoic acid (PFUnDA) and PFDA were found in wheat shoots; perfluorohexanoic (PFHxA), perfluoropentanoic acid (PFPeA), and PFDA

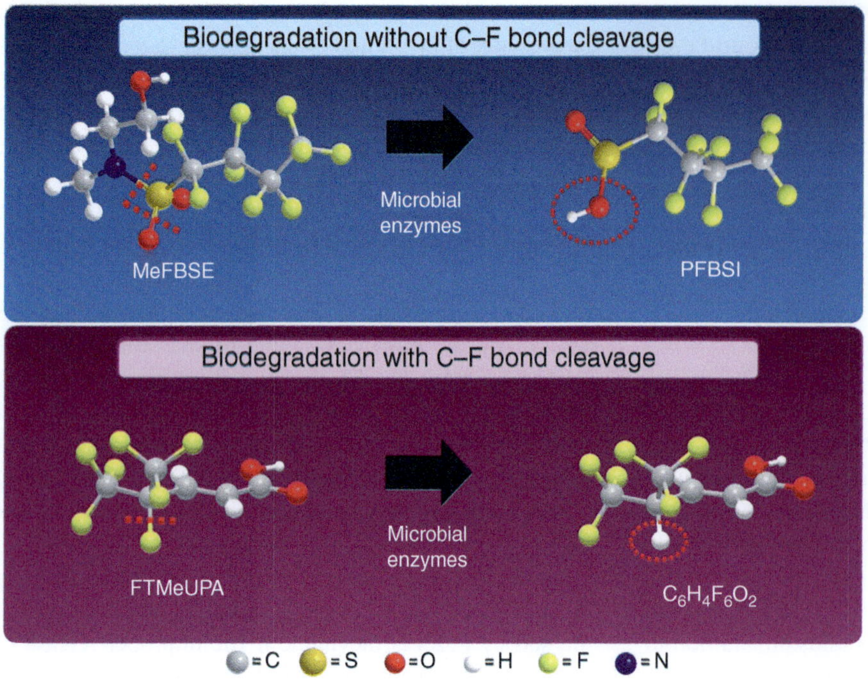

Figure 10.2 Major biotransformation pathways of PFAS. *Source:* Adapted from Zhang et al. (2022b).

were identified in wheat roots; and PFDA and PFNA were observed in earthworms, indicating the biotransformation of 10:2 FTOH via the metabolic pathways of wheat and earthworms. Furthermore, various derivatives of sulfonamide, such as *N*-ethylperfluorooctane sulfonamidoethanol (EtFOSE) and N-ethylperfluorooctane sulfonamide (EtFOSA), are reported to result in PFOS via biotransformation by bacteria, earthworms, and wheat plants (Bolan et al. 2021).

There are two main pathways involved in the biotransformation of PFAS: biodegradation with C—F bond cleavage and biodegradation without C—F bond cleavage (Figure 10.2). However, many of the studies are limited to the biodegradation of PFAS without C—F bond cleavage (Zhang et al. 2022b). PFAS compounds with shorter carbon chain lengths have higher environmental persistence due to their high resistance to biodegradation. However, it is possible to exist biodegradation pathways governed by certain enzymes with abilities to cleave the high-strength C—F bond of PFAS by either oxidation or reduction (Shahsavari et al. 2021). On the other hand, it is important to note that most of the biotransformation mechanisms for PFAS are experimentally explained and hypothesized while no confirmed pathways are exhibit (Zhang et al. 2022b). Therefore, further studies targeting to find out the exact mechanisms for PFAS biotransformation are essential to describe their environmental fate.

10.4 Transportation and Occurrence of PFAS in Water Resources

The transportation and occurrence of PFAS in water resources are closely related to the anthroposphere and the hydrological cycle. The high water solubility of PFAS further attributed to their greater mobility and occurrence in aquatic matrices. PFAS are water-soluble because of their hydrophilic groups, which increases their ability to contaminate water matrices (Zhou et al. 2021; Colomer-Vidal et al. 2022). The concentrations of PFAS occurring in surface and groundwater resources worldwide range from ng/l to μg/l levels.

10.4.1 PFAS in Surface Water Resources

PFAS contamination has been regularly reported in surface water resources that are located in close proximity to point sources such as firefighting training facilities, industrial sites, wastewater treatment plants, and landfill areas (Li et al. 2020a). Generally, PFAS manufacturing industries contribute to the highest amount of PFAS contamination in surface water sources. Therefore, limited data are available for the PFAS contamination status of water resources in countries with no established PFAS manufacturing industries (Lenka et al. 2022). The finding of Lenka et al. (2022) discussed the potential contribution of wastewater treatment plant effluent as well as other sources including airports, septic schemes, and industries for PFAS contamination in coastal waters of New Zealand. Another meta-analysis found that atmospheric depositions and direct emissions are the major sources of contamination in surface water bodies by short-chain PFAS compounds such as PFOS and PFOA (Podder et al. 2021).

PFAS with shorter carbon chain lengths are highly mobile, persistent, and regularly detected in water resources compared to PFAS compounds consisting of longer chain lengths (Li et al. 2020b). Therefore, short-chain PFAS, such as PFOS and PFOA, induce higher toxicity in aquatic environments. Podder et al. (2021) in their meta-analysis found that PFOS and PFOA in various surface water bodies are greater than the US EPA permissible limit for a lifetime exposure level in drinking water (70 ng/l). However, not only the dissolved portion of PFAS but also the PFAS absorbed into the suspended particulate matter should be considered because an adsorbed fraction is greatly attributed to the total PFAS loads in surface water bodies (Cookson and Detwiler 2022).

10.4.2 PFAS in Groundwater

A recent meta-analysis conducted by Johnson et al. (2022) depicted PFOA and PFOS as the most frequently reported PFAS compounds in groundwater sources in 20 countries throughout the world. The PFOA concentrations in groundwater sources were reported between <0.03 ng/l and ~7 mg/l, whereas the PFOS concentrations ranged between 0.01 ng/l and ~5 mg/l. However, 6 : 2 fluorotelomer sulfonate (6 : 2 FTS), which is a replacement for legacy PFAS compounds, occupied the highest reported concentration in groundwater (~15 mg/l) in 20 countries (Johnson et al. 2022). The findings of Dasu et al. (2022) indicated the occurrence of PFOA and PFOS at the highest average concentrations in the groundwater contaminated with AFFF. The same study found that landfill leachate is the second highest contributor to PFOA and PFOS presence in groundwater. Hepburn et al. (2019) determined the PFAS in groundwater sources surrounded by legacy landfill sites in Australia and detected PFOA, PFOS, perfluorobutane sulfonate (PFBS), and PFHxS in all samples. Among 14 PFAS detected, PFHxS had the highest average concentration (34 ng/l) and subsequently PFOS, PFOS, and PFOA detected respective concentrations of 26, 19, and 12 ng/l. Furthermore, the sum of the 14 PFAS compounds detected in the samples ranged between 26 and 5200 ng/l. Moreover, according to Xu et al. (2021), six PFAS compounds, namely PFOA, PFOS, PFBA (perfluorobutanoic acid), PFBS, PFNA, and PFHxS, are frequently found in groundwater up to a concentration of 21,000 ng/l.

Soil, surface water sources, landfill leachate plumes, ice and snow deposition, rainfall, and atmospheric depositions are the sources of groundwater contamination with PFAS. For instance, 90% of PFOA and PFOS contamination in groundwater is estimated to be due to migration from soil (Xu et al. 2021). Furthermore, PFBA, PFBS, PFOA, PFDA, PFPeA, PFHxA, and PFHpA (perfluoroheptanoic acid) in groundwater exhibited a significant correlation with their concentrations in soil, suggesting their shared source of origin (Cao et al. 2019).

Utilization of surface and groundwater contaminated with PFAS for irrigational purposes and industrial and household activities ultimately results in soil contamination in distant localities.

10.5 PFAS in Soil and Interactions

Brusseau et al. (2020) gathered data from more than 30,000 soil samples from over 2500 sites all over the world, and virtually every sample contained PFAS. PFOA and PFOS were the most frequently found PFAS compounds in soil. Johnson et al. (2022) in their meta-analysis emphasized the presence of PFAS compounds, especially PFOA and PFOS, in the soil at significantly higher concentrations compared to other environmental matrices such as surface water, groundwater, seawater, and precipitation. The reasons to report comparatively highest PFAS concentrations in soil include being the primary entry point for other environmental compartments and bearing higher PFAS retention capacities. Two main processes, namely sorption onto soil particles and adsorption at the water–air interface, are involved in the retention of PFAS in unsaturated soil (Brusseau 2018). However, the sorption process of PFAS onto soil particles could involve complex and multiple mechanisms, and it is further affected by the different head groups of various PFAS (Cáñez et al. 2021).

The transportation ability and bioavailability of PFAS in soil are affected by the migration efficiency of PFAS and are related to multiple factors such as soil organic matter, pH, surface-bound cations, and soil biota including worms and microbes (Oliver et al. 2020). Moreover, rainfall can also increase the migration and diffusion of PFAS in highly permeable amended soils (Eun et al. 2020; Zhang et al. 2016). Dauchy et al. (2019) studied the downward migration of PFAS in firefighter training facilities and found declining PFAS concentrations toward deeper components of the soil profile. Direct infiltration is the most influential governing factor for the downward movement of PFAS in soil. Brusseau et al. (2020) pointed out the same decreasing trend of PFAS concentrations in the unsaturated zone (vadose zone). The same study revealed higher concentrations of PFAS in soil and unsaturated zone compared to the PFAS concentrations in groundwater in many study sites, indicating soil and unsaturated zone as the primary long-term

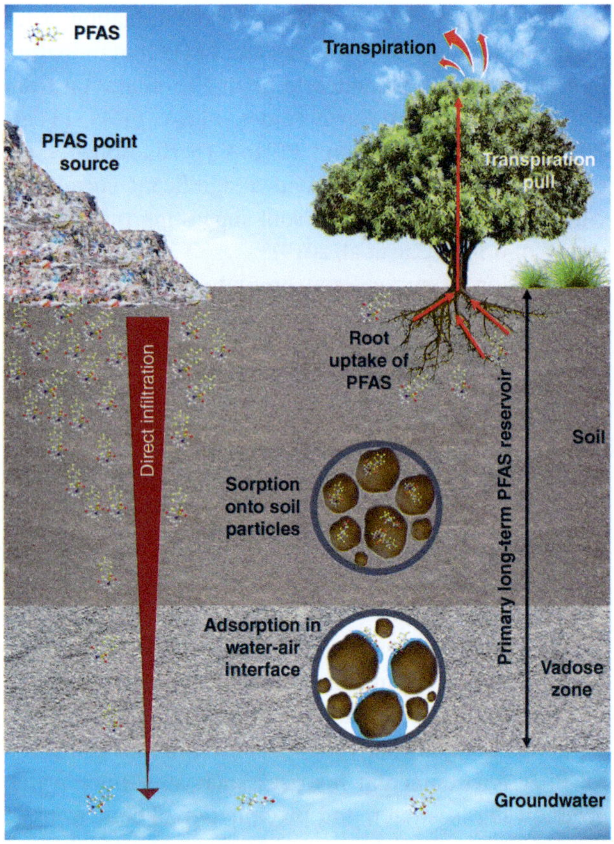

Figure 10.3 PFAS in soil–water systems.

PFAS reservoir in the environment. The migration behavior of PFAS in soil and unsaturated zone is influenced by the properties of soil and PFAS source, PFAS precursor compounds, infiltration rates, climatic factors, and geochemical and physical variations (Brusseau et al. 2020; Cáñez et al. 2021). Figure 10.3 further illustrates the mobilization and interactions of PFAS in soil–water systems.

10.5.1 PFAS and Soil Microbiome

The soil microbiome consists of taxonomically diverse microbes such as bacteria, nematodes, fungi, actinomycetes, and protozoans, each of which has its own contribution to the sustainability of soil systems (Ossowicki et al. 2021). Changes in the form and function of soil biota present a serious threat to plant growth, crop production, and consequently human health (Díaz-García et al. 2021). Studies show that PFAS compounds can negatively impact soil microbial activities and communities and change the rhizosphere structure and composition (Cai et al. 2021). Bioavailability and toxicity of PFAS further vary according to the soil type (i.e. high in sandy soil) (He et al. 2016). Among different types of soil microbes, bacteria predominantly form biofilms that are advantageous for plant growth (Ahmad et al. 2017). In the presence of PFAS compounds, toxic metals such as Cr can easily disrupt the activity of biofilm formation by *Bacillus subtilis*, expose the plant to diseases, and reduce its resistance to cope with environmental changes (Zhang et al. 2020b). Moreover, the abundance, structure, and composition of the microbial community have been greatly altered when the soil systems are exposed to sludge contaminated with PFAS (specifically PFOS) combined with heavy metals such as Cu (Liu et al. 2017). When anaerobic sludge is exposed to PFAS compounds (i.e. PFOS), the methanogenic activities may change significantly, so that it can have an adverse effect on the steps of the nitrogen cycle that are mediated by the soil bacteria (Lu et al. 2020a). Furthermore, PFOA substances inhibit nitrification and increase the denitrification processes, thus causing an imbalance in the nitrogen cycle (Chen et al. 2021). Both alive and dead bacteria have the affinity to bind PFOS, the latter in high concentrations. Studies that used the soil-dwelling bacterivorous nematode *Caenorhabditis elegans* to test the effects of PFAS reveal that when these nematodes feed on bacteria that contain PFOS (both dead and alive), these compounds were transferred to the nematodes, were concentrated in their bodies, and caused changes in gene expression, thus having the potential to transfer through food chains (Stylianou et al. 2019). In addition to bacteria and nematodes, fungi are an important group of soil microbes that play a vital role in decomposition. The white-rot fungi *Phanerochaete chrysosporium* found in the soil decompose wood and other materials have long been used by researchers to examine the effects of various toxic chemicals (Singh and Chen 2008). Studies on the white-rot fungi that were exposed to 100 mg/l PFOS show a significant decrease in their biomass (>75%) along with membrane and oxidative damages (Qiao et al. 2019). It is evident that the decomposition rates would in turn change the functionality of soil biota. Additionally, PFAS greatly inhibits the trophic level transferring efficiency of a plethora of soil microbes ranging from methanogenic archaea to protozoa. The tropic level transfer is an important factor that determines the length of food chains (Wu et al. 2022). However, the impact of PFAS pollution on soil biota is an emerging research area that has not been sufficiently explored (Melo et al. 2022). Figure 10.4 describes the various impacts of PFAS on soil microorganisms.

10.6 Plant Interactions and Uptake of PFAS

Plant uptake of PFAS can occur through water, soil, and sediments (Colomer-Vidal et al. 2022). PFAS contamination further depends on the physicochemical properties of PFAS (e.g. perfluorocarbon chain length, functional head

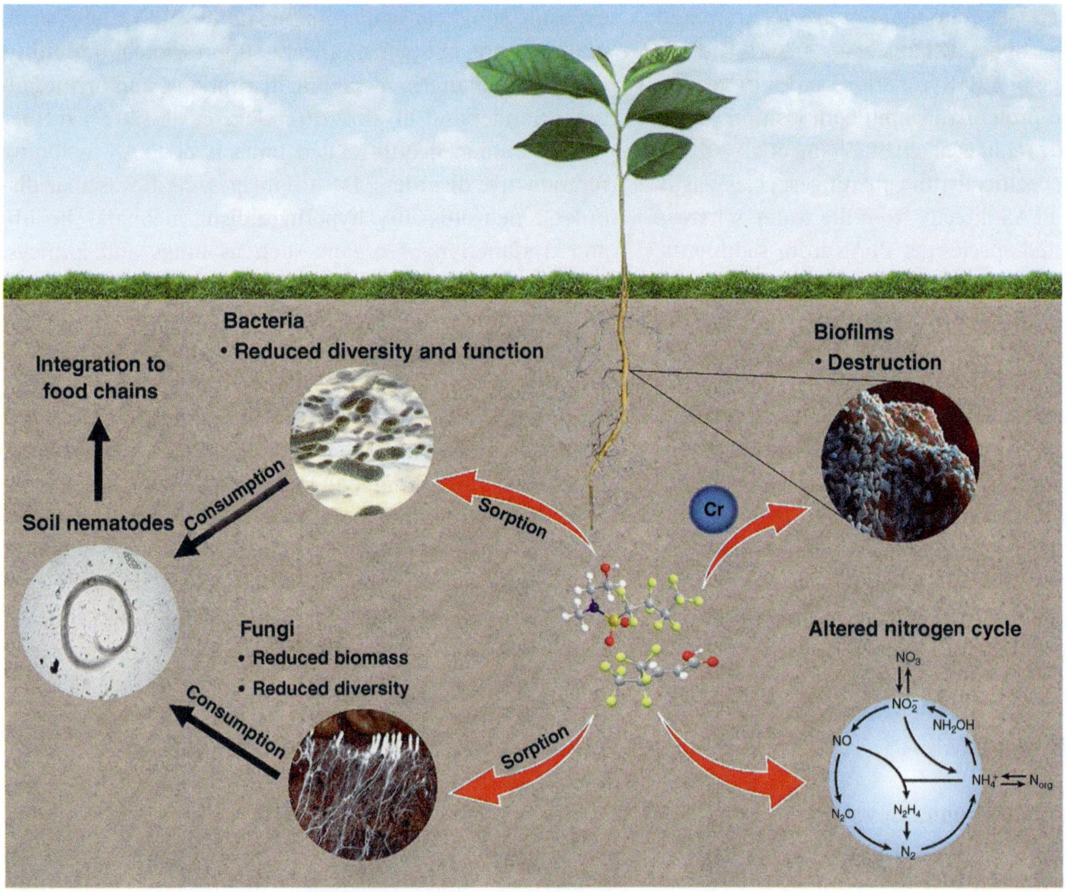

Figure 10.4 Influence of PFSA on soil microbiome.

group, water solubility, and volatility), plant physiology (e.g. transpiration rate, lipid content, and protein content), and abiotic factors (e.g. soil organic matter content, pH, salinity, and temperature) (Ghisi et al. 2019; Wang et al. 2020b; Colomer-Vidal et al. 2022).

Contamination of irrigation water, diffusion in soil, and atmospheric deposition are pathways of PFAS contamination in plant systems (Ghisi et al. 2019; Felizeter et al. 2021). However, the presence of PFAS in irrigation water is identified as one of the most prominent pathways to reach crop plants. The application of recycled water from wastewater treatment plants, landfill leachates, and biosolids applied to agricultural soil are all point sources of PFAS transmission to crops (Ghisi et al. 2019). PFAS can be incorporated into the root systems of plants such as cereals, fruits, and vegetables once they have been introduced to agricultural fields (Shahsavari et al. 2021).

Due to the hydrophilicity of PFAS, transpiration plays an important role in their accumulation and translocation provided by the upward mobility of water from roots to shoots of plants. Generally, the accumulation ability of PFAS in roots is higher than in shoots; however, this also depends on factors such as the plant species, carbon-chain length of PFAS compound, and microbial activity (Pullagurala et al. 2018). Evidence from studies shows that there is a significant relationship between the types and concentrations of PFAS in agricultural products and the irrigation water used (Zhang et al. 2016).

PFAS are absorbed by crops when grown in contaminated soil and accumulate in plant tissues, presenting a potential route for animal and human exposure through food chains (Huff et al. 2020). Studies show that in China, higher concentrations of PFAS have been detected in the soil and crops near fluorochemical industrial facilities as opposed to long-distance transmission (Ghisi et al. 2019; Liu et al. 2019; Zhang et al. 2020b; Zhou et al. 2021). The bioaccumulation and transport capacities of different PFAS in vegetables re determined by the structure of the compound, such as its carbon chain length and the type of polar group present. Furthermore, the ionizing ability of PFAS determines their capacity for transfer across the Casparian strip into the vascular root tissues (Felizeter et al. 2014). The ability of PFAS to transfer from roots to shoots is enhanced with a shorter carbon chain, allowing transpiration to occur (Wen et al. 2014). Long- chain carbon (C8–C14) components mainly adsorb to the root surfaces, while shorter ones (C4–C7) are more easily taken up and are translocated to the shoots (Zhang et al. 2020a). The distributional difference of PFAS in various types of vegetables depends on the protein and lipid composition of the different edible tissues (Liu et al. 2019; Zhang et al. 2020b). In aquatic plants, specifically, the floating species easily take up long-chain PFAS directly from the water, whereas submerged and rooted species get PFAS from sediments. Long-chain PFAS remains accumulated in the roots because of protein affinity, while short-chain PFAS were more mobile and translocated to the shoots (Colomer-Vidal et al. 2022).

Over the past decades, numerous studies have been carried out on the mechanisms of PFAS contamination in cultivated vegetables and crops, emphasizing distribution, pollution source assessment, and migration pathway confirmation of PFAS. However, many of these investigations were carried out only for PFOA and PFOS but not for emerging PFAS derivatives, which have become a threat to plants and cropping systems.

10.7 Health Risks of PFAS

PFAS exposure in humans is omnipresent in the world. For instance, PFOS and PFOA alone were detected in more than 90% human population in the United States (Kato et al. 2011). Together with their long environmental persistency, PFAS compounds exhibit greater capacities for bioaccumulation and biomagnification across trophic levels and ultimately reach humans with dietary components (Garg et al. 2020). For example, Reinikainen et al. (2022) calculated the average intake of collectively four PFAS (i.e. PFOA, PFOS, PFHxS, and PFNA) via fish consumption of a fisheries community living in Finland and the resulting value of 5.4–18.0 ng/kg/d surpasses the new group tolerable daily intake level demarcated by European Food Safety Authority (EFSA). On the other hand, ingestion of contaminated groundwater and surface water contributes to several health-related complications in humans. Contaminated air and dust account for smaller fractions of PFAS exposure to adult humans while breastfeeding and in utero transfer causes PFAS exposure in infants (Sunderland et al. 2019). However, the PFAS exposure route and the magnitude vary with lifestyle, drinking water consumption and dietary patterns, and distance to point and non-point PFAS sources (Blake and Fenton 2020). For example, the workers in PFAS manufacturing industries or industries that use PFAS as raw materials could have high exposure values.

PFAS have an extensively long half-life in the human body and accumulate in kidneys, brain, liver, lungs, and body serums (Pérez et al. 2013). A high level of PFAS exposure could cause disruptions in the endocrine system, malformation of organs, cancers, suppression of immunity, behavioral changes, metabolic disruptions, and organ failures (Sunderland et al. 2019). Garg et al. (2020) further specify human health-related impacts of PFAS including reproductive disorders, DNA damages, cardiovascular disorders, neurotoxicity, hypothyroidism, neonatal health, and dysfunction of organs such as lungs and kidneys. However, the results of Solan et al. (2022) obtained using in vitro human cell-based models indicated the disproportionate impacts of PFAS on different human tissue types. In their study, neural cell lines showed the highest sensitivity to short- and long-chain PFAS while colon and kidney cell lines demonstrated relatively less sensitivities. Furthermore, the brain, kidney, lung, and mucus cell lines exhibited viability loss within comparatively narrow range of PFAS exposure (EC_{50} = 1–70 μM). Therefore, the type of PFAS, daily exposure values and exposure period, and impacted tissue/organ type have significant relationship with the nature and extent of human health-related consequences.

10.8 Implications for Remediation

There are conventional as well as advanced techniques, such as ion exchange, adsorption, membrane filtration, photolysis, photocatalysis, thermolysis, sonolysis, oxidation–reduction, and electrochemical reactions, that have been studied for the effective and efficient removal and remediation of PFOS contamination (Li et al. 2020a) (Figure 10.5). One classical approach that is currently used to stabilize PFAS is sorption using adsorption materials such as biochar (Zhang et al. 2022a). Natural plant-based compounds such as *Moringa oleifera* seed powder coupled with calcium alginate are also known to be efficient adsorbents of PFAS but are not yet widely utilized in remediation (Militao et al. 2022). PFAS found in liquid forms can be mineralized into harmless compounds with sonolysis techniques using ultrasound. However, it is a very complex process where numerous parameters (e.g. frequency and temperature) need to be continuously monitored. Despite its complexity, it is known as an efficient treatment method that is often recommended by researchers (Sidnell et al. 2022). Membrane filtration of PFAS is usually carried out under high pressure using nanofiltration membranes. Oxidation of PFAS can be carried out through ex situ and in situ methodologies (Pilli et al. 2021). For example, under highly acidic conditions, permanganate ions have the ability to decompose more than 70% of PFOS over a period of 18 days (Liu et al. 2012). PFAS degradation can also be carried out using biological means, such as using *Pseudomonas* strain D2, and many other microbes, but this is not widely

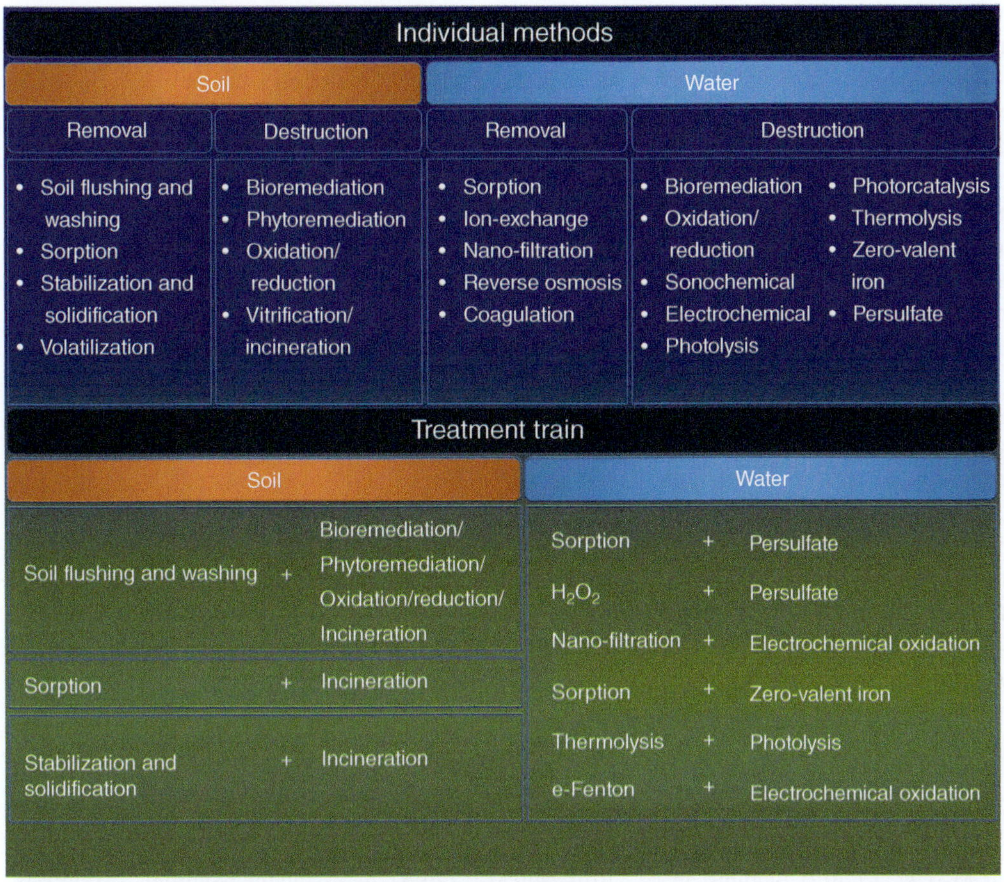

Figure 10.5 Remediation technologies for PFAS in environment.

practiced (Pilli et al. 2021). Moreover, treatment train approaches (i.e. use of two or more synergistic remediation methods) have been developed since 2015 to facilitate in situ remediation of PFAS in an effective manner (Lu et al. 2020b) (Figure 10.5). Furthermore, improving the current remediation methods and experimenting with environmentally friendly and economically sound novel integrated PFAS treatment methodologies are essential for sustainable management of the environment.

10.9 Recommendations and Future Research Directions

PFAS consists of an array of fluorinated, highly bioaccumulative compounds that are widespread in the environment and raise health issues for humans and other living organisms (Houck et al. 2021). Epidemiological studies suggest that there are numerous adverse health effects related to continuous exposure to PFAS (Fenton et al. 2021). However, there is a major challenge for PFAS exposure assessments since there are no sufficient statistically representative population surveys for both humans and wildlife. Additionally, there is still not enough data on how PFAS are translocated into the tissues of living organisms (De Silva et al. 2021). Therefore, as an initial step, it is essential to classify or group PFAS using unified methods to phase them out or reduce their impact on production chains and also to establish regulations to identify PFAS-related compounds from consumer products to minimize their future usage (Cousins et al. 2020). Thus, governments can implement regulations to restrict their manufacture and usage. Local sources of PFAS contamination, such as industrial units, sewage treatment facilities, and landfills, can be tested for point contamination of PFAS. If not tested appropriately, these high-volume emissions would affect large geographic areas and consequently impact larger populations of humans and wildlife (Herrick et al. 2017). Apart from identifying the hazardous effects and contamination pathways of PFAS, long-term continuous experiments are needed to understand their fate and their degradation products, along with the establishment of databases that can be used for environmental modeling (Sima and Jaffé 2021). Even though there are thousands of PFAS-containing compounds existing in the environment, only a few have been regulated internationally (i.e. PFAS, PFOA). There is an urgent need to find alternative replacements for PFAS and provide recommendations to reduce their usage. Day-to-day usage of PFAS, most of which are unidentified and unregulated, has largely contaminated plant-soil-water systems. Advanced research on PFAS compounds and their transportation to the soil–water systems and humans, backed with further regulatory activities, would help to reduce the environmental release of these compounds in the future.

Moreover, it is necessary to establish efficient, cost-effective, and environmentally friendly treatment methods to remediate PFAS-contaminated water sources and lands. Most widely utilized conventional treatment methods for aqueous media, such as membrane filtration and the use of ion-exchange materials, are effective against the removal of PFAS with longer C chains but showed relatively less performance toward the removal of shorter chain PFAS, such as PFOS and PFAS (Li et al. 2020b). The use of the aforementioned techniques for the removal of short-chain PFAS results in poor regeneration efficiencies of adsorptive materials as well as higher costs for waste residue disposal. Moreover, sophisticated techniques, such as advanced oxidation methods (e.g. sonolysis and thermolysis), demonstrated total mineralization of PFAS; however, they are associated with superior process costs. Therefore, low-cost, green adsorption materials such as biochar and biochar composite materials coupled with different activation and functionalization techniques should be further studied to unveil their PFAS removal capacities. In addition to the efficacy, the duration and dosage of the sorbent need to be clearly determined according to the concentration of PFAS compounds (Zhang et al. 2022a). Therefore, there is a current need for further research and development to make these compounds available for industrial and large-scale usage around the world. Furthermore, extensive research on phytoremediation and microbial-assisted degradation to remediate PFAS-contaminated lands should be carried out as cost-effective and environmentally friendly techniques. In this regard, identification of new plant varieties/microbial strains and their capacities to remove or degrade PFAS with different chain lengths and headgroups is essential. However, studies on the combined application of plants and microorganisms (i.e. microbial assisted phytoremediation) on PFAS-contaminated soil could be more appropriate to increase PFAS removal efficiency.

References

Ahmad, I., Khan, M.S., Altaf, M.M. et al. (2017). Biofilms: an overview of their significance in plant and soil health. *Biofilms in Plant and Soil Health* 1–25. https://doi.org/10.1002/9781119246329.ch1.

Al Amin, M., Sobhani, Z., Liu, Y. et al. (2020). Recent advances in the analysis of per-and polyfluoroalkyl substances (PFAS) – a review. *Environmental Technology & Innovation* 19: 100879. https://doi.org/10.1016/j.eti.2020.100879.

Ambaye, T.G., Vaccari, M., Prasad, S., and Rtimi, S. (2022). Recent progress and challenges on the removal of per-and poly-fluoroalkyl substances (PFAS) from contaminated soil and water. *Environmental Science and Pollution Research* 1–24. https://doi.org/10.1007/s11356-022-21513-2.

Blake, B.E. and Fenton, S.E. (2020). Early life exposure to per-and polyfluoroalkyl substances (PFAS) and latent health outcomes: a review including the placenta as a target tissue and possible driver of peri-and postnatal effects. *Toxicology* 443: 152565. https://doi.org/10.1016/j.tox.2020.152565.

Bolan, N., Sarkar, B., Yan, Y. et al. (2021). Remediation of poly- and perfluoroalkyl substances (PFAS) contaminated soils– to mobilize or to immobilize or to degrade? *Journal of Hazardous Materials* 401: 123892. https://doi.org/10.1016/j.jhazmat.2020.123892.

Brusseau, M.L. (2018). Assessing the potential contributions of additional retention processes to PFAS retardation in the subsurface. *Science of the Total Environment* 613: 176–185. https://doi.org/10.1016/j.scitotenv.2017.09.065.

Brusseau, M.L., Anderson, R.H., and Guo, B. (2020). PFAS concentrations in soils: background levels versus contaminated sites. *Science of the Total Environment* 740: 140017. https://doi.org/10.1016/j.scitotenv.2020.140017.

Buck, R.C., Franklin, J., Berger, U. et al. (2011). Perfluoroalkyl and polyfluoroalkyl substances in the environment: terminology, classification, and origins. *Integrated Environmental Assessment and Management* 7: 513–541. https://doi.org/10.1002/ieam.258.

Cai, Y., Wang, Q., Zhou, B. et al. (2021). A review of responses of terrestrial organisms to perfluorinated compounds. *Science of the Total Environment* 793: 148565. https://doi.org/10.1016/j.scitotenv.2021.148565.

Cáñez, T.T., Guo, B., Mcintosh, J.C., and Brusseau, M.L. (2021). Perfluoroalkyl and polyfluoroalkyl substances (PFAS) in groundwater at a reclaimed water recharge facility. *Science of the Total Environment* 791: 147906. https://doi.org/10.1016/j.scitotenv.2021.147906.

Cao, X., Wang, C., Lu, Y. et al. (2019). Occurrence, sources and health risk of polyfluoroalkyl substances (PFASs) in soil, water and sediment from a drinking water source area. *Ecotoxicology and Environmental Safety* 174: 208–217. https://doi.org/10.1016/j.ecoenv.2019.02.058.

Chen, H., Zou, M., Zhou, Y. et al. (2021). Monitoring the nitrous oxide emissions and biological nutrient removal from wastewater treatment: impact of perfluorooctanoic acid. *Journal of Hazardous Materials* 402: 123469. https://doi.org/10.1016/j.jhazmat.2020.123469.

Coggan, T.L., Moodie, D., Kolobaric, A. et al. (2019). An investigation into per-and polyfluoroalkyl substances (PFAS) in nineteen Australian wastewater treatment plants (WWTPs). *Heliyon* 5: e02316. https://doi.org/10.1016/j.heliyon.2019.e02316.

Colomer-Vidal, P., Jiang, L., Mei, W. et al. (2022). Plant uptake of perfluoroalkyl substances in freshwater environments (Dongzhulong and Xiaoqing Rivers, China). *Journal of Hazardous Materials* 421: 126768. https://doi.org/10.1016/j.jhazmat.2021.126768.

Cookson, E. and Detwiler, R.L. (2022). Global patterns and temporal trends of perfluoroalkyl substances in municipal wastewater: a meta-analysis. *Water Research* 118784. https://doi.org/10.1016/j.watres.2022.118784.

Cousins, I.T., Goldenman, G., Herzke, D. et al. (2019). The concept of essential use for determining when uses of PFASs can be phased out. *Environmental Science: Processes & Impacts* 21: 1803–1815. https://doi.org/10.1039/C9EM00163H.

Cousins, I.T., Dewitt, J.C., Glüge, J. et al. (2020). Strategies for grouping per-and polyfluoroalkyl substances (PFAS) to protect human and environmental health. *Environmental Science: Processes & Impacts* 22: 1444–1460. https://doi.org/10.1039/D0EM00147C.

Darlington, R., Barth, E., and Mckernan, J. (2018). The challenges of PFAS remediation. *The Military Engineer* 110: 58.

Dasu, K., Xia, X., Siriwardena, D. et al. (2022). Concentration profiles of per-and polyfluoroalkyl substances in major sources to the environment. *Journal of Environmental Management* 301: 113879. https://doi.org/10.1016/j.jenvman.2021.113879.

Dauchy, X., Boiteux, V., Colin, A. et al. (2019). Deep seepage of per-and polyfluoroalkyl substances through the soil of a firefighter training site and subsequent groundwater contamination. *Chemosphere* 214: 729–737. https://doi.org/10.1016/j.chemosphere.2018.10.003.

De Silva, A.O., Armitage, J.M., Bruton, T.A. et al. (2021). PFAS exposure pathways for humans and wildlife: a synthesis of current knowledge and key gaps in understanding. *Environmental Toxicology and Chemistry* 40: 631–657. https://doi.org/10.1002/etc.4935.

Díaz-García, L., Huang, S., Spröer, C. et al. (2021). Dilution-to-stimulation/extinction method: a combination enrichment strategy to develop a minimal and versatile lignocellulolytic bacterial consortium. *Applied and Environmental Microbiology* 87: e02427–e02420. https://doi.org/10.1128/AEM.02427-20.

Eun, H., Yamazaki, E., Taniyasu, S. et al. (2020). Evaluation of perfluoroalkyl substances in field-cultivated vegetables. *Chemosphere* 239: 124750. https://doi.org/10.1016/j.chemosphere.2019.124750.

Felizeter, S., Mclachlan, M.S., and De Voogt, P. (2014). Root uptake and translocation of perfluorinated alkyl acids by three hydroponically grown crops. *Journal of Agricultural and Food Chemistry* 62: 3334–3342. https://doi.org/10.1021/jf500674j.

Felizeter, S., Jürling, H., Kotthoff, M. et al. (2021). Uptake of perfluorinated alkyl acids by crops: results from a field study. *Environmental Science: Processes & Impacts* 23: 1158–1170. https://doi.org/10.1039/D1EM00166C.

Fenton, S.E., Ducatman, A., Boobis, A. et al. (2021). Per-and polyfluoroalkyl substance toxicity and human health review: current state of knowledge and strategies for informing future research. *Environmental Toxicology and Chemistry* 40: 606–630. https://doi.org/10.1002/etc.4890.

Gallen, C., Eaglesham, G., Drage, D. et al. (2018). A mass estimate of perfluoroalkyl substance (PFAS) release from Australian wastewater treatment plants. *Chemosphere* 208: 975–983. https://doi.org/10.1016/j.chemosphere.2018.06.024.

Garg, S., Kumar, P., Mishra, V. et al. (2020). A review on the sources, occurrence and health risks of per-/poly-fluoroalkyl substances (PFAS) arising from the manufacture and disposal of electric and electronic products. *Journal of Water Process Engineering* 38: 101683. https://doi.org/10.1016/j.jwpe.2020.101683.

Ghisi, R., Vamerali, T., and Manzetti, S. (2019). Accumulation of perfluorinated alkyl substances (PFAS) in agricultural plants: a review. *Environmental Research* 169: 326–341. https://doi.org/10.1016/j.envres.2018.10.023.

Hamid, H., Li, L.Y., and Grace, J.R. (2018). Review of the fate and transformation of per-and polyfluoroalkyl substances (PFASs) in landfills. *Environmental Pollution* 235: 74–84. https://doi.org/10.1016/j.envpol.2017.12.030.

He, W., Megharaj, M., and Naidu, R. (2016). Toxicity of perfluorooctanoic acid towards earthworm and enzymatic activities in soil. *Environmental Monitoring and Assessment* 188: 1–7. https://doi.org/10.1007/s10661-016-5416-y.

Hepburn, E., Madden, C., Szabo, D. et al. (2019). Contamination of groundwater with per-and polyfluoroalkyl substances (PFAS) from legacy landfills in an urban re-development precinct. *Environmental Pollution* 248: 101–113. https://doi.org/10.1016/j.envpol.2019.02.018.

Herrick, R.L., Buckholz, J., Biro, F.M. et al. (2017). Polyfluoroalkyl substance exposure in the mid-Ohio River

Valley, 1991–2012. *Environmental Pollution* 228: 50–60. https://doi.org/10.1016/j.envpol.2017.04.092.

Houck, K.A., Patlewicz, G., Richard, A.M. et al. (2021). Bioactivity profiling of per-and polyfluoroalkyl substances (PFAS) identifies potential toxicity pathways related to molecular structure. *Toxicology* 457: 152789. https://doi.org/10.1016/j.tox.2021.152789.

Huff, D.K., Morris, L.A., Sutter, L. et al. (2020). Accumulation of six PFAS compounds by woody and herbaceous plants: potential for phytoextraction. *International Journal of Phytoremediation* 22: 1538–1550. https://doi.org/10.1080/15226514.2020.1786004.

Janousek, R.M., Lebertz, S., and Knepper, T.P. (2019). Previously unidentified sources of perfluoroalkyl and polyfluoroalkyl substances from building materials and industrial fabrics. *Environmental Science: Processes & Impacts* 21: 1936–1945. https://doi.org/10.1039/C9EM00091G.

Johnson, G.R., Brusseau, M.L., Carroll, K.C. et al. (2022). Global distributions, source-type dependencies, and concentration ranges of per-and polyfluoroalkyl substances in groundwater. *Science of the Total Environment* 841: 156602. https://doi.org/10.1016/j.scitotenv.2022.156602.

Kato, K., Wong, L.-Y., Jia, L.T. et al. (2011). Trends in exposure to polyfluoroalkyl chemicals in the US population: 1999–2008. *Environmental science & technology* 45: 8037–8045. https://doi.org/10.1021/es1043613.

Kurwadkar, S., Dane, J., Kanel, S.R. et al. (2021). Per-and polyfluoroalkyl substances in water and wastewater: a critical review of their global occurrence and distribution. *Science of the Total Environment* 151003. https://doi.org/10.1016/j.scitotenv.2021.151003.

Lenka, S.P., Kah, M., and Padhye, L.P. (2021). A review of the occurrence, transformation, and removal of poly-and perfluoroalkyl substances (PFAS) in wastewater treatment plants. *Water Research* 199: 117187. https://doi.org/10.1016/j.watres.2021.117187.

Lenka, S.P., Kah, M., and Padhye, L.P. (2022). Occurrence and fate of poly-and perfluoroalkyl substances (PFAS) in urban waters of New Zealand. *Journal of Hazardous Materials* 428: 128257. https://doi.org/10.1016/j.jhazmat.2022.128257.

Li, F., Duan, J., Tian, S. et al. (2020a). Short-chain per-and polyfluoroalkyl substances in aquatic systems: occurrence, impacts and treatment. *Chemical Engineering Journal* 380: 122506. https://doi.org/10.1016/j.cej.2019.122506.

Li, J., Zheng, T., Yuan, D. et al. (2020b). Probing the single and combined toxicity of PFOS and Cr(VI) to soil bacteria and the interaction mechanisms. *Chemosphere* 249: 126039. https://doi.org/10.1016/j.chemosphere.2020.126039.

Liu, C.S., Shih, K., and Wang, F. (2012). Oxidative decomposition of perfluorooctanesulfonate in water by permanganate. *Separation and Purification Technology* 87: 95–100. https://doi.org/10.1016/j.seppur.2011.11.027.

Liu, X., Yin, H., Tang, S. et al. (2017). Effects of single and combined copper/perfluorooctane sulfonate on sequencing batch reactor process and microbial community in activated sludge. *Bioresource Technology* 238: 407–415. https://doi.org/10.1016/j.biortech.2017.04.045.

Liu, Z., Lu, Y., Song, X. et al. (2019). Multiple crop bioaccumulation and human exposure of perfluoroalkyl substances around a mega fluorochemical industrial park, China: implication for planting optimization and food safety. *Environment International* 127: 671–684. https://doi.org/10.1016/j.envint.2019.04.008.

Lu, B., Qian, J., Wang, P. et al. (2020a). Effect of perfluorooctanesulfonate (PFOS) on the rhizosphere soil nitrogen cycling of two riparian plants. *Science of the Total Environment* 741: 140494. https://doi.org/10.1016/j.scitotenv.2020.140494.

Lu, D., Sha, S., Luo, J. et al. (2020b). Treatment train approaches for the remediation of per-and polyfluoroalkyl substances (PFAS): a critical review. *Journal of Hazardous Materials* 386: 121963. https://doi.org/10.1016/j.jhazmat.2019.121963.

Martin, D., Munoz, G., Mejia-Avendaño, S. et al. (2019). Zwitterionic, cationic, and anionic perfluoroalkyl and polyfluoroalkyl substances integrated into total oxidizable precursor assay of contaminated groundwater. *Talanta* 195: 533–542. https://doi.org/10.1016/j.talanta.2018.11.093.

Mei, W., Sun, H., Song, M. et al. (2021). Per-and polyfluoroalkyl substances (PFASs) in the soil–plant system: sorption, root uptake, and translocation. *Environment International* 156: 106642. https://doi.org/10.1016/j.envint.2021.106642.

Melo, T.M., Schauerte, M., Bluhm, A. et al. (2022). Ecotoxicological effects of per- and polyfluoroalkyl substances (PFAS) and of a new PFAS adsorbing organoclay to immobilize PFAS in soils on earthworms and plants. *Journal of Hazardous Materials* 433: 128771. https://doi.org/10.1016/j.jhazmat.2022.128771.

Militao, I.M., Roddick, F., Bergamasco, R., and Fan, L. (2022). Rapid adsorption of PFAS: application of Moringa oleifera seed powder encapsulated in alginate beads. *Environmental Technology & Innovation* 28: 102761. https://doi.org/10.1016/j.eti.2022.102761.

Nakayama, S.F., Yoshikane, M., Onoda, Y. et al. (2019). Worldwide trends in tracing poly- and perfluoroalkyl substances (PFAS) in the environment. *TrAC Trends in Analytical Chemistry* 121: 115410. https://doi.org/10.1016/j.trac.2019.02.011.

Nguyen, H.T., Kaserzon, S.L., Thai, P.K. et al. (2019). Temporal trends of per- and polyfluoroalkyl substances

(PFAS) in the influent of two of the largest wastewater treatment plants in Australia. *Emerging Contaminants* 5: 211–218. https://doi.org/10.1016/j.emcon.2019.05.006.

Nickerson, A., Maizel, A.C., Kulkarni, P.R. et al. (2020). Enhanced extraction of AFFF-associated PFASs from source zone soils. *Environmental Science & Technology* 54: 4952–4962. https://doi.org/10.1021/acs.est.0c00792.

Oliver, D.P., Li, Y., Orr, R. et al. (2020). Sorption behaviour of per- and polyfluoroalkyl substances (PFASs) in tropical soils. *Environmental Pollution* 258: 113726. https://doi.org/10.1016/j.envpol.2019.113726.

Ossowicki, A., Raaijmakers, J.M., and Garbeva, P. (2021). Disentangling soil microbiome functions by perturbation. *Environmental Microbiology Reports* 13: 582–590. https://doi.org/10.1111/1758-2229.12989.

Pérez, F., Nadal, M., Navarro-Ortega, A. et al. (2013). Accumulation of perfluoroalkyl substances in human tissues. *Environment international* 59: 354–362. https://doi.org/10.1016/j.envint.2013.06.004.

Pilli, S., Pandey, A.K., Pandey, V. et al. (2021). Detection and removal of poly and perfluoroalkyl polluting substances for sustainable environment. *Journal of Environmental Management* 297: 113336. https://doi.org/10.1016/j.jenvman.2021.113336.

Podder, A., Sadmani, A.H.M.A., Reinhart, D. et al. (2021). Per and poly-fluoroalkyl substances (PFAS) as a contaminant of emerging concern in surface water: a transboundary review of their occurrences and toxicity effects. *Journal of Hazardous Materials* 419: 126361. https://doi.org/10.1016/j.jhazmat.2021.126361.

Pullagurala, V.L.R., Rawat, S., Adisa, I.O. et al. (2018). Plant uptake and translocation of contaminants of emerging concern in soil. *Science of the Total Environment* 636: 1585–1596. https://doi.org/10.1016/j.scitotenv.2018.04.375.

Qiao, W., Zhang, Y., Xie, Z. et al. (2019). Toxicity of perfluorooctane sulfonate on Phanerochaete chrysosporium: growth, pollutant degradation and transcriptomics. *Ecotoxicology and Environmental Safety* 174: 66–74. https://doi.org/10.1016/j.ecoenv.2019.02.066.

Reinikainen, J., Perkola, N., Äystö, L., and Sorvari, J. (2022). The occurrence, distribution, and risks of PFAS at AFFF-impacted sites in Finland. *Science of The Total Environment* 829: 154237. https://doi.org/10.1016/j.scitotenv.2022.154237.

Ruan, T., Lin, Y., Wang, T. et al. (2015). Methodology for studying biotransformation of polyfluoroalkyl precursors in the environment. *TrAC Trends in Analytical Chemistry* 67: 167–178. https://doi.org/10.1016/j.trac.2014.11.017.

Salice, C.J., Anderson, T.A., Anderson, R.H., and Olson, A.D. (2018). Ecological risk assessment of perfluooroctane sulfonate to aquatic fauna from a bayou adjacent to former fire training areas at a US Air Force installation. *Environmental Toxicology and Chemistry* 37: 2198–2209. https://doi.org/10.1002/etc.4162.

Shahsavari, E., Rouch, D., Khudur, L.S. et al. (2021). Challenges and current status of the biological treatment of PFAS-contaminated soils. *Frontiers in Bioengineering and Biotechnology* 8: 602040. https://doi.org/10.3389/fbioe.2020.602040.

Sharifan, H., Bagheri, M., Wang, D. et al. (2021). Fate and transport of per- and polyfluoroalkyl substances (PFASs) in the vadose zone. *Science of the Total Environment* 771: 145427. https://doi.org/10.1016/j.scitotenv.2021.145427.

Sidnell, T., Wood, R.J., Hurst, J. et al. (2022). Sonolysis of per- and poly fluoroalkyl substances (PFAS): a meta-analysis. *Ultrasonics Sonochemistry* 105944: https://doi.org/10.1016/j.ultsonch.2022.105944.

Sima, M.W. and Jaffé, P.R. (2021). A critical review of modeling poly- and perfluoroalkyl substances (PFAS) in the soil–water environment. *Science of the Total Environment* 757: 143793. https://doi.org/10.1016/j.scitotenv.2020.143793.

Singh, D. and Chen, S. (2008). The white-rot fungus *Phanerochaete chrysosporium*: conditions for the production of lignin-degrading enzymes. *Applied Microbiology and Biotechnology* 81: 399–417. https://doi.org/10.1007/s00253-008-1706-9.

Solan, M.E., Senthilkumar, S., Aquino, G.V. et al. (2022). Comparative cytotoxicity of seven per-and polyfluoroalkyl substances (PFAS) in six human cell lines. *Toxicology* 153281. https://doi.org/10.1016/j.tox.2022.153281.

Stylianou, M., Björnsdotter, M.K., Olsson, P.-E. et al. (2019). Distinct transcriptional response of *Caenorhabditis elegans* to different exposure routes of perfluorooctane sulfonic acid. *Environmental Research* 168: 406–413. https://doi.org/10.1016/j.envres.2018.10.019.

Sunderland, E.M., Hu, X.C., Dassuncao, C. et al. (2019). A review of the pathways of human exposure to poly-and perfluoroalkyl substances (PFASs) and present understanding of health effects. *Journal of Exposure Science & Environmental Epidemiology* 29: 131–147. https://doi.org/10.1038/s41370-018-0094-1.

Wang, Z., Cousins, I.T., Scheringer, M. et al. (2014). Global emission inventories for C4–C14 perfluoroalkyl carboxylic acid (PFCA) homologues from 1951 to 2030, part I: production and emissions from quantifiable sources. *Environment International* 70: 62–75. https://doi.org/10.1016/j.envint.2014.04.013.

Wang, Y., Chang, W., Wang, L. et al. (2019). A review of sources, multimedia distribution and health risks of novel fluorinated alternatives. *Ecotoxicology and Environmental Safety* 182: 109402. https://doi.org/10.1016/j.ecoenv.2019.109402.

Wang, T.-T., Ying, G.-G., He, L.-Y. et al. (2020a). Uptake mechanism, subcellular distribution, and uptake process of perfluorooctanoic acid and perfluorooctane sulfonic acid by wetland plant *Alisma orientale*. *Science of the Total Environment* 733: 139383. https://doi.org/10.1016/j.scitotenv.2020.139383.

Wang, W., Rhodes, G., Ge, J. et al. (2020b). Uptake and accumulation of per- and polyfluoroalkyl substances in plants. *Chemosphere* 261: 127584. https://doi.org/10.1016/j.chemosphere.2020.127584.

Wen, B., Li, L., Zhang, H. et al. (2014). Field study on the uptake and translocation of perfluoroalkyl acids (PFAAs) by wheat (*Triticum aestivum* L.) grown in biosolids-amended soils. *Environmental Pollution* 184: 547–554. https://doi.org/10.1016/j.envpol.2013.09.040.

Wu, J.-Y., Ding, F.-G., Shen, Z.-W. et al. (2022). Linking microbiomes with per-and poly-fluoroalkyl substances (PFASs) in soil ecosystems: microbial community assembly, stability, and trophic phylosymbiosis. *Chemosphere* 305: 135403. https://doi.org/10.1016/j.chemosphere.2022.135403.

Xu, B., Liu, S., Zhou, J.L. et al. (2021). PFAS and their substitutes in groundwater: occurrence, transformation and remediation. *Journal of Hazardous Materials* 412: 125159. https://doi.org/10.1016/j.jhazmat.2021.125159.

Zhang, Y., Tan, D., Geng, Y. et al. (2016). Perfluorinated compounds in greenhouse and open agricultural producing areas of three provinces of China: levels, sources and risk assessment. *International Journal of Environmental Research and Public Health* 13: 1224. https://doi.org/10.3390/ijerph13121224.

Zhang, D.Q., Wang, M., He, Q. et al. (2020a). Distribution of perfluoroalkyl substances (PFASs) in aquatic plant-based systems: from soil adsorption and plant uptake to effects on microbial community. *Environmental Pollution* 257: 113575. https://doi.org/10.1016/j.envpol.2019.113575.

Zhang, M., Wang, P., Lu, Y. et al. (2020b). Bioaccumulation and human exposure of perfluoroalkyl acids (PFAAs) in vegetables from the largest vegetable production base of China. *Environment International* 135: 105347. https://doi.org/10.1016/j.envint.2019.105347.

Zhang, W., Jiang, T., and Liang, Y. (2022a). Stabilization of per- and polyfluoroalkyl substances (PFAS) in sewage sludge using different sorbents. *Journal of Hazardous Materials Advances* 100089. https://doi.org/10.1016/j.hazadv.2022.100089.

Zhang, Z., Sarkar, D., Biswas, J.K., and Datta, R. (2022b). Biodegradation of per-and polyfluoroalkyl substances (PFAS): a review. *Bioresource Technology* 344: 126223. https://doi.org/10.1016/j.biortech.2021.126223.

Zhao, S. and Zhu, L. (2017). Uptake and metabolism of 10: 2 fluorotelomer alcohol in soil-earthworm (*Eisenia fetida*) and soil–wheat (*Triticum aestivum* L.) systems. *Environmental Pollution* 220: 124–131. https://doi.org/10.1016/j.envpol.2016.09.030.

Zhou, Y., Zhou, Z., Lian, Y. et al. (2021). Source, transportation, bioaccumulation, distribution and food risk assessment of perfluorinated alkyl substances in vegetables: a review. *Food Chemistry* 349: 129137. https://doi.org/10.1016/j.foodchem.2021.129137.

11

One Health Relationships in Microbe–Human Domain

Nimroth Ambanpola, Kapila N. Seneviratne, and Nimanthi Jayathilaka

Department of Chemistry, Faculty of Science, University of Kelaniya, Kelaniya, Sri Lanka

11.1 Microbial Domain in Human

All animals and plants consist of an abundant and diverse microbiota. In many cases, the number of symbiotic microorganisms and their combined genetic information far exceed that of their host. A popular way of explaining host–microbiome ecology and evolution is by the "Hologenome" concept (Rosenberg and Zilber-Rosenberg 2020). The hologenome concept posits that the holobiont (the host with its endocellular and extracellular microbiota) can function as a distinct biological entity, which maintains that the physiology of any macroscopic organism derives from the integrated activities of its own genome and all the microbiomes. All animals and plants are holobionts. Holobionts' microbiota is varied based on genetics, gender, developmental stage, aging, lifestyle (including diet), various environmental exposures, host physiologic status (including properties of the innate and adaptive immune system), the transient microbiota, and diseases. Microbiotas are transferred over the generations by a variety of methods, including cytoplasmic inheritance, direct contact, via insect vectors, and via the environment (Rosenberg and Zilber-Rosenberg 2013).

The human microbiota is composed of communities of a variety of microorganisms including eukaryotes, archaea, bacteria, and viruses that reside in different body habitats, including the skin, oral cavity, respiratory tract, gastrointestinal tract, and urinary tract. The microbiota outnumbers human somatic and germ cells by an estimated 10-fold. The development of various new technologies, namely meta-transcriptomics, metagenomics, metabolomics, and other bioinformatics tools, has aided in the understanding of the contribution of the different microbiomes and their importance in human health and diseases.

11.2 Normal Bacterial Makeup of the Body

The Human Microbiome Project (HMP) and the Metagenomics of the Human Intestinal Tract (MetaHIT) project have initiated massive programs aimed at surveying the human microbiome (Peterson et al. 2009; Ehrlich 2011). The core human microbiome is consisted of a set of shared genes found in each habitat in all humans. The total human microbiome also consists of a set of variably represented genes. There is a possibility that over the course of human "micro-evolution," new genes may have been added to the core microbiome while others may have been lost.

According to dominance, the predominant bacterial phyla in the human body are the Actinobacteria, Bacteroidetes, Firmicutes, and Proteobacteria, and more than 90% of all bacterial phylogenetic types belong to the Bacteroidetes and the Firmicutes. The abundance and diversity of these different bacterial species vary significantly among individuals, and the composition of the bacterial community appears to primarily depend on the different habitats in the body. The bacterial diversity for different sites in the human body is presented in Table 11.1.

11.2.1 Skin Microbiota

The skin is colonized by a discrete group of microorganisms associated with moist, dry, and sebaceous microenvironments. A recent analysis of 16S rRNA gene sequences obtained from 20 different skin sites of healthy humans identified 19 bacterial phyla, but most sequences were assigned to 4 phyla: Actinobacteria (51.8%), Firmicutes (24.4%), Proteobacteria (16.5%), and Bacteroidetes (6.3%). Sebaceous sites were dominated by lipophilic *Propionibacterium*

One Health: Human, Animal, and Environment Triad, First Edition. Edited by Meththika Vithanage and Majeti Narasimha Vara Prasad.

Table 11.1 Bacteria commonly associated with different sites of the human body.

	Bacteria	
Site in the human body	**Principal phyla**	**Principal genera**
Skin	Actinobacteria	*Actinobacter, Corynebacterium, Propionibacterium, Micrococcus, Brevibacterium, Dermobacter*
	Firmicutes	*Staphylococcus, Streptococcus, Veillonella*
	Proteobacteria	*Enhydrobacter*
	Bacteroidetes	*Bacteroides, Prevotella*
Oral cavity	Proteobacteria	*Haemophilus, Lautropia, Neisseria*
	Actinobacteria	*Actinomyces, Corynebacterium, Propionibacterium, Rothia*
	Firmicutes	*Eubacteria, Gemella, Lactobacillus, Peptostreptococcus, Staphylococcus, Streptococcus, Veillonella*
	Bacteroidetes	*Porphyromonas, Prevotella*
	Fusobacteria	*Fusobacterium, Leptotrichia*
Respiratory tract	Firmicutes	*Dolosigranulum, Megasphaera, Staphylococcus, Streptococcus, Veillonella*
	Bacteroidetes	*Prevotella*
	Actinobacteria	*Corynebacterium, Propionibacterium*
	Proteobacteria	*Acinetobacter, Haemophilus, Moraxella, Neisseria, Pseudomonas, Sphingomonas*
	Fusobacteria	*Fusobacterium, Leptotrichia*
Esophagus, stomach	Firmicutes	*Bacillus, Streptococcus, Veillonella*
	Bacteroidetes	*Prevotella*
	Proteobacteria	*Enterobacter, Haemophilus, Helicobacter, Pseudomonas*
	Actinobacteria	*Rothia*
	Fusobacteria	*Leptotrichia*
Small intestine and colon	Bacteroidetes	*Alistipes, Bacteroides, Prevotella*
	Firmicutes	*Streptococcus, Clostridium, Enterococcus, Lachnospiraceae, Lactobacillus, Ruminococcus, Veillonella*
	Proteobacteria	*Enterobacter, Escherichia*
	Actinobacteria	*Bifidobacterium*
	Verrucomicrobia	*Akkermansia*
Male urethra	Firmicutes	*Enterococcus, Mollicute, Staphylococci, Streptococcus*
	Actinobacteria	*Corynebacterium*
	Proteobacteria	*Citrobacter, Shigella*
	Bacteroidetes	*Prevotella*
Vagina	Firmicutes	*Anaerococcus, Coprococcus, Enterococcus, Lactobacillus, Peptococcus, Peptoniphilus, Peptostreptococcus, Ruminococcus, Sarcina, Staphylococci, Veillonella*
	Proteobacteria	*Burkholderia, Citrobacter, Klebsiella, Proteus, Enterobacter, Escherichia, Shigella*
	Bacteroidetes	*Bacteroides, Prevotella*
	Actinobacteria	*Corynebacterium*
	Fusobacteria	*Fusobacterium*

spp. The lipophilic bacteria are able to metabolize sebum lipids into short-chain fatty acids (SCFAs), which leads to a decrease in pH. The decrease in pH promotes the growth of *Staphylococcus* and *Corynebacterium* species (Skowron et al. 2021).

11.2.2 Oral Microbiota

Oral microbiota is complex and about 700 kinds of microorganisms exist in the human mouth. The average temperature of the oral cavity is 37 °C and the pH ranges from 6.5–7, which provides bacteria a stable environment to survive (Deo and Deshmukh 2019). Saliva hydrates the bacteria, and the hydrated environment is important as a medium for nutrient transportation. Diet has minimal effect on the composition of oral bacteria compared to gut microbiota. The oral microbiome is dominated by *Haemophilus*, *Neisseria*, *Rothia*, *Streptococcus*, and *Veillonella*, which make up 85.4% (Burcham et al. 2020).

11.2.3 Respiratory System Microbiota

The conducting zone (nose along with pharynx, larynx, trachea, and bronchi) of the respiratory system is heavily colonized by microorganisms. However, the respiratory part (bronchioles, alveolar duct, alveolar sacs, and alveoli) is free from microbes and is generally sterile. The composition of the microbial community is influenced by environmental factors (humidity, temperature, relative oxygen concentration, and type of epithelial cells), the interactions of microbes, and the host immune system. The closest part to the external environment includes serous and sebaceous glands, which enrich lipophilic species (Dekaboruah et al. 2020).

11.2.4 Gut Microbiota

The gut microbiota varies taxonomically and functionally in each part of the gastrointestinal tract (GI) tract and undergoes variations in the same individual due to infant transitions, age, pH, O_2 tension, digestion flow rates (rapid in the mouth to the caecum, slower afterward), host secretions, and environmental factors such as diet, medication, and GI infection. The stomach, along with the small intestine, contains very few species of bacteria in comparison to the large intestine. The small intestine is a more challenging environment for microbial colonization due to short transit times (three to five hours) and high bile concentrations. The large intestine, which is characterized by slow flow rates and neutral to mildly acidic pH, harbors by far the largest microbial community dominated by obligate anaerobic bacteria (Rinninella et al. 2019).

11.2.5 Urogenital Microbiota

This is distinctive between men and women due to differences in anatomical structures and hormones. In females, the kidney, ureters, and bladder are normally sterile, but the urethra is usually colonized by a heterogeneous bacterial population. The lactic-acid–producing bacteria such as lactobacillus (almost 70%) in the vagina are dominated in women, resulting in a lower pH, varying between 3 and 4.5. The vaginal microbiota is modulated by pH levels, which results in an acidic environment that helps prevent the invasion of pathogenic species (Perez-Carrasco et al. 2021).

11.3 How Microbiome Impact on Human Health and Homeostasis

Homeostasis is a self-regulating, dynamic process by which biological systems maintain stability while changing internal conditions as adjusting to changing external conditions. All homeostatic regulation mechanisms must function properly for the health of an organism. The human microbiome impacts human health and homeostasis through mechanisms such as metabolism of nutrients and other food components, drug metabolism, synthesis of essential vitamins, defense against pathogens, bile acids and cholesterol metabolism, immune modulation, and resistance and susceptibility against infection (Trinh et al. 2018). The most commonly associated bacterial species in the identified major infectious diseases are listed in Table 11.2 (Dekaboruah et al. 2020).

11.3.1 Metabolism of Nutrients and Other Food Components

The gut microbiota contributes to the metabolism of dietary carbohydrates, bile acids, proteins, plant polyphenols, and vitamins (Rowland et al. 2018).

The saccharolytic gut microbiota ferments nonenzyme-digested oligo- and polysaccharides and results in SCFAs (acetate, propionate, and butyrate), hydrogen (H_2), and carbon dioxide (CO_2) gases, which are then rapidly absorbed, while producing intermediate fermentation products such as fumarate, succinate, and lactate using extracellular enzymes. Intermediate fermentation products are normally detected at low levels in the feces of healthy individuals due to their extensive utilization by other bacteria. The main saccharolytic genera in the gut microbiota are *Bacteroides, Bifidobacterium, Clostridium, Eubacterium, Lactobacillus*, and *Ruminococcus*. The obligate anaerobic species belonging to the families Lachnospiraceae and Ruminococcaceae produce butyrate.

Table 11.2 Bacteria commonly associated with major microbial infections of different sites in the human body.

Body site	Disease	Commonly associated bacterium/bacterial genera
Skin	Acne	*Propionibacterium acnes*
	Atopic dermatitis (eczema)	*Staphylococcus aureus*
	Wound infections	*Staphylococcus, Streptococcus, Proteobacteria*
	Trichomycosis	*Corynebacterium*
	Erythrasma	*Corynebacterium minutissimum*
	Erysipelas, impetigo	*Streptococcus pyogenes, S. aureus*
	Cellulitis	*Streptococcus, Staphylococcus*
Oral cavity	Dental caries	*Prevotella, Lactobacillus, Dialister, Filifactor*
	Periodontitis	*Fusobacterium nucleatum, Porphyromonas gingivalis, Treponema denticola, Tannerella forsythia, Filifactor alocis, Parvimonas micra, Aggregatibacter actinomycetemcomitans*
	Oral cancer	*Streptococcus mutans, Capnocytophaga gingivalis, Prevotella melaninogenica and Streptococcus mitis*
	Esophageal cancer	*T. forsythia, P. gingivalis*
Respiratory tract	Pharyngitis (sore throat)	*S. pyogenes, Corynebacterium diptheriae, Haemophilus influenza, Legionella pneumophilia, Neisseria gonorrhoeae, Neisseria meningitides*
	Sinusitis	*Haemophilus influenzae, Streptococcus pneumoniae, S. pyogenes, Branhamella catarrhalis, Staphylococci, Peptostreptococcus, Fusobacterium, Prevotella, Porphyromonas*
	Pneumonia	*Legionella pneumophila, S. pneumoniae, Haemophilus influenza, S. aureus, Mycoplasma pneumonia, Chlamydophila pneumoniae, Pseudomonas aeruginosa, Enterobacteriaceae, Actinobacter*
	Asthma	*Proteobacteria* (*Haemophilus, Neisseria, Pseudomonas, Moraxella*) and *Firmicutes* (*Lactobacilus*)
	Chronic obstructive pulmonary disease (COPD)	*Proteobacteria* (*Pseudomonas, Haemophilus*)
	Cystic fibrosis	*Rothia, Prevotella, Streptococcus, Actinomyces, Veillonella*
Gastrointestinal tract	Irritable bowel syndrome	Increase – *Veillonella, Streptococci, Ruminococcus, Enterobacteriaceae*
		Decrease – *Lactobacilli, Faecalibacterium, Bifidobacteria, Collinsella*
	Inflammatory bowel diseases	Increase – *Fusobacterium, Pasturellaceae, Proteobacteria, Ruminococcus gnavus, Veillonellaceae*
		Decrease – *Bacteroides, Bifidobacterium, Clostridium XIVa, Clostridium IV, Faecalibacterium prausnitzii, Roseburia, Suterella*
	Celiac disease	Increase – *Bacteroides and E. coli*
		Decrease – *Bifidobacterium, Bifidobacterium longum, Clostridium histolyticum, Clostridium lituseburense, F. prausnitzii*
	Colorectal cancer	Increase – *Bacteroides fragilis, Enterococcus, Escherichia, Shigella, Klebsiella, Streptococcus, Peptostreptococcus, Dorea, Faecalibacterium*
		Decrease – *Roseburia, Lachnospiraceae, Bacteroides, Coprococcus*
Urinary system	Urinary tract infection	*Escherichia coli, Enterococcus, Staphylococcus, Lactobacillus crispatus, Gardnerella vaginalis*
	Urothelial cancer	*Acinetobacter, Anaerococcus, Sphingobacterium, Herbaspirillum, Porphyrobacter, Bacteroides, Staphylococcus*
	Bacterial vaginosis	*G. vaginalis, Prevotella, Peptostreptococci, G. vaginalis, Mycoplasma hominis, Ureaplasma, Mobiluncus.*

Propionate is produced by *Bacteroides* and some *Clostridium* species. Certain Bacteroidetes and Firmicutes species produce propionate and butyrate from peptide and amino acid fermentation (Rowland et al. 2018).

Butyrate is important as the key energy source for human colonocytes, a potential anti-colon cancer molecule, and an activator of intestinal gluconeogenesis (Coppola et al. 2021). Propionate is an energy source for the epithelial cells, a G protein-mediated signaling molecule, and an activator of intestinal gluconeogenesis (Nwe 2021). Acetate is the most abundant SCFA. It is an essential cofactor for the growth of other bacteria. Acetate is transported to the peripheral tissues and used in cholesterol metabolism, lipogenesis, and central appetite regulation.

Colonic microbiota has proteolytic activity, converting ingested dietary protein, host endogenous proteins, and mucin into shorter peptides, amino acids and derivatives, SCFAs, and gases (including NH_3, H_2, CO_2, and H_2S). *Bacteroides* and *Propionibacterium* species are the predominant proteolytic species. Other proteolytic bacteria belong to the genera *Bacillus, Clostridium, Staphylococcus*, and *Streptococcus*. Recently, studies revealed that aromatic amino acids (phenylalanine, tyrosine, and tryptophan) can be fermented to phenylpropanoid-derived metabolites. It is important to note that the relative concentrations of some of the existing amino acids in the intestinal microbiota greatly affect overall amino acid utilization (Rowland et al. 2018).

Most polyphenols (phenolic acids, flavonoids, stilbenes, lignans, and secoiridoids) from fruits and vegetables are poorly absorbed in the small intestine and metabolized by the colonic microbiota. The polyphenols can exert both antimicrobial activity and growth inhibition. Microbial species involved in polyphenol metabolism include *Bacteroides, Clostridium, Enterococcus, Eubacterium, Lachnospiraceae*, and *Lactobacillus* species (Makarewicz et al. 2021). Gut dysbiosis is an imbalance in the gut microbiota associated with unhealthy outcomes. It can cause several diseases including inflammatory bowel disease and colorectal cancer (Table 11.2).

11.3.2 Synthesis of Essential Vitamins

Vitamins are the main organic micronutrients needed for bacterial metabolism, which primarily act as enzymatic cofactors or precursors of cofactors. All gut microbes belonging to the phyla Bacteroidetes, Fusobacteria, and Proteobacteria have the necessary B-vitamin biosynthetic pathways. Some Firmicutes and Actinobacteria can biosynthesize vitamin B. The major fraction of the microbially produced vitamins is utilized by other non-vitamin producing bacteria. Vitamin K (menaquinone) is also synthesized by certain intestinal bacteria. Lactic acid bacteria species such as *Lactococcus lactis, Lactobacillus gasseri, Lactobacillus reuteri*, and *Bifidobacterium adolescentis* produce these vitamins often in large quantities. These bacteria are often found in fermented foods (Yoshii et al. 2019).

Butyrate production directly depends on the presence of two vitamins: thiamine and riboflavin. Final forms or precursors of vitamin-related cofactors are commonly shared by microbial community members. The abundance of certain vitamin pathway genes within the microbiota has been changing over the life course of humans. For example, folate synthesis genes are enriched in the gut microbiota of babies, while cobalamin and thiamine biosynthesis genes increase with age.

11.3.3 Host Bile Acids and Cholesterol Metabolism

The host-derived primary bile acids (including colic acid and chenodeoxycholic acid) are saturated sterols produced from cholesterol in the liver. These are stored in the gallbladder, then released into the small intestine after food intake to aid in lipid and lipophilic vitamin emulsification and absorption. Primary bile acids are metabolized by the gut microbiota into secondary bile acids (deoxycholic acid and lithocholic acid). Secondary bile acids are important for energy production and altering enteric pathogen virulence. The different bacterial species belonging to *Bacteroides, Bifidobacterium, Clostridium, Enterococcus Lactobacillus, Listeria*, and *Ruminococcus* genera produce different secondary bile acids in the adult human (Winston and Theriot 2020).

About 1–2.4 g/day of cholesterol (including dietary cholesterol and cholesterol biosynthesized in the liver) enters the intestine. Some of intestinal cholesterol is absorbed and the rest can be lost from the body as the fractions of bile salts, with feces, and sebum. All cholesterol received by the large intestine can be metabolized mainly to coprostanol and minorly to coprostanone by the colonic microbiota of the genera *Bacteroides* and *Eubacterium* (Gérard 2013).

11.3.4 Drug Metabolism

Intestinal microbes affect the metabolism of drugs and toxicants. The probiotics (genera *Bifidobacterium, Lactobacillus*, and *Streptococcus*) have an effect on the mRNA and protein expression levels of many detoxifying enzymes and drug-metabolizing enzymes (Nichols et al. 2019). The intestinal microbiota modulates the gene expression of the host via numerous mechanisms including the ability of the gut microbiome to generate metabolites (vitamin B12 and vitamin K), metabolize endogenous metabolites (dehydroxylation of bile acids), and modify xenobiotic compounds. Relationships between drugs such as levodopa (L-DOPA), lactulose, irinotecan, and digoxin and the intestinal microbiome have been identified to some extent (Sun et al. 2019).

Fecal microbiota transplants (FMT) treatment is used to introduce the healthy intestinal microbiome into an eligible patient with resilient *C. difficile* infections (Wortelboer et al. 2019). FMT is being developed as a potential treatment for ulcerative colitis and obesity.

Research on the human microbiome will be useful in personalized medicine development depending on a combination of the complete human microbiome composition, the individual genetic makeup, environmental factors, and dietary plans.

11.3.5 Defense Against Pathogens

The human immune system encompasses innate and adaptive components and plays a vital role in host defense against various harmful external agents. Humans and their commensal microorganisms co-evolved toward symbiosis and homeostasis. Commensal bacteria protect humans from other pathogenic bacteria by producing antibiotics, bacteriocin, toxic metabolites, and protein complexes that have an antagonistic effect on pathogenic organisms. The products of these bacteria are helpful in pH modification, cell signaling, and regulation of the function of innate and adaptive immune cells. They also compete with other strains of a similar species for the available resources such as binding sites, nutrients, and niches.

Early-life colonization of the commensal microorganisms plays an important role in the maturation of the host's immune system without intestinal defects of lymphoid tissue architecture and immune functions. Therefore, dysbiosis of the gut increases the susceptibility to pathogenic invasion, the risk of "non-communicable" GI diseases, and abnormal immune responses (Zheng et al. 2020). The intestinal tract is an active immunological organ with more resident immune cells (IgA-producing plasma cells, intraepithelial lymphocytes, and $\gamma\delta$T cell receptor-expressing T cells) than anywhere else in the body. In this system, bacterial-derived metabolites serve as signals for the proper function of the epithelial barrier and immune cells. Some metabolites are produced by bacteria directly from dietary components, while others are produced by the host and biochemically modified by gut bacteria (Table 11.3) (Postler and Ghosh 2017).

Recent research has identified that purposeful modulation of the skin microbiome may be an effective treatment for some skin disorders such as atopic dermatitis and psoriasis. The skin and vaginal microbiome can affect host gene expression just as the gut microbiome can. Some extrapolations of microbiota regarding different body sites can be made by using the existing exposures of the gut microbiome (Zhou et al. 2020).

Table 11.3 Immunomodulatory metabolites produced by intestinal bacteria.

Metabolite	Source	Effects on immune system
Short-chain fatty acids	Polysaccharides	Anti-inflammatory activity (protect from colitis, inhibit production of cytokines by innate immune cells, inhibit maturation of dendritic cells, and promote production and differentiation of regulatory T cells Tregs, etc.)
Indole derivatives	Dietary tryptophan	Activation of aryl hydrocarbon receptor (AHR), promoting type 3 innate lymphoid cells (ILC3)
Polyamines (putrescine, spermidine, spermine)	Arginine	Inhibit the production of pro-inflammatory cytokines by monocytes and macrophages
Secondary bile acids	Host-derived hepatic bile acids	Inhibit pro-inflammatory cytokine secretion by dendritic cells and macrophages
Taurine	Host-derived primary bile salts	Enhances epithelial barrier function and maintenance by promoting epithelial production of IL-18

Several studies of the oral microbiome have focused on probiotics as a means of microbiome modulation. For example, *Streptococcus* sp. A12 has increased arginine deiminase system activity, which inhibits *S. mutans* in the oral microbiome. *Lactobacillus* spp. could drastically reduce the acid production of a high-sugar environment, which could be used as a protective treatment for dental caries. The harmful biofilms that grow in the gingival margin affect the host gene expression, particularly via the inflammasome (Nichols et al. 2019).

11.3.6 Immune Modulation

The human immune system has evolved to recognize and eradicate pathogenic microbes while having a symbiotic relationship with multiple species of bacteria. Many studies have shown that individual species of the microbiota can induce very different types of immune cells (e.g. Th1 cells, Th17 cells, and Foxp3+ regulatory T cells) and responses. External factors such as diet or antibiotic treatment can alter the gut microbiota balance. The gut microbiota shapes the immune response at both intestinal and extra-intestinal sites and affects in controlling the development of some types of autoimmune allergic diseases and some forms of cancer. Activation of the innate immune response during the primary colonization involves the induction of toll-like receptors (TLRs), which increases gut permeability to the colonizing microbes and their metabolites. The recognition of the gut microbes via TLRs is crucially important in early life, and it avoids the risk of attack against the commensals (Lo et al. 2021).

Several members of pioneer gut colonizers such as *Escherichia* spp. and *Streptococcus* spp. produce neurotransmitters norepinephrine and serotonin, while *Lactobacillus* and *Bifidobacterium* species produce GABA and acetylcholine. It is believed that colonization of a "healthy" microbiota decreases susceptibility to diseases and ensures normal development of the mucosal and systemic immunity, metabolism, and the development of hypothalamic–pituitary–adrenal (HPA) axis, which impacts the gut through its action on the enteric nervous system, immune system, and the central nervous system (Lo et al. 2021).

11.4 Factors That Influence the Microbial Domain Due to Interactions Between Humans, Animals, Plants, and Our Environment

The health of people is closely connected to the health of animals and their shared environment. Global changes include human population expansion into new geographic areas, climate changes, anthropogenic activities, development of international travel and trade movements, urbanization, and chemical pollution.

11.4.1 Human Population Expansion into New Geographic Areas

People have close contacts with wild and/or domestic animals through international trade of exotic animals and increased human encroachment into wildlife habitats. Animals play an important role in our lives, whether for food, companionship, fiber, livelihoods, travel, education, and sport; more contacts with animals and their environments mean greater opportunities for the transfer of zoonotic diseases (zoonoses). According to the World Organization for Animal Health (OIE), 60% of the identified human infectious diseases have originated in animals.

11.4.2 Climate Changes and Anthropogenic Activities

The earth is undergoing climate and land use changes. Climate changes such as global warming have an impact on Earth's weather patterns posing multiple risks to health and well-being through increased risk of extreme weather events such as floods, landslides, droughts, and heatwaves. According to the Food and Agriculture Organization of the United Nations (FAO), livestock farming generates 18% of human-produced greenhouse gas emissions worldwide. This amount is higher than the greenhouse gas emissions by the global transport sector. The effects of livestock farming include high water consumption, deforestation, and soil contamination via feces (release microorganisms, antibiotics, and other waste), ammonia from animal feed, acid rain, and coral reef degeneration. Deforestation has many negative effects on the environment such as habitat loss and loss of biodiversity. This forces species to seek out new niches closer and closer to human settlements, bringing them into contact with people and increasing the risk of zoonoses.

11.4.3 Development of International Travel and Trade Movements

Global and local movements of people, animals, and food products have increased dramatically due to international travel and trade. As a result, diseases and vectors of transmission can spread quickly across borders and around the world. Therefore, outbreaks of new or emerging infectious diseases in one country can become a health emergency of great concern to the entire world.

11.4.4 Urbanization

Rapid and unplanned urbanization leads to high population density, poverty, and a lack of sufficient infrastructure. These factors increase the risk of zoonotic diseases by increasing contact between humans and wild animals.

11.4.5 Chemical Pollution

Animal illnesses due to toxicological disasters often lead to adverse health effects in humans. In 1956, the outbreak in Minamata Bay, Japan, was one of the best examples of this situation. The toxin-producing harmful algal blooms generated as the result of anthropogenic activities lead to chemical pollution. The common route of toxin exposure is through shared sources of food and water between humans and animals and consumption of contaminated animal products. Therefore, the outbreak settings should include consideration of the common environments and food sources shared by humans and animals and the potential for contamination.

11.5 One Health Threats

One Health threats include zoonotic diseases, antimicrobial resistance, food safety and food security, vector-borne diseases, and other health threats shared by people, animals, and the environment.

11.5.1 Zoonotic Diseases

Zoonoses are caused by an infectious agent, such as a bacterium, virus, parasite, or prion, that spreads between animals (usually vertebrates) and humans. Then, the infected human spreads the infectious agent among thc population. Endemic zoonoses lead to millions of people dying, suffering from debilitating, and chronic conditions that reduce their quality of life and economic prospects.

Zoonoses can spread to humans via direct contact with the body fluids of infected animals, direct contact with areas where animals live and roam, and objects or surfaces that have been contaminated with pathogens. Vector-borne diseases also spread through ticks, mosquitoes, or fleas, or through food or water. Places selling raw meat or by-products of wild animals are particularly at high risk, as many new and undocumented pathogens exist in some wild animal populations. In agricultural areas with high use of antibiotics for farm animals, contaminated soil and water may be at increased risk of antimicrobial resistance. People living adjacent to wilderness areas or in semi-urban areas with higher numbers of wild animals are at risk of disease from animals such as rats, bats, pigs, monkeys, foxes, and raccoons.

Prevention methods for zoonotic diseases differ from one another. Practicing appropriate animal care guidelines in the agricultural sector helps reduce the potential for food-borne zoonoses. Standards for clean drinking water, waste removal, and protection of surface water are also important. Handwashing practice after contact with animals and other behavioral adjustments can reduce the community's spread of zoonotic diseases when they occur.

11.5.2 Antimicrobial Resistance

Antimicrobial resistance is a global health crisis that threatens the ability to treat bacterial infections. The use and overuse of antimicrobials in multiple sectors, poor infection control, environmental contamination, and the geographical movement of infected humans are important drivers. Microorganisms faced with antibiotics give rise to resistant strains with enhanced fitness by expressing resistance genes. The sharing of those genes with other bacterial populations increases the threat. Eliminating inappropriate use of antimicrobials and limiting the spread of an infection preserve the continued effectiveness of antimicrobials. A few antimicrobial classes are reserved for humans, and a few others are limited to veterinary use. However, most antimicrobial classes are used to treat bacterial infections in humans as well as in animals. Third-generation cephalosporins, fluoroquinolones, colistin, tetracyclines, and macrolides, which are widely used in animals and the agriculture sector are critically important for the treatment of a wide variety of frequently serious infections in humans. Tetracyclines, streptomycin, and some other antimicrobials are used in horticulture for the treatment of bacterial infections of fruits. Antimicrobial resistance reduces the effectiveness of antimicrobial treatment. There is considerable evidence that antimicrobial use in animals is an important contributor to antimicrobial resistance in human pathogens such as *Campylobacter* spp., *E. coli*, *Enterococcus* spp., and *Salmonella* spp. Exposure of bacteria to heavy metals and biocides such as disinfectants and antiseptics may also lead to antimicrobial resistance (Mcewen and Collignon 2018).

It is essential to take suitable actions to prevent infections, reduce over-prescribing, improve sanitation and hygiene, and provide adequate treatment of waste to control antimicrobial resistance. Numerous international agencies and countries have included necessary actions to overcome this threat. WHO has launched new guidelines on the use of medically important antimicrobials in food-producing animals with the aim to help preserve the effectiveness of antimicrobials by reducing their use in animals.

11.5.3 Vector-Borne Diseases

Many vector-borne diseases are transmitted through the bite of arthropod vectors, such as mosquitoes, ticks, and fleas. Popular examples of vector-borne diseases include dengue fever (virus), lymphatic filariasis (nematode worm), leishmaniasis (protozoan), and malaria (protozoan). Vector-borne diseases account for 17% of all global infectious diseases. Vector-borne diseases spread increasingly in Asia, Africa, and the American regions. High population growth rates, deforestation, and loss of biodiversity contribute to the increase of host–vector contact rates. Vector-borne pathogens could spread more readily within a disrupted ecosystem than a diverse ecosystem. Climate change will develop both short- and long-term impacts on vector-borne pathogen transmission. It is estimated that global temperatures will increase by 1.0–3.5 °C by 2100 and proportionally increase the likelihood of many vector-borne diseases (Faburay 2015). Combating vector-borne diseases is a challenging endeavor that will require involving both medical and veterinary personnel, as well as sustained investments in research and development for the rapid pathogen detection and vaccine technologies.

11.6 Animals as Early Warning Signs of Potential Human Illness

Animals also share human susceptibility to some diseases and environmental hazards because they share the same environment and spend more time outdoors compared to humans. Because of this, wild or domestic animals can sometimes serve as early warning signs of potential human illness prior to humans. Furthermore, the biologically short lifespans of some animals may allow them to develop clinical signs more effectively after exposure to specific pathogens, and they do not share some human behaviors such as smoking that may confound investigation results. Proactive surveillance of domestic or wild animals facilitates the identification of infectious diseases and other zoonoses. The observed data can be used to identify disease trends and potential outbreaks (Pei et al. 2017).

11.7 Tools for Studying the Shared Microbiome

11.7.1 Sequencing Methods, Technological Advances for Studying the Microbiome

Recent molecular microbiology studies have focused on the investigation of the composition of the microbiota in any given specific body site, habitat, or ecosystem using metagenomics. Metagenomic experiments bypass in vitro studies. Classic infectious diseases and pathology have focused on one pathogen causing one disease. However, the current understanding is that reduction in microbial diversity and outgrowth of specific species are also associated with many different diseases. Microbiome studies produce big data which need sophisticated computational tools and technologies for the analysis. Moreover, most of those tools available provide assessments, but not causation. Therefore, classical in vitro techniques and in vivo model experimentation should be used to determine the cause and effect.

There are several technologies available to study the microbiome. Some of the fundamental methods are marker-based microbiome profiling, shotgun metagenomics metatranscriptomics, metabolomics, and metaproteomics. These technologies can provide strain-level taxonomic resolution of the taxa present in microbiomes, assess the potential functions encoded by the microbiota, and quantify the metabolic activities occurring within the microbiome (Hanson et al. 2021).

11.7.1.1 Marker-Based Microbiome Profiling

16S rRNA and 18S rRNA or Internal Transcribed Spacer (ITS) region are commonly used marker genes for bacterial and fungal profiling, respectively. Highly conserved genes provide a unique barcode, which can be used to identify each member within the microbial community.

11.7.1.1.1 16S rRNA Sequencing 16S rRNA subunit gene consists of eight highly conserved regions and nine hypervariable regions (V1–V9), which are ubiquitous in bacteria and archaea. The 16S rRNA gene is around 1550 base pairs (bp) long. When conducting a 16S rRNA sequencing study, one or several hypervariable regions are amplified using broad-range primers (Kamble et al. 2020).

Various bioinformatics tools have been developed to analyze the 16S rRNA sequencing data. There are three core steps to microbiome profiling: data preprocessing and quality control, taxonomic assignment, and community characterization. The taxonomic assignment is conducted based on either operational taxonomic unit (OTU) or amplicon sequence variant (ASV). In the OTU-based analysis, first clusters sequence into different OTUs using either reference-free OTU clustering (de novo clustering) or reference-based OTU clustering method. OTUs are determined by the sequence similarity according to a predefined similarity threshold, most commonly 97% (Gao et al. 2021). ASV approach attempts to go in the opposite direction of the OTU approach. It will be started by determining which sequences were read and how many times each sequence was read. These data will be combined to infer the biological sequences in the sample, enabling the comparison of similar reads to determine the probability that a given read at a given frequency is not due to sequencing error as little as a single nucleotide. Therefore, an ASV approach can provide a higher-resolution taxonomic result. Both OTU- and ASV-based methods provide the phylogenetic information. However, these methods do not provide the functional gene composition. Phylogeny is strongly correlated with biomolecular function, which leads to predicting metagenome functional content from 16S data using software tools such as PICRUSt (phylogenetic investigation of communities by reconstruction of unobserved states) and Tax4Fun (Gao et al. 2021).

11.7.1.1.2 18S rRNA Sequencing and Internal Transcribed Spacer (ITS) Sequencing Here also, DNA is amplified with specific primers and then moved to sequence processing, sequence analyzing, and comparing with the known database to identify the species of fungi. 18S rRNA has nine hypervariable regions. The eukaryotic ITS region is a 500–700 base pair long nuclear ribosomal DNA sequence, which is separated into two regions: ITS1 (between 18S and

5.8S) and ITS2 (between 5.8S and 28S). ITS2 is less taxonomically biased than ITS1. The 18S rRNA sequencing allows alignment across taxa above the species level, but the ITS sequencing is not able to do so due to lack of reference sequences. The ITS sequencing can provide lower-taxonomical level information (species and subspecies), as there is more variation in the ITS1 and ITS2 regions than 18S rRNA regions (Gao et al. 2021).

11.7.1.2 Shotgun Metagenomics

Marker gene sequencing methodologies only focus on a small portion of microbial genomes, but shotgun metagenomics approaches capture the full genetic information from a microbiome sample allowing the study of bacteria, fungi, DNA viruses, and other microbes. This information can be used to identify the composition and the relative abundance of each taxon, identify gene coding sequences, and perform functional analysis of the microbial community.

The steps of the shotgun metagenomic sequencing process include sample collection and storage, nucleic acid extraction, library preparation, quality control of reads, and data analysis. Quality control is the first step in the shotgun metagenomic analysis pipeline. It involves tools such as MultiQC. The resulted quality reads can have either mapped to reference genomes (alignment-based approach) or assembled with assembly tools (assembly-based approach). The combination of both approaches can get the most accurate results. In the alignment-based approach, sequence reads are identified through known microbial reference genomes or sequence databases. Different marker gene databases and protein-encoding gene databases are available for taxonomic and functional annotation. KEGG (Kyoto Encyclopedia of Genes and Genomes), PFAM (protein family annotations), COG (clusters of orthologous groups), and eggnog (evolutionary genealogy of genes: Non-supervised Orthologous Groups) are examples of reference databases. The shotgun metagenomic data are assembled either de novo, based on reference genomes, or a hybrid of both. Similar to whole genome sequencing, short read data are joined, based on overlapping reads to construct contigs. Then the contigs are classified using k-mers and coverage statistics to form draft genome sequences. Commonly associated bioinformatics platforms for shotgun metagenomic sequencing are IDBA (Iterative De Bruijn Graph De Novo Assembler), SPAdes, MEGAHIT, MetaPhlAn, MG-RAST, and HUMAnN2 (Gao et al. 2021).

11.7.1.3 Metatranscriptomics, Metabolomics, and Metaproteomics

Different human body sites consist of host and microbial cells, secreted proteins, metabolites, and exosomes. All of these interact with each other and impact human health. Integrating the data from multi-omic approaches provides additional insight into microbiome functions.

Metatranscriptomics enables understanding of how the microbiota respond to their environment by gene expression. It also allows whole gene expression profiling of complex microbial communities. The major difference between metagenomics and metatranscriptomics relies on the type of biomolecules studied in each discipline. Metagenomics studies DNA, while metatranscriptomics studies the transcribed DNA, mRNA sequences. The first step of the metatranscriptome is the isolation of total RNA from bacteria. Prokaryotic mRNA content is about 1–5% of total RNA species, the majority being 16S and 23S rRNAs as well as tRNAs. Prokaryotic mRNA lacks a poly-A tail and, therefore, cannot be selected by synthesizing cDNA using oligo-d(T) primers. Removal of rRNA is carried out with the use of probes attached to magnetic beads, which target specific rRNA regions. The remaining population of mRNAs is representative of transcriptionally active genes. Then these mRNAs are enriched and fragmented; cDNA is synthesized; and adapters are ligated to the cDNA ends and then sequenced. Sequence reads can be mapped to reference genomes and pathways (KEGG) to identify the taxonomy of active organisms and the function of their expressed genes (Bashiardes et al. 2016).

Metabolomics analyses focus on the profile of the secreted or modulated metabolite composition of the microbiota, which enable the understanding of the functional dynamics influencing community and host interactions. These methods are used to quantify small molecules such as antibiotics, antibiotic byproducts, and host and/or bacterial metabolism intermediates. Metabolomics often utilizes nuclear magnetic resonance (NMR) or liquid chromatography/gas chromatography–mass spectrometry (LC/GC–MS) to identify known metabolites. Metaproteomics also uses LC/GC–MS but focuses instead on the entire protein profile of the microbiota communities studied under different conditions. Metaproteomics and metabolomics are both rapidly developing technologies for studying the microbiota. Bioinformatics programs, such as MetaLab, MetaProteomeAnalyzer, and Galaxy, have been used to analyze metaproteomic data (Hanson et al. 2021).

11.7.2 Bioinformatic Tools for Studying the Microbiome

11.7.2.1 Microbial Diversity Measurements

A variety of biodiversity indices have been used to express quantitative estimates of biological variability in the space/time of biological entities. Richness and evenness are the two main factors that should be taken into account when measuring diversity. Richness is the number of different kinds of organisms present in a certain niche. Evenness describes the uniformity of the community and size of each of the species present. Generally, when increasing the species richness and evenness, diversity also increases. A number of statistical approaches have been developed to compare species richness-evenness between samples.

The rarefaction method is used to adjust the differences in sample sizes to compare diversity indices based on OTUs or ASVs. It involves selecting a specified number of samples that is equal to or less than the number of OTUs/ASVs in the smallest sample, and then randomly discarding reads from larger samples until the number of remaining samples is equal to this threshold.

The taxonomic relation between different organisms in a community is evaluated by comparing alpha and beta diversity metrics. Alpha diversity metrics quantify diversity within samples and across groups. The Chao Index, Simpson Index, Shannon-Weaver Index, and ACE Index have been traditionally used to measure the alpha diversity of communities. The Shannon Index is more influenced by rare OTUs, while the Inverse Simpson Index is more influenced by abundant OTUs. Beta diversity compares diversity between samples and is often calculated by comparing feature dissimilarity, resulting in a distance matrix between all pairs of samples (Kim et al. 2017). The Bray-Curtis, Euclidean, Unifrac, Jaccard, and Aitchison are such distance matrices that are then used to perform Principal Coordinates Analysis (PCoA) or other scaling techniques to visualize the data. In order to compare the bacterial diversity of samples of microorganisms, a variety of bioinformatics tools (QIIME, Mothur, VEGAN, phloseq, packages in R) have been developed (Hanson et al. 2021).

11.7.2.2 Functional Analysis of Microbiome

The differences between functional profiles of microbial populations can be identified by using programs such as PICRUSt (Langille et al. 2013) or Tax4Fun (Wemheuer et al. 2020) based on the marker-assistant microbiome profiling, shotgun metagenomics, and metatranscriptomics. Using the relative abundance of taxa, those programs can predict the gene content and potential functionality as a rough approximation.

Once the metagenome is assembled, MetaGeneMark can be used for identifying protein-coding regions in metagenomic sequences. Then functional annotation is carried out using homology searches in UBLAST and USEARCH algorithms against databases. UCLUST is used to assign sequences to clusters (Edgar 2010). Several open submission automated pipelines have been developed for phylogenetics, functional annotation, basic statistics, and visualization of metagenomes, such as MG-RAST and MEGAN-CE. Novel bioinformatics platforms compatible with Linux, Mac, or Windows operational systems are developed worldwide to support easier and deeper analysis without having much programming knowledge.

11.7.2.3 Statistical Analysis and Data Visualization

The microbiome data sets are multidimensional as they have many taxonomic units and differences in sequencing depth. Most of the time, visualizing data reveals potential associations or markers, which can then be further tested via more advanced statistical tools. Due to the complexity of microbiome data, often used multivariate analysis visualization methods are PCoA or principal component analysis (PCA). This allows the investigator to visualize potential clustering based on metadata.

ANalysis Of SIMilarities (ANOSIM) is used for a non-parametric test of significant difference between two or more groups. The Permutational multivariate analysis of variance (PERMANOVA) is a non-parametric permutation test that performs multivariate analysis of variance based on distance matrices to test the overall difference in microbiome community structure between different clusters or groups. Analysis Of Composition Of Microbiomes (ANCOM) is used for comparing the composition of microbiomes in two or more populations. Heat maps are also used to visualize microbiome data to detect potential clusters or differences between groups (Khomich et al. 2021).

Conventional statistical methods, such as the mean, t-test, and ANOVA, are often used to compare simpler features. When comparing the lower-level taxonomic differences (genus, species), these conventional tests give false positives due to the large number of variables.

11.7.3 Systems for Studying the Microbiome

11.7.3.1 Considerations in Sampling the Human Microbiome

The first step in studying a microbiome is the collection of microbial biomass specimens that will be used in various assays. The gut microbiome is most commonly sampled from stool, which has an extreme microbial density and minimal human genetic contamination and contains material that can be assayed with a variety of molecular techniques. In a clinical setting, sequencing technologies are usually based on samples collected from feces, intestinal fluid, mucosal biopsy, mucosal brushing, rectal swabs, etc. The Brisbane Aseptic Biopsy Device and the intelligent capsule are novel sampling technologies (Tang et al. 2020). Swab sampling is the easiest skin microbial biomass sampling method but retrieves the smallest amount of biomass. But the combination of razor scraping and swabbing is the most practical for retrieving samples with greater biomass. Skin biopsies recovered the greatest microbial and human biomass. However, skin microbiome requires more extensive sequencing and care during analysis due to the low biomass of skin microbiome. Different sampling approaches such as swabs, aspirates, sputum, lavage, and brushings have been used to obtain material from the nasal passages, sinus cavities, oral cavity and pharyngeal region, and the tracheobronchial tree. However, differences in the techniques of sample collection and processing can strongly influence any microbiome assays (Aagaard et al. 2013).

11.7.3.2 Culture Systems for Characterizing the Human Microbiome

Culturing of microorganisms is the conventional in vitro technique for studying microorganisms. Culture-based techniques have been developed to capture a wider array of organisms under accurately controlled conditions. Bioreactors have also been developed to test specific microorganism interactions, metabolite production, chemical transformations and kinetics, and effects of chemicals on microbiome structure and functions. The knowledge of optimal environmental conditions for the desired microorganism, such as pH, redox potential, temperature, and nutrients, is important for the success of any culturing technique. Moreover, in vitro host–microbiome simulator devices or bioreactors are used to understand specific microbial changes. For example, simulator of the human intestinal microbial ecosystem (SHIME), which is a continuous culture system, mimics the human small and large intestines microbiota (Verhoeckx et al. 2015). Recent advancements in culturing techniques enhanced by sequencing and metabolomics techniques have increased the percentage of host-associated cultivable microorganisms.

11.7.3.3 Understanding the Human Microbiome by Using Model Organisms

Insights into the human microbiome and its interactions with hosts and their environments can be recapitulated to some extent by using diverse nonhuman model systems. Animal models are used to study the human microbiome, as such systems are much easier to manipulate than human subjects, allowing the careful control of experimental variables, scalability, and reproducibility that is often impossible in human studies. However, physiologic attributes of the animal body are highly complex and dynamic and, therefore, cannot be recapitulated in vitro or in silico models.

Gnotobiotic animal models (an animal that has no microorganisms or an animal whose composition of associated microorganisms is fully defined by experimental methods) or germ-free mice are frequently used to test the effects in the absence of the microbiome or in the presence specific communities/strains (Martín et al. 2016). Commonly used gnotobiotic animals are mice, rats, *Caenorhabditis elegans*, *Drosophila melanogaster*, zebrafish, and piglets.

11.7.3.4 Engineered Systems for Studying Human–Microbiome Interactions (*in vitro* and *ex vivo* Models)

Rather than using model organisms, studies conducted in vitro or ex vivo give greater opportunity for manipulation of experimental conditions and the ability to examine interactions that are too complex to study in vivo. In vitro systems typically rely on such samples as cell lines or laboratory microbial strains, and ex vivo systems typically rely on samples that are directly isolated from a host organism. The main experimental systems currently used to study microbial interaction with the host include co-culturing microorganisms with or without host primary epithelial cells, tissues, or cell lines; microfluidic co-culture with or without engineered tissue; and intestinal enteroids or organoids (Hanson et al. 2021).

11.8 Concluding Remarks

One Health approaches often encourage comparing the changes in human microbiomes with multiple animal or environmental factors. The rapid development of high throughput DNA sequencing technology and bioinformatics tools has expanded the study of both pathogenic and non-pathogenic microbial transfer between entities of One Health triad. Those studies enhance the understanding of innovative interventions to prevent and manage a variety of human diseases, providing a positive impact on the future of human health.

References

Aagaard, K., Petrosino, J., Keitel, W. et al. (2013). The Human Microbiome Project strategy for comprehensive sampling of the human microbiome and why it matters. *The FASEB Journal* 27 (3): 1012–1022.

Bashiardes, S., Zilberman-schapira, G., and Elinav, E. (2016). Use of metatranscriptomics in microbiome research. *Bioinformatics and Biology Insights* 10: 19–25.

Burcham, Z.M.,Garneau, N.L., Comstock, S.S. et al. (2020). Patterns of oral microbiota diversity in adults and children: A crowdsourced population study. *Scientific Reports* 10 (1): 1–15.

Coppola, S., Avagliano, C., Calignano, A. et al. (2021). The protective role of butyrate against obesity and obesity-related diseases. *Molecules* 26 (3): 682.

Dekaboruah, E., Suryavanshi, M.V., Chettri, D. et al. (2020). Human microbiome: an academic update on human body site specific surveillance and its possible role. *Archives of Microbiology* 202 (8): 2147–2167.

Deo, P.N. and Deshmukh, R. (2019). Oral microbiome: unveiling the fundamentals. *Journal of Oral and Maxillofacial Pathology* 23 (1): 122–128.

Edgar, R.C. (2010). Search and clustering orders of magnitude faster than BLAST. *Bioinformatics* 26 (19): 2460–2461.

Ehrlich, S.D. (2011). MetaHIT: the European Union project on metagenomics of the human intestinal tract. In: *Metagenomics of the Human Body* (ed. K.E. Nelson), 307–316. New York: Springer.

Faburay, B. (2015). The case for a "one health" approach to combating vector-borne diseases. *Infection Ecology & Epidemiology* 5: 1–4.

Gao, B. et al. (2021). An introduction to next generation sequencing bioinformatic analysis in gut microbiome studies. *Biomolecules* 11 (4): 1–22.

Gérard, P. (2013). Metabolism of cholesterol and bile acids by the gut microbiota. *Pathogens* 3 (1): 14–24.

Hanson, B., Health, E., and Genomics, M. (2021). Tools for analysis of the microbiome. *Digestive Diseases and Sciences* 65 (3): 674–685.

Kamble, A., Sawant, S., and Singh, H. (2020). 16S ribosomal RNA gene-based metagenomics: a review. *Biomedical Research Journal* 7 (1): 5–11.

Khomich, M. et al. (2021). Analysing microbiome intervention design studies: comparison of alternative multivariate statistical methods. *PLoS One* 16 (11 November): 1–20.

Kim, B. et al. (2017). Deciphering diversity indices for a better understanding of microbial communities. *Journal of Microbiology and Biotechnology* 27 (12): 2089–2093.

Langille, M.G.I. et al. (2013). Predictive functional profiling of microbial communities using 16S rRNA marker gene sequences. *Nature Biotechnology* 31 (9): 814–821.

Lo, B.C. et al. (2021). Gut microbiota and systemic immunity in health and disease. *International Immunology* 33 (4): 197–209.

Makarewicz, M. et al. (2021). The interactions between polyphenols and microorganisms, especially gut microbiota. *Antioxidants* 10 (2): 1–70.

Martín, R., Bermúdez-Humarán, L.G., and Langella, P. (2016). Gnotobiotic rodents: an in vivo model for the study of microbe–microbe interactions. *Frontiers in Microbiology* 7 (Mar): 1–7.

Mcewen, S.A. and Collignon, P.J. (2018). Antimicrobial resistance: a one Health perspective. *Veterinary World* 15: 1–26. https://doi.org/10.1128/microbiolspec.ARBA-0009-2017.Correspondence.

Nichols, R.G., Peters, J.M., and Patterson, A.D. (2019). Interplay between the host, the human microbiome, and drug metabolism. *Human Genomics* 13 (1): 27.

Nwe, P.K. (2021). Decoding gut microbial metabolites through G-protein coupled receptor (GPCR) activation. EliScholar – a digital platform for scholarly publishing at Yale.

Pei, J., Neo, S., and Tan, B.H. (2017). The use of animals as a surveillance tool for monitoring environmental health hazards, human health hazards and bioterrorism. *Veterinary Microbiology* 203: 40–48.

Perez-Carrasco, V. et al. (2021). Urinary microbiome: Yin and Yang of the urinary tract. *Frontiers in Cellular and Infection Microbiology* 11 (May): 1–17.

Peterson, J. et al. (2009). The NIH human microbiome project. *Genome Research* 19 (12): 2317–2323.

Postler, T.S. and Ghosh, S. (2017). Review understanding the holobiont: how microbial metabolites affect human health and shape the immune system. *Cell Metabolism* 1–21.

Rinninella, E. et al. (2019). What is the healthy gut microbiota composition? A changing ecosystem across age, environment, diet, and diseases. *Microorganisms* 7 (1): 14.

Rosenberg, E. and Zilber-Rosenberg, I. (2013). Variation in holobionts. In: *The Hologenome Concept: Human, Animal and Plant Microbiota* (ed. I.Z. Rosenberg), 81–94. Cham: Springer.

Rosenberg, E. and Zilber-Rosenberg, I. (2020). The hologenome concept of evolution: do mothers matter most? *BJOG: An International Journal of Obstetrics and Gynaecology* 127 (2): 129–137.

Rowland, I. et al. (2018). Gut microbiota functions: metabolism of nutrients and other food components. *European Journal of Nutrition* 57 (1): 1–24.

Skowron, K. et al. (2021). Human skin microbiome: impact of intrinsic and extrinsic factors on skin microbiota. *Microorganisms* 9 (3): 1–20.

Sun, C., Chen, L., and Shen, Z. (2019). Mechanisms of gastrointestinal microflora on drug metabolism in clinical practice. *Saudi Pharmaceutical Journal* 27 (8): 1146–1156.

Tang, Q. et al. (2020). Current sampling methods for gut microbiota: a call for more precise devices. *Frontiers in Cellular and Infection Microbiology* 10: 151.

Trinh, P. et al. (2018). One health relationships between human, animal, and environmental microbiomes: a mini-review. *Frontiers in Public Health* 6 (August): 1–9.

Verhoeckx, K. et al. (2015). The impact of food bioactives on health: in vitro and ex vivo models. In: *in vitro and ex vivo Models*, 1–327. Springer.

Wemheuer, F. et al. (2020). Tax4Fun2: prediction of habitat-specific functional profiles and functional redundancy based on 16S rRNA gene sequences. *Environmental Microbiomes* 15 (1): 1–12.

Winston, J.A. and Theriot, C.M. (2020). Diversification of host bile acids by members of the gut microbiota. *Gut Microbes* 11 (2): 158–171.

Wortelboer, K., Nieuwdorp, M., and Herrema, H. (2019). Fecal microbiota transplantation beyond *Clostridioides difficile* infections. *eBioMedicine* 44: 716–729.

Yoshii, K. et al. (2019). Metabolism of dietary and microbial vitamin B family in the regulation of host immunity. *Frontiers in Nutrition* 6 (April): 1–12.

Zheng, D., Liwinski, T., and Elinav, E. (2020). Interaction between microbiota and immunity in health and disease. *Cell Research* 30: 492–506.

Zhou, H. et al. (2020). Applications of human skin microbiota in the cutaneous disorders for ecology-based therapy. *Frontiers in Cellular and Infection Microbiology* 10 (October): 1–12.

12

Biomedical Waste During COVID-19

Status, Management, and Treatment

Sanchayita Rajkhowa[1] *and Jyotirmoy Sarma*[2]

[1] *Department of Chemistry, The Assam Royal Global University, Guwahati, India*
[2] *Department of Chemistry, Assam Don Bosco University, Guwahati, India*

12.1 Introduction

Biomedical waste (BMW) or healthcare waste is one of the hazardous wastes produced in tons at the global level every year. They include both hazardous and non-hazardous wastes that fall under sharps, chemical wastes, medical devices, pharmaceutical wastes, blood, and human body parts. These wastes are produced from various healthcare units such as hospitals, nursing homes, mortuaries, blood banks, autopsy centers, COVID care centers, and other medical locations. These wastes are generated during the medical processes that include treatment, diagnosis, research, and biological testing. A proper handling of such wastes must be assured; otherwise, they would create havoc. During infectious disease outbreaks like the COVID-19 pandemic, there is an exponential increase in the wastes produced from health sectors, and therefore utmost care should be attended to avoid the toxic impacts of such wastes. The first case of outbreak of COVID-19 disease from SARS-CoV-2 virus causing acute respiratory illness was reported in Wuhan, China, in December 2019 (Mol and Caldas 2020; Wang et al. 2020). With the highly contagious rate of this virus, COVID-19 was immediately declared as a Public Health Emergency of International Concern (PHEIC) (Wilder-Smith and Osman 2020). Within a few months, the entire globe was hit by the coronavirus and continues to be under the threat of the virus for the next couple of years. The rapid augmentation in COVID-19-infected patients has led to an increase in hospitalizations. Accordingly, there is a sudden rise in the generation of solid waste from healthcare sectors. For instance, the demand for personal protective equipment (PPE) shoots up during the pandemic vis-à-vis the ordinary days, which ultimately contributes to high healthcare solid waste generation (Haji et al. 2020; Wei and Manyu 2020; WHO 2020). It has become prime concern to manage and treat the waste to restrict the further spread of the disease.

Improper disposal and mismanagement of medical waste take at least 5.2 million lives annually at a global level, out of which 4 million are children (Star 2020). With the rapid transmission of the COVID-19 virus, there is an additional burden on the society and environment to combat against the threat imposed by excessive BMWs production during this pandemic. Health of frontline workers, like doctors, nurses, waste management workers, and laboratory technicians, was at stake, although they were protected by wearing proper PPE kit and gloves and using sanitizers. Any solid wastes, such as sharps, glass waste, chemical waste, anatomical waste, and laboratory waste, produced during the pandemic are considered as infectious wastes. There is thus an urgent need of proper installation of waste collection mechanism for such wastes by skilled person to place the waste in designated color-coded bins. In situ treatment is another effective measure that could be employed before final disposal of BMWs (WHO, water, sanitation, hygiene, and waste management for the COVID-19 virus: 2020). Several reports claim that storage of these wastes in a disinfected environment for continuous nine days eventually disinfects the waste for safe disposal (Ilyas et al. 2020). Non-hazardous solid BMWs produced must also be collected in specific containers or bag and properly sealed prior to transportation and final disposal by skilled workers. It is also suggested to treat these wastes via alternative methods such as autoclave, incinerations, chemical treatment, to minimize their ill impacts on the environmental, human, and animal health. In fact, the chemical treatment is expected not to produce any harmful by-products during the waste decomposition processes. During COVID-19 pandemic, each nation was combating the worsening situation due to rapid spreading

One Health: Human, Animal, and Environment Triad, First Edition. Edited by Meththika Vithanage and Majeti Narasimha Vara Prasad.

of the contagious novel virus along with the proper handling of waste produced with their own strategies and guidelines. World Health Organization has formulated a set of guidelines to measure the BMW management to be adopted at global level (WHO 2020). With each new variant of the virus and lack of understanding of its mutation processes, the world has faced a challenge in handling as well as constructing the management strategies of the waste. Therefore, different countries and organizations adopted separate management strategies during the COVID-19 outbreak (HCWH 2020; IGES 2020; Sarkodie and Owusu 2021; Sinha et al. 2020).

For the sake of protecting the human race against the coronavirus, the use of PPE kits, masks, gloves, sanitizers, soaps, etc., has also suddenly increased. For instance, China has 450% increment in the production of face masks in a single month (Bown 2020). An estimation of 65 million gloves and 129 billion face masks has already been made in a month (Prata et al. 2020). The use of PPE items augments in plastic and other wastes in the environment. These are often termed as PPE litter or COVID-19 litter that comprises single-use plastic gloves, face masks made up of polypropylene fabric attached to rubber strings, safety goggles, face-shields, gowns, head covers, and shoe covers. After making face mask obligatory, PPE litter especially the gloves and face masks was located on the beaches (~30%) and inland (more than 69%) as reported in the Great British Beach Clean 2020 (Riglen 2020). About 70 discarded masks were found on the uninhabited Soko Islands beach, Hong Kong (Kassam 2020). Nevertheless, there is growing concern on such litter among the public, which is evident from the Google News search data during the month of March–Aril 2020 for the keywords "PPE" and "litter" along with the news articles containing these phrases (Canning-Clode et al. 2020). Countries like the United States have imposed/raised fines on PPE littering in response to their increasing amount up to $5500 in Massachusetts (O'Laughlin 2020) and $250 in Florida (Erbla and Baittinger 2021).

There is a continuous challenge to protect human, animal, and environment health by adopting an integrated approach. The objective toward One Health: Human, animal, and the environment triad has brought the international organizations viz. Food and Agriculture Organization of the United Nations (FAO), the World Health Organization (WHO), the World Organization for Animal Health (OIE), and the UN Environment Programme (UNEP) under one umbrella to become the quadripartite by signing a memorandum of understanding (OIE 2022). The One Health approach is an attempt to balance and harmonize human, animal, and environmental health sustainably. It brings together many regions, communities, and disciplines to work in collaboration to promote sustainability and addresses the threats to human–animal health and ecosystems. It also fosters a collective urgency to fulfill the demands for clean and safe water, air, and food, as well as equal energy distribution, in spite of the continuous climate, by adopting sustainable routes for progress and development.

12.2 Composition of Healthcare Waste

In general, the BMWs produced from different sources are composed of ~70–90% solid waste. This solid waste may be considered as "non-hazardous" or "general healthcare" waste usually produced from administration, housekeeping practices, the kitchen of hospitals, medicals, and other healthcare units. The remaining 10–25% of the waste is regarded as "hazardous waste" that can impose serious health and environmental risks. Ironically, the waste produced during the COVID-19 pandemic has drastically increased in the amount of BMW with enhanced risk factor for being a medium for spreading the highly contagious coronavirus. For proper handling and management of BMWs, their composition must be identified prior to segregating them into various categories as given in Figure 12.1.

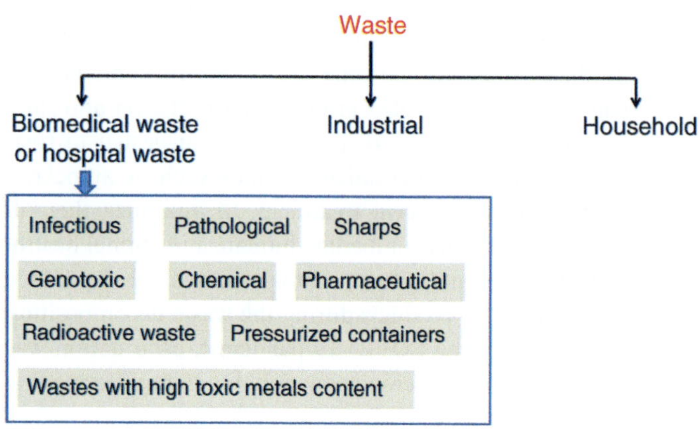

Figure 12.1 Classification of wastes and BMWs. *Source:* Adapted from WHO (2018).

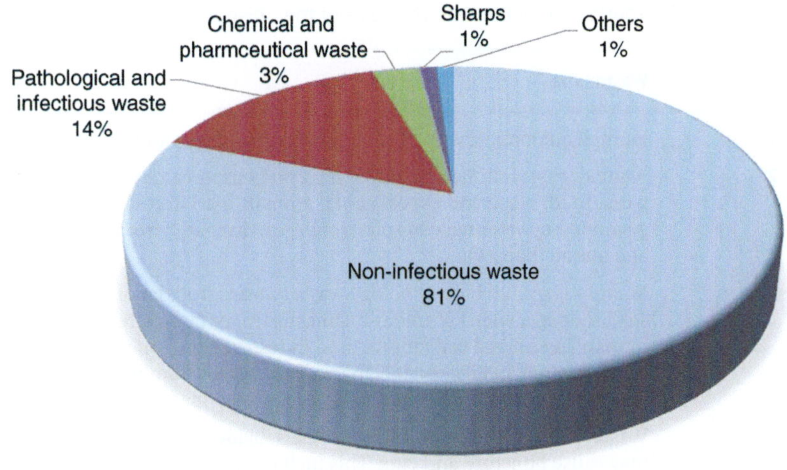

Figure 12.2 Distribution of BMWs.
Source: Adapted from BMW MANAGEMENT By – ppt download (slideplayer.com).

Different categories of BMWs have their own share of distribution worldwide. Figure 12.2 shows their distribution as reported by the WHO.

12.3 Waste Management Strategies During COVID-19 Pandemic

BMW management program should address the strategies of (i) compliance with regulations, (ii) responsibilities of health workers, (iii) segregation of BMW, (iv) proper handling of waste, (v) train the front-line health workers, and (vi) educate common public to segregate BMWs from other waste. Although separate countries adopt and follow their own unique set of rules for managing and treating these wastes, the common goal is to minimize the level of infections through them. The management strategies also vary according to the amount of waste produced and the capability of a country to handle such wastes. Table 12.1 represents the possible production of BMW by several countries. There must be an observatory measurement on the excessive amount of wastes produced and guidelines to deal with these additional wastes beyond the expected volume.

Table 12.1 Probable volumes of wastes production.

City	Population (world population review)	Additional medical waste (t/d = tons per day)	Total possible production over 60 days (tons)
Manila	14 million	280	16,800
Jakarta	10.6 million	212	12,750
Kuala Lumpur	7.7 million	154	9,240
Bangkok	10.5 million	210	12,600
Ha Noi	8 million	160	9,600

Source: ADB (2020)/Asian Development Bank/CC BY 3.0 IGO.

The process of disposal and treatment of BMWs must follow proper guidelines for effective measures. Depending upon the treatment method adopted, these wastes can be further categorized as mentioned in Table 12.2. There are several steps universally followed for BMW management.

Step 1: Segregation of different types of waste
Step 2: Collection of these wastes separately in proper color-coded and labeled containers and store them.
Step 3: Safe transportation
Step 4: Treatment and management
Step 5: Final disposal of waste

Although the classification of wastes may not be uniform in all countries, most countries follow the guidelines and criteria narrated by the WHO. Nevertheless, segregation of BMWs plays a significant role in the overall management process. This step involves the separation of various kinds of wastes as per the classification mentioned in Table 12.2. Segregation must be done as soon as the wastes are collected from the waste producing sites. Segregation of recyclable and non-hazardous wastes is an effective way to minimize the amount of BMW. At first, segregation of BMW is done by separating the wastes into appropriately labeled containers to distinguish various types of infectious waste. For keeping infectious waste, generally leak-proof plastic bags or plastic boxes are used to meet the performance standards by eliminating fluids and sharps. Specific color coding is followed to segregate or identify the waste types. In general, transparent or black color bags are used to collect BMWs. For collecting infectious wastes, the containers should be labeled properly with the international biohazard symbol in color contrast. Sharps, needles, blades, etc., are carefully disposed of in high-resistant rigid plastic

Table 12.2 Categorization of BMW on the basis of their disposal and treatment techniques.

Category no.	Waste type	Treatment and/or disposal mechanism
1	Human anatomical waste (human tissues, organs, and body parts)	Incineration, deep burial
2	Animal waste (animal tissues, organs, body parts carcasses, bleeding parts, fluid, blood and experimental animals used in research, waste generated by veterinary hospitals colleges, discharge from hospitals, and animal houses)	Incineration, deep burial
3	Microbiology and biotechnology waste (wastes from laboratory cultures, stocks, or specimens of micro-organisms live or attenuated vaccines, human and animal cell culture used in research and infectious agents from research and industrial laboratories, wastes from production of biologicals, toxins, and dishes and devices used for transfer of cultures)	Local autoclaving, microwaving, incineration
4	Waste sharps (needles, syringes, scalpels, blades, glass, etc., that may cause puncture and cuts. This includes both used and unused sharps.)	Disinfection (chemical treatment, autoclaving, microwaving and mutilation, shredding)
5	Discarded medicines and cytotoxic drugs (wastes comprising outdated, contaminated, and discarded medicines)	Incineration, destruction, and drug disposal in secured landfills
6	Solid waste (items contaminated with blood and body fluids including cotton, dressings, soiled plaster casts, lines, beddings, and other material contaminated with blood)	Incineration, autoclaving, microwaving
7	Solid waste (wastes generated from disposable items other than the waste sharps such as tubings, catheters, and intravenous sets)	Disinfection by chemical treatment, autoclaving, microwaving and mutilation, shredding
8	Liquid waste (waste generated from laboratory and washing, cleaning, housekeeping, and disinfecting activities)	Disinfection by chemical treatment and discharge into drains
9	Incineration ash (ash from incineration of any biomedical waste)	Disposal in municipal landfill
10	Chemical waste (chemicals used in the production of biologicals and chemicals used in disinfection, such as insecticides)	Chemical discharge into drains for liquids and secured landfill for solids

containers without any leakage and puncture. In order to prevent any mishaps due to leakage or spilling during transportation, secondary leak-proof containers must be used. Appropriate labelling, accurate number, and proper placement of waste collecting containers ensure efficient segregation of these wastes that finally improves their overall management. Hoardings and posters illustrating schemes/guidelines for the proper steps of segregation and disposal will not only serve as reminders to the health workers but also create awareness among the common public. Handling and managing a large volume of such wastes, especially produced during the COVID-19 pandemic, has created the biggest challenge worldwide. Nevertheless, the temporary waste management centers and temporary transportation facilities have lessened this burden and also helped in restricting the transmission of the coronaviruses to a certain extent. Wastes produced from various healthcare units are collected and transferred to these centers where they are treated and then finally transferred to disposal centers. Since an unpredictable amount of waste is generated every day, these temporary treatment and transit centers collectively helped in mitigating the wastes and combating against the disease (Yu et al. 2020).

12.4 Treatment of BMW During COVID-19

The first step in treatment strategies is the disinfection technology (DT) of the BMW for safer and better handling of these wastes. These wastes should undergo preliminary disinfection treatment technologies during the storage of the wastes in the healthcare centers prior to their transportation and further disposal on a large scale (Barcelo 2020). DT could be classified into incineration, chemical, and physical disinfection techniques. Incineration is the most widely used technique among others due to its simple procedure with higher effectiveness. Incineration is generally adopted for large amount of wastes.

In addition to these techniques, the waste management strategies must keep several other measures into consideration for ensuring proper disinfection. These measures are subject to change with the economic status of a country, its resources, amount of waste generated, and the strength of the manpower at work. Various organizations are offering different set of guidelines for managing and handling such wastes that provide an appropriate DT in a sustainable way (WHO 2020). According to the guidelines released by European Union (EU), any solid BMW produced during the COVID-19 pandemic must be considered as infectious wastes, and thus, the management capacity of these wastes are amplified. Temporary storage facilities are provided if there is a lack of incineration or other treatment techniques. The wastes should always be stored in sealed, leak-proof containers with proper labelling or color coding under the supervision of authorized person. Each worker handling such materials should follow the protocols of safety measures. During COVID-19, China has adopted to the strategy to ply special vehicles for transportation of BMW with proper maintenance of the database. The waste disposal locations are separated from any connection to water bodies, locked, and disinfected to prevent further dissemination (ADB 2020). Centers for Disease Control and Prevention (CDC), USA, announced to consider BMW produced by COVID-19-infected patients similar to any wastes generated by ordinary patients, and therefore, all the BMWs are treated uniformly (Commendatore 2020). On the other hand, the Philippine Government has adopted special amendments for handling COVID-19 BMW by providing separate vehicles for transportation, storage, treatment, and disposal. The waste is collected with a special permit that segregated the infectious and other pathological wastes, while the treated infectious wastes were disposed of on Luzon Island (EMB 2020). The healthcare waste management system of Jordan has emphasized on the reduction of additional waste, segregation and isolation of infectious wastes, and adequate treatment to minimize the risk to the environment, human, and animal health. The use of PPE, nanomasks, protective glasses, face shields, gloves, fluid-protective gowns, etc., was made mandatory while handling such wastes. Authorities are endowed with the responsibility to supervise and be vigilant of the implementation of these guidelines. The infectious wastes were collected and disposed of on a regular basis. Sanitization of storage areas and healthcare units was carried out to prevent the spread of the COVID-19 virus (Das et al. 2021).

From these examples, it is evident that different countries have adopted separate set of rules and guidelines to combat against the novel virus. The healthcare units across the globe were overburdened with a greater number of COVID-19 patients than their accommodation facilities. Meanwhile, the frontline health workers were also infected and some died during this pandemic, which made the situation worse. Ironically, there were no proper management strategies for such wastes produced from households. A special management strategy was the need of the hour; however, country's economy has a crucial role in the development and management strategies of the wastes with environmental sustainability.

12.5 Healthcare Solid Waste Treatment Techniques

Although the classification of solid waste varies with the country, the most commonly practiced waste treatment methods are listed in the following sections.

12.5.1 On-Site Medical Waste Treatment

12.5.1.1 Autoclaving

Autoclaving or thermal treatment is typically preferred for small-scale on-site waste treatment, which primarily includes sharps and other infectious wastes. An autoclave is analogous to a pressure cooker but much bigger in size that works at a high temperature to produce steam, which ultimately kills the microorganisms. The size of the autoclaving machine varies as per the type and size of waste sterilized. These machines can efficiently be used for wastes of size ranging from 100 l to more than 4000 l (Rutberg et al. 2002). Latest autoclaves require less manpower to be operated, eliminating the number of accidents and injuries while handling the needles, sharps, etc., along with less chances of contamination. Disinfected wastes are then safely disposed of as non-infectious waste or can be treated further to completely perish their existence. However, chemical wastes, pharmaceutical wastes, and chemotherapy wastes cannot be introduced into autoclaves. Pre-vacuum autoclaves are also available, which requires lesser time for disinfection as compared to conventional ones. The pre-release of steam in such autoclaves makes it necessary to use high-efficiency particulate air (HEPA) filters at the vents. Autoclaving between 15 and 30 psi (or, 540 and 2280 mmHg) pressure, optimum temperature of 121 °C for at least 30 minutes is recommended for effective disinfection. Efficacy of disinfection technique depends on pressure, temperature, size of waste, time, sequence of steps/stacking configuration involved, packing density, physical state of the waste, air, and moisture content in the waste material.

12.5.1.2 Chemical Treatment

Chemical treatment is another on-site method that is often used to deactivate or decontaminate liquid wastes. These wastes are not preferred to be packed and transported to another facility as they could spill over the place. Chemical treatment is also used for disinfecting several solid wastes. Such solid wastes must be shredded prior to introducing into the treatment plant so that all sections of the waste are uniformly exposed to the chemical reagents. Chemicals like chlorinated acids, bases, alcohols, spirits, and calcium hydroxide are the common reagents for such treatments. The COVID-19 virus is proved to be killed by a solution containing 70% alcohol, 1% hypochlorite, and hydrogen peroxide or a soap solution. According to BMW management rules 2016, a freshly prepared solution of 1% sodium hypochlorite is used for about 30 minutes to disinfect any waste. For animal/human tissue or cytotoxic wastes, alkaline hydrolysis should be carried out.

12.5.1.3 Microwave Treatment

Microwave treatment is similar to an autoclave that works on high heat to disinfect and decontaminate BMW. In this technique, semi-dry solid wastes are heated by microwave (frequency ~ 2450 MHz, wavelength of 12.24 cm). The moisture present in the waste allows it to penetrate through the shredded parts, and steam produced from water in which the waste is mixed sterilizes the waste completely. Shredding reduces the waste volume making it easier to be landfilled after treatment. A batch system microwave can treat 30–100 l waste within 1 hour. while a semicontinuous system can treat up to 250 kg/hr waste. Microwave treatment is also used for pathological tissue wastes. However, inflammable and radioactive wastes should be avoided in this process.

12.5.2 Off-Site Medical Waste Disposal

12.5.2.1 Incineration

It is a high-temperature, dry oxidation process used for waste with a high calorific value of more than 2000 kcal/kg. This process actually burns the wastes to reduce its volume to a minimum. Incineration of BMW is carried out in a controlled environment that ensures absolute combustion with minimum pollution. The significance of this process is that it is possible to kill 99% of microorganisms without producing large amounts of waste.

12.5.2.2 Land Disposal

Land disposal is a typical or most commonly employed method used for shredded, treated, and decontaminated waste in developing countries due to its low costs. Sometimes, it is also used for hazardous or untreated waste that cannot be disinfected/decontaminated by any other techniques. Extra care should be taken in choosing the landfill site so that no further soil and water contamination occurs from disposal of such wastes.

12.5.2.3 Plasma Pyrolysis

This is a modern technique where suitable wastes are directly used as fuel or converting them into another fuel. This approach is based on the principles of green chemistry that emphasizes the minimization of fossil fuel consumption by using alternate sources. Pyrolysis is defined as the process of heating organic substances, like biomass, in the absence of air or oxygen. Pyrolysis is also regarded as a thermal process for waste treatment at elevated temperatures with a limited supply of air (or oxygen). The plasma pyrolysis is carried out at much higher temperature that ensures complete disinfection and burning of the BMW.

12.5.2.4 Encapsulation and Inertization

If no suitable method is available or feasible on-site or off-site, then wastes must be kept in properly sealed metallic containers, stored in isolated sites, or filled in landfill areas. This method is particularly suitable for BMW or other chemical wastes.

12.5.3 Other Emerging Technologies

Novel technologies and treatment methods, like superheated steam, ozone, and promession, are the emerging processes that can overpass the conventional waste treatment methods in the near future.

12.6 Future Aspects and Conclusion

The COVID-19 pandemic has made every individual realize their participation in and responsibility toward BMW handling as well as management. This also urges the policymakers to frame the guidelines of BMW management at various stages. BMW generated from home-isolated patients or chronically ill patients has also increased during this period that accounts for the enhanced total BMW. Awareness and importance of appropriate handling of BMW should not only be limited to health workers but also be addressed among the general public at local and national level. BMW generated at household level can be considered as different category and treated accordingly based on their amount and type. However, BMW produced at household level was minimum due to limited medical activities carried out at home. Interestingly, production of such wastes drastically increased during the COVID-19 outbreak as a result of home isolation of infected patients, door-to-door sample collection facilities, self-administered medicines and medical devices, excessive use of mask and gloves, etc. Collection, treatment, and disposal of BMW during COVID-19 require efficient and prompt measures to handle the highly infectious wastes. Separate, double-sealed bins or bags are used to keep these wastes in medical, home quarantine, and public quarantine centers. The role of local bodies plays a crucial role in timely collection and disposal of wastes, especially in the lockdown period. The unregulated management of solid and BMW creates a major issue during the pandemic. This pose a great threat to human, animal, and environmental health. Safe handling of COVID-19 BMW by following environmentally accepted principles must be paid paramount attention. Strategies involving "identify, isolate, disinfect, and safe treatment practices" are effective for safer management of COVID-19 waste. Segregation of COVID-19 BMW at the source, then awareness, use of sustainable technologies, and precautions at all stages of the entire waste-cycle are the only way to address this crisis.

References

ADB (2020). Managing infectious medical waste during the COVID-19 pandemic. *Asian Development Bank*. https://www.adb.org/publications/managing-medical-waste-covid19 (accessed 15 March 2022).

Barcelo, D. (2020). An environmental and health perspective for COVID-19 outbreak: meteorology and air quality influence, sewage epidemiology indicator, hospitals disinfection, drug therapies and recommendations. *J. Environ. Chem. Eng.* 8 (4): 104006.

Bown, C. P. (2020). COVID-19: China's exports of medical supplies provide a ray of hope. *Peterson Institute for International Economics*. https://www.piie.com/blogs/trade-and-investment-policy-watch/covid-19-chinas-exports-medical-supplies-provide-ray-hope (accessed 23 March 2022).

Canning-Clode, J., Sepúlveda, P., Almeida, S., and Monteiro, J. (2020). Will COVID-19 containment and treatment measures drive shifts in marine litter pollution? *Front. Mar. Sci.* 7: 691.

Commendatore, C. (2020). Waste and recycling industry stakeholders are closely monitoring developments surrounding COVID-19 as well as the medical waste being generated. *Waste360*. https://www.waste360.com/medical-waste/coronavirus-impacts-hit-solid-waste-managers-generators (accessed 13 March 2022).

Das, A.K., Islam, M.N., Billah, M.N., and Sarker, A. (2021). COVID-19 pandemic and healthcare solid waste management strategy – a mini-review. *Sci. Total Environ.* 778: 146220.

EMB (2020). Management of infectious healthcare waste during Covid-19 pandemic. *EMB*. https://emb.gov.ph/management-of-infectious-healthcare-waste-during-covid-19-pandemic (accessed 25 March 2022).

Erblat, A. and Baittinger, B. (2021). Boca Raton among first in Florida to increase fines for littering masks. *Sun Sentinel*. https://www.sun-sentinel.com/local/palm-beach/boca-raton/fl-ne-boca-raton-ppe-litter-fines-follow-20210323-cse3pqe7cvh2zdgmdv3yjfrn6e-story.html (accessed 5 April 2022).

Haji, J.Y., Subramaniam, A., Kumar, P. et al. (2020). State of personal protective equipment practice in indian intensive care units amidst COVID-19 pandemic: a nationwide survey. *Ind. J. Crit. Care Med.* 24: 809–816.

HCWH (2020). Health care waste management: coronavirus update. http://*noharm.org*. https://noharm-global.org/sites/default/files/documents-files/6339/HCWH%20Covid-19%20Waste%20Facts_0.pdf (accessed 23 March 2022).

IGES (2020). *Waste Management during the COVID-19 Pandemic from Response to Recovery*. United Nations Environment Programme.

Ilyas, S., Srivastava, R.R., and Kim, H. (2020). Disinfection technology and strategies for COVID-19 hospital and bio-medical waste management. *Sci. Total Environ.* 749: 141652.

Kassam, A. (2020). More masks than jellyfish': coronavirus waste ends up in ocean. *The Guardian*. https://www.theguardian.com/environment/2020/jun/08/more-masks-than-jellyfish-coronavirus-waste-ends-up-in-ocean.

Mol, M.P. and Caldas, S. (2020). Can the human coronavirus epidemic also spread through solid waste? *Waste Manag. Res.* 38 (5): 485–486.

OIE (2022). UN Environment Programme joins alliance to implement one health approach. *OIE World Organisation forAnimalHealth*. https://www.oie.int/en/un-environment-programme-joins-alliance-to-implement-one-health-approach.

O'Laughlin, F. (2020). Mass. Police warn public that dumping used gloves, masks in parking lots is punishable by $5K fine. *News Boston*. https://whdh.com/news/mass-police-warn-public-that-dumping-used-gloves-masks-in-parking-lots-is-punishable-by-5k-fine (accessed 9 April 2022).

Prata, J.C., Silva, A.L., Walker, T.R. et al. (2020). COVID-19 pandemic repercussions on the use and management of plastics. *Environ. Sci. Technol.* 54: 7760–7765.

Riglen, V. (2020). Great British Beach Clean 2020 results: PPE pollution on the rise on UK's beaches. *Marine Conservation Society*. https://www.mcsuk.org/news/great-british-beach-clean-results-2020 (accessed 9 April 2022).

Rutberg, P.G., Bratsev, A.N., Safronov, A.A. et al. (2002). The technology and execution of plasmachemical disinfection of hazardous medical waste. *IEEE Nucl. Plasma Sci.* 30 (4): 1445–1448.

Sarkodie, S.A. and Owusu, P.A. (2021). Impact of COVID-19 pandemic on waste management. *Environ. Dev. Sustain.* 23: 7951–7960.

Sinha, R., Michelsen, J. D., and Akcura, E. (2020). COVID-19's impact on the waste sector. *International Finance Corporation (IFC).* https://www.ifc.org/wps/wcm/connect/dfbceda0-847d-4c16-9772-15c6afdc8d85/202006-COVID-19-impact-on-waste-sector.pdf?MOD=AJPERES&CVID=na-eKpI (accessed 23 March 2022).

Star, T. D. (2020). Poor medical waste management will increase infections. *The Daily Star.* https://www.thedailystar.net/editorial/news/poor-medical-waste-management-will-increase-infections-1909561 (accessed 11 March 2022).

Wang, C., Horby, P.W., Hayden, F.G., and Gao, G.F. (2020). A novel coronavirus outbreak of global health concern. *The Lancet* 395 (10223): 470–473.

Wei, G. and Manyu, L. (2020). The hidden risks of medical waste and the COVID-19 pandemic. *Waste360.* https://www.waste360.com/medical-waste/hidden-risks-medical-waste-and-covid-19-pandemic (accessed 11 March 2022).

WHO (2018). Health-care waste. *World Health Organization.* https://www.who.int/news-room/fact-sheets/detail/health-care-waste (accessed 28 March 2022).

WHO (2020). Water, sanitation, hygiene, and waste management for the COVID-19 virus. *WHO.* https://www.who.int/publications/i/item/WHO-2019-nCoV-IPC-WASH-2020.4 (accessed 11 March 2022).

Wilder-Smith, A. and Osman, S. (2020). Public health emergencies of international concern: a historic overview. *J. Travel Med.* 27 (8): 1–13.

Yu, H., Sun, X., Solvang, W., and Zhao, X. (2020). Reverse logistics network design for effective management of medical waste in epidemic outbreaks: insights from the coronavirus disease 2019 (COVID-19) outbreak in Wuhan (China). *Int. J. Environ. Res. Public Health* 17 (5): 1770.

13

Spatiotemporal Dynamics of Disease Transmission

Learning from COVID-19 Data

Naleen Chaminda Ganegoda[1], Dipo Aldila[2], and Karunia Putra Wijaya[3]

[1] *Department of Mathematics, University of Sri Jayewardenepura, Nugegoda, Sri Lanka*
[2] *Department of Mathematics, University of Indonesia, Depok, Indonesia*
[3] *Mathematical Institute, University of Koblenz, Koblenz, Germany*

13.1 Introduction

COVID-19 became a global crisis in a rapid phase that no one expected. The World Health Organization (WHO) announced it as a pandemic in March 2020, alarming on its ability to overwhelm healthcare capacity (World Health Organization 2022). COVID-19 spreads quickly due to high transmissibility of the causing virus, SARS-CoV-2, and extensive mobility of humans that creates contacts for contracting the virus. Revealing the global burden, approximately 290 million total cases and 5.5 million deaths have been reported by the end of 2021 (Worldometer 2022a).

Transmission and subsequent control measures of infectious diseases are based on both temporal and spatial aspects. During a pandemic, different variants of pathogens are inevitable, spreading in different time–space combinations (Piret and Boivin 2021). In the temporal aspect, vaccination and health guidelines are important for mitigating further transmission. Meanwhile, spatial spread, for instance from one city to another, can be reduced by imposing travel restrictions and lockdown. Many governments have been struggling to make decisions when to impose mobility restrictions and in which scale. This is apparent due to trade-off between healthcare cost and economic downturn (Lasaulce et al. 2021).

Spatial characteristics of COVID-19 should be frequently investigated for better healthcare preparedness (Ghorbanzadeh et al. 2021; Ma et al. 2021). Higher human mobility and population density are key spatial factors for COVID-19 transmission (Jia et al. 2020; Ram'ırez and Lee 2020). These factors are worth to analyze in terms of both prevalence and mortality (Kianfar et al. 2022). However, unavailability of region-wise mobility data often hinders comprehensive analyses covering a whole country. Nonetheless, it is possible to trial with approximate structures based on the central locations of spatial units. For instance, distance between main city centers of districts might be in charge of mobility between those districts. Gravity model and radiation model are extensively used to mimic human mobility, which encounter a decaying connectivity as distance increases (Hong et al. 2019). Such a decaying effect is expected in spatial autocorrelation as well. Since the appearance of COVID-19 as a global threat, researchers have introduced many mathematical models, especially those related to forecasting incidence in various countries using compartmental models (de León et al. 2020; Ghosh et al. 2022; Kassa et al. 2020) and time series analysis (Chyon et al. 2022; Kibria et al. 2022). However, the knowledge of spatial attributes is yet to be established in a comprehensive manner. Many of the studies are restricted to short time periods and to limited space. In addition, many other confounding factors create gaps between reality and what models explain (Han et al. 2021). This chapter aims at interpreting spatial association covering the whole country of Sri Lanka, choosing districts as spatial units. Sri Lanka is a country with high household size, day-to-day community activities, congested living conditions in urban areas, and extensive use of public transport; all these aspects bring out high contact rates, and a substantial effort had been made earlier to control human mobility (Department of Census and Statistics – Sri Lanka 2022; Erandi et al. 2020). A period of three months with no designated travel restrictions was chosen as the study period. It is a period worth to test as mobility dominated the spread (Srinivasan 2021b).

Spatial autocorrelation is the technique executed in this work. In the sequel, Moran's I index was selected as the autocorrelation measure, which is a predominant tool in

One Health: Human, Animal, and Environment Triad, First Edition. Edited by Meththika Vithanage and Majeti Narasimha Vara Prasad.

spatial analyses (Rendana et al. 2021). Subsequently, the concept of spatial lag was attributed via Moran scatter plot, in which one can identify spatial units in four categories as per the similar or dissimilar incidence of neighboring units (Anselin 2020). Finally, a comprehensive profile for spatiotemporal dynamics was produced that can be converted to a risk map.

13.2 Data Processing

13.2.1 Study Area and Study Period

Total confirmed cases of COVID-19 in Sri Lanka reached nearly 600,000 by the end of 2021. The number of deaths by that time was nearly 15,000 (Worldometer 2022b). Sri Lanka is located in the Indian Ocean between latitudes 5°55′ and 9°50′N and longitudes 79°31′ and 81°53′E. The country has a population of about 21.9 million, and it consists of 25 administrative districts that belong to 9 provinces (Central Bank of Sri Lanka 2020; Department of Census and Statistics – Sri Lanka 2022). There are 26 Regional Director of Health Services (RDHS) divisions covering health administration across the country. Ampara district consists of two RDHS divisions (Ampara and Kalmunai), while other divisions coincide with the administrative districts. These RDHS divisions are further divided into 356 primary units called Medical Officer of Health (MOH) areas (Department of Census and Statistics – Sri Lanka 2022).

The number of confirmed cases of COVID-19 is reported to a main unit called Epidemiology Unit of the Ministry of Health from each MOH area (Epidemiology Unit – Ministry of Health Sri Lanka 2021). In addition, the number of deaths and recovered cases is also recorded daily. In this study, the number of daily confirmed cases in RDHS areas was used as the main data stream. The study period is from 1 May to 31 July 2021, which is after the Sinhala-Hindu new year festival season. A new wave of cases had occurred during this period (Srinivasan 2021b; Farzan 2021), and later it was suppressed by the major wave of the delta variant (Srinivasan 2021a). Cases arisen due to the festival season are categorized as "New year cluster" by the Epidemiology Unit (Epidemiology Unit – Ministry of Health Sri Lanka 2021). The mobility of the general public can be considered as the main cause of the spread of COVID-19 during this period, giving an ideal platform for a spatial analysis where no designated travel restrictions are imposed. However, the general public is always advised to refrain from unessential traveling, in addition to emphasizing health guidelines (National Operation Centre for Prevention of COVID – 19 Outbreak 2021).

13.2.2 Data Visualization

Figure 13.1(a) shows the total confirmed cases during the study period, indicating the overall situation across the country. Data of two days (30 and 31 May 2021) were interpolated using nearby data to rectify a mismatch in the recorded data. Hereafter, RDHS areas are referred by their administrative counterparts, simply the district names (recall that 26 RDHS divisions correspond to 25 administrative districts; the divisions Ampara and Kalmunai correspond to one administrative district, Ampara). A higher number of total cases were reported in Colombo and Gampaha of the Western province, which is the commercial and industrial hub of Sri Lanka. Figure 13.1(b) illustrates the total confirmed cases normalized by the population, giving cases per million individuals. Interestingly, Kalutara acquires the highest normalized cases, although it has not exceeded Colombo and Gampaha in Figure 13.1(a). Such variations are evident in some other districts too. For instance, several districts in the northern and middle parts of the country (e.g. Mannar, Jaffna, Kilinochchi, Matale, and Badulla) show more prominence via normalized illustration. Such districts should also be given the priority in controlling irrespective of lower incidence in numbers.

From now on, investigations have been carried out using normalized data (cases per million). Figure 13.2 reflects the epidemiological situation over the timeline for each district. It is evident that higher values occur in the period from mid-May to mid-June (days 15–45).

The behavior of monthly total cases (normalized per million) is illustrated in Figure 13.3. A clear dominance is shown by the three districts: Colombo, Gampaha, and Kalutara, while Gampaha takes prominence in July from Kalutara that had the highest in May and June. Many of the other districts also show different prominence in different months, motivating toward further spatiotemporal analysis.

13.3 Spatial Autocorrelation

Spatial autocorrelation simply refers to systematic spatial variation, describing how far spatial units associate with other spatial units with respect to an observation (Haining 2001). Observations might be gathered as raw data or statistical measures. In this chapter, daily COVID-19 cases (normalized) of districts and respective medians over the study period were observed with the aim of revealing spatial associations. As further instances other than to the incidence of diseases, one might consider weather data, incidence of crimes, measures of agricultural production, econometric measures, etc.

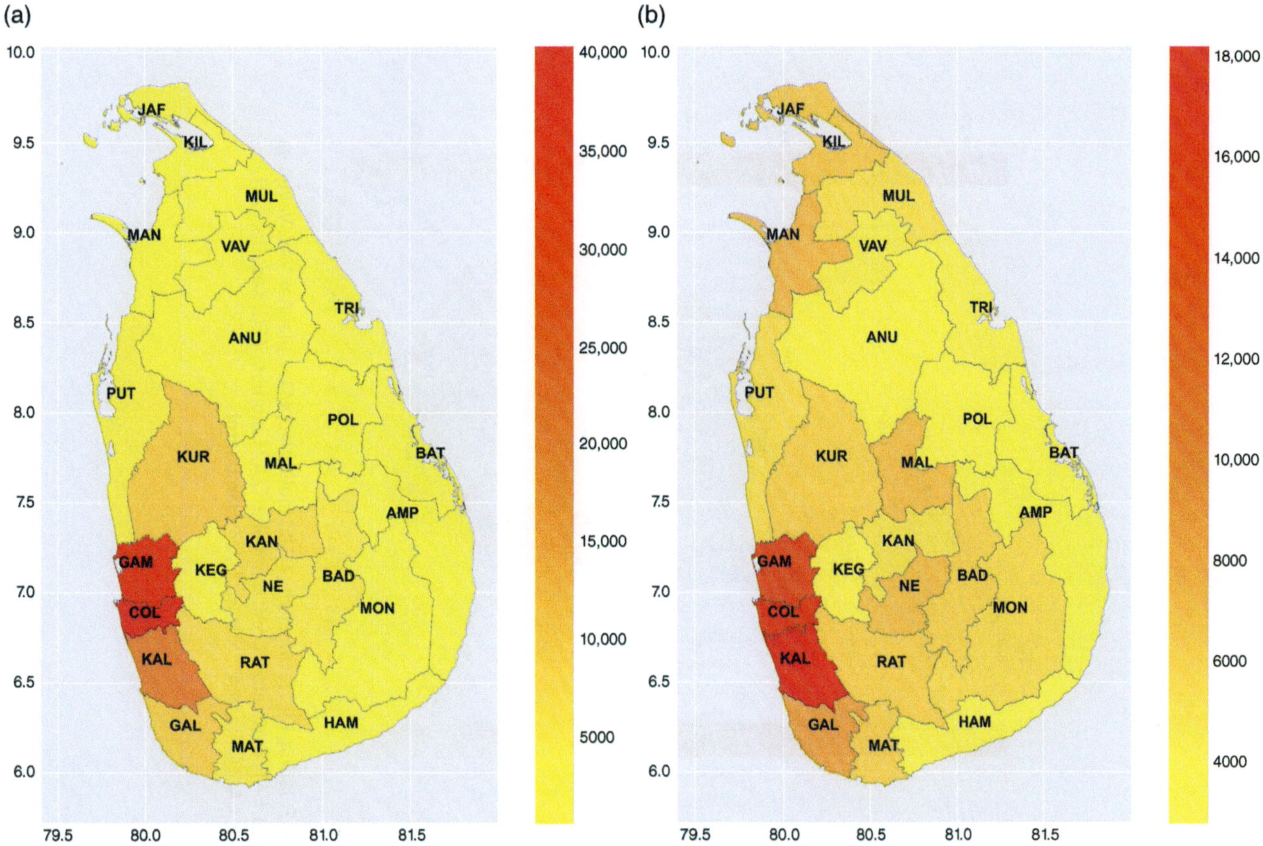

Figure 13.1 District-wise distribution of total cases and normalized total cases. (a) Total cases. (b) Normalized total cases (per million). JAF: Jaffna, KIL: Kilinochchi, MUL: Mullaitivu, MAN: Mannar, VAV: Vavuniya, PUT: Puttalam, ANU: Anuradhapura, TRI: Trincomalee, KUR: Kurunegala, MAL: Matale, POL: Polonnaruwa, BAT: Batticaloa, GAM: Gampaha, COL: Colombo, KEG: Kegalle, KAN: Kandy, NE: Nuwara Eliya, BAD: Badulla, AMP: Ampara, KAL: Kalutara, RAT: Ratnapura; MON: Monaragala, GAL: Galle, MAT: Matara, HAM: Hambantota.

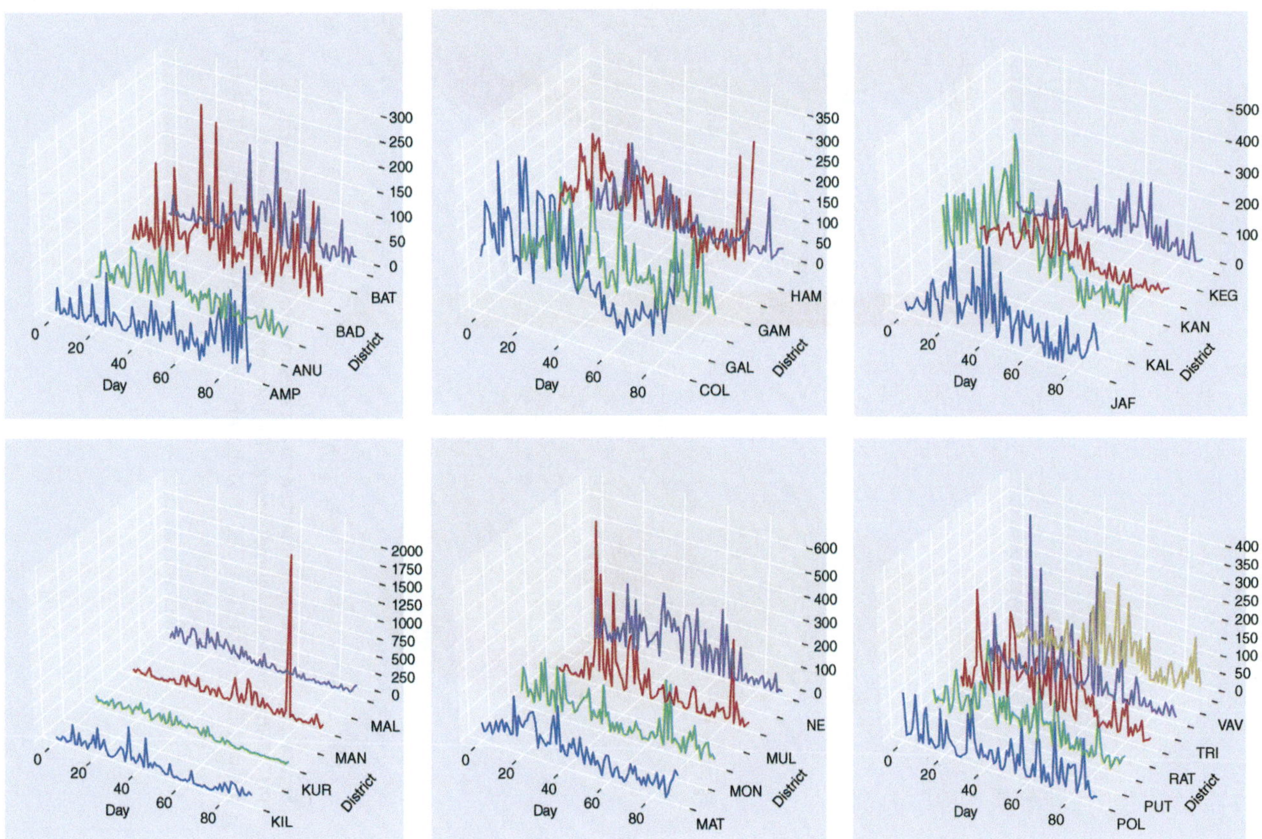

Figure 13.2 Normalized daily cases (per million).

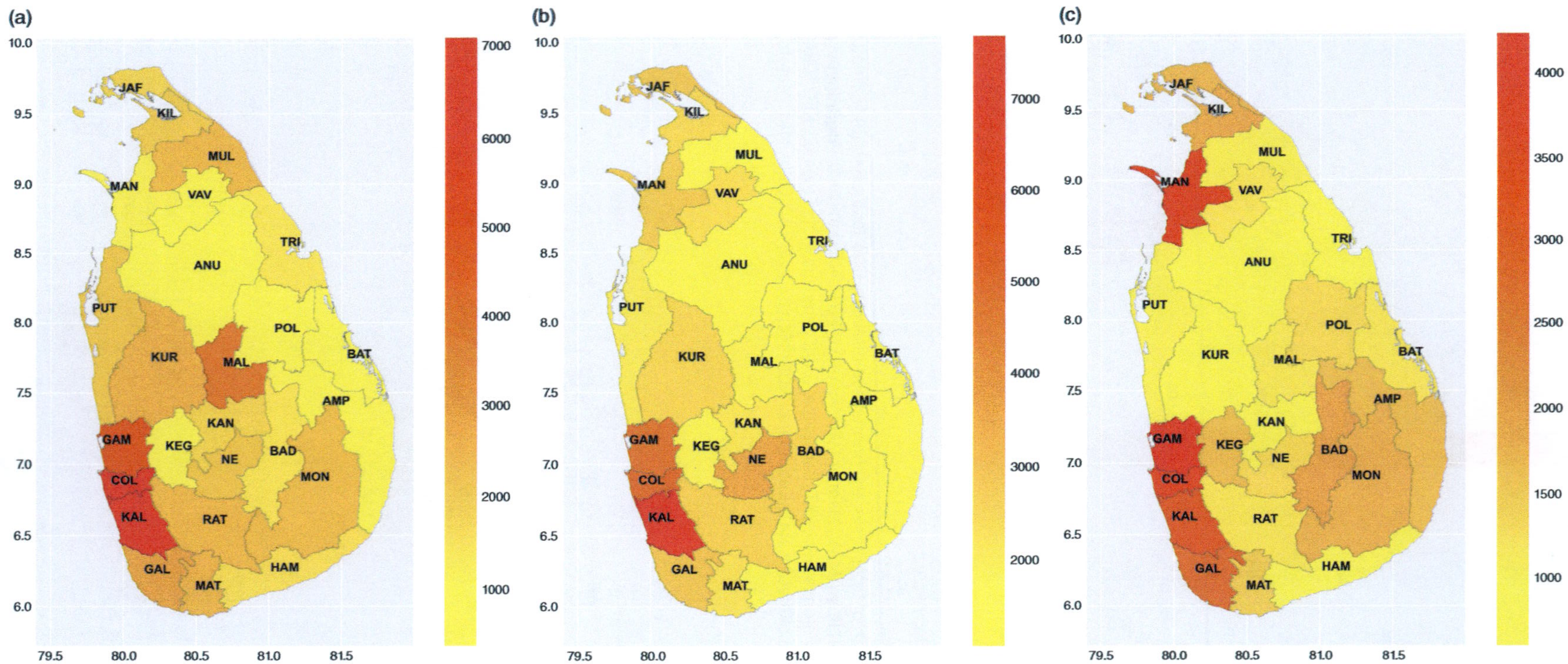

Figure 13.3 Monthly normalized total cases (per million). (a) May 2021, (b) June 2021, (c) July 2021. JAF: Jaffna, KIL: Kilinochchi, MUL: Mullaitivu, MAN: Mannar, VAV: Vavuniya, PUT: Puttalam, ANU: Anuradhapura, TRI: Trincomalee, KUR: Kurunegala, MAL: Matale, POL: Polonnaruwa, BAT: Batticaloa, GAM: Gampaha, COL: Colombo, KEG: Kegalle, KAN: Kandy, NE: Nuwara Eliya, BAD: Badulla, AMP: Ampara, KAL: Kalutara, RAT: Ratnapura; MON: Monaragala, GAL: Galle, MAT: Matara, HAM: Hambantota.

Analogous to working with time-dependent data with time lag in time series autocorrelation, spatial autocorrelation lines up with a series of spatial data with so-called spatial lag. In spatial data, a strong positive autocorrelation refers to a locally clustered setting of spatial units with similar values (Haining 2001). Then units having higher observations tend to cluster together, whereas the units with lower observations are also clustered. A strong negative autocorrelation arises when higher and lower observations reported one after the other, almost like black and white squares dispersed on a chess board. A random dispersion would occur if there is no significant correspondence to positive or negative autocorrelation.

Moran's I, Geary's C, and Getis-Ord G_*^i are frequently used as spatial autocorrelation measures (Chen 2013; Getis and Ord 1995). Moran's I and Geary's C are closely related to each other that allow further investigations with only one measure (Chen 2013). Geary's C and Getis-Ord G_*^i are oriented toward local association between each pair of spatial units, whereas Moran's I is comprised of central features as well via the deviation from the mean (Getis and Ord 1992; Zhou and Lin 2008).

13.3.1 Moran's I

Global Moran's I was developed by Patrick Alfred Pierce Moran in 1948, and it gained much popularity due to the work of Cliff and Ord in 1973 (Anselin 2020; Moran 1948). The formula for Moran's I is given in (13.1).

$$I = \frac{N}{W} \frac{\sum_{i=1}^{n} \sum_{j=1}^{n} w_{ij}\left(x_i - \bar{x}\right)\left(x_j - \bar{x}\right)}{\sum_{i=1}^{n}\left(x_i - \bar{x}\right)^2} \tag{13.1}$$

Here, N stands for the number of spatial units indexed as $S_i; i = 1, 2, \ldots, n$. x_i is the observation of interest of the spatial unit S_i and $\bar{x}$ is the mean of x_i's. The product $\left(x_i - \bar{x}\right)\left(x_j - \bar{x}\right)$ leads to a positive contribution when both the observations x_i and x_j are higher or lower than $\bar{x}$. Otherwise, a negative contribution occurs. Thus, the deviations of the form $\left(x_i - \bar{x}\right)$ resemble a notion of lag, but with a spatial connectivity infused by the weight w_{ij}. The term w_{ij} is a bidirectional measure that connects two units S_i and S_j. One of the simplest approach is to set $w_{ij} = 1$, if the two units are adjacent neighbours, and 0 otherwise. The mobility of people can be attributed to w_{ij} via distance measures or number of commuters traveling to and fro. W is the sum of all w_{ij}'s. For computational convenience, one would use row-standardized weights giving $\sum_{j=1}^{n} w_{ij} = 1$ for each i, and hence the term N/W can be removed from (13.1). The other summation $\sum_{i=1}^{n}\left(x_i - \bar{x}\right)^2$ also brings a normalization upon all deviations.

Moran's I usually lie in $[-1, 1]$ indicating a strong positive and a negative correlation when I is close to 1 and -1, respectively. Further mathematical outlook on this range is given in Ganegoda et al. (2022). $I = 1$ indicates perfect clustering, while $I = -1$ indicates perfect dispersion. $I = 0$ refers to perfect randomness (Glen 2022). The expected value of Moran's I is $E(I) = -1/(N-1)$, which indicates a tendency for random spatial pattern when the number of spatial units (N) increases. (Note that $-1/(N-1) \rightarrow 0$ as $N \rightarrow \infty$.) Moran's I is an inferential statistic that needs statistical significance for corresponding claims. This is carried out through a hypothesis testing investigated with z-scores and p-val. Random spatial pattern is assumed for the null hypothesis, and the alternate hypothesis stands for locally clustered patterns with similar values or dispersed with dissimilar values (Glen 2022). The p-val brings the evidence against the null hypothesis. The smaller p-val than the significance level direct to reject the null hypothesis.

The weights w_{ij} can be formulated by boundary-based and distance-based approaches. Usually, adjacency-based case refers $w_{ij} = 1$ when two spatial units S_i and S_j are adjacent (sharing a common boundary), and $w_{ij} = 0$ otherwise. This approach caters connectivity only with adjacent neighbours, which is weak in representing a countrywide mobility. Often, self-influence can be excluded by $w_{ii} = 0$ (Smith 2017). In distance-based approaches, appropriate centers should be located for each spatial unit, and a method such as standard Haversine formula can be used to measure the distance between centers. Centroid of the polygon representing the shape of each district is a fair enough choice for centers. Haversine formula provides great-circle distance between two points on a sphere located by their longitudes and latitudes (Sohrabinia 2022). Usually, the spatial connectivity should be deteriorated as the distance increases. For this purpose, the power functional form (13.2) and the exponential form (13.3) can be implemented (Kondo 2018). Here, d_{ij} is the distance between the centers of S_i and S_j and the parameter $\delta(>0)$ controls the decaying effect. The criterion $d_{ij} < d$ brings a threshold d for the connectivity of two spatial units. Smaller values of d allow connectivity only with close neighbors and large enough values clear the way for more spatial units, however, with decaying effect. Both of the formulas (13.2, 13.3) are in row-standardized form. More options for weights w_{ij} are available in (Smith 2017).

$$w_{ij} := \begin{cases} \dfrac{d_{ij}^{-\delta}}{\sum_{j=1}^{n} d_{ij}^{-\delta}}; d_{ij} < d, i \neq j \\ 0; \text{otherwise} \end{cases} \tag{13.2}$$

$$w_{ij} := \begin{cases} \dfrac{e^{-\delta d_{ij}}}{\sum_{j=1}^{n} e^{-\delta d_{ij}}}; d_{ij} < d, i \neq j \\ 0; \text{otherwise} \end{cases} \tag{13.3}$$

13.3.2 Moran Scatter Plot

Moran scatter plot is an effective way of illustrating the autocorrelation given by Moran's I. This was introduced by Luc Anselin in the 1990s, and it locates each spatial unit in support of or against to claim positive/negative autocorrelation (Anselin 1995). To conveniently approach Moran scatter plot, the following version (13.4) of the Moran's I is introduced. Here, $z_i = x_i - \bar{x}$ and $z_j = x_j - \bar{x}$.

$$I = \frac{\sum_{i=1}^{n}\left(z_i \times \sum_{j=1}^{n} w_{ij} z_j\right)}{\sum_{i=1}^{n} z_i^2} \tag{13.4}$$

Note that I represents the slope of linear regression of $\sum_{j=1}^{n} w_{ij} z_j$ on z_i, resembling the slope $\sum_i x_i y_i / \sum_i x_i^2$ given by the linear regression of bivariate data (x_i, y_i). By positioning z_i and $\sum_{j=1}^{n} w_{ij} z_j$ into x-axis and y-axis, respectively, and setting the origin as their mean values (0, 0), four quadrants are located in the Moran scatter plot (Anselin 2020). Each spatial unit has a corresponding scatter in the plot. RHS ($z_i > 0$) and LHS ($z_i < 0$) of the y-axis indicate whether x_i is higher or lower than the mean $\bar{x}$. The term $\sum_{j=1}^{n} w_{ij} z_j$ often referred as spatial lag locates its values with respect to their mean, in the upper and lower halves of the plot. Now the four quadrants appear as: Q_1 upper-right (high-high or hotspots) – high values surrounded by high values, Q_2 upper-left (low-high) – low values surrounded by high values, Q_3 lower-left (low-low or cold-spots) – low values surrounded by low values, and Q_4 lower-right (high-low) – high values surrounded by low values (see Figure 13.4). Thus, Q_1 and Q_3 associate with positive spatial autocorrelation indicating similar neighbors in nature. In contrast, Q_2 and Q_4 adhere to negative spatial autocorrelation suggesting dissimilar neighbors.

Corresponding units in four quadrants can easily be transferred to a color map that can underpin space-related decisions such as closing district borders. Spatial units in Q_2 and Q_4 are worth to recognize, since the disease may diffuse into low incidence units from high incidence units.

13.3.3 Optimal Weight Function

Different forms of weight function (e.g. power functional form, exponential form, etc.) and different combinations of parameters (δ and d) yield different values of Moran's I and different clustering of Moran scatters. Thus, a systematic choice is required for informative illustrations. This was carried out via a sensitivity analysis of Moran's I

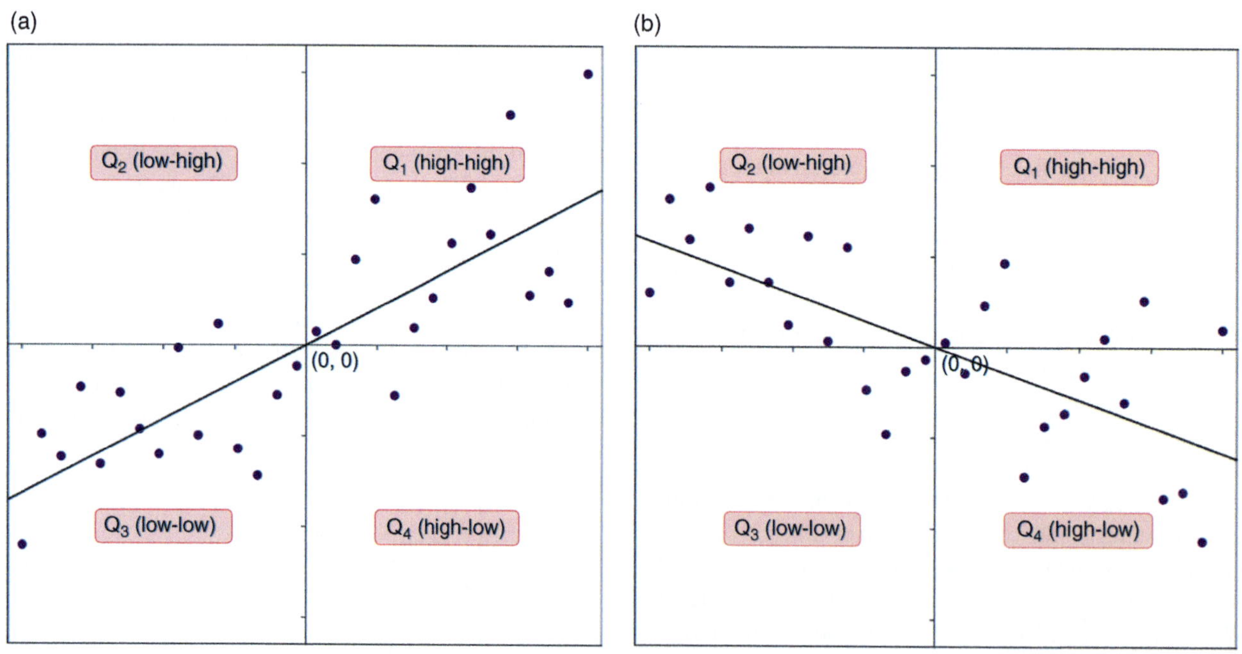

Figure 13.4 Moran scatter plot. (a) Positive autocorrelation $I > 0$. (b) Negative autocorrelation $I < 0$.

corresponding to δ and d in Ganegoda et al. (2022). However, it is also important to see the distribution of distances between spatial units in choosing d. Often, sensitivity analysis on Moran I is carried out upon δ and d to pick the values that produce less variation in I (Ganegoda et al. 2022). In this work, sensitivity analysis is replaced by a discrete optimization with the objective of seeing a spatial unit in one quadrant as much as possible over the timeline.

In the sequel, the objective function is designed using a basis function upon the corresponding quadrant of the spatial unit and the observation date. The basis function $l_{ij}^{(k)}$ of spatial unit S_i; $i = 1, 2, \ldots, N$ that corresponds to quadrant Q_k; $k = 1, 2, 3, 4$ on jth day is given in (13.5).

$$l_{ij}^{(k)} := \begin{cases} 1; S_i \text{ belongs to } Q_k \\ 0; \text{otherwise} \end{cases} \tag{13.5}$$

Next, an index m_{ij} is defined to be used later in the objective function.

$$m_{ij} = l_{ij}^{(1)} \times 1 + l_{ij}^{(2)} \times 2 + l_{ij}^{(3)} \times 3 + l_{ij}^{(4)} \times 4 \tag{13.6}$$

The objective function is given in (13.7). It should be minimized over δ and d to achieve the objective of keeping a spatial unit in one quadrant in most of the days. Here, J is the number of days in the study period.

$$f(\delta, d) = \sum_i \left(1 - \max_k \left(T_i^{(k)}\right)\right), \text{where } T_i^{(k)} = \frac{1}{J} \sum_{j(m_{ij}=k)} 1 \tag{13.7}$$

Note that the minimum $f(\delta, d) = 0$ occurs if all spatial units remain in similar quadrants for the whole study period, for instance say S_1 remains in Q_2, S_2 remains in Q_4, etc. If each S_i is in a particular quadrant in 50% of days, then $f(\delta, d) = (1-0.5)\times 25 = 12.5$. For a summarized inspection, the observation x_i of S_i is taken as the median of normalized cases over the study period. Figure 13.5 illustrates the behavior of $f(\delta, d)$ over the range of [28, 398] for d aligning with the minimum and maximum distances for our study area which are 28.55 and 397.65 km, respectively. The range for δ is set from 0 to an arbitrary value. Function values are obtained in a 100×100 grid of (δ, d) coordinates.

According to Figure 13.5, $f(\delta, d)$ is lesser when d is lesser. This occurs due to many of the weights are zero, resembling a situation of no spatial connectivity. The same scenario is noticeable when δ is high that refers to a high decaying effect. The power functional form was used for further computations since the exponential form is much steepest in decay, which might also be sensitive to small changes of δ.

To proceed with a fair enough coverage of d, it was fixed approximately to the first, second, and third quartiles (92.0028, 145.3069, and 213.2553 km, respectively) of pairwise distances between districts. In addition, d was set to exceed the maximum distance of 397.65 km, allowing spatial connectivity between all spatial units. All the quartiles

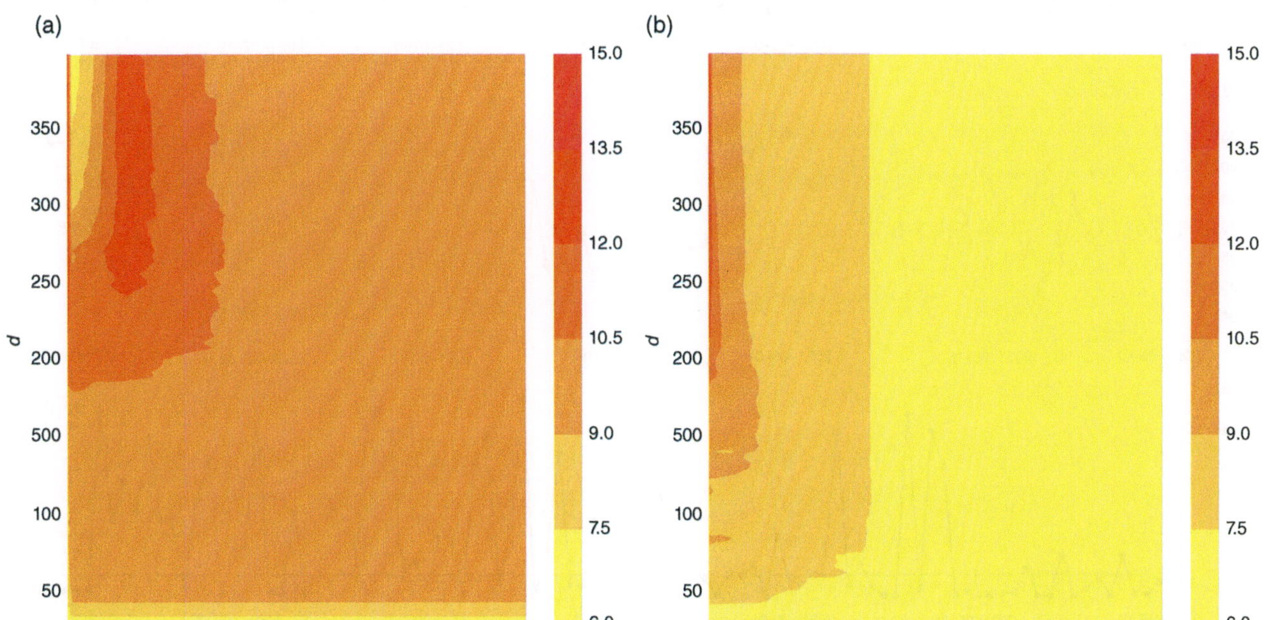

Figure 13.5 Objective function $f(\delta, d)$. Color represents function values: (a) power functional form of w_{ij} and (b) exponential form of w_{ij}.

and the maximum were rounded up to the nearest integer and denoted as $q_1 = 93$ (≈first quartile), $q_2 = 146$ (≈second quartile), $q_3 = 214$ (≈third quartile), and max = 398 (≈maximum). δ was set to 1, which gives no change of $f(\delta, d)$ over the above choices of d. For this choice, it can be estimated that roughly 64% of days are aligned with one quadrant ($f(1, d) = 9 \rightarrow (1-9/25)\times 100\% = 64\%$).

13.4 Spatiotemporal Analysis

This section contains the findings of Moran's I and Moran scatters according to the parametrization in Section 13.3.3.

13.4.1 Dynamics of Moran's I

Moran's I was computed for normalized cases on a daily basis (Figure 13.6). I lies in positive trajectory, but close to zero, which suggests a random spatial pattern. Statistical evidence given by p-val also supports the claim as null hypothesis of random pattern cannot be rejected (p-val $> \alpha = 0.05$) for considerable number of days. Claiming random pattern is further strengthened as no rejection appears in all the four cases of d. Therefore, the whole country should be scrutinized in designing control measures rather than focusing only on hotspots.

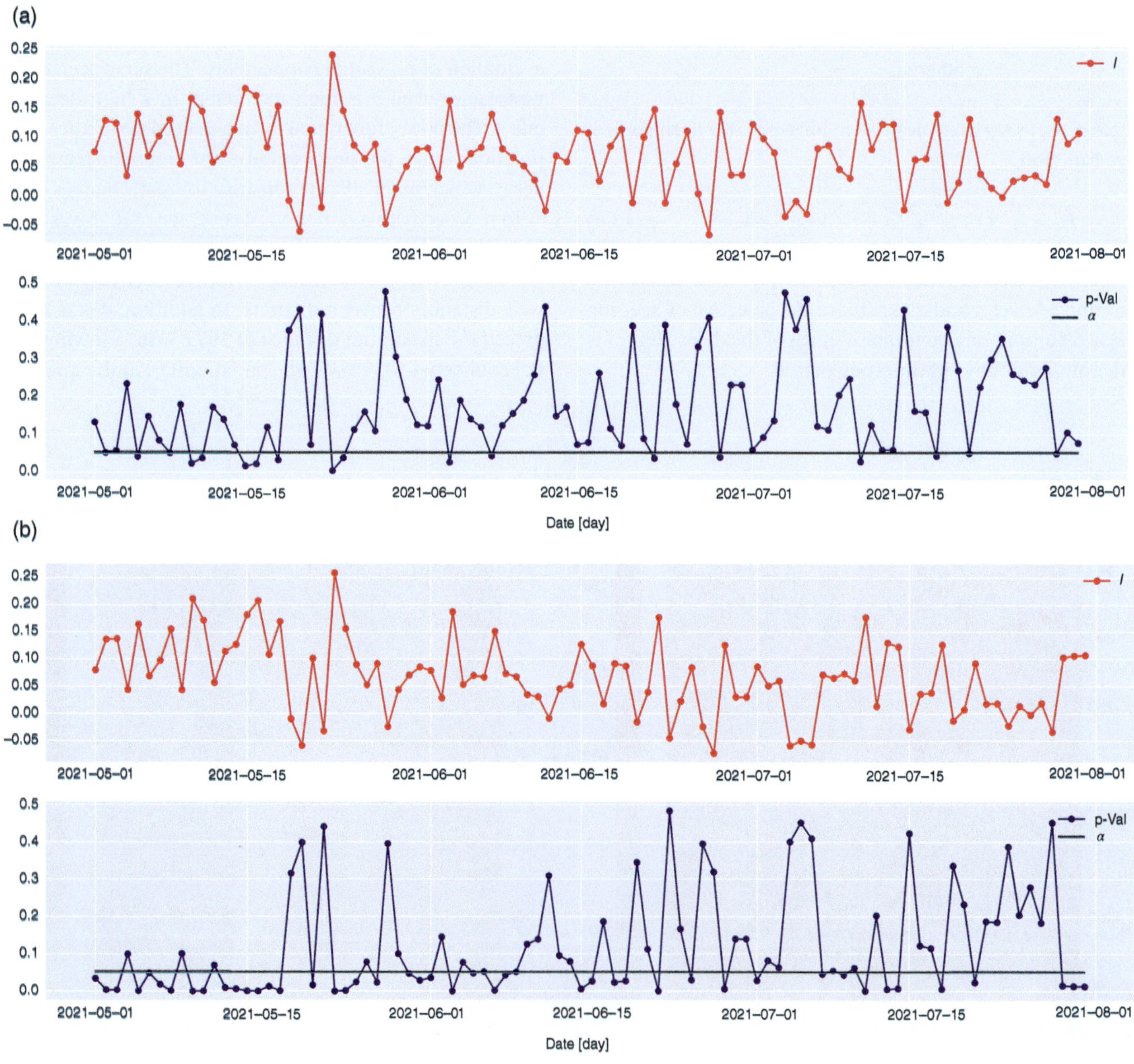

Figure 13.6 Daily Moran's I and p-val. (a) $d = q_1$ (b) $d = q_2$ (c) $d = q_3$ (d) d = max.

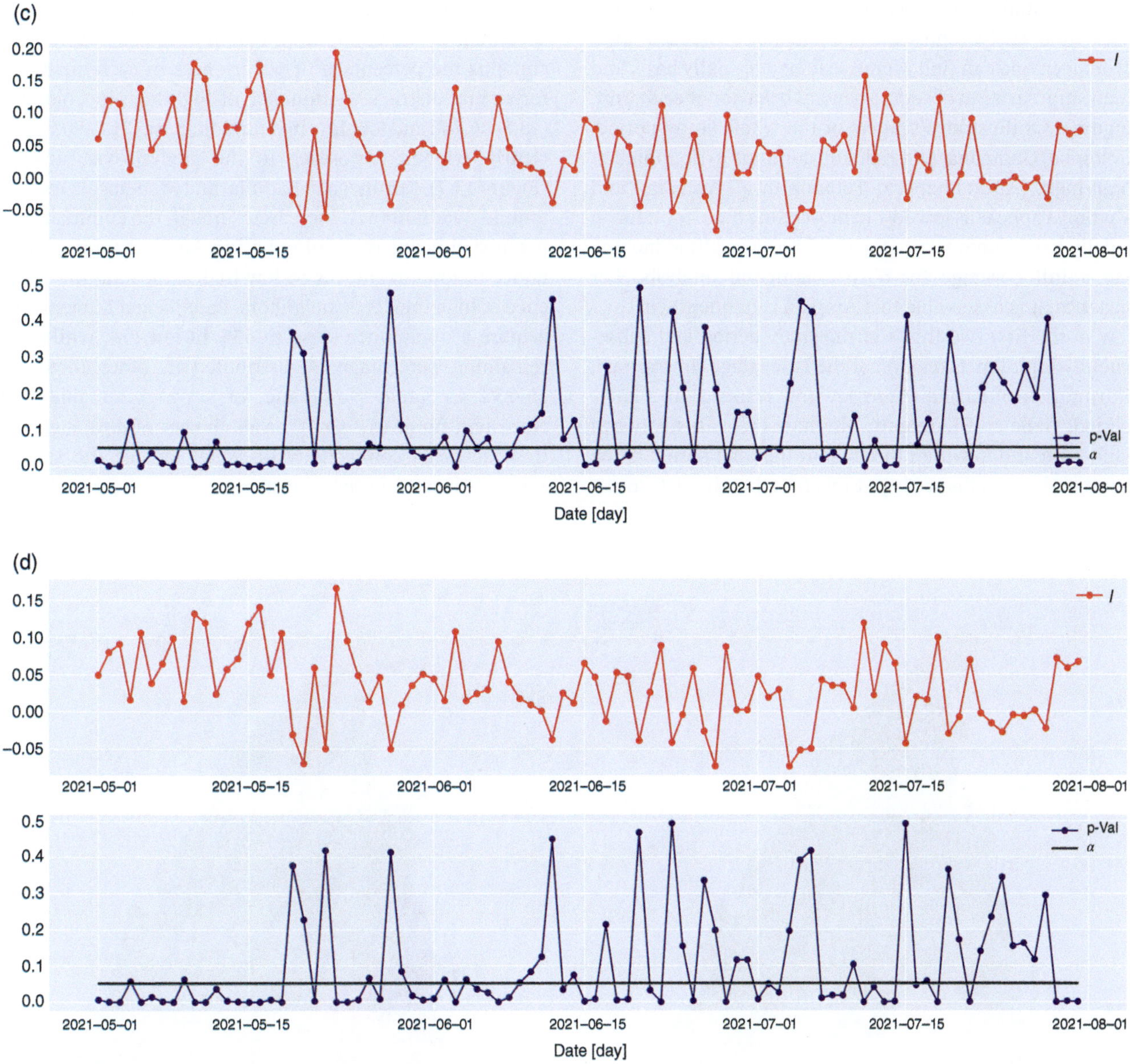

Figure 13.6 (Continued)

13.4.2 Illustrations of Moran Scatters

Figure 13.7 shows Moran scatters for the median of normalized cases. The median is used here since the mean would be biased on rapid escalations at times in some districts (e.g. Mannar, Mullaitivu, and Trincomalee; see Figure 13.2). Such outliers might occur due to inconsistencies in testing and reporting in some areas.

Colombo, Gampaha, Kalutara, Galle, Matara, Ratnapura, and Nuwara-Eliya remain as high-high hotspots irrespective of the choices of d. This is apparent as a result of closer neighbors showing higher incidence (in normalized sense). Kurunegala and Badulla move from high-low to high-high when d increases from q_1 to q_2. It claims that higher connectivity established by an increase of d forms more neighbors of high incidence. Indeed, the districts in the south-western part of the country reinforce that influence. The same reasoning prevails for moving Puttalam from low-low to low-high. However, Badulla moves to high-low as d increases to q_3 and max indicating the influence of low incidence districts. For Kurunegala, such a swap is not evident, probably due to higher influence from high-high neighbors. Moneragala needs more connectivity to show a risk of diffusing in, which moves to low-high only in $d = \text{max}$ from previous low-low status.

Interpretations should be cautiously made since median data occur at different time points. Thus, one should reflect on the spatial autocorrelation, assuming that the median over time fairly represents the incidence of each unit. Moreover, one can find Moran scatters on a daily basis and then summarize to observe a general behavior of each unit. Figure 13.8 illustrates scatters of the whole study period. Colombo, Gampaha, and Kalutara continue to dominate in high-high. Anuradhapura, Polonnaruwa, Ampara, and Vavuniya appear as low-low in most of the days. Scatters on a daily basis demonstrate the dynamics over timeline giving a full coverage for a spatiotemporal analysis. For instance, it is observable that Ampara is frequently in low-low in the first two-thirds of the study period and subsequently high-low takes over at the latter stage. In contrast, Kurunegala often maintains low-low status at the latter period. Galle and Ratnapura alternate the status between high-high and low-high throughout the time period. Such a full-scale surveillance is possible for other districts too.

The full profile given by Figure 13.8 can be summarized according to the dominating quadrant (color). Table 13.1 contains the percentage of occurrences in each quadrant for several districts. Dominance of high-high in Colombo (93.5–96.7%) and low-low in Anuradhapura (71.7–90.2%) is clearly evident. According to the analysis via median (Figure 13.7), Kurunegala, Badulla, and Moneragala moved around quadrants as d increases. Though the dominance is not as significant as in Colombo and Anuradhapura, dominance of low-low moves to low-high indicating the presence of high incidence neighbors. Badulla and Moneragala acquire a dominance close to 45% in low-low, while the remaining percentage is distributed in other three by 15–25%. In Kandy, dominance of low-high remains in a consistent range (51–54%) for all choices of d. It suggests that increased connectivity does not change the status. Kandy is located in the central region, and there is almost

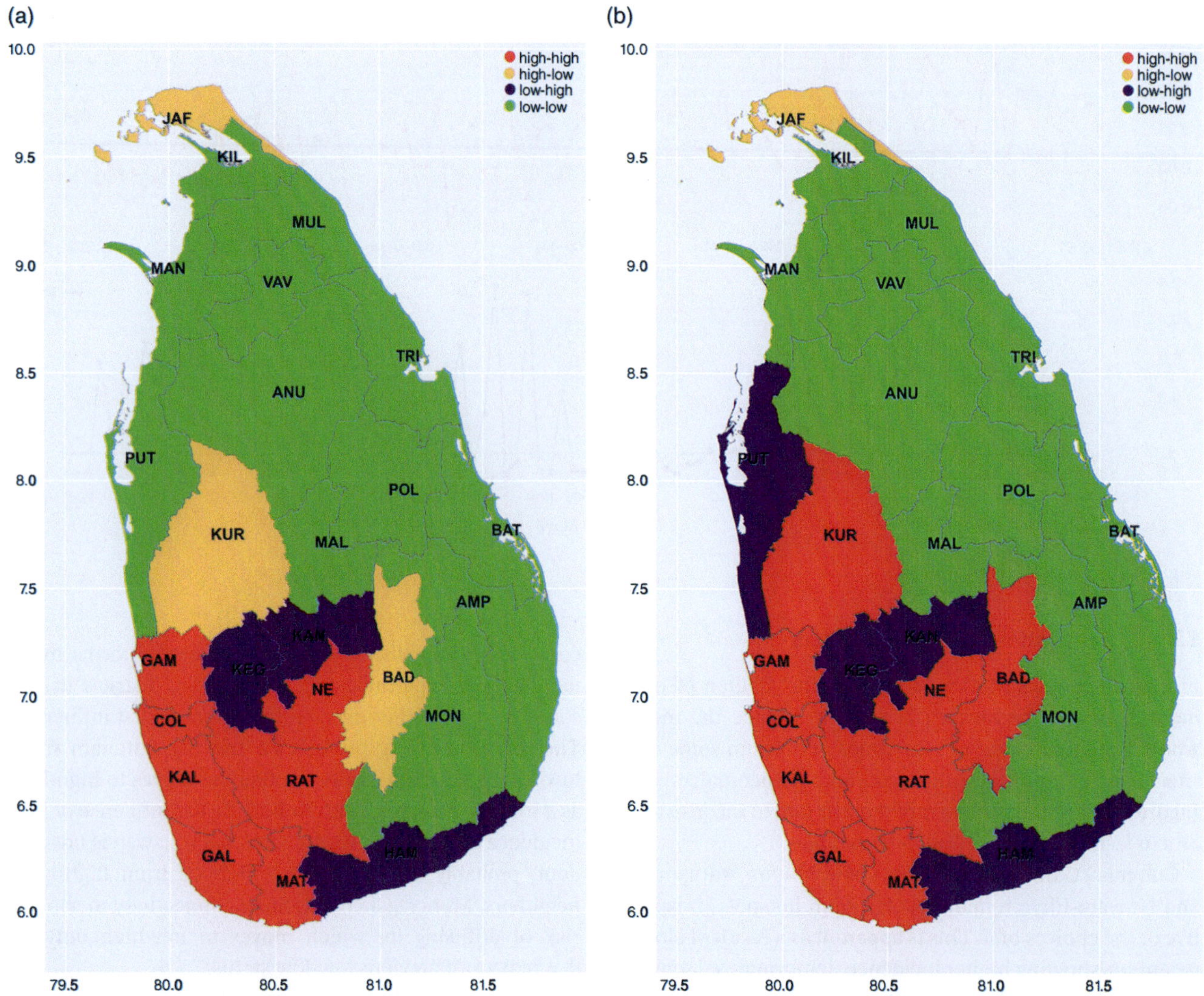

Figure 13.7 Mapping from Moran scatter of median. (a) $d = q_1$ (93 km), (b) $d = q_2$ (146 km), (c) $d = q_3$ (214 km), and (d) $d = \max$ (398 km).

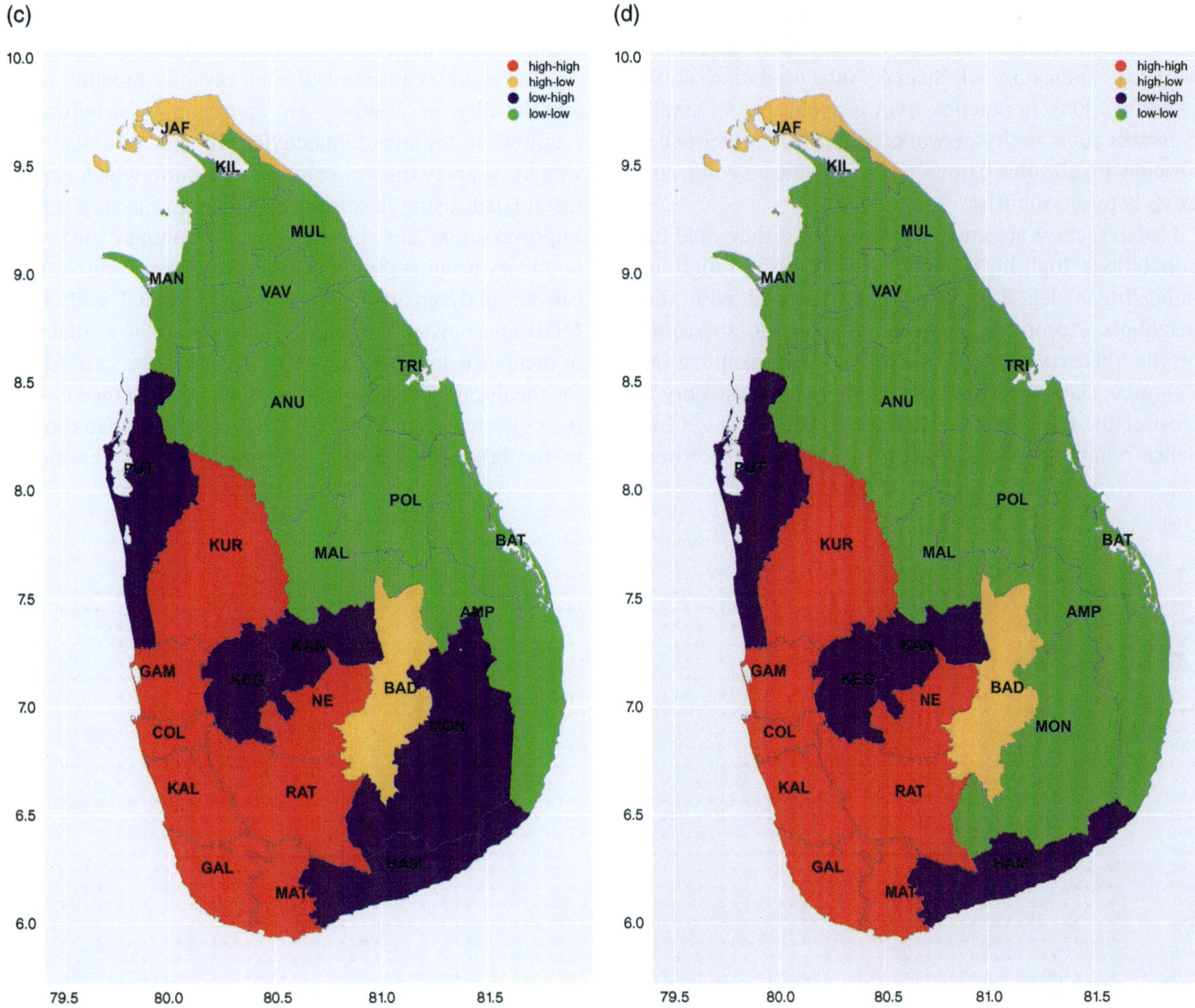

Figure 13.7 (Continued)

an equal chance of connecting neighbors of low incidence (from north-east) and high incidence (from south-west) when d increases.

13.4.3 Risk Mapping

Figure 13.9 directs us to observe crucial district borders that should be controlled in possible outbreaks in the future. This map was obtained using highest percentage quadrants with $d = \text{max}$ to be aligned with a new normal situation of no travel restrictions.

Borders between high-high (red) and low-high (blue) districts should be given priority to mitigate further diffusion from higher incidence areas to comparatively low incidence areas. Appearance of low-high districts near to high-high shows clear diffusion across those borders. Next, the borders between low-high (blue) and low-low (green) must be controlled to again suppress diffusion, though it might occur in a low phase. Such guidelines on prioritizing districts can be implemented in administering vaccines and enhancing healthcare capacity too.

13.5 Discussion

It is always worth to analyze how the spatial connectivity influences the spread of a disease, particularly in a pandemic situation (Franch-Pardo et al. 2020). In this chapter, a full profile representing the spatiotemporal dynamics of COVID-19 was produced via Moran scatters, and a random pattern was found for spatial autocorrelation using Moran's I. Moran's I interprets an overall spatial pattern instead of reflecting the status of individual spatial units (Oliveau and Guilmoto 2005). This measure was selected ahead of more locally oriented measures, Geary's C and Getis-Ord $G^* i$. In fact, Moran's I also has a local counterpart known as Local Indicators of Spatial Autocorrelation (LISA) (Anselin 1995). In practice, LISA is applicable for smaller networks such as city networks, where city center is connected with all suburb units, but no significant connection exists between suburbs.

Moran scatters are much instructional as they yield four possibilities: high-high, low-high, low-low, and high-low, indicating a degree of similarity compared with their neighbors. According to the findings of Moran scatters profile, districts in the Western part of the country (e.g. Colombo, Gampaha, Kalutara) are in hotspot category for most of the days showing high incidence with high incidence neighbors. In contrast, districts in the northern, eastern, and north-eastern parts (e.g. Mullaitivu, Trincomalee, Anuradhapura) remain in low-low category. As it is complex to monitor each person's mobility from one locality to another, an approximate structure is required to mimic connectivity of spatial units. The weights w_{ij} play the key role in this regard, which can be formulated using a distance-based approach. Further improvements are possible via combined distance-boundary weights (Smith 2017). Alternatively, correlation can be analyzed using much smaller spatial units (e.g. MOH areas instead of districts) subject to the availability of incidence data. A discrete optimization was carried out for the decaying rate δ and the threshold distance d with the objective of maximizing the presence of spatial units in similar quadrants over the study period. This novel

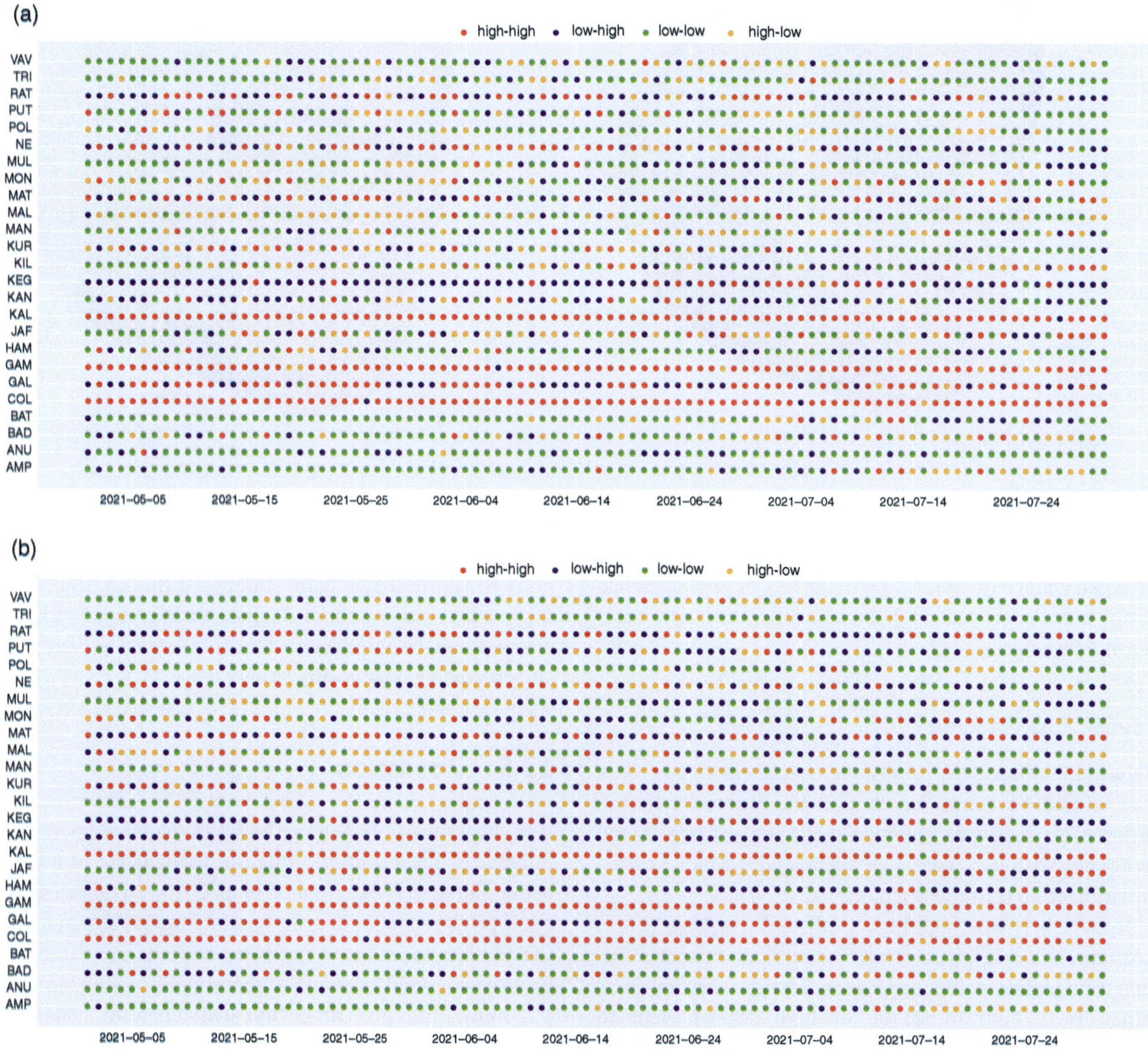

Figure 13.8 Moran scatters on a daily basis. (a) $d = q_1$ (93 km), (b) $d = q_2$ (146 km), (c) $d = q_3$ (214 km), (d) $d = \max$ (398 km).

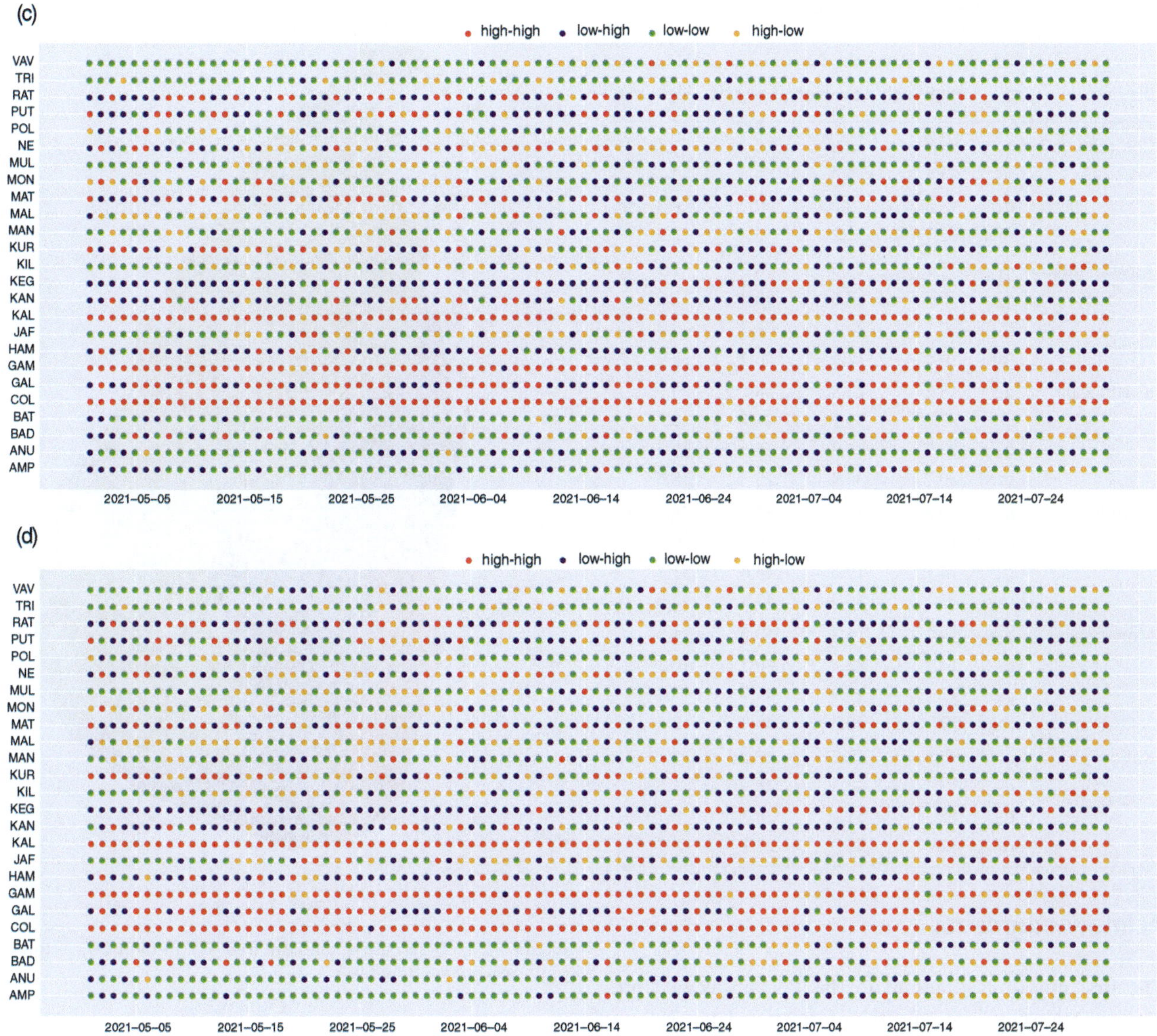

Figure 13.8 (Continued)

approach was chosen instead of usual sensitivity analysis, giving more realistic options on *d*.

In epidemics, incidence of infected persons is population driven. This is predominant in diseases having person-to-person transmission like COVID-19. According to the situation reports, highly populated districts (e.g. Colombo and Gampaha) shared largest number of confirmed cases (Epidemiology Unit – Ministry of Health Sri Lanka 2021). Normalized data are used for better comparisons in population-driven circumstances, which was closely monitored in earlier studies too (Ganegoda et al. 2021, 2022). This is the case for this study as well, as highly populated districts (e.g. Colombo and Gampaha) shared largest number of confirmed cases (Epidemiology Unit – Ministry of Health Sri Lanka 2021). Findings of normalized data facilitate unbiased decision making, where even less-populated areas might experience a relatively high risk of transmission. Normalized data attribute some intra-connections also within a spatial unit. If the spread is random across a country as observed in this work, control measures should be planned without too much of bias on case numbers. It is preferable to administer vaccinations for each district by a target percentage instead of a target number. Then many of the less-populated rural districts can benefit even amidst poor access to healthcare. Risk maps based on the frequency of Moran scatters are useful to prioritize border controls instead of imposing complete shutdown. Accordingly, a comprehensive decision support system can be designed with the aid of spatial autocorrelation measures for mitigating disease transmission, particularly in pandemic situations similar to COVID-19.

Table 13.1 Percentage of time points according to the quadrant of Moran scatters.

District	*d*	High-high	Low-high	Low-low	High-low
Colombo	q_1	96.7	2.2	0	1.1
	q_2	94.6	2.2	0	3.3
	q_3	93.5	2.2	0	4.3
	max	95.7	2.2	0	2.2
Anuradhapura	q_1	1.1	19.6	78.3	1.1
	q_2	0	7.6	90.2	2.2
	q_3	0	26.1	71.7	2.2
	max	0	17.4	80.4	2.2
Kurunegala	q_1	15.2	22.8	38	23.9
	q_2	27.2	39.1	21.7	12
	q_3	20.7	35.9	25	18.5
	max	20.7	35.9	25	18.5
Badulla	q_1	9.8	12	52.2	26.1
	q_2	15.2	26.1	38	20.7
	q_3	14.1	19.6	44.6	21.7
	max	13	16.3	47.8	22.8
Moneragala	q_1	14.1	16.3	53.3	16.3
	q_2	14.1	22.8	46.7	16.3
	q_3	13	23.9	45.7	17.4
	max	12	20.7	48.9	18.5
Kandy	q_1	7.6	52.2	27.2	13
	q_2	13	54.3	25	7.6
	q_3	12	51.1	28.3	8.7
	max	12	53.3	26.1	8.7

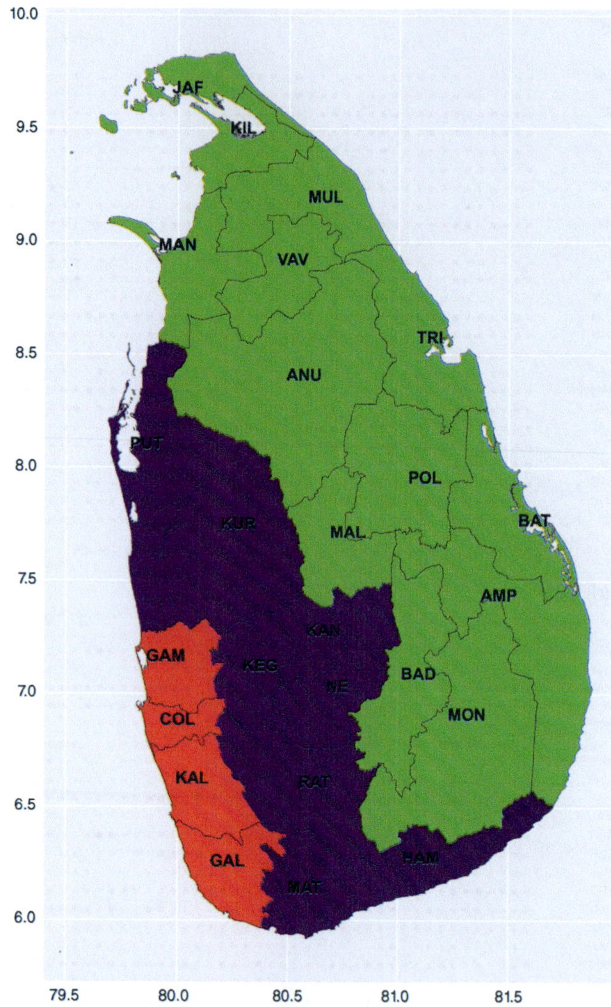

Figure 13.9 Dominating quadrant (red – high-high, blue – low-high, and green – low-low).

Acknowledgments

The first author is thankful to the Epidemiology Unit, Medical Statistics Unit, Health Information Unit, Health Promotion Bureau of the Ministry of Health – Sri Lanka for ensuring free access to data and the National Science Foundation of Sri Lanka for facilitating collaborations with the above units. The authors are grateful to the editors and reviewers of the book *One Health: Human, Animal, and Environment Triad.*

References

Anselin, L. (1995). Local indicators of spatial association-LISA. *Geographical Analysis* 27: 93–115.

Anselin, L. (2020). Global spatial autocorrelation. https://geodacenter.github.io/workbook/5a_global_auto/lab5a.html (accessed 3 January 2022).

Central Bank of Sri Lanka (2020). Annual Report 2020. https://www.cbsl.gov.lk/en/publications/economic-and-financial-reports/annual-reports/annual-report-2020 (accessed 20 August 2021).

Chen, Y. (2013). New approaches for calculating moran's index of spatial autocorrelation. *PLoS One* 8: e68336–e68314.

Chyon, F.A., Suman, M.N.H., Fahim, M.R.I., and Ahmmed, M.S. (2022). Time series analysis and predicting covid-19 affected patients by arima model using machine learning. *Journal of Virological Methods* 301: 114433–114436.

Department of Census and Statistics – Sri Lanka (2022). Population and housing. http://www.statistics.gov.lk/ (accessed 12 January 2022).

Epidemiology Unit – Ministry of Health Sri Lanka (2021). COVID – 19 Daily Situation Report. https://www.epid.gov.lk/web/index.php?option=com_content&view=article&id=225&lang=en (accessed 20 December 2021).

Erandi, K.K.W.H., Mahasinghe, A.C., Perera, S.S.N., and Jayasinghe, S. (2020). Effectiveness of the strategies implemented in Sri Lanka for controlling the covid-19 outbreak. *Journal of Applied Mathematics* 2020: 2954519–2954510.

Farzan, Z. (2021). New year cluster continues to climb as SL hits another daily record high with 1891 cases. *News First*. https://www.newsfirst.lk/2021/05/02/new-year-cluster-continues-to-climb-as-sl-hits-another-daily-record-high-with-1891-cases/ (accessed 10 February 2022).

Franch-Pardo, I., Napoletano, B.M., Rosete-Verges, F., and Billa, L. (2020). Spatial analysis and GIS in the study of covid-19. A review. *Science of the Total Environment* 739: 140033–140010.

Ganegoda, N.C., Wijaya, K.P., Amadi, M. et al. (2021). Interrelationship between daily covid-19 cases and average temperature as well as relative humidity in Germany. *Scientific Reports* 11: 11302–11316.

Ganegoda, N.C., Wijaya, K.P., Chavez, J.P. et al. (2022). Reassessment of contact restrictions and testing campaigns against covid-19 via spatio-temporal modeling. *Nonlinear Dynamics* 107: 3085–3109.

Getis, A. and Ord, J.K. (1992). The analysis of spatial association by use of distance statistics. *Geographical Analysis* 24: 189–206.

Getis, A. and Ord, J.K. (1995). Local spatial autocorrelation statistics: distributional issues and an application. *Geographical Analysis* 27: 286–306.

Ghorbanzadeh, M., Kim, K., Erman Ozguven, E., and Horner, M.W. (2021). Spatial accessibility assessment of covid-19 patients to healthcare facilities: a case study of Florida. *Travel Behaviour and Society* 24: 95–101.

Ghosh, J.K., Biswas, S.K., Sarkar, S., and Ghosh, U. (2022). Mathematical modelling of covid-19: a case study of italy. *Mathematics and Computers in Simulation* 194: 1–18.

Glen, S. (2022). Moran's I: definition, examples. https://www.statisticshowto.com/morans-i/ (accessed 15 January 2022).

Haining, R. (2001). Spatial sampling. In: *International Encyclopedia of the Social & Behavioral Sciences* (ed. N.J. Smelser and P.B. Baltes), 14822–14827. Pergamon.

Han, Y., Yang, L., Jia, K. et al. (2021). Spatial distribution characteristics of the covid-19 pandemic in beijing and its relationship with environmental factors. *Science of the Total Environment* 761: 144257–144211.

Hong, I., Jung, W.S., and Jo, H.H. (2019). Gravity model explained by the radiation model on a population landscape. *PLoS One* 14: e0218028–e0218013.

Jia, J.S., Lu, X., Yuan, Y. et al. (2020). Population flow drives spatio-temporal distribution of covid-19 in china. *Nature* 582: 389–394.

Kassa, S.M., Njagarah, J.B., and Terefe, Y.A. (2020). Analysis of the mitigation strategies for covid-19: from mathematical modelling perspective. *Chaos, Solitons and Fractals* 138: 109968–109926.

Kianfar, N., Mesgari, M.S., Mollalo, A., and Kaveh, M. (2022). Spatio-temporal modeling of covid-19 prevalence and mortality using artificial neural network algorithms. *Spatial and Spatio-temporal Epidemiology* 40: 100471–100416.

Kibria, H.B., Jyoti, O., and Matin, A. (2022). Forecasting the spread of the third wave of covid-19 pandemic using time series analysis in Bangladesh. *Informatics in Medicine Unlocked* 28: 100815–100818.

Kondo, K. (2018). Testing for global spatial autocorrelation in stata. MORANSI: Stata module to compute Moran's I. Stratistical Software Components S458473. Boston College Department of Economics (Revised 14 Jun 2021).

Lasaulce, S., Zhang, C., Varma, V., and Mor˘arescu, I.C. (2021). Analysis of the tradeoff between health and economic impacts of the Covid-19 epidemic. *Frontiers in Public Health* 9: 620770–620713.

de León, U.A.P., Pérez, Á.G., and Avila-Vales, E. (2020). An SEIARD epidemic model for COVID-19 in Mexico: mathematical analysis and state-level forecast. *Chaos, Solitons & Fractals 140*: 110165.

Ma, Q., Gao, J., Zhang, W. et al. (2021). Spatio-temporal distribution characteristics of covid-19 in china: a city-level modeling study. *BMC Infectious Diseases* 21: 816–814.

Moran, P.A.P. (1948). The interpretation of statistical maps. *Journal of the Royal Statistical Society B* 10: 243–251.

National Operation Centre for Prevention of COVID – 19 Outbreak (2021). Official website for Sri Lanka's response to COVID-19 response. https://covid19.gov.lk/news/health.html (accessed 10 November 2021).

Oliveau, S. and Guilmoto, C.Z. (2005). Spatial correlation and demography: exploring India's demographic patterns. In: *XXV International Population Conference*. Tours, France: Office of Population Research at Princeton University.

Piret, J. and Boivin, G. (2021). Pandemics throughout history. *Frontiers in Microbiology* 11: 631736.

Ram´ırez, I.J. and Lee, J. (2020). Covid-19 emergence and social and health determinants in Colorado: a rapid spatial analysis. *International Journal of Environmental Research and Public Health* 17: 3856–3815.

Rendana, M., Idris, W.M.R., and Rahim, S.A. (2021). Spatial distribution of covid-19 cases, epidemic spread rate, spatial pattern, and its correlation with meteorological factors during the first to the second waves. *Journal of Infection and Public Health* 14: 1340–1348.

Smith, T.E. (2017). Spatial weight matrices. ACM SIGSPATIAL International Workshop on Advances in Geographic Information Systems. https://doi.org/10.1007/978-3-319-17885-1_101296.

Sohrabinia, M. (2022). MATLAB central file exchange – LatLon distance. www.mathworks.com/matlabcentral/fileexchange/38812-latlon-distance (accessed 12 January 2022).

Srinivasan, M. (2021a). Sri Lanka reports delta variant amid a daunting third wave. *The Hindu*. https://www.thehindu.com/news/international/coronavirus-sri-lanka-reports-delta-variant-amid-a-daunting-third-wave/article34843288.ece (accessed 15 February 2022).

Srinivasan, M. (2021b). Sri lanka braces for third covid-19 wave. *The Hindu*. https://www.thehindu.com/news/international/sri-lanka-braces-for-imminent-third-covid-19-wave/article34417392.ece (accessed 10 February 2022).

World Health Organization (2022). Timeline: WHO's COVID-19 response. https://www.who.int/emergencies/diseases/novel-coronavirus-2019/interactive-timeline#! (accessed 4 January 2022).

Worldometer (2022a). Coronavirus worldwide graphs. https://www.worldometers.info/coronavirus/worldwide-graphs/ (accessed 1 February 2022).

Worldometer (2022b). COVID-19 coronavirus pandemic: Sri Lanka. https://www.worldometers.info/coronavirus/country/sri-lanka/ (accessed 15 January 2022).

Zhou, X. and Lin, H. (2008). Geary's c. In: *Encyclopedia of GIS* (ed. S. Shekhar and H. Xiong), 329–330. Boston: Springer.

14

Organic Farming: The Influence on Soil Health

Jithya Wijesinghe, Shermila M. Botheju, Bhagya Nallaperuma, and Niwantha Kanuwana

Department of Indigenous Medical Resources, Faculty of Indigenous Health Sciences and Technology, Gampaha Wickramarachchi University of Indigenous Medicine, Yakkala, Sri Lanka

14.1 Introduction

14.1.1 Concept of Organic Farming

Learn the language of the soil; the soil will speak to us.

According to the International Federation of Organic Agriculture Movements (IFOAM), organic agriculture is a production system that sustains the health of soils, ecosystems, and people. It relies on ecological processes, biodiversity, and cycles adapted to local conditions rather than inputs with adverse effects. Organic agriculture combines tradition, innovation, and science to benefit the shared environment and promote fair relationships and good quality of life for all involved. Organic farming is derived from four basic principles: principles of health, ecology, fairness, and care (Alsanius et al. 2019).

14.1.1.1 Principles of Health

According to the World Health Organization (WHO), health is a state of complete physical, mental, and social well-being and not merely the absence of disease or infirmity. Further added by IFOAM, organic agriculture is intended to produce high-quality, nutritious food that contributes to preventive health care and well-being. This principle points out that the health of individuals and communities cannot be separated from the health of ecosystems and healthy soils produce healthy crops that foster the health of animals and people. With this focus on health, it should avoid fertilizers, pesticides, animal drugs, and food additives that may have adverse health effects.

14.1.1.2 Principles of Ecology

As the basics of ecology state, energy and materials recycle, and organic farming facilitates the ecological process and recycling. It is promoted to reduce inputs by reuse, recycling, and efficient management of materials and energy to maintain and improve environmental quality and conserve resources.

14.1.1.3 Principles of Fairness

The fairness in organic farming exhibits fairness along the agriculture value chain, including value chain actors, activities, and functions. Besides, the fairness should be stretched to natural and environmental resources used for production and consumption, managed in a socially and ecologically sound way, and held in trust for future generations.

14.1.1.4 Principles of Care

Organic farming is a natural and living farming system focused on a healthy, safe, and ecologically sound system. The productivity enhancement strategies of organic farming should never be overstepped beyond the well-being of the human or ecological system.

14.1.2 Global Scenario of Organic Farming

When organic farming and affiliated actors, actives, and functions are considered, IFOAM has been a vital organization for the regulation and promotion of organic farming. IFOAM was founded in 1972 and initiated the articulation of private standards for organic agriculture in the 1980s. Because of the site-specific character of organic agricultural practices and the worldwide engagement of IFOAM, the standards of IFOAM are "standards for standards" and are therefore called the IFOAM Basic Standards (IES) (Anonymous 2005).

Organic farming was considered a niche portion of agriculture until recent times. Organic food accounts for 1–2% of food sales worldwide (FiBL 2021). In the future, growth is expected to range from 10 to 50% annually depending on the country (Amarjit 2015). The important point is the growth rate rather than the existing sales percentage.

One Health: Human, Animal, and Environment Triad, First Edition. Edited by Meththika Vithanage and Majeti Narasimha Vara Prasad.

Amarjit (2015) predicts a USD150 billion market for organic foods and drinks based on the present figures. In 2008, the global organic market reached USD 50 billion, and within 10 years, it surpassed the USD100 billion margins.

FiBL (2021) records a categorical description of organic products traded in 2019, putting tropical fruits, nuts, and spices on top with 27% of total organic sales. In some product categories, such as olive oil, 20% of sales have been recorded as organic, making a promising future. The organic land extension increased by 1.1 Mn ha in 2019, with significant increases in India and Kazakhstan. More importantly, it has recorded a rise in almost all world regions in 2019 (FiBL 2021). The number of organic producers was nearly 3.1 Mn in 2019, which is an increment of 12.5% compared to 2018. Kirchner et al. (2021) stated that 72 countries had fully implemented organic regulations by 2020, while another 22 countries implementing them. To mitigate the cost factor of third-party certification, Participative Guarantee Scheme (PGS) has emerged as an affordable alternative among small-scale farmers. When the present situation of organic farming is analyzed, an increase in land extends, producers, trade volume, and supportive regulatory infrastructure could be observed.

14.1.3 Organic Farming vs. Conventional Farming

Organic agriculture is a production system that regenerates soil health, ecosystems, and people, while organic farmers rely on natural processes, biodiversity, and natural cycles adapted to local conditions rather than synthetic inputs such as chemical fertilizers, pesticides, and herbicides.

Conventional agriculture practices have contributed to increased greenhouse gas emissions, soil erosion, water pollution, and threats to human health. Organic farming ensures a smaller carbon footprint, safeguards and builds soil health, and replenishes natural ecosystems for cleaner water and air, all without contaminating toxic pesticide residues. It is evident that organic and conventional farming differ because conventional farming relies on chemical intervention to fight pests and weeds and provide plant nutrition with synthetic pesticides, herbicides, and fertilizers, respectively. Organic farming instead relies on natural principles such as biodiversity and composting to produce healthy food. Organic production is not the mere avoidance of chemical inputs but the substitution of natural inputs for synthetic ones. Organic farmers apply inherent techniques used by their ancestors, such as seasonal cropping, auspicious timing, dynamics of solar and lunar, crop rotations, composted animal manures, and green manure crops, in ways that are economically sustainable in today's world. In organic production, overall system health is emphasized, and the interaction of management practices is the primary concern.

14.1.3.1 Biodynamic Agriculture

Biodynamic agriculture is also a method of organic farming that was introduced by Dr. Rudolf Steiner in 1924. The biodynamic agriculture is a holistic view of a farm as an organism, with the plant and animal communities of a natural habitat striving for a certain balance where the number of species and individuals is constant. Any such activity that disturbs the balance is considered as an unbalance and leads to destroying the harness and balance that existed. More frequently used agronomic practices such as clearing, tilling, plowing, and mono-cropping are considered unbalancing activities. The usage of pesticides, herbicides, and chemical fertilizers are also in the same manner considered as unbalancing activities.

Biodynamic farming includes crop diversification and the use of green manures, compost, and manures improved by biodynamic preparations (Smith and Collins 2007). Studies have shown that biodynamically managed fields maintain higher soil C levels, microbial respiration, mineralizable N, earthworm populations, microbial biomass C and N, and greater enzyme activities. Biodynamic farms have better soil quality, primarily due to enhanced microbial decomposition and stabilization of organic matter (Smith et al. 2014). The main difference between biodynamic agriculture and organic agriculture is determined by the preparations done in biodynamic agriculture, such as fermentation of plant and animal substances.

The safer usage of inputs in organic farming has contributed a lot to the health benefits of consumers. Multiple studies have shown that organic varieties provide significantly greater levels of vitamin C, iron, magnesium, and phosphorus than non-organic varieties of the same foods (Timsina 2018) while they are higher in these nutrients, they are also significantly lower in nitrates and pesticide residues. In addition, organic foods typically provide greater levels of several important antioxidant phytochemicals (anthocyanins, flavonoids, and carotenoids). Although, in vitro studies of organic fruits and vegetables consistently demonstrate that organic foods have greater antioxidant activity, are more potent suppressors of the mutagenic action of toxic compounds, and inhibit the proliferation of certain cancer cell lines.

14.2 Soil Health

Feed the soil; the soil will feed the plant.

Soil is a composite material made up of minerals, gases, water, organic matter, and living organisms. It serves as the primary medium for plant growth, regulates water supplies, modifies the atmosphere through various physical, chemical, and biological processes, provides habitats for various organisms, and acts as a major engineering medium for human-built structures. Thus, the soil is a major ecosystem in its own right. The soil quality, soil health, or its current status determines the nature of the plant ecosystems and the capacity of the land to support animal life and society.

Historically, soils have been classified as "good," "bad," "worn-out," "fertile," or "infertile." However, scientists and land managers needed a better tool to understand and evaluate the processes that improved soil conditions in recent years and thus developed the two concepts of *soil quality* and *soil health*. Although these two terms are frequently used interchangeably, they refer to two distinct concepts.

14.2.1 Soil Health vs. Soil Quality

Soil health refers to the "capacity of soil to function as a vital living system, within the ecosystem and land-use boundaries, to sustain plant and animal productivity, maintain or enhance water and air quality, and promote plant and animal health" (USDA-NRCS 2019) (Figure 14.1), and it bridges agricultural and soil science to policy, stakeholder needs, and sustainable supply chain management (Lehmann et al. 2020). Historically, soil assessments were primarily concerned with crop production; however, soil health now encompasses the role of the soil in water quality, climate change, and human health. The concept of soil health emerged in the early

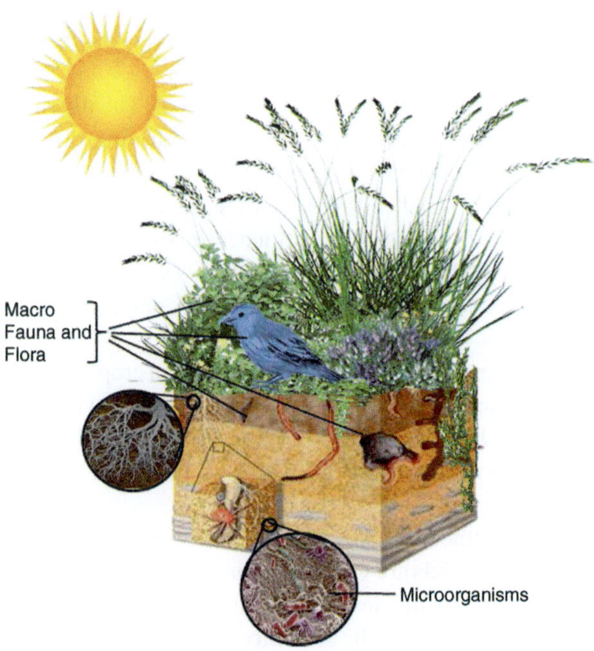

Figure 14.1 Healthy soil ecosystem, with organisms living within and above the soil surface. *Source:* Carlyn Iverson and USDA-SARE.

2000s and has since developed connections to the emerging "One Health" concept, which connects the health of humans, animals, and the environment.

"Soil quality" predates the term soil health and refers to the "ability of soils to function for agriculture and its immediate environmental context" (Lehmann et al. 2020). Thus, soil quality encompasses the effects of soils on water quality, plant and animal health, and the overall health of entire ecosystems. Inherent soil quality refers to the aspects of soil quality relating to a soil's natural composition and properties that are influenced by the natural long-term factors and processes of soil formation. These are generally unaffected by human management. Dynamic soil quality, which is synonymous with soil health, refers to soil properties that change over time as a result of soil use and management. Soil health evokes the notion that soil is a living ecosystem that must be carefully managed in order to reclaim and maintain its ability to function optimally. Farmers have generally preferred the term soil health, while scientists have preferred the term soil quality.

14.2.1.1 Soil Health Indicators

Soil health has a qualitative nature. The physical, chemical, and biological characteristics of soil can all be used to determine its "healthiness." Farmers and scientists have developed their own set of soil health indicators, including color, tilth, drainage, the presence of macrofauna and weeds, and crop yield, etc. Numerous soil properties have been examined to determine soil health by examining the response of specific soil functions to a practical change in the soil property and its ease of use (Norris et al. 2020). The health indicators that have been widely accepted as a common set of metrics for measuring and monitoring soil health over time, combining soil chemical, physical, and biological metrics are called Tier 1 indicators (Figure 14.2) (Soil Health Institute 2018).

14.2.1.2 Soil Health Management and Soil Health Principles

Soils are integral components of all terrestrial ecosystems, whether urban, agricultural, marshy, or grassland, because they interact with physical, chemical, and biological components in the ecosystem. It cannot alter land use practices without affecting the soil and its constituents. Inappropriate land use, crop cultivation, animal grazing, and fertilization all contribute to the degradation of soil health and function. The way we manage plant communities affects the long-term stability and health of the soil. As a result, effective soil management practices are required to preserve and improve soil health, particularly on agricultural lands. Therefore, five principles have been introduced by the USDA-NRCS to maintain and promote soil health, i.e. soil

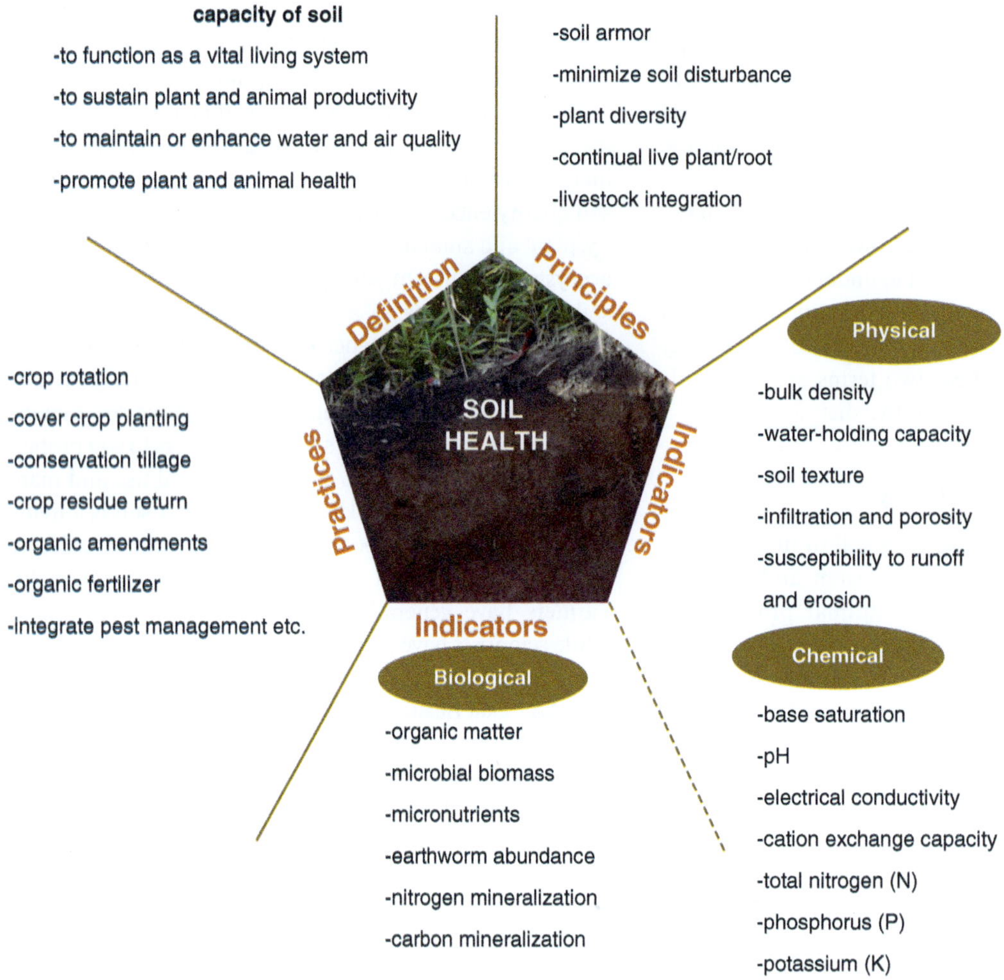
capacity of soil
-to function as a vital living system
-to sustain plant and animal productivity
-to maintain or enhance water and air quality
-promote plant and animal health
-soil armor
-minimize soil disturbance
-plant diversity
-continual live plant/root
-livestock integration
Definition
Principles
SOIL HEALTH
Practices
Indicators
Physical
-bulk density
-water-holding capacity
-soil texture
-infiltration and porosity
-susceptibility to runoff and erosion
-crop rotation
-cover crop planting
-conservation tillage
-crop residue return
-organic amendments
-organic fertilizer
-integrate pest management etc.
Indicators
Biological
-organic matter
-microbial biomass
-micronutrients
-earthworm abundance
-nitrogen mineralization
-carbon mineralization
Chemical
-base saturation
-pH
-electrical conductivity
-cation exchange capacity
-total nitrogen (N)
-phosphorus (P)
-potassium (K)

Figure 14.2 Soil health as a comprehensive expression of various principles, indicators, and management practices.

armor, minimizing soil disturbance, plant diversity, continual live plant/root, and livestock integration (USDA-NRCS 2021). Furthermore, a variety of available soil management practices (e.g. crop rotation, cover crop planting, conservation tillage, crop residue return, land application of manure and compost, and biochar amendment) have been recommended and practiced for promoting the health of agricultural soils (Guo 2020; Williams et al. 2020).

14.3 Organic Farming Affecting Soil Health: Soil Physical, Chemical, and Biological Properties

Organic farming practices help minimize the negative environmental impacts of modern agriculture by applying the best soil management practices, including proper land use, appropriate cropping systems, conservation tillage, land application of organic residues, organic fertilization, based on soil health principles (Figure 14.2). The different management strategies used in organic farming directly affect the chemical, physical, and biological soil properties, thus affecting soil health as well (Jernigan et al. 2020). Tully and McAskill (2020) identified four key organic farming practices that improve soil health, i.e. use of cover crops, organic amendments, crop rotation, and reduce soil disturbances.

Cover crops are plants grown between cash crop cycles to protect the land from erosion and enrich the soil with root exudates and biomass. For the soil health benefit to be fully realized, cover crop biomass must be returned to the soil following the desired growing period.

Soil amendments made from naturally occurring plant or animal materials are widely used in organic farming that provide essential nutrients maintaining while improving yields and soil health. The sequence of crops grown on the same land in succession is a critical component of maintaining healthy soils and has the important benefit of interrupting the disease cycle as a new crop cannot serve as a host for the existing pathogen. Tillage is occasionally used to control weeds in organic farms, but it can degrade soil structure and result in loss of soil organic carbon (SOC). As a result, conservation tillage practices such as no-till or reduced tillage have long been established to conserve soil and sequester carbon in the soil by minimizing soil disturbance and maintaining residue soil cover.

In this chapter, we focused on Tire 1 soil health indicators available in recent literature with the four key organic farming practices mentioned earlier.

14.3.1 Effect of Organic Farming on Soil Physical Properties

The application of compost, green manure, animal manure, mulches, and vermicomposting are all common practices in organic farming that help increase soil organic matter and improve the abiotic and biotic properties of the soil. These nontoxic organic fertilizers are rich in organic matter, humus, and beneficial microorganisms as well (De Corato 2020). Organic matter is crucial for the health and fertility of the soil. In general, increased soil organic matter accumulation improves soil structure, fertility, and health, allowing for better water infiltration and moisture retention, ultimately increasing crop yield. Therefore, organic amendments and fertilizers have the potential to alter the physicochemical properties of soil as well as the activity of various soil enzymes, thereby alleviating the negative impact of long-term excessive inorganic fertilizer application on soil health (Qaswar et al. 2020).

According to Sheoran et al. (2019), applying an appropriate organic fertilizer to the soil can reduce the bulk density, increase the porosity, and increase the aggregates of the soil by improving its physical properties. Reduced soil bulk density by organic fertilizer application aids plant roots in anchoring the plants and acquiring and transporting water, mineral nutrients, and oxygen from the soil pores to the leaves. When root penetration and elongation are increased as a result of low bulk density, the volume of soil that can be exploited for essential nutrients and water is increased, resulting in an increase in overall plant growth. Devarajan et al. (2021) also advocated for the widespread use of compost to alleviate soil compaction. Composting on a yearly basis over time develops a desirable soil structure and subsequent alteration in pore size distribution, making it much easier to work, lowering bulk density, reducing soil erosion, and increasing soil fertility. The high biological activities facilitated by organic farming contain a large number of biopores, which will enhance water infiltration rates and the water-holding capacity of the soil.

Tillage is a critical practice in agricultural systems that heavily affects soil health. A 34-year study conducted in the cotton field in the USA supported evidence for the increase of SOC, wet aggregate stability, water availability, and hydraulic conductivity yield in the non-tillage system compared with conventional tillage and, thus, the high yield of cotton with the above improvements in soils (Nouri et al. 2019).

The phenomenon of holding greater water in soils with high crop residue retention is due to the larger quantity of plant residues and organic matter, which contribute to retaining water in soil pore spaces. Al-Busaidi et al. (2020) reported that soils amended with biochar have a greater capacity to retain water than soils devoid of biochar. Biochar has properties that affect the porosity and surface area of the soil, which are the most critical physical properties for soil improvement. Compost, in general, is said to improve soil functions by increasing the capacity of amended soils to hold water. In contrast, Al-Busaidi et al. (2020) observed no effect of the compost on the water-holding capacity of the organic matter contained in the compost. However, the addition of compost did not alter the texture of the soil but altered its structure (Al-Busaidi et al. 2020; Devarajan et al. 2021).

With the addition of crop residues and organic amendments, the soil tilth (structure and aggregation) and its associated benefits of drainage, aeration, moisture-holding capacity, rooting depth, and resistance to erosion and compaction are maintained and enhanced by fungal hyphae, earthworms, and the glue-like metabolites of microbes feeding on fresh residues. Stable soil organic matter also contributes to tilth by helping to hold aggregates together. Fresh residues on the soil surface aid in erosion control, moisture conservation, and aggregate protection as well. However, the amount and chemical composition of crop residues are important, as they determine their degradation and transformation in soils. Al-Busaidi et al. (2020) confirmed the ability of soil organic amendments to increase the soil organic matter, water-holding capacity, and total organic carbon. Therefore, they suggest that the application of soil organic supplements is worthy for soil health progression and sustainable agriculture due to their ability to improve soil physical, chemical, and biological properties. However, the effectiveness of specific amendments will depend on the type and quality of amendments, the soil type, and the crop type. For example, recently the quality of the compost, biosolids, and manure was questionable as it was identified as a vector of microplastics, pharmaceuticals, and personal care products into the soil. Introducing these types of contaminants into soil negatively influence the soil structure and bulk density, which can affect root penetration resistance, changes in water-holding capacity and carbon storage (Rillig et al. 2021), and, finally, overall plant growth and primary production (Rillig et al. 2019).

14.3.2 Effect of Organic Farming on Soil Chemical Properties

Conservation tillage practices, such as no-till organic farming, could favor SOC accumulation by reducing soil disturbance and increasing crop residue retention. Hati et al. (2020) and Jha et al. (2020) observed an increase in SOC in no-tillage systems as a result of residue retention being greater than in conventional tillage systems. Therefore, residue retention can be considered as another critical factor that can impact the rate of SOC accumulation in organic agriculture. The results of a 36-year experiment conducted in a sorghum production field in the USA have demonstrated unequivocally that adopting a non-tillage system with crop residue retention increases soil carbon storage and decreases carbon loss (Govindasamy et al. 2021). Therefore, conservation tillage practices have the potential to increase SOC concentrations in organic farming systems and thereby result in net positive effects on soil health. Furthermore, tillage has a significant effect on the increase in the rate of carbon mineralization by mixing crop residues in the soil, breaking larger macroaggregates, and exposing the protected SOC in the aggregates to soil microorganisms (Kan et al. 2020; Singh et al. 2020). Decomposition of soil organic matter initiates carbon mineralization, which has a direct effect on soil nutrient supply and CO_2 emissions. Govindasamy et al. (2021) observed the slow mineralization of stable carbon in non-tillage organic systems, which contributes to soil health enhancement. Similarly, Szostek et al. (2022) reported that soils with simplified tillage systems contained the highest levels of organic carbon (C) and total nitrogen (N), regardless of the type of fertilizer applied (organic or mineral) or the crop cultivated. For example, they found that organic farms with plowing had the lowest total C and N content. This means regardless of the type of natural fertilization applied to soils, disturbance of the soil surface layers by plowing may result in a higher rate of C and N transformation and mineralization, which likely affects organic C and N losses, providing additional evidence for the effect of tillage practices on soil health.

The addition of organic amendments and fertilizer has an effect on the soil chemical properties. When organic amendments are incorporated, soil organisms initiate the decomposition of applied materials and release nutrients quickly, thereby meeting the nutrient requirements of the growing cash crops in organic fields. Kranz et al. (2020) observed the long-term maintenance nutrient levels in soil with the addition of compost. Active soil organic matter acts as a reservoir for slow-release nutrients, particularly N, phosphorus (P), sulfur (S), and boron (B), and also acts as a buffer for micronutrient levels, mitigating both deficiency and toxicity and thereby improving soil health. Organic fertilizer application increases not only the total amount of nutrients in the soil but also the amount of available nutrients such as alkali N, available P, and K (Qaswar et al. 2020). In addition to the increase in nutrients, a significant improvement in cation exchange capacity, catalase and phosphatase were reported under organic fertilizer treatments in rice fields (Liu et al. 2021), indicating that organic fertilizer can be used to comprehensively improve the soil environment in terms of total nutrients, available nutrients, and enzyme activities. Devarajan et al. (2021) also reported increased levels of micronutrients, organic matter, and initial moisture content in soils amended with compost and cover crops, as well as a decrease in soil pH. Simultaneously, organic fertilizer can help reduce N, P, and K losses through leaching and improve soil fertilizer retention performance.

Finally, all of these soil health improvements result in increased crop yields. There has been evidence of a direct positive relationship between SOC content, soil nutrient status, and crop yield as well (Xu et al. 2019). The study conducted by Liu et al. (2021) also revealed the contribution of soil nutrients and bacteria to increase rice yield in long-term organic fertilizer substitution treatment. In addition, organic fertilizer application has a positive effect on crop quality with the increased amount of available soil N, P, and K (Gondwe et al. 2020). For example, after organic fertilizer replacement treatment, an increase in accumulation of N, P, and K levels in rice leaves, sheaths, panicles, and seeds and the dry matter content of the plants were observed by Moe et al. (2019).

According to the meta-analysis carried out by Crystal-Ornelas et al. (2021), organic amendments showed the largest mean increase of in-depth weighted SOC concentration among the management practices in organic farming while greater increase of SOC with conservation tillage and long-term cover crop maintenance. Regardless of the time period of management, organic amendments increased depth-weighted SOC concentrations in comparison to control groups, providing strong evidence to support organic farming as a means of improving soil health and suggesting it as a best management practice in organic farming to achieve agricultural sustainability. Therefore, applying organic amendments would be a long-term investment in soil health improvement.

In contrast to the benefits, aforementioned in Section 14.3.2, the quality of the organic fertilizer or amendments would negatively affect soil chemical properties. In support of this claim, de Souza Machado et al. (2019) reported significant changes in the carbon cycle in numerous ways with the application of compost containing impurities such as microplastics by being carbon themselves and by influencing soil microbial processes, litter decomposition, nutrient availability, and terrestrial biodiversity following exposure to microplastics. Similarly, phosphorous, dissolved organic carbon, cation exchange capacity, and pH have been observed to decrease significantly with the addition of microplastics in compost (Yu et al. 2020).

Until now, we discussed the effect on soil health indicators of incorporating a single conservation practice (cover crops, organic amendments, crop rotation, tillage, etc.). Organic farmers, on the other hand, are increasingly integrating multiple practices into their cropping systems. Combining several soil health-enhancing practices, referred to as "stacked" practices, such as reducing tillage and combining multiple organic amendment sources (e.g. mixing compost and manure) can result in greater soil health benefits than either practice alone (Tully and McAskill 2020). Additionally, stacking practices may enable farmers to gain multiple benefits while mitigating the negative consequences of adopting these practices alone. For example, although most organic farmers use conventional tillage to control weeds, such practices can deplete SOC and microbial biomass C, increase runoff and erosion, and reduce earthworm abundance and biomass. By incorporating cover crops into a crop rotation, they can effectively suppress weeds and provide a source of carbon that can help offset some of the SOC losses associated with conventional tillage systems. Therefore, employing stacking practices in organic farming systems would help to maximize soil health.

14.3.3 Effect of Organic Farming on Soil Biological Properties

The diversity of the living organisms in the soil, including microorganisms, which are a countless number of organisms not visible to the naked eye, mesofauna, and macrofauna together with the plant roots reflect the term soil biodiversity. The major functions of the soil organisms are acting as the primary driving agents of nutrient cycling, balancing the changes of soil organic matter, soil carbon sequestration and greenhouse gas emission, amending and improving the soil physical structure and water systems, escalating the amount and the efficiency of nutrient acquisition by the vegetation, and improving the plant health (FAO 2020).

Compost is one of the effective forms of nutrition used in organic agriculture to improve both soil health and soil biota. Humic materials add microorganisms such as bacteria, actinomycetes, and fungi to the soil systems, stimulate their proliferation, and increase the activity of the soil enzymes, which are responsible for converting the nutrients from unavailable to available forms (Sanathara and Vibhute 2020). Rich microbial diversity is positively correlated with the soil functions, including soil nutrient turnover by decomposition and nutrient mineralization, and it acts as a better resilience to disturbances (Kharti and Sharma 2021). The soils of the organic farming system were characterized by the highest enzymatic activity and an increase in biochemical activity due to the limitations of the chemization of agriculture (Szostek et al. 2022). Organic fertilizer application has been shown to be directly correlated with the activities of soil urease, invertase, catalase, phosphatase, and other enzymes, which can improve the living environment for microorganisms.

As reported by various studies, the appropriate application of organic fertilizer can regulate the structure of the soil microbial community including number and diversity, form the most stable interactions between plants and microbial communities, and improve the soil microecological environment in different soil types and for different plant types (Liu et al. 2021). For example, Ikoyi et al. (2020) discovered that the relative abundances of bacteria involved in nutrient cycling and/or plant growth promotion, such as *Burkholderia*, *Allorhizobium*, *Terrimonas*, *Chryseolinea*, *Terrimonas*, and *Ohtaekwangia*, were significantly greater in grassland soil columns treated with organic fertilizer than in those treated with inorganic fertilizer. The introduction of cover crops and composts as soil amendments could increase soil macronutrients, organic matter, and soil moisture, in turn causing marked shifts in the bacterial community (Devarajan et al. 2021). Furthermore, heterogeneous distribution of species inside the bacterial community and a higher fungal diversity have been reported under organic farming processes (Cuartero et al. 2021). In addition to enhancing the beneficial soil microorganisms, reducing the harmful pathogen population in the soil is another significant impact of the organic fertility amendments that improve soil health (Anyango et al. 2020). For example, composts can help suppress crop pests and pathogens by altering soil characteristics and microbial diversity (De Corato 2020). The greatest diversity of soil microbiota contributes to a higher abundance and antagonists, resource competitors, and predators of pathogens in soil, the rhizosphere, plants, and animals (Bongiorno et al. 2019). Soil with rich microbial diversity contains plant growth-promoting microorganisms in the rhizosphere and plant endosphere, leading to significantly induced systemic resistance throughout the plants. Root exudates act as a signal to initiate symbiotic association of microbes as well as attack harmful pathogens. Therefore, the pathogens may not be able to ascertain the roots, and the damage to the plants by the pathogen is turned down (Kharti and Sharma 2021). The production of antifungal agents, including siderophores and volatile metabolites, secreted by the soil microbial community present under organic farming management systems has been reported to manifest a suppressive role in the progression of plant diseases (Kharti and Sharma 2021).

Termites, together with ants and earthworms, are considered a major part of the soil macrofauna who play an important role in improving soil health. As Anyango et al. (2020) described, termite populations, diversity, and activities were higher under the organic farming system than the other farming systems due to the use of a large number of organic inputs.

14.4 Organic Farming Toward One Health

> Healthy soils generate healthy crops which lead to healthy livestock and humans.
>
> — *Sir Albert Howard*

Following the discussion over the effects of organic farming on soil health, it is worth appraising organic farming referring to the concept of One Health. The concept of One Health simply depends on a connection between human, animal, and environmental health with respect to zoonotic pathogens, antibiotic resistance, and pathogen vectors (Alsanius et al. 2019; Bruggen et al. 2019). Recently, the socioeconomic, cultural, and ecological aspects were also included in One Health concept (Queenan et al. 2016). It encourages the synergies, collaborations, and cross-fertilization of all the professional sectors and actors generally whose activities may impact health. According to the One Health perspectives, reducing hazards, making the harvested products sterile, and lowering the contamination of the crop or production are some of the fundamental critical points. In short, the concept of One Health is useful for achieving goals including controlling and combating diseases, ensuring food security, safeguarding and enhancing environmental quality, and upholding humane values in society (Garcia et al. 2020). Failure to do so may pose a public health issue.

There are several motives behind the consumers' inclination toward organic farming, as it promotes the values of health-promoting properties of organic produces, concerns about pesticide residuals, genetically modifies organisms, and food additives (Alsanius et al. 2019). Moreover, in his exploration of the factors driving the process of purchasing organic produces, Hjelmar (2011) states several complex psychological motives related to egoism and altruism. Therefore, the clear communication of technical aspects of organic farming and its effects on human health under the theme of One Health concept become a matter of paramount importance in the case of substantiating popular claims resounded among the public. This section is dedicated to serve this purpose in a bid to highlight the salient points referring to environmental and food safety.

The use of waste materials derived from animal biomasses in organic farming poses a potential risk of zoonoses especially for fruits and vegetables that are consumed raw or with minimal processing. In general, these products are not subjected to any unit operation of pathogen elimination before they come to the shelf. Thus, organically produced fruits and vegetables deem critical points in the transmission of biological hazards (especially fecal pathogens) from animal to human and then human to human (Alsanius et al. 2019). The reported outbreak caused by the shigatoxigenic *E. coli* strain O104:H4 that originated from organically produced sprouts in Germany and France in 2011 exemplifies this risk. Further, there are several other common biological hazards in relation to the foodborne diseases transmitted mainly through the fecal-oral route: *Salmonella* spp., *Yersinia enterocolitica, Listeria monocytogenes, Shigella* spp., *Bacillus cereus, Cyclospora cayetanensis,* and *Cryptosporidium parvum.*

While organic farming and healthy nutrition have become increasingly popular in recent years, the application of organic fertilizer poses a risk to human health due to the toxic substances it may contain. For example, unsystematic waste management practices allow for significant contamination of compost with plastic debris, which is one of the primary sources of microplastics in agricultural soil (Braun et al. 2021; Gui et al. 2021; Vithanage et al. 2021). It has been reported that an excessive amount of microplastics in compost, manure, and biosolids originate from domestic and municipal wastes. Braun et al. (2021) reported that according to the common recommendations in composting practice, which range from 7 to 35 t compost/ha, the compost application to agricultural fields is accompanied by plastic loads of 84,000–1,610,000 plastic items/ha/a, respectively, amounting to 0.34–47.53 kg plastic/h/a. Toxic metals such as cadmium (Cd), lead (Pb), arsenic (As), and chromium (Cr) that have been included in the production process of the plastics can end up in the compost and leach from the microplastics into the surrounding soil during the disintegration process of plastics in compost (Duan et al. 2021). Further, microplastics can simultaneously adsorb toxic trace metals onto their surface, providing a medium for surface metal complexation (Bradney et al. 2019; Zou et al. 2020). Therefore, microplastics can function as a vector by providing a surface for heavy metals to bind and release in the soil (Wang et al. 2020), and the released heavy metals would be bioavailable and could potentially be absorbed by plants, posing food safety risks. Ugulu et al. (2021) investigated the accumulation of trace metals in pepper (*Capsicum annuum* L.) grown with organic fertilizers and reported on the potential health risk associated with Cd, Co, and Pd accumulation in pepper. Wajid et al. (2020) also discovered the presence of potentially toxic elements in maize when organic fertilizers such as press mud, poultry waste, and farmyard manure were used. Further, long-term application of livestock manure compost may cause severe heavy metal pollution, endangering crop quality and human health (Awasthi et al. 2021), as it contains dissolved organic matter, the most active ingredient in compost, which directly determines the speciation and environmental behavior of heavy metals by complexation, ion exchange, and reduction and alters the bioavailability and fate of heavy metals in soil. For example, Laurent et al. (2020) discovered that the increase in dissolved organic matter concentration was the primary cause of the increase in total Cu content as opposed to total Zn content in the soil following long-term application of organic manure compost. Cui et al. (2020) also demonstrated that in dissolved organic matter derived from various composts, including chicken manure, dairy cattle manure, and kitchen waste, only the ligands of the humic-like component have Hg^{2+} binding capacity.

Moreover, compost, biosolids, and manure applications in organic farming systems are identified as the prime sources of addition of emerging contaminants such as pharmaceutical and personal care products (PPCPs) into the soil, which may result in the uptake of PPCPs into crops (Madikizela et al. 2018; Christou et al. 2019; Keerthanan et al. 2021). The dietary intake of PPCPs contaminated with vegetables and fruits can cause a potentially harmful impact on human health. For example, the daily consumption of PPCPs, particularly vegetables contaminated with antibiotics, can lead to the development of antibiotic-resistant pathogens in the human body, thereby increasing the risk of complex health complications. As investigated by Zhao et al. (2019) the long-term application of manure under realistic farming conditions introduced antibiotics to peanut plants. As a result, verifying the quality and origin of organic fertilizer is critical before applying it to the field.

In contrast to the health risks mentioned earlier, Zou et al. (2020) reported the positive side of the presence of microplastics in the soil, as they play an important role as an adsorbent that immobilizes toxic metals and reduces their bioavailability through various mechanisms including precipitation, adsorption process, and redox reactions. Further, it has been observed that microplastics enhance microbial activity and ensure the production of essential soil enzymes, thereby increasing nutrient availability (Vithanage et al. 2021).

As organic farming and postharvest handling of its produces do not foster reactive disinfections or chemical eradications of pathogens, the fruits and vegetables of organic origin bear an inherent associated risk of contamination with pathogens and dirt. The possible routes of such contaminations can be water resources of crops (surface waters, treated or non-treated wastewaters, stored waters), organic manures, zoonotic pest infestations, farm animals involved in on-site or off-site operations, poor hygiene and sanitation of handlers and facilities, etc. (Alsanius et al. 2019). These contaminations become harder-to-fix when it comes to more delicate and perishable commodities like berries, tomatoes, broccoli, and peaches. In the resolution of potential problems, the employment of microbiocidal and/or microbiostatic hurdle technologies can be recommended by way of proactive measures in organic farming of fruits and vegetables. A foundational guideline for such an initiative can be drawn from what has been developed and published for other agricultural produces (dairy products) (Codex Alimentarius Commission 2004). The exclusion of animal-derived manure (vegan organic produces) also remains as an option to evade the risk of zoonotic contamination (Vegan Organic Network 2007). However, its case-based technical feasibility and economic viability should be well analyzed as it is a challenging task to be accomplished in real practice.

In contrast to the above-discussed cautious perspective, van Bruggen et al. (2019) point out the pathogen-suppressive effect of organic farming on biological communities. The microbial diversity and species richness preserved in organically managed soils are believed to exert pathogen suppression through bacterial antagonism, competition for resources, and bacterial predation in all the spheres of soil, plants, and animals (Gómez Expósito et al. 2017). Further, the diverse microbiome maintained in plants inoculates animals through feed, and it may enhance the vigor of their immunity through the synergy of microbial diversity and the host's immune response (Leung and Weitz 2017). On the basis of this argument of microbial connectedness of soil, plants, and animals, the agroecosystems rich in diverse microbial communities have a lesser risk of contamination and dissemination of enteric pathogens (Franz and van Bruggen 2008). In support of this claim, Motta et al. (2018) have demonstrated the negative effect of glyphosate on both soil and gut microflora referring to the plant and animal pathogenicity. The susceptibility to pathogens, especially of animals, is assumed to be due to glyphosate's dual effects of direct toxicity and perturbation of friendly gut microflora (Kelly et al. 2010; van Bruggen et al. 2018).

Considering all these, the current development of research on organic farming divulges reciprocal and complementary benefits between soil, plant, and animal domains in the overall ecosystem through microbial interconnectedness. Thus, the promotion of organic farming is recommended to move forward with rather integrated and harmonized well-being of the overall ecosystem advancing beyond the human-health centric point of view. Accordingly, the One Health concept provides a solid platform for organic farming to progress along a scientifically sound, technically feasible, and economically viable avenue.

14.5 Challenges, Trends, and Prospects

Organic farming is an excellent sustainable agricultural system. A sustainable agriculture system ensures that nutritious food is accessible for everyone, and the natural resources are managed in a way that maintains the ecosystem functions to support current and future human needs. As the global population grows, we will need to produce more food that maintains or enhances its nutrient content on essentially the same land area, as arable lands are always limited. One of the main challenges in organic farming is to increase production since the crop yield gained from organic farming is lower than conventional farming. Modifying the current practices in organic agriculture systems can improve productivity, and the productivity will need to continue to increase in the future to secure sufficient food and other agricultural products supply. Further, as water scarcity worsens and agriculture seeks to cut greenhouse gas emissions and water, energy-efficient production technologies will become increasingly crucial. Therefore, organic farming systems should fulfill future requirements as well.

There are potential areas that should investigate in organic farming and its interaction with soil health. Only a few research outcomes are available on stacked practices. For example, researchers should focus on investigating and assessing soil health benefits that organic fields can gain from stacking multiple management practices within organic farming systems. Furthermore, there is a research gap on the effect of crop rotation length and diversity, organic amendment types and rates, cover crop species, quantity, and quality on soil health matrices in soil organic farming. Studies on the environmental impact, especially water and air quality effects of organic farming and weed management options, particularly under climate change by nonchemical and biological methods are other critical topics to be focused on in future research. In addition, the accumulation of toxic elements including heavy metals, and antibiotics with the application of organic fertilizers containing contaminants such as microplastics, pharmaceutical, and personal care products, and evolving of foodborne pathogens are a potential risk for plant and human health. Therefore, more research is needed to forecast these events, find the technical solutions to minimize their impacts on human health, and continue these practices as important options to secure soil health.

One Health together with organic agriculture can be used to build a revolutionary strategy to enhance the total health and well-being of humans, animals, and the environment by boosting sustainable agricultural methods. Therefore, a multidisciplinary team comprised of experts from academic, government, public, and private institutions would be more effective in achieving meaningful changes in public awareness, legislation, and practices that promote the implementation of sustainable agricultural practices, which are the expected outcomes from the One Health concept. As a result, we need agronomists, biologists, chemists, communications specialists, medical doctors, public health specialists, toxicologists, sociologists, and soil scientists to collaborate on common soil and human health goals. In some cases, establishing these collaborations will necessitate a paradigm shift in our current approach to human health issues.

Epidemiological data and laboratory information should be shared to successfully detect, respond, and prevent outbreaks of zoonoses and food safety problems. Thereby, the government officials, researchers, and workers across the local, national, regional, and global level sectors can implement joint responses to health threats. Promoting the multisectoral responses to food safety hazards, risks from zoonoses, and other public health threats at the human–animal–ecosystem interface and providing guidance on reducing these risks are essential for maintaining the One Health in organic farming systems. Therefore, a multidisciplinary research approach is required to face the upcoming challenges in organic farming to direct toward the human, animal, and plant health.

References

Al-Busaidi, W., Khan, M., Janke, R., and Al-Sheriqi, M. (2020). Efficacy of soil amendments in organic farming systems. *Agrociencia* 54 (1): 1–31.

Alsanius, B.W., von Essen, E., Hartmann, R. et al. (2019). The "one health" – concept and organic production of vegetables and fruits. *Acta Hortic.* 1242: 1–14.

Amarjit, S. (2015). The global market for organic food and drink. In: *World of Organic Agriculture-Statistics and Emerging Trends 2021* (ed. H. Willer, J. Trávníček, C. Meier and B. Schlatter), 140–157. Germany: Helga.

Anonymous (2005). *The IFOAM Norms for Organic Production and Processing (Version 2005S)*, 132.

Bonn: International Federation of Organic Agriculture Movements (IFOAM).

Anyango, J.J., Bautze, D., Fiaboe, K.K.M. et al. (2020). The impact of conventional and organic farming on soil biodiversity conservation: a case study on termites in the long-term farming systems comparison trials in Kenya. *BMC Ecol.* 20: 13. https://doi.org/10.1186/s12898-020-00282-x.

Awasthi, S.K., Duan, Y., Liu, T. et al. (2021). Sequential presence of heavy metal resistant fungal communities influenced by biochar amendment in the poultry manure composting process. *J. Clean. Prod.* 291: 125947.

Bongiorno, G., Postma, J., Bünemann, E.K. et al. (2019). Soil suppressiveness to *Pythium ultimum* in ten European long-term field experiments and its relation with soil parameters. *Soil Biol. Biochem.* 133: 174–187. https://doi.org/10.1016/j.soilbio.2019.03.012.

Bradney, L., Wijesekara, H., Palansooriya, K.N. et al. (2019). Particulate plastics as a vector for toxic trace-element uptake by aquatic and terrestrial organisms and human health risk. *Environ. Int.* 131: 104937.

Braun, M., Mail, M., Heyse, R., and Amelung, W. (2021). Plastic in compost: prevalence and potential input into agricultural and horticultural soils. *Sci. Total Environ.* 15 (760): 143335. https://doi.org/10.1016/j.scitotenv.2020.143335.

van Bruggen, A.H.C., He, M.M., Shin, K. et al. (2018). Environmental and health effects of glyphosate. *Sci. Total Environ.* 616–617: 255–268.

Bruggen, A.H.C., Goss, E.M., Havelaar, A. et al. (2019). One health – cycling of diverse microbial communities as a connecting force for soil, plant, animal, human and ecosystem health. *Sci. Total Environ.* 664: 927–937. https://doi.org/10.1016/j.scitotenv.2019.02.091.

Christou, A., Kyriacou, M.C., Georgiadou, E.C. et al. (2019). Uptake and bioaccumulation of three widely prescribed pharmaceutically active compounds in tomato fruits and mediated effects on fruit quality attributes. *Sci. Total Environ.* 647: 1169–1178. https://doi.org/10.1016/j.scitotenv.2018.08.053.

Codex Alimentarius Commission, 2004. Code of hygienic practice for milk and milk products. CAC/RCP 57-2004. Food and Agriculture Organization, Rome

Crystal-Ornelas, R., Thapa, R., and Tully, K.L. (2021). Soil organic carbon is affected by organic amendments, conservation tillage, and cover cropping in organic farming systems: a meta-analysis. *Agric. Ecosyst. Environ.* 312: 107356.

Cuartero, J., Özbolat, O., Sánchez-Navarro, V. et al. (2021). Changes in bacterial and fungal soil communities in long-term organic cropping systems. *Agriculture* 11: 445. https://doi.org/10.3390/agriculture11050445.

Cui, H.Y., Zhang, S.B., Zhao, M.Y. et al. (2020). Parallel faction analysis combined with two-dimensional correlation spectroscopy reveal the characteristics of mercury-composting-derived dissolved organic matter interactions. *J. Hazard. Mater.* 384: 121395. https://doi.org/10.1016/j.jhazmat.2019.121395.

De Corato, U. (2020). Disease-suppressive compost enhances natural soil suppressiveness against soil-borne plant pathogens: a critical review. *Rhizosphere* 13: 100192.

Devarajan, N., McGarvey, J.A., Scow, K. et al. (2021). Cascading effects of composts and cover crops on soil chemistry, bacterial communities and the survival of foodborne pathogens. *J. Appl. Microbiol.* 131: 1564–1577. https://doi.org/10.1111/jam.15054.

Duan, J., Bolan, N., Li, Y. et al. (2021). Weathering of microplastics and interaction with other coexisting constituents in terrestrial and aquatic environments. *Water Res.* 196: 117011.

FAO, ITPS, GSBI, CBD & EC (2020). State of Knowledge of Soil Biodiversity – Status, Challenges and Potentialities, Report 2020. FAO: Rome. https://doi.org/10.4060/cb1928en.

FiBL. (2021). *The World of Organic Agriculture Statistics and Emerging Trends 2021*. Germany: Plump Druck and Median CmbH.

Franz, E. and van Bruggen, A.H.C. (2008). Ecology of *E. coli* O157:H7 and *Salmonella enterica* in the primary vegetable production chain. *Crit. Rev. Microbiol.* 34: 143–161.

Garcia, S.N., Osbium, B.I., and Jay-Russell, T. (2020). One health for food safety, food security, and sustainable food production. *Front. Sustain. Food Syst.* 4 (1): https://doi.org/10.3389/fsufs.2020.00001.

Gómez Expósito, R., de Bruijn, I., Postma, J., and Raaijmakers, J.M. (2017). Current insights into the role of rhizosphere bacteria in disease suppressive soils. *Front. Microbiol.* 8: 2529. https://doi.org/10.3389/fmicb.2017.02529.

Gondwe, R.L., Kinoshita, R., Suminoe, T. et al. (2020). Available soil nutrients and NPK application impacts on yield, quality, and nutrient composition of potatoes growing during the main season in Japan. *Am. J. Potato Res.* 97: 234–245.

Govindasamy, P., Liu, R., Provin, T. et al. (2021). Soil carbon improvement under long-term (36 years) no-till sorghum production in a sub-tropical environment. *Soil Use Manag.* 37: 37–48. https://doi.org/10.1111/sum.12636.

Gui, J., Sun, Y., Wang, J. et al. (2021). Microplastics in composting of rural domestic waste: abundance, characteristics, and release from the surface of macroplastics. *Environ. Pollut.* 274: 116553. https://doi.org/10.1016/j.envpol.2021.116553.

Guo, M. (2020). The 3R principles for applying biochar to improve soil health. *Soil Syst.* 4: 9. https://doi.org/10.3390/soilsystems4010009.

Hati, K.M., Biswas, A.K., Somasundaram, J. et al. (2020). Soil organic carbon dynamics and carbon sequestration under conservation tillage in tropical vertisols. In: *Carbon Management in Tropical and Sub-Tropical Terrestrial Systems* (ed. P.K. Ghosh, S.K. Mahanta, D. Mandal, et al.), 201–212. Singapore City: Springer.

Hjelmar, U. (2011). Consumers' purchase of organic food products. A matter of convenience and reflexive practices. *Appetite* 56 (2): 336–344.

Ikoyi, I., Egeter, B., Chaves, C. et al. (2020). Responses of soil microbiota and nematodes to application of organic and inorganic fertilizers in grassland columns. *Biol. Fertil. Soils* 56: 647–662.

Jernigan, A.B., Wickings, K., Mohler, C.L. et al. (2020). Legacy effects of contrasting organic grain cropping systems on soil health indicators, soil invertebrates, weeds, and crop yield. *Agric. Syst.* 177: 102719. https://doi.org/10.1016/j.agsy.2019.102719.

Jha, P., Hati, K.M., Dalal, R.C. et al. (2020). Soil carbon and nitrogen dynamics in a vertisol following 50 years of no-tillage, crop stubble retention and nitrogen fertilization. *Geoderma* 358: 113996.

Kan, Z.R., Ma, S.T., Liu, Q.Y. et al. (2020). Carbon sequestration and mineralization in soil aggregates under long-term conservation tillage in the North China Plain. *Catena* 188: 104428. https://doi.org/10.1016/j.catena.2019.104428.

Keerthanan, S., Jayasinghe, C., Biswas, J.K., and Vithanage, M. (2021). Pharmaceutical and personal care products (PPCPs) in the environment: plant uptake, translocation, bioaccumulation, and human health risks. *Crit. Rev. Environ. Sci. Technol.* 51: 1221–1258. https://doi.org/10.1080/10643389.2020.1753634.

Kelly, D.W., Poulin, R., Tompkins, D.M., and Townsend, C.R. (2010). Synergistic effects of glyphosate formulation and parasite infection on fish malformations and survival. *J. Appl. Ecol.* 47: 498–504.

Kharti, S. and Sharma, S. (2021). How does organic farming shape the soil and plant associated microbiota? *Symbiosis* 84: 391–398. https://doi.org/10.1007/s13199-021-00767-3.

Kirchner, C., Andrighetto, J.K., and Castro, M.E. (2021). *Organic agriculture regulations worldwide: Current situation in In World of Organic Agriculture-Statistics and Emerging Trends 2021* (ed. H. Willer, J. Trávníček, C. Meier and B. Schlatter), 152–157. Germany.

Kranz, C.N., McLaughlin, R.A., Johnson, A. et al. (2020). The effects of compost incorporation on soil physical properties in urban soils: a concise review. *J. Environ. Manag.* 261: 110209.

Laurent, C., Bravin, M.N., Crouzet, O. et al. (2020). Increased soil pH and dissolved organic matter after a decade of organic fertilizer application mitigates copper and zinc availability despite contamination. *Sci. Total Environ.* 709: 135927. https://doi.org/10.1016/j.scitotenv.2019.135927.

Lehmann, J., Bossio, D.A., Kögel-Knabner, I., and Rillig, M.C. (2020). The concept and future prospects of soil health. *Nat. Rev. Earth Environ.* 1: 544–553. https://doi.org/10.1038/s43017-020-0080-8.

Leung, C.Y. and Weitz, J.S. (2017). Modeling the synergistic elimination of bacteria by phage and the innate immune system. *J. Theor. Biol.* 429: 241–252.

Liu, J., Shu, A., Song, W. et al. (2021). Long-term organic fertilizer substitution increases rice yield by improving soil properties and regulating soil bacteria. *Geoderma* 404: 115287. https://doi.org/10.1016/j.geoderma.2021.115287.

Madikizela, L.M., Ncube, S., and Chimuka, L. (2018). Uptake of pharmaceuticals by plants grown under hydroponic conditions and natural occurring plant species: a review. *Sci. Total Environ.* 636: 477–486. https://doi.org/10.1016/j.scitotenv.2018.04.297.

Moe, K., Moh, S.M., Htwe, A.Z. et al. (2019). Effects of integrated organic and inorganic fertilizers on yield and growth parameters of rice varieties. *Rice Sci.* 26 (5): 309–318.

Motta, E.V.S., Raymann, K., and Moran, N.A. (2018). Glyphosate perturbs the gut microbiota of honeybees. *Proc. Natl. Acad. Sci.* 2018: https://doi.org/10.1073/pnas.1803880115.

Norris, C.E., Bean, G.C., Cappellazzi, S.B. et al. (2020). Introducing the North American project to evaluate soil health. *Agron. J.* 112: 3195–3215.

Nouri, A., Lee, J., Yin, X. et al. (2019). Thirty four years of no-tillage and cover crops improve soil quality and increase cotton yield in Alfisols, Southeastern USA. *Geoderma* 337: 998–1008. https://doi.org/10.1016/j.geode rma.2018.10.016.

Qaswar, M., Jing, H., Ahmed, W. et al. (2020). Yield sustainability, soil organic carbon sequestration and nutrients balance under long-term combined application of manure and inorganic fertilizers in acidic paddy soil. *Soil Tillage Res.* 198: 1–6.

Queenan, K., Häsler, B., and Rushton, J. (2016). A one health approach to antimicrobial resistance surveillance: is there a business case for it? *Int. J. Antimicrob. Agents* 48 (4): 422–427. https://doi.org/10.1016/j.ijantimicag.2016.06.014.

Rillig, M.C., Lehmann, A., de Souza Machado, A.A., and Yang, G. (2019). Microplastic effects on plants. *New Phytol.* 223: 1066–1070.

Rillig, M.C., Leifheit, E., and Lehmann, J. (2021). Microplastic effects on carbon cycling processes in soils. *PLoS Biol.* 19: e3001130.

Sanathara, M. and Vibhute, B. (2020). *A Review of Organic Farming for Soil Conservation Towards Sustainable & Natural Farming in India*. Annual Technical Volume of Agricultural Engineering Division Board.

Sheoran, H.S., Kakar, R., Kumar, N., and Seema (2019). Impact of organic and conventional farming practices on soil quality: a global review. *Appl. Ecol. Environ. Res.* 17: 951–968.

Singh, S., Nouri, A., Singh, S. et al. (2020). Soil organic carbon and aggregation in response to thirty-nine years of tillage management in the southeastern US. *Soil Tillage Res.* 197: 104523. https://doi.org/10.1016/j.still.2019.104523.

Smith, J.L. and Collins, H.P. (2007). Management of organisms and their processes in soils. In: *Soil Microbiology, Ecology, and Biochemistry* (ed. E.A. Paul), 471–502. Academic Press.

Smith, J.L., Collins, H.P., Crump, A.R., and Bailey, V.L. (2014). Management of soil biota and their properties. In: *Soil Microbiology, Ecology, and Biochemistry* (ed. E.A. Paul), 539–565. Academic Press.

Soil Health Institute (2018). National Soil Health measurements to accelerate agricultural transformation. https://soilhealthinstituteorg/national-soil-healthmeasurements-accelerate-agricultural-transformation/ (accessed 20 January 2022).

de Souza Machado, A.A., Lau, C.W., Kloas, W. et al. (2019). Microplastics can change soil properties and affect plant performance. *Environ. Sci. Technol.* 53: 6044–6052.

Szostek M, Szpunar-Krok E, Pawlak R, Stanek-Tarkowska J, Ilek A. Effect of different tillage systems on soil organic carbon and enzymatic activity. *Agronomy* 2022; 12(1):208. https://doi.org/https://doi.org/10.3390/agronomy12010208

Timsina, J. (2018). Can organic sources of nutrients increase crop yields to meet global food demand? *Agronomy* 8 (10): 214.

Tully, K.L. and McAskill, C. (2020). Promoting soil health in organically managed systems: a review. *Org. Agric.* 1–20: https://doi.org/10.1007/s13165-019-00275-1.

Ugulu, I., Akhter, P., Iqbal Khan, Z. et al. (2021). Trace metal accumulation in pepper (*Capsicum annuum* L.) grown using organic fertilizers and health risk assessment from consumption. *Food Res. Int.* 140: 109992. https://doi.org/10.1016/j.foodres.2020.109992.

USDA-NRCS (2019). *Soil Health.* Washington, DC: Natural Resources Conservation Service, U.S. Department of Agriculture. https://www.nrcs.usda.gov/wps/portal/nrcs/main/soils/health (accessed 26 January 2022).

USDA-NRCS (2021). *Soil Health Management.* Washington, DC: Natural Resources Conservation Service, U.S. Department of Agriculture. https://www.nrcs.usda.gov/wps/portal/nrcs/main/soils/health/mgnt (accessed 17 August 2021).

Vegan Organic Network (2007). The stockfree organic standards (UK). www.veganorganic.net (accessed 20 January 2022).

Vithanage, M., Ramanayaka, S., Hasinthara, S., and Navaratne, A. (2021). Compost as a carrier for microplastics and plastic-bound toxic metals into agroecosystems. *Curr. Opin. Environ. Sci. Health* 24: 100297. https://doi.org/10.1016/j.coesh.2021.100297.

Wajid, K., Ahmad, K., Khan, Z.I. et al. (2020). Effect of organic manure and mineral fertilizers on bioaccumulation and translocation of trace metals in maize. *Bull. Environ. Contam. Toxicol.* 104: 649–657. https://doi.org/10.1007/s00128-020-02841-w.

Wang, C., Zhao, J., and Xing, B. (2020). Environmental source, fate, and toxicity of microplastics. *J. Hazard. Mater.* 124357.

Williams, H., Colombi, T., and Keller, T. (2020). The influence of soil management on soil health: an on-farm study in southern Sweden. *Geoderma* 360: 114010. https://doi.org/10.1016/j.geoderma.2019.114010.

Xu, J., Han, H., Ning, T. et al. (2019). Long-term effects of tillage and straw management on soil organic carbon, crop yield, and yield stability in a wheat-maize system. *Field Crop Res.* 233: 33–40. https://doi.org/10.1016/j.fcr.2018.12.016.

Yu, H., Hou, J., Dang, Q. et al. (2020). Decrease in bioavailability of soil heavy metals caused by the presence of microplastics varies across aggregate levels. *J. Hazard. Mater.* 395: 122690.

Zhao, F., Yang, L., Chen, L. et al. (2019). Bioaccumulation of antibiotics in crops under long-term manure application: occurrence, biomass response and human exposure. *Chemosphere* 219: 882–895. https://doi.org/10.1016/j.chemosphere.2018.12.076.

Zou, J., Liu, X., Zhang, D., and Yuan, X. (2020). Adsorption of three bivalent metals by four chemical distinct microplastics. *Chemosphere* 248: 126064.

15

Chronic Kidney Disease with Uncertain Etiology in Sri Lanka

Selected Case Studies

Saranga Diyabalanage[1,2] and Rohana Chandrajith[3]

[1] *Instrument Centre, Faculty of Applied Sciences, University of Sri Jayewardenepura, Nugegoda, Sri Lanka*
[2] *Ecosphere Resilience Research Center, Faculty of Applied Sciences, University of Sri Jayewardenepura, Nugegoda, Sri Lanka*
[3] *Department of Geology, Faculty of Science, University of Peradeniya, Peradeniya, Sri Lanka*

15.1 Introduction

Chronic Kidney Disease (CKD) is a condition characterized by the gradual decline of kidney function over time and associated with reduced glomerular filtration rate, increased albumin excretion, or both. It is a worldwide public health issue, with adverse outcomes leading to end-stage kidney failure, cardiovascular disease, and even death. It is estimated that around 8–16% of the world population suffers from CKD (Jha et al. 2013). Traditionally, factors that lead to impairment of kidney function are diabetes mellitus, hypertension, snake bite with envenomation, chronic glomerulonephritis, or obstructive nephropathy. In the early 1990s, an increasing number of kidney patients was reported among the agricultural communities of Sri Lanka and Central America. Initially, it was found among paddy farmers in the dry zone of Sri Lanka and sugarcane workers in Central America (Weaver et al. 2015). In both localities, the agricultural community, which has a common socioeconomic status and occupational determinants, are the principal victim of the disease. The disease is relatively rapid progressing and is not related to the traditional known risk factor, thus named "Chronic Kidney Disease of Unknown Etiology" (CKDu). The pathogenesis has been identified as a nonspecific chronic interstitial nephritis and is progressive and irreversible (Anand et al. 2019). In the end stages, renal failure and death may occur unless regular dialysis or kidney transplant is performed (Vlahos et al. 2021). A similar epidemic has also been reported in some regions in India (Tatapudi et al. 2019), the Balkan Peninsula, and Egypt (Pearce et al. 2019). Although the clinical, pathological, and epidemiological expressions of the disease are comparable, the disease has been defined in several terms based on the location, such as Chronic Kidney Disease of uncertain etiology (CKDu) in Sri Lanka, Meso-American Nephropathy (MeN) in the Central American region, Salvadoran Agricultural Nephropathy in El-Salvador, and Uddanam Endemic Nephropathy in India (Jayasinghe and Zhu 2020; Vervaet et al. 2020) (Figure 15.1). One of the important aspects of CKDu is the asymptomatic nature in its early stages. Symptoms such as diabetes and hypertension are initially absent in CKDu patients; however, later with the disease progression, patients exhibit fatigue, nausea, poor appetite, and anemia (Elledge et al. 2014; Nyachoti et al. 2022). CKDu has become a significant burden on the public healthcare system in affected countries, as it is a medical mystery responsible for tens of thousands of annual death counts worldwide.

15.2 Prevalence of CKDu in Sri Lanka

The disease is first recorded in Sri Lanka during the early 1990s among the rural population of the North Central Province (Chandrajith et al. 2011b). The disease prevalence is common in dry zone regions including the North Central, North Western, Uva, and Eastern provinces of Sri Lanka, where the estimated prevalence rate is between 15.1 and 22.9% (Kafle et al. 2019; Vlahos et al. 2021) (Figure 15.2). Particularly in the North Central Province, it has been identified that 10% of the adult population is affected by CKD/CKDu of which nearly 27% are CKDu cases (Ranasinghe et al. 2019). A recent investigation on CKDu prevalence in the dry zone of Sri Lanka with 8049 households has revealed at least one CKDu patient in 1238 households (Kafle et al. 2019). However, the distribution of CKDu cases in those regions shows an unusual mosaic

One Health: Human, Animal, and Environment Triad, First Edition. Edited by Meththika Vithanage and Majeti Narasimha Vara Prasad.

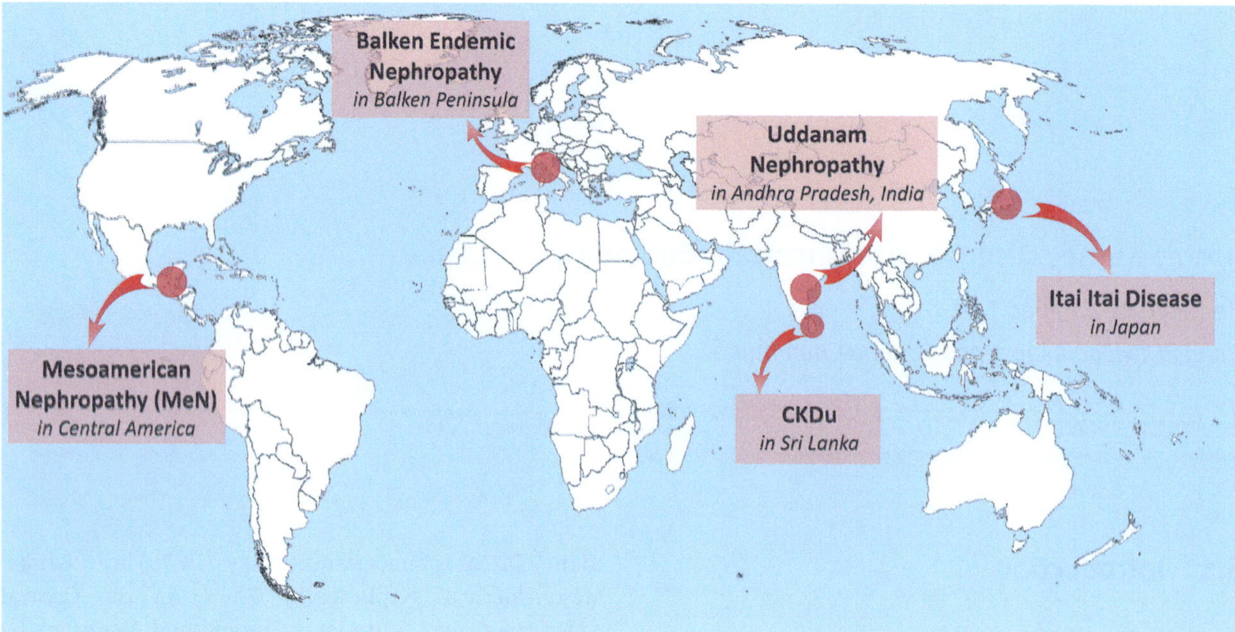

Figure 15.1 Regional kidney epidemics that have occurred throughout the world in the past.

distribution pattern, which depicts highly endemic regions with clusters of disease prevalence and non-endemic regions nearby (Balasooriya et al. 2020). Girandurukotte, Medawachchiya, Nikawewa, Wilgamuwa, Padaviya, Sripura, Dehiattakandiya, Mahiyanganaya, Medirigiriya, Welioya, Mahawa, and Horowpathana areas have been identified as CKDu hotspots (Chandrajith et al. 2011b; Balasooriya et al. 2020). The disease often contributes significantly to morbidity and mortality rates among dry zone farming communities due to its rapid progression and lack of dialysis and kidney transplant facilities (Abeyagunawardena and Shroff 2021). Since its emergence, approximately 180,000 patients have been identified, and nearly 50,000 deaths have been reported (Hettithanthri et al. 2021). As the disease progression reaches an epidemic level, it has been identified as a national health issue in the country, which accounts for approximately $19.7 million in expenditure per annum for the management of CKDu patients (Wimalawansa 2019). Although it has been reported for almost 30 years, no specific causes have yet been found to date to define CKDu; hence, the etiology remains unknown.

In Sri Lanka, farming communities with low socioeconomic backgrounds and those who are exposed to a high degree of occupational and environmental hazards are the victims of CKDu. Initially, only male farmers in the age group of 30–50 years were identified as the primary victims of the disease. Once diagnosed, the estimated survival rate is five years, while most deaths occur within three years (Rajapakse et al. 2016). However, currently, the disease has also been reported among the less exposed individuals, including nonagricultural workers, women, and children.

15.3 Etiology of CKDu

Histopathological investigations in CKDu patients have revealed tubular interstitial lesions, suggesting a potential involvement of a toxin in the causation of CKDu (Nanayakkara et al. 2014). Accordingly, over 30 hypotheses have been proposed for the etiology of CKDu in Sri Lanka, while most of which are linked with the agricultural lifestyle of the community. Previous case–control, cross-sectional, and cohort studies have suggested several hypotheses as the causes of CKDu such as excess fluoride in drinking water (Chandrajith et al. 2011b), the influence of agrochemicals (Wanigasuriya et al. 2007), contamination of toxic heavy metals such as As, Cd, and Pb in drinking water and food (Bandara et al. 2010; Jayasumana et al. 2014; Ananda Jayalal et al. 2019), high ionocity in groundwater (Dharma-Wardana 2018), the combined effect of fluoride and hardness in water (Chandrajith et al. 2011a; Dissanayake and Chandrajith 2019; Balasooriya et al. 2020; Liyanage et al. 2022), cyanobacteria toxins (Liyanage et al. 2016), and heat stress and associated dehydration (Jayasekara et al. 2013; Herath et al. 2018) (Figure 15.3). Other than that, sociological factors such as poverty and malnutrition (Abeywickrama et al. 2020) and genetic factors (Nanayakkara et al. 2014) are also proposed as possible influencing reasons for CKDu. Among those,

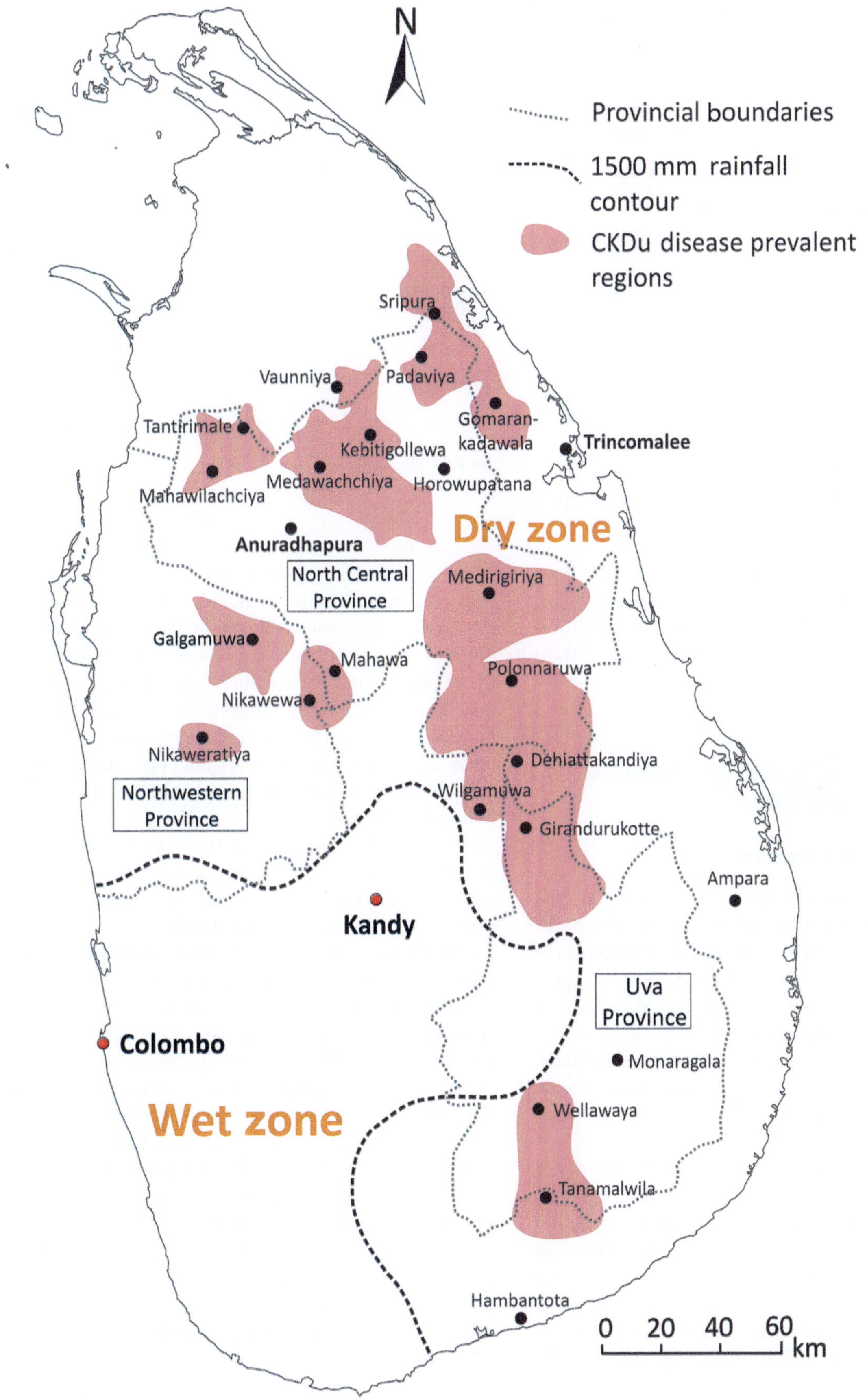

Figure 15.2 Identified CKDu hotspots in Sri Lanka.

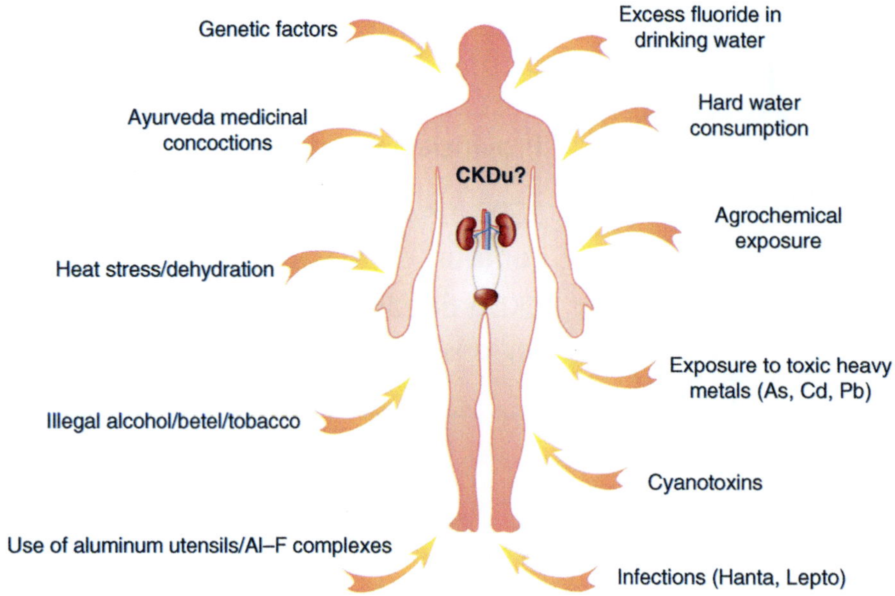

Figure 15.3 Hypothesized causes for CKDu occurrence in Sri Lanka.

hypotheses focused on geo-environmental factors have gained wider attention because of the peculiar geographical distribution and the absence of the disease in the wet zone regions of the island (Chandrajith et al. 2011b) (Figure 15.2).

15.4 Influence of Hydro-geochemical Quality of Drinking Water

15.4.1 Fluoride and Hardness

Majority of people living in CKDu-affected areas consume water obtained from domestic shallow or deep (tube) wells. Previous studies highlighted the possible significant contribution of groundwater to the etiology or disease progression (Chandrajith et al. 2011b; Wickramarathna et al. 2017). Chronic exposure to inorganic contaminants such as fluoride, toxic heavy metals (As, Cd, and Pb), water hardness, and cyanobacterial toxins through drinking water are the main suggested factors that could contribute to the onset of CKDu.

The major solute composition of the dry zone water is dominated by Na^+, K^+, Ca^{2+}, Mg^{2+}, HCO_3^-, Cl^-, and SO_4^{2-}. In most wells, anion abundances followed the sequence $HCO_3^- > Cl^- > SO_4^{2-} > NO_3^-$ (Chandrajith and Diyabalanage 2022). Groundwater found in CKDu-affected regions normally contains high fluoride concentrations and higher hardness with high ionicity (Chandrajith et al. 2011b; Balasooriya et al. 2020). Geologically, over 90% of the island of Sri Lanka is underlain by Precambrian high-grade metamorphic rocks, and groundwater is mainly extracted from weathered overburden or structural discontinuities in crystalline hard rocks (Dissanayake and Chandrajith 2018). Higher fluoride levels in groundwater may be attributed to the dissolution of fluoride-bearing minerals in high-grade metamorphic rocks such as apatite, micas, and amphibolite (Chandrajith et al. 2020). In many cases, dry zone groundwater in Sri Lanka contained higher fluoride levels than the WHO drinking water guideline value of 1.5 mg/l (WHO 2011). However, this limit is not always applicable and may depend on the local environmental conditions; thus, the limit of 0.8 mg/l has been defined for tropical climatic regions (WHO 2011).

Fluoride is a known nephrotoxic element (Ananda Jayalal et al. 2019), and many previous studies showed higher fluoride in CKDu-affected regions (Table 15.1). Due to its nephrotoxic nature, damage can happen to the kidneys at the molecular level during the excretion process. Compared to plasma fluoride levels, 50 times higher fluoride levels can be expected in excreted urine, making kidney cells more vulnerable to damage (Jiménez-Córdova et al. 2018). Further, higher fluoride levels in serum and urine have also been reported in biopsy-proven CKDu patients compared to the control population living in the same endemic area (Fernando et al. 2020). Interestingly, both groundwater fluoride distribution and prevalence of CKDu show a heterogeneous distribution, and both hotspots are mostly overlapping each other (Figures 15.2 and 15.4).

Table 15.1 Concentrations of major constituents of groundwater from identified CKDu hotspot regions (HD; total hardness)

Identified CKDu hotspot region	Parameters							References
	HD (mg/L)	F (mg/L)	Na (mg/L)	Ca (mg/L)	Mg (mg/L)	As (μg/L)	Cd (μg/L)	
Girandurukotte ($n = 180$)								
Min	5.64	0.01	0.08	2.07	0.05	<0.02	<0.01	(Balasooriya et al. 2020; Chandrajith and Diyabalanage 2022; Wickramarathna et al. 2017)
Max	516	5.20	157	394	76.2	2.54	43.0	
Mean	135	0.74	24.7	31.8	11.2	0.24	0.94	
Median	107	0.54	18.5	19.5	7.17	0.16	0.02	
Wilgamuwa ($n = 344$)								
Min	8.00	0.01	1.31	3.70	0.26	0.02	<0.01	(Chandrajith and Diyabalanage 2022; Wickramarathna et al. 2017)
Max	830	4.40	495	1451	472	4.80	11.4	
Mean	158	0.71	35.3	94.6	19.6	0.47	0.20	
Median	124	0.60	24.4	31.6	13.5	0.28	0.03	
Nikawewa ($n = 11$)								
Min	236	0.16	14.6	13.8	3.06	0.05	<0.01	(Wickramarathna et al. 2017)
Max	628	3.44	157	152	74.3	0.30	0.44	
Mean	397	1.03	64.5	71.1	35.1	0.15	0.11	
Median	426	0.79	43.9	36.4	35.3	0.15	0.08	
Moneragala ($n = 30$)								
Min	16.6	0.28	4.6	12.3	4.23	0.06	<0.01	(Liyanage et al. 2021)
Max	162	6.80	204	131	44.2	0.62	0.12	
Mean	82.4	2.02	35.0	57.7	24.8	0.24	0.03	
Median	81.8	1.70	22.7	53.1	27.1	0.17	0.03	
Medawachchiya/Medirigiriya ($n = 97$)								
Min	NA	0.08	0.75	3.76	0.15	<1.0	<0.14	(Levine et al. 2016)
Max	NA	2.05	156	161	58.4	1.55	0.17	
Mean	NA	0.60	39.8	55.4	20.5	NA	NA	
Median	NA	NA	NA	NA	NA	NA	NA	
Medawachchiya ($n = 30$)								
Min	NA	0.07	10.9	8.3	5.6	0.005	NA	(McDonough et al. 2020)
Max	NA	3.70	234	140	95.2	0.005	NA	
Mean	NA	1.24	82.3	74.1	39.7	0.005	NA	
Median	NA	1.11	33.9	71.7	33.9	0.005	NA	
Padaviya ($n = 34$)								
Min	70	0.02	2.09	2.35	2.08	NA	NA	(Chandrajith et al. 2011)
Max	816	1.33	188	113	41.6	NA	NA	
Mean	443	0.62	58.3	35.0	20.1	NA	NA	
Median	NA	NA	NA	NA	NA	NA	NA	
Padaviya ($n = 6$)								
Min	NA	0.33	29.9	28.0	20.4	<1	NA	(Nikagolla et al. 2020)
Max	NA	1.01	94.4	75.0	54.5	<1	NA	
Mean	NA	0.67	52.3	49.3	31.0	<1	NA	

(Continued)

Table 15.1 (Continued)

Identified CKDu hotspot region	Parameters							References
	HD (mg/L)	F (mg/L)	Na (mg/L)	Ca (mg/L)	Mg (mg/L)	As (μg/L)	Cd (μg/L)	
Median	NA	NA	NA	NA	NA	NA	NA	
Mahiyanganaya ($n = 7$)								
Min	NA	0.15	6.93	7.66	4.68	<1	NA	Nikagolla et al. 2020
Max	NA	1.18	59.0	107	22.9	<1	NA	
Mean	NA	0.65	26.5	26.1	12.6	<1	NA	
Median	NA	NA	NA	NA	NA	NA	NA	
Anuradhapura ($n = 102$)								
Min	NA	<0.01	0.50	0.41	0.20	<0.02	<0.01	Paranagama et al. 2018
Max	NA	1.75	393	208	76.3	<0.02	<0.01	
Mean	NA	0.52	78.8	61.3	27.8	<0.02	<0.01	
Median	NA	0.42	68.2	48.8	24.7	<0.02	<0.01	
Polonnaruwa ($n = 90$)								
Min	NA	0.04	9.90	24.4	5.27	<0.02	<0.01	Paranagama et al. 2018
Max	NA	1.14	89.0	120	77.3	<0.02	<0.01	
Mean	NA	0.49	40.2	69.4	28.7	<0.02	<0.01	
Median	NA	0.46	35.8	71.0	25.6	<0.02	<0.01	
	HD	F	Na	Ca	Mg	As	Cd	
	300	1.5	200	75	50	10	3	WHO Permissible Limit (WHO 2022)

A recent case–control study on water quality carried out in Moneragala District, one of the CKDu hotspot in Sri Lanka, showed that over 87% of the sampled wells in the CKDu prevalent area contained higher fluoride levels than the recommended level (>0.8 mg/l) for the dry zone of Sri Lanka (Udeshani et al. 2020; Liyanage et al. 2022). In this region, the mean fluoride content was reported as 2.02 ± 1.50 mg/l (median: 1.70 mg/l) in CKDu hotspots, while it was 0.31 ± 0.16 mg/l (median: 0.30 mg/l) in endemic control samples (Table 15.1). Girandurukotte is another CKDu hotspot region where CKDu-affected villages are found close to the non-affected villages. Similar water quality study by Balasooriya et al. (2020) reported groundwater fluoride levels varied from 0.26 to 5.00 mg/l with a mean of 0.92 mg/l (median: 0.63 mg/l) in CKDu areas. In contrast, it varied from 0.12 to 5.20 mg/l in non-CKDu areas with a mean of 0.74 mg/l (median: 0.49 mg/l) with a significant difference to CKDu areas. Wickramarathna et al. (2017) outlined the groundwater quality in three CKDu hotspots in Sri Lanka (Girandurukotte, Wilgamuwa, and Nikawewa) and found higher fluoride levels that varied from 0.02 to 5.47 mg/l with a mean of 0.86 mg/l. Nikagolla et al. (2022) also reported higher fluoride levels in groundwater from CKDu regions, exceeding the permissible limits for consumption. These results suggest a possible influence of fluoride on the CKDu onset or the disease progression.

Most of the groundwater in the dry zone of Sri Lanka can be categorized as moderately hard (61–121 mg/l) and hard (121–180 mg/l) (Rubasinghe et al. 2015; Chandrajith and Diyabalanage 2022). Previous studies have revealed that the groundwater hardness is comparatively higher in CKDu endemic regions than the non-endemic regions (Balasooriya et al. 2020, Liyanage et al. 2022). For instance, Wickramarathna et al. (2017) reported groundwater hardness in CKDu regions varied from 10 to 560 mg/l with a mean of 181 mg/l. Liyanage et al. (2022) have identified significantly higher groundwater hardness in the CKDu region, which varied from 16.6 to 162 mg/l (mean: 82.4 ± 35.7 mg/l), compared to the control region, which varied from 5.15 to 105 mg/l (mean: 37.7 ± 30.6 mg/l) (Table 15.1). The same study signifies a possible influence of Mg^{2+} ions on CKDu progression as drinking water from CKDu regions contained higher Mg^{2+} together with fluoride compared to the endemic controls. The dominance of Mg^{2+} ions in hard water has been suggested as a possible

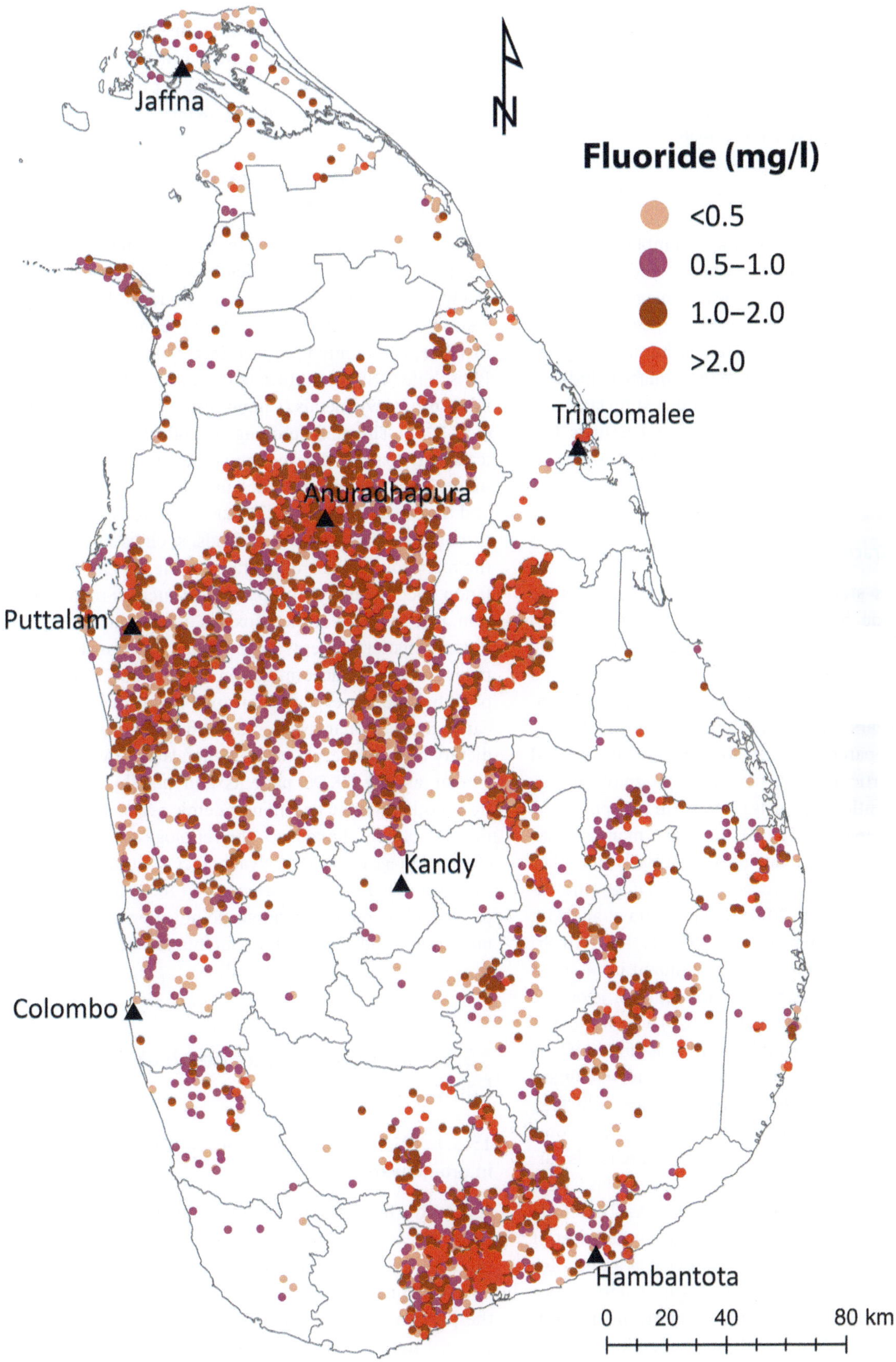

Figure 15.4 Distribution of the groundwater fluoride in Sri Lanka. *Source:* Chandrajith et al. (2020)/with permission of Elsevier.

influencing parameter for CKDu (Dharma-Wardana 2018; Balasooriya et al. 2020; Liyanage et al. 2022). The presence of low Na^+/Ca^{2+} ratios in hard groundwater with elevated fluoride content could lead to CKDu in Sri Lanka (Chandrajith et al. 2011a). In a recent animal model study, Perera et al. (2020) showed the possibility of occurring tubular injury due to the consumption of water with higher fluoride and hardness for a longer time.

A Hofmeister-type action of anions and ion pair formation explains the formation of MgF^+ complex, which is nephrotoxic and can disrupt the structure and functionality of proteins leading to kidney damage (Dharma-Wardana 2018). Therefore, it could be postulated that long-term exposure to hard water, that is dominated by Mg ion with high fluoride may enhance the damage to kidneys and may lead to renal failure. Another interesting fact to be noted is the incidence and prevalence of CKDu is low among people who consume surface water such as natural springs, rivers, streams, lakes, and reservoirs.

15.4.2 Toxic Trace Metals

Several previous studies have emphasized the possible influence of toxic heavy metal/s (e.g. As, Cd, and Pb) through contaminated groundwater could be a possible cause of CKDu (Bandara et al. 2010; Jayasumana et al. 2015). Besides geogenic sources, the use of agrochemicals and fertilizers containing higher amounts of toxic heavy metals apparently could contaminate the natural environment. Particularly, As content in groundwater has gained wider attention due to its presence in phosphate fertilizers (Jayasumana et al. 2015). However, many studies have reported lower availability of As ($<10\,\mu g/l$) and other nephrotoxic heavy metals such as Cd and Pb in groundwater (Wickramarathna et al. 2017; Nanayakkara et al. 2019; Chandrajith and Diyabalanage 2022) (Table 15.1). In Sri Lanka, As-bearing minerals are not abundant in underlying metamorphic rocks; hence, the influence of geogenic As is implausible (Chandrajith et al. 2020). Chronic exposure to arsenic mainly causes skin manifestations such as skin lesions and pigmentation, gangrene and malignant neoplasm, hard patches on the palms, and soles of the feet, but it could also effect on kidney, liver, and lung functions. A case–control study on trace element exposure levels carried out by Diyabalanage et al. (2017) revealed that CKDu patients were not exposed to higher levels of As. Therefore, it is quite unlikely that As is contributing to the onset of CKDu. Further, Cd in water is also suspected as a causative factor for CKDu (Bandara et al. 2010). Later studies have noted excessively lower Cd contents in groundwater from both endemic and non-endemic localities (Balasooriya et al. 2020; Liyanage et al. 2022; Nanayakkara et al. 2019). However, a significantly higher Cd content has been identified in urine samples from CKDu patients compared to a control population (Jayatilake et al. 2013). Convincing evidence is still lacking to prove groundwater contamination with toxic heavy metals.

15.4.3 Agrochemical Usage and Food Contamination

To meet the growing demand for foods, farmers use fertilizers and agrochemicals (pesticides and weedicides) extensively in agricultural fields to obtain a higher yield, resulting in possible heavy metal contamination. For instance, commonly used fertilizers, such as Triple Super Phosphate (TSP) and Muriate of Potash (MOP), may contain toxic heavy metals (Chandrajith et al. 2010; Nyachoti et al. 2022). Therefore, prolonged application of agrochemicals may lead to the accumulation of certain toxic elements and pesticide residues in soil and water (Sirisena and Suriyagoda 2018). Toxic heavy metals can then ingest through the consumption of foods, such as rice, which is the main source of carbohydrates in the Sri Lankan population. Depending on soil properties such as redox condition, pH, presence of metal oxides, microbial activity, and organic matter content, trace metals are translocated in plant tissues and accumulate in rice grains. This leads to potential dietary exposure to toxic metals and thus may cause renal tubular dysfunction. Studies showed that the dietary exposure levels to those metals are lower and also similar among CKDu patients and healthy populations from both endemic and non-endemic regions, hence cannot be clearly linked to the etiology of the disease (Diyabalanage et al. 2016; Nyachoti et al. 2022). This is further supported by Balasooriya et al. (2020) indicating that paddy soils in endemic regions do not show excessive contamination and total metal contents are generally below the recommended threshold values.

15.5 Influence of Biochemical Factors on CKDu

15.5.1 Dissolved Organic Carbon (DOC) in groundwater

A potential link between Dissolved Organic Carbon (DOC) in groundwater and the endemicity of CKDu has also been proposed recently (Makehelwala et al. 2020). DOC originates from natural and anthropogenic sources and acts as the primary carbon source for most biogeochemical processes (Shin et al. 2016). According to the suggested hypothesis, once ingested, proteins such as tyrosine and tryptophan are metabolized by gut microbiota to form uremic toxins (e.g. indoxyl sulfate, p-cresylsulfate, phenyl sulfate), which can cause oxidative stress in kidney tissues (Wang and Zhao 2018). It has been identified that groundwater in CKDu high-risk zones, particularly in the Anuradhapura district, is highly enriched with aromatic, nonbiodegradable DOC and correlates with major solutes such as Mg^{2+}, Ca^{2+}, and SO_4^{2-} (Makehelwala et al. 2019). Further, enrichment of such organic matter can govern the interaction of heavy metals and their mobility through complexation and adsorption, facilitating their availability in groundwater (Makehelwala et al. 2019, 2020).

15.5.2 Cyanotoxins

It has been hypothesized that ingestion of toxins and pollutants either directly or via food or drinking water could significantly contribute to CKDu (Liyanage et al. 2016). For instance, certain cyanobacteria can produce toxins that lead to detrimental health effects, hence their presence in drinking water sources could make the community more susceptible to those toxins. Jayasekara et al. (2013) disclosed cyanobacteria in reservoirs in CKDu endemic regions. Their growth has been facilitated by the application of fertilizer in surrounding regions of reservoirs. Cyanotoxins can damage kidney tissues, leading to kidney failures thus considered a possible causative factor for CKDu. Different cyanotoxins, such as microcystins, cylindrospermopsis, and nodularin, have been found in the reservoirs in CKDu endemic regions (Liyanage et al. 2016).

15.5.3 Heat Stress

Due to the lack of easy access to drinking water and the prevailing high ambient temperature in the dry zonal regions in Sri Lanka, farming communities are always at severe risk of getting dehydrated (Nanayakkara et al. 2020). Since it can affect kidney function, heat stress and repeated episodes of dehydration are other causative factors suggested for CKDu. However, heat stress and dehydration cannot explain the mosaic geographical distribution of the disease. Sometimes, high and low or no prevalence villages are located next to each other and share the same lifestyle and socioeconomic conditions (Balasooriya et al. 2020). In addition, it does not explain the gender and age distribution of the disease since women, children, and adolescents who are not engaged in agricultural work also suffer from CKDu. Therefore, heat stress and dehydration cannot be identified as the main causative factors of CKDu, but they may trigger factors of kidney damage, and the other environmental conditions exaggerate the disease progression.

15.6 Future Directions

Despite two decades of intensive research and debate, the etiological factor or factors causing CKDu remain elusive to date. This is mainly due to the uneven distribution of disease and variation of exposure for suggested environmental causative factors across geographic areas. Up to current understanding, the disease is associated with a multifactorial origin where the individual factors may interact and cause adverse effects. The suggested geochemical, environmental, and sociological factors may interrelate with each other and systematically control the emergence of CKDu. However, current evidence suggests a significant contribution of groundwater quality to the pathogenesis and/or progression of the disease. Renal injuries were identified among children who are less exposed to most other causative factors except drinking water quality. Therefore, attention should be paid to supplying drinking water with improved quality to the community, especially for the community that lives in CKDu hotspot regions. Further, attention should be paid to applying specific and sensitive biomarker/s for early diagnosis of the disease, and then the interventions would be more workable.

References

Abeyagunawardena, A.S. and Shroff, R. (2021). CKDu: the known unknowns. *Pediatric Nephrology* 36: 219–221. https://doi.org/10.1007/s00467-020-04596-2.

Abeywickrama, H.M., Wimalasiri, S., Koyama, Y. et al. (2020). Quality of life and symptom burden among chronic kidney disease of uncertain etiology (CKDu) patients in Girandurukotte, Sri Lanka. *International Journal of Environmental Research and Public Health* 17: 4041. https://doi.org/10.3390/ijerph17114041.

Anand, S., Montez-Rath, M.E., Adasooriya, D. et al. (2019). Prospective biopsy-based study of CKD of unknown etiology in Sri Lanka. *Clinical Journal of the American Society of Nephrology* 14: 224–232. https://doi.org/10.2215/cjn.07430618.

Ananda Jayalal, T.B., Jayaruwan Bandara, T.W.M.A., Mahawithanage, S.T.C. et al. (2019). A quantitative analysis of chronic exposure of selected heavy metals in a model diet in a CKD hotspot in Sri Lanka. *BMC Nephrology* 20: 208. https://doi.org/10.1186/s12882-019-1371-5.

Balasooriya, S., Munasinghe, H., Herath, A.T. et al. (2020). Possible links between groundwater geochemistry and chronic kidney disease of unknown etiology (CKDu): an investigation from the Ginnoruwa region in Sri Lanka. *Exposure and Health* 12: 823–834. https://doi.org/10.1007/s12403-019-00340-w.

Bandara, J.M.R.S., Wijewardena, H.V.P., Liyanege, J. et al. (2010). Chronic renal failure in Sri Lanka caused by elevated dietary cadmium: Trojan horse of the green revolution. *Toxicology Letters* 198: 33–39. https://doi.org/10.1016/j.toxlet.2010.04.016.

Chandrajith, R. and Diyabalanage, S. (2022). Geo-environmental assessment of geochemistry of groundwater and associated human health risks in the dry zone terrain of Sri Lanka. *Journal of the National Science Foundation of Sri Lanka* 50: 213–229.

Chandrajith, R., Seneviratna, S., Wickramaarachchi, K. et al. (2010). Natural radionuclides and trace elements in rice field soils in relation to fertilizer application: study of a chronic kidney disease area in Sri Lanka. *Environmental Earth Sciences* 60: 193–201. https://doi.org/10.1007/s12665-009-0179-1.

Chandrajith, R., Dissanayake, C.B., Ariyarathna, T. et al. (2011a). Dose-dependent Na and Ca in fluoride-rich drinking water – another major cause of chronic renal failure in tropical arid regions. *Science of the Total Environment* 409: 671–675. https://doi.org/10.1016/j.scitotenv.2010.10.046.

Chandrajith, R., Nanayakkara, S., Itai, K. et al. (2011b). Chronic kidney diseases of uncertain etiology (CKDue) in Sri Lanka: geographic distribution and environmental implications. *Environmental Geochemistry and Health* 33: 267–278. https://doi.org/10.1007/s10653-010-9339-1.

Chandrajith, R., Diyabalanage, S., and Dissanayake, C.B. (2020). Geogenic fluoride and arsenic in groundwater of Sri Lanka and its implications to community health. *Groundwater for Sustainable Development* 10: 100359. https://doi.org/10.1016/j.gsd.2020.100359.

Dharma-Wardana, M.W.C. (2018). Chronic kidney disease of unknown etiology and the effect of multiple-ion interactions. *Environmental Geochemistry and Health* 40: 705–719. https://doi.org/10.1007/s10653-017-0017-4.

Dissanayake, C.B. and Chandrajith, R. (2018). The hydrogeological and geochemical characteristics of groundwater of Sri Lanka. In: *Groundwater of South Asia* (ed. A. Mukherjee), 405–428. Springer https://doi.org/10.1007/978-981-10-3889-1_25.

Dissanayake, C.B. and Chandrajith, R. (2019). Fluoride and hardness in groundwater of tropical regions-review of recent evidence indicating tissue calcification and calcium phosphate nanoparticle formation in kidney tubules. *Ceylon Journal of Science* 48: 197–207. https://doi.org/10.4038/cjs.v48i3.7643.

Diyabalanage, S., Navarathna, T., Abeysundara, H.T.K. et al. (2016). Trace elements in native and improved paddy rice from different climatic regions of Sri Lanka: implications for public health. *Springerplus* 5: 1864. https://doi.org/10.1186/s40064-016-3547-9.

Diyabalanage, S., Fonseka, S., Dasanayake, D.M.S.N.B., and Chandrajith, R. (2017). Environmental exposures of trace elements assessed using keratinized matrices from patients with chronic kidney diseases of uncertain etiology (CKDu) in Sri Lanka. *Journal of Trace Elements in Medicine and Biology* 39: 62–70. https://doi.org/10.1016/j.jtemb.2016.08.003.

Elledge, M.F., Redmon, J.H., Levine, K.E. et al. (2014). Chronic kidney disease of unknown etiology in Sri Lanka: quest for understanding and global implications. *RTI Press Research Brief* https://doi.org/10.3768/rtipress.2014.rb.0007.1405.

Fernando, W.B.N.T., Nanayakkara, N., Gunarathne, L., and Chandrajith, R. (2020). Serum and urine fluoride levels in populations of high environmental fluoride exposure with endemic CKDu: a case–control study from Sri Lanka. *Environmental Geochemistry and Health* 42: 1497–1504. https://doi.org/10.1007/s10653-019-00444-x.

Herath, C., Jayasumana, C., De Silva, P.M.C.S. et al. (2018). Kidney diseases in agricultural communities: a case against heat-stress nephropathy. *Kidney International Reports* 3: 271–280. https://doi.org/10.1016/j.ekir.2017.10.006.

Hettithanthri, O., Sandanayake, S., Magana-Arachchi, D. et al. (2021). Risk factors for endemic chronic kidney disease of unknown etiology in Sri Lanka: retrospect of water security in the dry zone. *Science of the Total Environment* 795: 148839. https://doi.org/10.1016/j.scitotenv.2021.148839.

Jayasekara, J.M., Dissanayake, D.M., Adhikari, S.B., and Bandara, P. (2013). Geographical distribution of chronic kidney disease of unknown origin in North Central Region of Sri Lanka. *Ceylon Medical Journal* 58: 6–10.

Jayasinghe, S. and Zhu, Y.-G. (2020). Chronic kidney disease of unknown etiology (CKDu): using a system dynamics model to conceptualize the multiple environmental causative pathways of the epidemic. *Science of the Total Environment* 705: 135766. https://doi.org/10.1016/j.scitotenv.2019.135766.

Jayasumana, C., Gunatilake, S., and Senanayake, P. (2014). Glyphosate, hard water and nephrotoxic metals: are they the culprits behind the epidemic of chronic kidney disease of unknown etiology in Sri Lanka? *International Journal of Environmental Research and Public Health* 11: 2125–2147. https://doi.org/10.3390/ijerph110202125.

Jayasumana, C., Fonseka, S., Fernando, A. et al. (2015). Phosphate fertilizer is a main source of arsenic in areas affected with chronic kidney disease of unknown etiology in Sri Lanka. *Springerplus* 4: 1–8. https://doi.org/10.1186/s40064-015-0868-z.

Jayatilake, N., Mendis, S., Maheepala, P., and Mehta, F.R. (2013). Chronic kidney disease of uncertain aetiology: prevalence and causative factors in a developing country. *BMC Nephrology* 14: 180. https://doi.org/10.1186/1471-2369-14-180.

Jha, V., Garcia-Garcia, G., Iseki, K. et al. (2013). Chronic kidney disease: global dimension and perspectives. *The Lancet* 382: 260–272. https://doi.org/10.1016/S0140-6736(13)60687-X.

Jiménez-Córdova, M.I., Cárdenas-González, M., Aguilar-Madrid, G. et al. (2018). Evaluation of kidney injury biomarkers in an adult Mexican population environmentally exposed to fluoride and low arsenic levels. *Toxicology and Applied Pharmacology* 352: 97–106. https://doi.org/10.1016/j.taap.2018.05.027.

Kafle, K., Balasubramanya, S., and Horbulyk, T. (2019). Prevalence of chronic kidney disease in Sri Lanka: a profile of affected districts reliant on groundwater. *Science of the Total Environment* 694: 133767. https://doi.org/10.1016/j.scitotenv.2019.133767.

Levine, K.E., Redmon, J.H., Elledge, M.F., Wanigasuriya, K.P., Smith, K., Munoz, B., Waduge, V.A., Periris-John, R.J., Sathiakumar, N., Harrington, J.M. and Womack, D.S. (2016) Quest to identify geochemical risk factors associated with chronic kidney disease of unknown etiology (CKDu) in an endemic region of Sri Lanka—a multimedia laboratory analysis of biological, food, and environmental samples. *Environmental Monitoring and Assessment*, 188(10), 548. https://doi.org/https://doi.org/10.1007/s10661-016-5524-8.

Liyanage, M., Magana-arachchi, D., Priyadarshika, C. et al. (2016). Cyanobacteria and cyanotoxins in well waters of the Girandurukotte, CKDu endemic area in Sri Lanka; do they drink safe water? *Journal of Ecotechnology Research* 18: 17–21. https://doi.org/10.11190/jer.18.17.

Liyanage, D.N.D., Diyabalanage, S., Dunuweera, S.P. et al. (2022). Significance of mg-hardness and fluoride in drinking water on chronic kidney disease of unknown etiology in Monaragala, Sri Lanka. *Environmental Research* 203: 111779. https://doi.org/10.1016/j.envres.2021.111779.

Makehelwala, M., Wei, Y., Weragoda, S.K. et al. (2019). Characterization of dissolved organic carbon in shallow groundwater of chronic kidney disease affected regions in Sri Lanka. *Science of the Total Environment* 660: 865–875. https://doi.org/10.1016/j.scitotenv.2018.12.435.

Makehelwala, M., Wei, Y., Weragoda, S.K., and Weerasooriya, R. (2020). Ca^{2+} and SO_4^{2-} interactions with dissolved organic matter: implications of groundwater quality for CKDu incidence in Sri Lanka. *Journal of Environmental Sciences* 88: 326–337. https://doi.org/10.1016/j.jes.2019.09.018.

McDonough, L.K., Meredith, K.T., Nikagolla, C. et al. (2020). The water chemistry and microbiome of household wells in Medawachchiya, Sri Lanka, an area with high prevalence of chronic kidney disease of unknown origin (CKDu). *Scientific Reports* 10 (1): 1–12.

Nanayakkara, S., Stmld, S., Abeysekera, T. et al. (2014). An integrative study of the genetic, social and environmental determinants of chronic kidney disease characterized by tubulointerstitial damages in the North Central Region of Sri Lanka. *Journal of Occupational Health* 56: 28–38. https://doi.org/10.1539/joh.13-0172-OA.

Nanayakkara, S., Senevirathna, S.T.M.L.D., Harada, K.H. et al. (2019). Systematic evaluation of exposure to trace elements and minerals in patients with chronic kidney disease of uncertain etiology (CKDu) in Sri Lanka. *Journal of Trace Elements in Medicine and Biology* 54: 206–213. https://doi.org/10.1016/j.jtemb.2019.04.019.

Nanayakkara, I., Dissanayake, R.K., and Nanayakkara, S. (2020). The presence of dehydration in paddy farmers in an area with chronic kidney disease of unknown aetiology. *Nephrology* 25: 156–162. https://doi.org/10.1111/nep.13605.

Nikagolla, C., Meredith, K.T., Dawes, L.A. et al. (2022). Dietary exposures to metals in relation to chronic kidney disease of unknown cause (CKDu) in Sri Lanka. *Exposure and Health* 14: 63–73. https://doi.org/10.1007/s12403-021-00418-4.

Nyachoti, S., Godebo, T.R., Okwori, O.F., Jeuland, M.A. and Manthrithilake, H. (2022) Dietary exposures to metals in relation to chronic kidney disease of unknown cause (CKDu) in Sri Lanka. *Expo Health* 14, 63–73. https://doi.org/https://doi.org/10.1007/s12403-021-00418-4

Paranagama, D.G., Bhuiyan, M.A., and Jayasuriya, N. (2018). Factors associated with chronic kidney disease of unknown aetiology (CKDu) in North Central Province of Sri Lanka: a comparative analysis of drinking water samples. *Applied Water Science* 8 (6): 1–16.

Pearce, N., Caplin, B., Gunawardena, N. et al. (2019). CKD of unknown cause: a global epidemic? *Kidney International Reports* 4: 367. https://doi.org/10.1016/j.ekir.2018.11.019.

Perera, T., Ranasinghe, S., Alles, N., and Waduge, R. (2020). Experimental rat model for acute tubular injury induced by high water hardness and high water fluoride: efficacy of primary preventive intervention by distilled water administration. *BMC Nephrology* 21: 103. https://doi.org/10.1186/s12882-020-01763-3.

Rajapakse, S., Shivanthan, M.C., and Selvarajah, M. (2016). Chronic kidney disease of unknown etiology in Sri Lanka.

International Journal of Occupational and Environmental Health 22: 259–264. https://doi.org/10.1080/10773525.2016.1203097.

Ranasinghe, A.V., Kumara, G.W.G.P., Karunarathna, R.H. et al. (2019). The incidence, prevalence and trends of chronic kidney disease and chronic kidney disease of uncertain aetiology (CKDu) in the North Central Province of Sri Lanka: an analysis of 30,566 patients. *BMC Nephrology* 20: 1–11. https://doi.org/10.1186/s12882-019-1501-0.

Rubasinghe, R., Gunatilake, S.K., and Chandrajith, R. (2015). Geochemical characteristics of groundwater in different climatic zones of Sri Lanka. *Environmental Earth Sciences* 74: 3067–3076. https://doi.org/10.1007/s12665-015-4339-1.

Shin, Y., Lee, E.-J., Jeon, Y.-J. et al. (2016). Hydrological changes of DOM composition and biodegradability of rivers in temperate monsoon climates. *Journal of Hydrology* 540: 538–548. https://doi.org/10.1016/j.jhydrol.2016.06.004.

Sirisena, D. and Suriyagoda, L.D.B. (2018). Toward sustainable phosphorus management in Sri Lankan rice and vegetable-based cropping systems: a review. *Agriculture and Natural Resources* 52: 9–15. https://doi.org/10.1016/j.anres.2018.03.004.

Tatapudi, R.R., Rentala, S., Gullipalli, P. et al. (2019). High prevalence of CKD of unknown etiology in Uddanam, India. *Kidney International Reports* 4: 380–389. https://doi.org/10.1016/j.ekir.2018.10.006.

Udeshani, W.A.C., Dissanayake, H.M.K.P., Gunatilake, S.K., and Chandrajith, R. (2020). Assessment of groundwater quality using water quality index (WQI): a case study of a hard rock terrain in Sri Lanka. *Groundwater for Sustainable Development* 11: 100421. https://doi.org/10.1016/j.gsd.2020.100421.

Vervaet, B.A., Nast, C.C., Jayasumana, C. et al. (2020). Chronic interstitial nephritis in agricultural communities is a toxin-induced proximal tubular nephropathy. *Kidney International* 97: 350–369. https://doi.org/10.1016/j.kint.2019.11.009.

Vlahos, P., Schensul, S.L., Anand, S. et al. (2021). Water sources and kidney function: investigating chronic kidney disease of unknown etiology in a prospective study. *NPJ Clean Water* 4: 1–7. https://doi.org/10.1038/s41545-021-00141-2.

Wang, Z. and Zhao, Y. (2018). Gut microbiota derived metabolites in cardiovascular health and disease. *Protein & Cell* 9: 416–431. https://doi.org/10.1007/s13238-018-0549-0.

Wanigasuriya, K.P., Peiris-John, R.J., Wickremasinghe, R., and Hittarage, A. (2007). Chronic renal failure in North Central Province of Sri Lanka: an environmentally induced disease. *Transactions of the Royal Society of Tropical Medicine and Hygiene* 101: 1013–1017. https://doi.org/10.1016/j.trstmh.2007.05.006.

Weaver, V.M., Fadrowski, J.J., and Jaar, B.G. (2015). Global dimensions of chronic kidney disease of unknown etiology (CKDu): a modern era environmental and/or occupational nephropathy? *BMC Nephrology* 16: 145. https://doi.org/10.1186/s12882-015-0105-6.

WHO (World Health Organization) (2011). *Guidelines for Drinking-Water Quality*. Geneva: World Health Organization.

WHO (World Health Organization) (2022). *Guidelines for Drinking-Water Quality: Fourth Edition Incorporating the First and Second Addenda*. Geneva: World Health Organization.

Wickramarathna, S., Balasooriya, S., Diyabalanage, S., and Chandrajith, R. (2017). Tracing environmental aetiological factors of chronic kidney diseases in the dry zone of Sri Lanka – a hydrogeochemical and isotope approach. *Journal of Trace Elements in Medicine and Biology* 44: 298–306. https://doi.org/10.1016/j.jtemb.2017.08.013.

Wimalawansa, S.J. (2019). Public health interventions for chronic diseases: cost–benefit modelizations for eradicating chronic kidney disease of multifactorial origin (CKDmfo/CKDu) from tropical countries. *Heliyon* 5: e02309. https://doi.org/10.1016/j.heliyon.2019.e02309.

16

Waste in One Health

Building Resilient Communities Through Sustainable Waste Management

Randika Jayasinghe[1], Pabasari Arundathi Koliyabandara[1], and Meththika Vithanage[2]

[1] *Faculty of Technology, University of Sri Jayewardenepura, Nugegoda, Sri Lanka*
[2] *Ecosphere Resilience Research Center, Faculty of Applied Sciences, University of Sri Jayewardenepura, Nugegoda, Sri Lanka*

16.1 Introduction

Waste and its adverse effects on the health of humans, animals, and the environment have become one of the most pressing global challenges today. According to a World Bank report, 2 billion tons of municipal solid waste are generated globally, with 33% of that being disposed of through open dumping. The report also forecasts that global waste generation will increase by 70% by 2050 (Kaza et al. 2018). Disposing of waste – out of sight, out of mind – is not an option anymore as many urban cities worldwide have reached their limits to capacity. Despite this urgent and recognized need, implementing waste management systems critical to a safer environment and better quality of life for humans and other living organisms has been inadequate, particularly in developing countries.

Poor waste management can cause severe environmental degradation, negatively impacting the environment and community resilience in an area. In most developing countries, solid waste is often disposed of in open dumpsites, along roadsides, on vacant lands, and in waterways (Kaza et al. 2018). Open burning of waste is also widely practiced to reduce the volume (Nanda and Berruti 2021). These unsustainable practices lead to unsanitary conditions, environmental pollution, and poor quality of life for both humans and animals alike. Haphazard waste disposal could lead to serious environmental issues such as soil and water pollution due to leachate runoff and waste accumulation. Open burning of waste causes air pollution and contributes to climate change due to greenhouse gas (GHG) emissions (Etea et al. 2021). Further, poor waste management could amplify social issues such as undesirable living conditions due to odor and open dumpsites overflowing with wastes. Recently, greater attention has also been given to the pollution of soil, freshwater, and marine ecosystems due to microplastics (Golwala et al. 2021).

A holistic waste management approach based on integrated waste management and circular economy principles working locally, nationally, and globally is imperative to attain the health of humans, animals, and the environment. An integrated waste management system contains measures to avoid unnecessary waste generation, reduce waste at source, and reuse products to prolong their lifecycles. Moreover, it encourages recycling materials and products, recovering energy and other materials from waste (Hosseinalizadeh et al. 2021), and finally, the safe disposal of residual waste (Nanda and Berruti 2021).

Sustainable waste management could address many of the sustainable development goals (SDGs) related to resilient communities and safer environment including but not limited to Good Health and Well-being (Goal 3), Sustainable Cities and Communities (Goal 11), Climate Action (Goal 13), Life Below Water (Goal 14), and Life on Land (Goal 15) (Elsheekh et al. 2021). With these thoughts in mind, this chapter aims to assess the current and potential impact of waste management on One Health at the human–animal–environmental interface. The chapter will also delve into the current challenges related to waste management amidst a global pandemic and discuss some futuristic approaches to building a resilient community through sustainable waste management.

16.2 Waste and Environmental Health

Healthy environments create a smooth relationship between biotic and abiotic systems, and it is a prerequisite for good health. Clean air, clean water and sanitation,

One Health: Human, Animal, and Environment Triad, First Edition. Edited by Meththika Vithanage and Majeti Narasimha Vara Prasad.

proper waste disposal, safe agricultural practices, and conserved natural resources are vital for the delicate functioning of the ecosystems.

Differently originated waste, such as municipal solid waste (MSW), clinical solid waste (CSW), industrial waste, electronic waste (e-waste), and biomedical waste (BMW), generates varied types of pollutants. The environmental burden caused by these wastes is considerably high. The waste generation keeps on the rise, while the inadequate infrastructure to effectively manage the waste is a concern (Peter et al. 2019). Environmental hazards from open dumping are a severe problem around the world. Prolonged incomplete handling of solid waste and lack of management at disposal sites have caused significant environmental and social challenges, such as pollution of nearby surface and groundwater water sources (Ferronato and Torretta 2021), unintentional landfill gas fires, atmospheric contaminants creating unpleasant and highly toxic gases and volatile organic carbons (VOCs), emission of GHGs, damage to vegetation, and air pollution leading to global warming (Ferronato et al. 2019).

Among the sources of water pollution, open dumpsites have been identified as one of the most significant threats. Open dumping releases heavy metals, such as Cd, As, Cr, and Fe, into the environment (Mohan and Joseph 2021). Moreover, landfills that have been constructed without engineered liners and leachate collection systems also create environmental pollution. Groundwater and surface water resources polluted with landfill leachate pose a substantial risk to the natural environment and human health. Toxic substances may be present in variable concentrations and are associated with the nature of the waste deposited. Pollution intensity is determined by the concentration of contaminants, groundwater flow direction, and depth of the water table. Typically, waste is deposited in non-engineered dumpsites, from which leachates receive heavy metals such as Hg, As, Cd, Pb, Zn, Ni, Cu, Cr, and Mn (Iqbal et al. 2022). High metal concentrations occur in leachate due to the slow release of these metals in an acidic environment.

The generation of gases from dumpsites also creates many environmental and health consequences. Biodegradation of organic matter during anaerobic acid fermentation generates volatile organic acids and CO_2. VOCs are converted to CH_4 and CO_2 in the methanogenic phase. Open dumpsites are known for releasing CH_4, CO_2, N_2O, bioaerosol emissions, and other GHGs into the environment (Njoku et al. 2019; Zhang et al. 2019). As the temperature increases in the landfill after placing waste, gases like H_2S and organic compounds containing sulfur like mercaptans tend to release. The objectionable odor that arises from dumpsites is due to the presence of ammonia and hydrogen sulfide. Open burning and spontaneous fires that occur in landfills produce particulate matter (PM), polyaromatic hydrocarbons (PAHs), and hazardous pollutants such as dioxins. Climatic conditions such as rainfall and wind direction increase the distribution of these pollutants and odors from landfills (Zhang et al. 2019).

Open dumping and open burning of waste directly contribute to GHG emissions. A comparative study has shown that open dumpsites generate 1000 kgCO_2-eq./t of GHG emissions, while landfills with low organic carbon waste generate only 70 kgCO_2-eq./t (Ferronato et al. 2019). Furthermore, open dumps are identified as a significant source of bioaerosols. Recorded values in Olusosun open dumpsite, Nigeria, for indicator groups are approximately 4.8–105 CFU/m^3 total bacteria and 1.4–106 CFU/m^3 gram-negative bacteria in 96 m^3 of air (Akpeimeh et al. 2019). Moreover, dumpsites are commonplace for the disposal of fire retardants, disinfectants, preservatives, pharmaceuticals, personal care products, persistent organic chemicals, etc. These are sources of emerging contaminants (ECs) that have a high potential for causing damage to ecosystems and human health (Anand et al. 2021; Antunes et al. 2021).

Haphazard disposal of waste into waterways is another global environmental issue. The intrusion of waste, including elevated quantities of plastics, into aquatic bodies, has threatened the biodiversity and the health of ecosystems. The waste dumped into land environments, drainages, and other water sources are carried to oceans via rivers (Gonzalez-Fernandez et al. 2021). About 80% of marine litter is generated on land and reaches the ocean through river inflows. These waste materials can alter the micro- and macroenvironment of aquatic systems and create unfavorable conditions for biota (Soto-Navarro et al. 2021).

Plastics are versatile materials; however, the production, use, and disposal of plastics have created a number of health, socioeconomic, and environmental issues. Mismanagement of plastic waste is a pressing socio-environmental issue around the world. Plastics do not biodegrade. When exposed to environmental conditions, they break down into smaller particles and generate micro- and nanoplastics. According to the U.S. National Oceanic and Atmospheric Administration (NOAA) and the European Chemicals Agency, microplastics are small fragments of plastics less than 5 mm in size (Ellen MacArthur Foundation and World Economic Forum 2016). Microplastics have been widely reported in marine, freshwater, and terrestrial environments, including the arctic ice and high alpine lakes (Allen et al. 2019; Bellasi et al. 2020).

Furthermore, a recent study reported that fragmentation of plastics in landfills could occur with time due to adverse environmental conditions, including pH and temperature gradients and microbial degradation in landfills, making landfills a long-term potential source of microplastics (He et al. 2019). Microplastics in the environment and food chains are of growing concern. While the evidence on the health implications of microplastics is not conclusive, there are sufficient indications that warrant further research and action. Attention has also been given to additives and chemical contaminants adsorbed by microplastics that may negatively affect human and animal health (Blackburn and Green 2022).

16.3 Waste and Human Health

The health of individuals is directly affected by environmental quality. Polluted waterways, soil, and air pose serious health risks to humans and can lead to various diseases. For example, the open dumping of waste has the potential to create detrimental effects on human health. Long-term exposure to gaseous emissions and chemicals from landfills may affect people with flu, asthma, skin irritations, lung problems, urinary issues, digestive concerns, etc. (Njoku et al. 2019; Doron 2021). Healthcare waste (HCW) can predispose victims to respiratory problems and anomalies (Aluko et al. 2021). Furthermore, vector-borne diseases such as dengue and malaria are related to poor waste management (Akmal and Jamil 2021).

Poor management of hazardous waste can cause adverse health risks for humans. Exposure to hazardous waste can be toxic or even fatal in some instances. Some of the negative health effects of hazardous waste include cancer, respiratory conditions, behavioral abnormalities, genetic mutations, and physiological malfunctions (Tekade 2021). In particular, children exposed to hazardous wastes can develop severe acute and chronic health problems as they are highly vulnerable to the toxic effects of chemicals (Ibrahim et al. 2021). Previous studies report that hazardous wastes are illegally dumped in some countries, threatening the environment and human health (Ibrahim et al. 2021; Otwong et al. 2021).

Many studies have been conducted on e-waste recycling and its impact on human health. E-waste recycling can cause severe health risks as these processes release diverse groups of pollutants. These include heavy metals, dioxins, polycyclic aromatic hydrocarbons, polychlorinated biphenyls (PCBs), brominated flame retardants (BFRs), perfluoroalkyl and polyfluoroalkyl substances (PFASs), polychlorinated dibenzo-p-dioxins (PCDDs), and polychlorinated dibenzofurans (PCDFs). The emitted pollutants have been reported to be present in surface soils, drainages, and waterways (Ahirwar and Tripathi 2021). Exposure routes for e-waste pollutants can be listed as inhalation, dermal contact, and digestion through the soil, air, water, and food. Cellular level exposure to the e-waste recycling derived pollutants can cause loss of enzyme activity, protein disfunction, depletion of antioxidants, and impaired membrane function (Rautela et al. 2021). It was also reported that carcinogenic risks could threaten people who live near e-waste processing plants (Ngo et al. 2021).

There is also a growing concern about microplastics and their impact on human health. However, it is important to note that there is currently no evidence for the direct adverse effects of microplastics on human health (Prata et al. 2021). Although the health effects of microplastics are debatable, there is evidence that microplastics significantly disturb the organ's homeostasis in the presence of sorbed contaminants, as demonstrated in animal models (Prata et al. 2021).

16.4 Waste and Animal Health

Improper disposal of waste leads to pollution, which directly and indirectly threatens all life forms. Terrestrial animals, birds, and marine species are prone to the risks due to swallowing of debris, direct and indirect ingestion of chemicals released from waste, and accidental consumption of hazardous waste. Intestinal block injuries in outer and inner body parts, malnutrition, infections, reduction in growth, anomalies in reproduction, and deaths have been widely reported in different animal species (Wang et al. 2020). Terrestrial animals such as cows, elephants, and dogs have been affected due to consuming plastics and synthetic waste mixed with food waste (Consoli et al. 2019). Another study has reported that camels in the United Arab Emirates show a regional mortality rate of 1% due to the consumption of plastic bags and ropes (Eriksen et al. 2021). Direct and indirect ingestion of litter by aquatic species and physical damage to reefs and mangroves could be stated as some of the critical problems associated with marine debris (Consoli et al. 2019).

The plastic waste degraded into micro- and nanoparticles can negatively impact both terrestrial and aquatic organisms. Microplastics can bioaccumulate and also act as a source and sink for toxic chemicals as well as pathogenic microorganisms (Bellas and Gil 2020; Xie et al. 2020). These can combine with organic, inorganic, and microbial pathogens present in aquatic environments. Marine life is heavily challenged by the intrusion of microplastics into the food web. Biomagnification can pose a serious threat to the trophic levels of the food chain as microplastics get bioaccumulated in a varied range of living organisms (Krause et al. 2021). The magnitude of the impact of microplastics in marine biota has not been fully identified, but the adverse effects can occur on the life span, reproduction, and feeding behaviors. Furthermore, due to the persistent nature and fragmentation tendency, microplastics can pose a threat to living organisms as they can be bioaccumulated by bacteria, fungi, phytoplankton, zooplankton, etc. Heavy metals, namely As, Cu, and Pb, have been reported to be adsorbed to microplastics in large concentrations and interfere with the metabolism of organisms (Xu et al. 2020). Microplastics binding to persistent organic pollutants can act as endocrine disruptors (Grova et al. 2019).

16.5 Waste Management During and Post-COVID-19 Pandemic

The COVID-19 pandemic has created additional challenges for waste management throughout the world, especially in developing countries (United Nations Environment Programme 2020). It has exacerbated waste pollution mainly due to the high usage of personal protective equipment (PPE) (Sharma et al. 2020; Das et al. 2021; Hantoko et al. 2021). An increasing trend in online shopping has also given rise to high volumes of packaging materials. Managing large volumes of waste generated during this period was challenging as waste systems have been disrupted during lockdown periods (United Nations Environment Programme 2020).

There has been a considerable increase in demand, consumption, and disposal of single-use plastics (SUPs) globally, including facemasks, face shields, gloves, protective medical gear, hand sanitizer bottles, and medical test kits since the COVID-19 pandemic began (Jennifer et al. 2020; Vanapalli et al. 2021; Yousefi et al. 2021). Health guidelines advise that medical gowns, gloves, and face masks should be disposed of after use regularly or at the end of the day. These mandatory health guidelines to curb the spread of the COVID-19 pandemic have reversed the momentum and global efforts to reduce single-use plastics. Moreover, system and behavioral changes caused by the pandemic have also led to an increase in takeaway food and beverage containers, plastic packaging for delivering goods, and plastic water bottles (Nzediegwu and Chang 2020; Hantoko et al. 2021).

According to a recent research study, around 3.4 billion single-use facemasks and face shields were discarded daily as a result of the COVID-19 pandemic during 2020 (Benson et al. 2021). In 2020, when the pandemic was fast spreading, there were new challenges and concerns on managing the large volumes of medical wastes generated in healthcare facilities, quarantine facilities, and even households where infected patients were receiving treatment (Sangkham 2020). These issues are still not fully addressed, leading to open dumping and open burning of wastes.

Waste management primarily depends on manual labor and low-tech equipment in low- and middle-income countries. The informal sector also plays a vital role in collecting and delivering recyclables to recycling facilities. These waste management systems were disrupted during the pandemic due to lockdowns and restricted movements (United Nations Environment Programme 2020). As a result, people have resorted to improper disposal methods, including burning solid waste to reduce volumes in the absence of regular waste collection (Oyedotun et al. 2020). Furthermore, the large volumes of PPE waste generated are not adequately recycled or disposed of properly. These wastes are often openly disposed of into the environment, dumped in uncontrolled dumpsites, or thrown into the waterways, rivers, and oceans (Sangkham 2020; Yousefi et al. 2021).

The effective management of medical wastes during the COVID-19 pandemic is a major challenge, especially in developing countries (Sangkham 2020). Generally, all used PPE should be put into designated clinical waste bins and sent to clinical waste treatment facilities (Das et al. 2021). These wastes can enter the marine and terrestrial ecosystems and lead to far more significant issues such as blocking waterways, increasing the risks of urban flash floods, and providing breeding grounds for vector-borne diseases. Moreover, the burning of polymeric wastes such as plastics and rubber releases harmful emissions, contributing to air pollution and decreased health. Once the PPEs are haphazardly disposed of into the environment, they slowly degrade into smaller particles, adding to the presence of micro- and nanoplastics in the environment (Fadare and Okoffo 2020).

Epidemiological studies have reported that the surface stability of SARS-CoV-2 and SARS-CoV-1 is high on a range of surfaces. COVID-19, an infectious disease caused by the SARS-CoV-2 virus, shows more surface stability and could remain viable on many different surfaces, including plastics, stainless steel, and glass for several hours up to days (Chin et al. 2020). Furthermore, nondegradable wastes such as plastics that remain in the environment for a more extended period can accumulate various toxic pollutants and pathogens on their surfaces, thus posing a threat to humans, animals, and marine organisms (Benson et al. 2021). As governments are overburdened with managing the pandemic, these negative consequences of unsustainable waste management are often overlooked.

An inadequate waste management system can deepen inequalities and vulnerabilities in urban communities and lead to serious public health concerns and a significant impact on the environment. Waste management during and post-pandemic requires best practices for waste management, including proper identification, efficient collection, source segregation, safe storage, proper treatment, and safe disposal of waste to reduce the negative impacts on human and animal health and the environment (Vanapalli et al. 2021). There is a timely requirement to analyze existing waste management processes and develop more robust systems to better manage waste during and post-COVID-19 pandemic and similar pandemic situations in the future (Hantoko et al. 2021). It is equally important to provide adequate awareness and training to the public on managing solid waste, especially infectious waste during a pandemic.

16.6 Futuristic Approaches in Waste Management

Waste is often considered a disposal problem in conventional waste management approaches. However, in recent times, attention has been given to more holistic approaches where waste is regarded as a resource with value rather than a liability that needs to be managed. Concepts such as the circular economy and Life Cycle approaches, smart IT-based solutions, and novel waste management technologies have paved the path toward this transition.

16.6.1 Waste Management in a Circular Economy

The circular economy is a sustainable alternative to the linear "take-make-dispose" economic model. It closes the loop by reusing, repairing, repurposing, and recycling materials and products, thereby reducing waste that will end up in the environment. A circular economy offers a new way of doing business, promoting sustainable and resource-efficient policies and practices (Ajwani-Ramchandani et al. 2021). An essential first step toward achieving a circular economy and sustainable living is starting to value resources. There has to be an understanding of limited resources and the repercussions of unsustainable production and consumption (Brydges 2021). Therefore, a transition to a circular economy will encourage more efficient use of resources, including waste materials.

The Ellen MacArthur Foundation is one of the leading organizations advocating and disseminating knowledge, tools, and case studies to accelerate a global transition to a circular economy. According to EMF, new technology innovations in waste management will play a major role in the circular economy (Ellen MacArthur Foundation 2020). Transitioning toward a CE will lead to less waste being disposed of haphazardly into the environment, thus contributing to a number of SDG goals (Sharma et al. 2021), namely Good Health and Well-being (Goal 3), Clean Water and Sanitation (Goal 6), Sustainable Cities and Communities (Goal 11), Responsible Consumption and Production (Jail 12), Climate Action (Goal 13), Life Below Water (Goal 14), and Life on Land (Goal 15).

A critical component in any waste management program is public awareness and participation. Recognizing the importance of the local context and knowledge is key to building resilient communities and sustainable waste management systems (Salmenperä et al. 2021). The success of any waste management initiative depends on the general public's engagement and how well local knowledge is leveraged. The community must understand how waste management systems work, the benefits they will gain from them, and how their active participation is crucial for the sustainability of these systems. With this in mind, some organizations have moved beyond 3R (Reduce, Reuse, Recycle) to develop a 10R approach to waste management (Figure 16.1). This approach calls for simple yet effective measures that communities should actively practice, including repairing, replacing, and regifting items to increase a product's life cycle. Furthermore, it highlights the importance of rethinking our current resource consumption and sharing the best waste management practices across communities.

The waste management hierarchy provides a general guide to select the best waste management option. However, specific local conditions such as availability of resources and technology, waste generation patterns, and sociocultural and political perspectives often influence the "best" option. Life Cycle approaches provide a scientifically sound approach based on factual evidence to ensure that the best option for the community and the environment can be identified and put in place (Iqbal et al. 2020). It takes the entire life cycle of a product or a process into account – from the extraction of resources to material processing, manufacturing, distribution, consumption, and finally, the reuse, recycling, energy and material recovery, and final disposal of any remaining waste. Life Cycle thinking looks at the impacts created throughout the product's life cycle. Life Cycle Assessment quantifies the impacts by assessing the emissions, resources consumed, and pressures on the environment ascribed to a product. These tools are increasingly becoming useful in decision making related to waste management (Camana et al. 2021; Zhang et al. 2021).

16.6.2 Waste Management in Smart Cities

The concept of smart cities has evolved from the need for sustainable development and a better future for people and the planet. Environmental issues, especially waste management, require innovative solutions to keep the cities clean. The challenges associated with the current waste

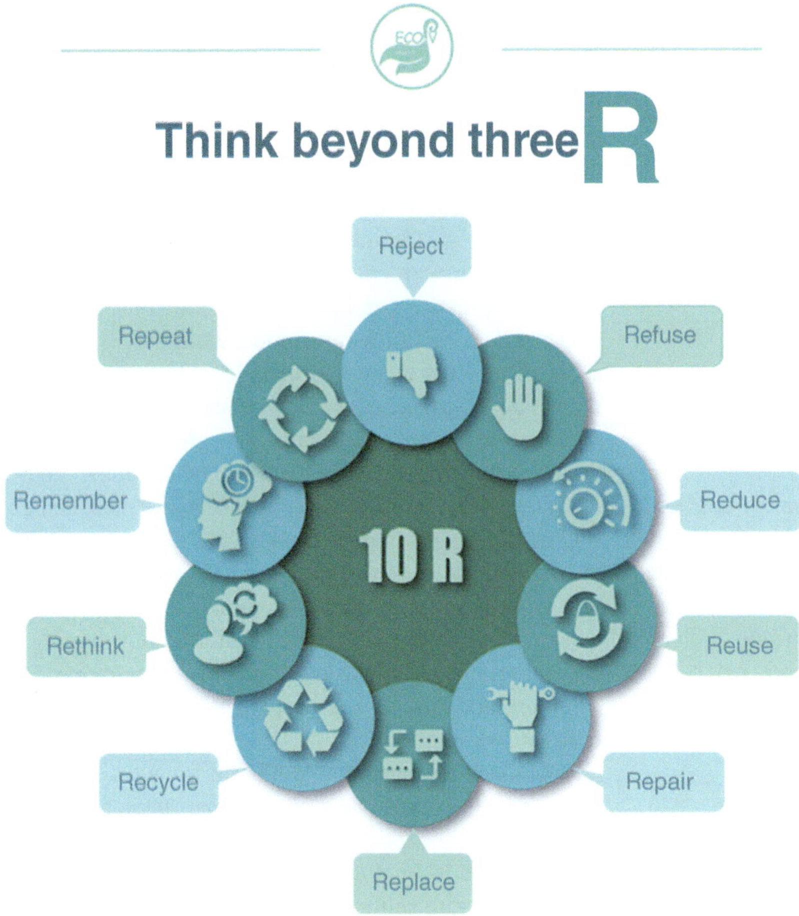

Figure 16.1 10R approach to waste management. *Source:* Eco Friendly Volunteers.

management systems need integrated solutions. New tools such as "blockchain", "internet of things" (IoT), "artificial intelligence" (AI), "cloud computing," and "smart transportation systems" can be introduced and integrated with the existing waste management systems and infrastructure to improve the efficiency of the waste management systems (Ajwani-Ramchandani et al. 2021; Shukla and Hait 2022). Furthermore, waste storage using smart bins, separate recycling bins, underground bins, etc., allows more waste to be stored securely until the collection.

Smart tools, such as GIS and remote sensing, are now widely used to determine and track the collection routes to reduce the number of vehicles, human resources, fuel consumption, and collection time (Abdallah et al. 2020). The tracking of waste collection vehicles is particularly important for hazardous waste transportation to ensure the safety of people and the environment en route and reduce any risks that can be caused due to accidents. Further, radio-frequency identification (RFID) techniques, embedded systems, and wireless mobile communication technologies are used for waste segregation, real-time collection, and optimal transportation, leading to higher waste recovery and recycling rates supporting a circular economy in smart cities (Kang et al. 2020). However, it is equally important to understand that these state-of-the-art techniques might be challenging to implement at once in developing countries due to their high cost, the need for advanced technology, and high maintenance.

16.6.3 New and Emerging Technologies in Waste Management

The need for better waste management processes that align with circular economy principles calls for developing and introducing novel technologies for waste management. The primary emphasis of conventional waste management technologies is to reduce environmental and human health risks to acceptable levels. In contrast, new and emerging technologies in waste management focus on reducing the amount of waste disposed of by recovering valuable materials and directing them for other end uses or converting waste into value-added products. Refused derived fuel, rapid composting, bioreactor landfill, etc., are some of the examples for new and emerging technologies in waste management (Govani et al. 2021).

New and emerging technologies in waste management can add value to different types of waste. Fruit and vegetable wastes are a potential source to produce and extract value-added natural products and chemicals. These perishable wastes are generally managed through composting, anaerobic digestion, animal feeding, or disposal in a landfill. Recently, there has been a growing interest in using emerging valorization technologies to convert fruit and vegetable wastes into bioactive compounds, enzymes, exopolysaccharides, biopolymers, and biofuels (Esparza et al. 2020). Similarly, chemical recycling of waste plastics can be used to transform waste plastics into value-added chemicals (Thiounn and Smith 2020). Other emerging plastic waste conversion technologies include photoreforming, plasma- and supercritical water-assisted gasification, and microwave-assisted pyrolysis (Zhao et al. 2022).

16.7 Final Remarks

Sustainable waste management is critical in planning resilient, healthy, and inclusive communities. However, the complex interconnectedness between human, animal, and environmental health necessitates a holistic waste management approach. Employing a holistic approach acknowledges that waste can be considered both an opportunity and a challenge. If it is not managed correctly, waste will cause adverse impacts on all three facets of the One Health triad. On the other hand, if it is managed properly, waste could be a valuable source of raw materials and energy. Therefore, implementing sustainable waste management systems in the One Health approach requires well-coordinated, multidisciplinary, and multi-stakeholder partnerships supported by national and international policies. The active participation of all stakeholders, especially the general public, is essential for the long-term success of waste management programs.

References

Abdallah, M., Abu Talib, M., Feroz, S. et al. (2020). Artificial intelligence applications in solid waste management: a systematic research review. *Waste Management* 109: 231–246. https://doi.org/10.1016/J.WASMAN.2020.04.057.

Ahirwar, R. and Tripathi, A.K. (2021). E-waste management: a review of recycling process, environmental and occupational health hazards, and potential solutions. *Environmental Nanotechnology Monitoring & Management* 15: 100409. https://doi.org/10.1016/J.ENMM.2020.100409.

Ajwani-Ramchandani, R., Figueira, S., Torres de Oliveira, R. et al. (2021). Towards a circular economy for packaging waste by using new technologies: the case of large multinationals in emerging economies. *Journal of Cleaner Production* 281: 125139. https://doi.org/10.1016/J.JCLEPRO.2020.125139.

Akmal, T. and Jamil, F. (2021). Assessing health damages from improper disposal of solid waste in metropolitan Islamabad–Rawalpindi, Pakistan. *Sustainability* https://doi.org/10.3390/su13052717.

Akpeimeh, G.F., Fletcher, L.A., and Evans, B.E. (2019). Exposure to bioaerosols at open dumpsites: a case study of bioaerosols exposure from activities at Olusosun open dumpsite, Lagos Nigeria. *Waste Management* 89: 37–47. https://doi.org/10.1016/j.wasman.2019.03.058.

Allen, S., Allen, D., Phoenix, V.R. et al. (2019). Atmospheric transport and deposition of microplastics in a remote mountain catchment. *Nature Geoscience* 12 (5): 339–344. https://doi.org/10.1038/s41561-019-0335-5.

Aluko, O.O., Obafemi, T.H., Obiajunwa, P.O. et al. (2021). Solid waste management and health hazards associated with residence around open dumpsites in heterogeneous urban settlements in Southwest Nigeria. *International Journal of Environmental Health Research* 1–16. https://doi.org/10.1080/09603123.2021.1879738.

Anand, U., Reddy, B., Singh, V.K. et al. (2021). Potential environmental and human health risks caused by antibiotic-resistant bacteria (ARB), antibiotic resistance genes (ARGs) and emerging contaminants (ECs) from municipal solid waste (MSW) landfill. *Antibiotics* https://doi.org/10.3390/antibiotics10040374.

Antunes, E., Vuppaladadiyam, A.K., Sarmah, A.K. et al. (2021). Application of biochar for emerging contaminant mitigation. *Advances in Chemical Pollution, Environmental Management and Protection* 7: 65–91. https://doi.org/10.1016/BS.APMP.2021.08.003.

Bellas, J. and Gil, I. (2020). Polyethylene microplastics increase the toxicity of chlorpyrifos to the marine copepod Acartia tonsa. *Environmental Pollution* 260: 114059. https://doi.org/10.1016/j.envpol.2020.114059.

Bellasi, A., Binda, G., Pozzi, A. et al. (2020). Microplastic contamination in freshwater environments: a review, focusing on interactions with sediments and benthic organisms. *Environments* https://doi.org/10.3390/environments7040030.

Benson, N.U., Bassey, D.E., and Palanisami, T. (2021). COVID pollution: impact of COVID-19 pandemic on global plastic waste footprint. *Heliyon* 7 (2): e06343. https://doi.org/10.1016/j.heliyon.2021.e06343.

Blackburn, K. and Green, D. (2022). The potential effects of microplastics on human health: what is known and what is unknown. *Ambio* 51 (3): 518–530. https://doi.org/10.1007/s13280-021-01589-9.

Brydges, T. (2021). Closing the loop on take, make, waste: investigating circular economy practices in the Swedish fashion industry. *Journal of Cleaner Production* 293: 126245. https://doi.org/10.1016/J.JCLEPRO.2021.126245.

Camana, D., Manzardo, A., Toniolo, S. et al. (2021). Assessing environmental sustainability of local waste management policies in Italy from a circular economy perspective. An overview of existing tools. *Sustainable Production and Consumption* 27: 613–629. https://doi.org/10.1016/J.SPC.2021.01.029.

Chin, A.W.H., Chu, J.T.S., Perera, M.R.A. et al. (2020). Stability of SARS-CoV-2 in different environmental conditions. *The Lancet Microbe* 1 (1): e10. https://doi.org/10.1016/S2666-5247(20)30003-3.

Consoli, P., Romeo, T., Angiolillo, M. et al. (2019). Marine litter from fishery activities in the Western Mediterranean sea: the impact of entanglement on marine animal forests. *Environmental Pollution* 249: 472–481. https://doi.org/10.1016/j.envpol.2019.03.072.

Das, A.K., Islam, M.N., Billah, M.M. et al. (2021). COVID-19 pandemic and healthcare solid waste management strategy – a mini-review. *Science of the Total Environment* 778: 146220. https://doi.org/10.1016/J.SCITOTENV.2021.146220.

Doron, A. (2021). Stench and sensibilities: on living with waste, animals and microbes in India. *The Australian Journal of Anthropology* 32 (S1): 23–41. https://doi.org/10.1111/taja.12380.

Ellen MacArthur Foundation (2020). The circular economy: a transformative Covid-19 recovery strategy: how policymakers can pave the way to a low carbon, prosperous future. https://emf.thirdlight.com/link/gx5sj8wvtaji-jhm1ww/@/preview/1?o (accessed 8 February 2022).

Ellen MacArthur Foundation and World Economic Forum (2016). *The New Plastics Economy: Rethinking the Future of Plastics*. Ellen MacArthur Foundation Publishing.

Elsheekh, K.M., Kamel, R.R., Elsherif, D.M. et al. (2021). Achieving sustainable development goals from the perspective of solid waste management plans. *Journal of Engineering and Applied Science* 68 (1): 9. https://doi.org/10.1186/s44147-021-00009-9.

Eriksen, M., Lusher, A., Nixon, M. et al. (2021). The plight of camels eating plastic waste. *Journal of Arid Environments* 185: 104374. https://doi.org/10.1016/J.JARIDENV.2020.104374.

Esparza, I., Jiménez-Moreno, N., Bimbela, F. et al. (2020). Fruit and vegetable waste management: conventional and emerging approaches. *Journal of Environmental Management* 265: 110510. https://doi.org/10.1016/J.JENVMAN.2020.110510.

Etea, T., Girma, E., and Mamo, K. (2021). Risk perceptions and experiences of residents living nearby municipal solid waste open dumpsite in Ginchi Town, Ethiopia: a qualitative study. *Risk Management and Healthcare Policy* 14: 2035–2044. https://doi.org/10.2147/RMHP.S309295.

Fadare, O.O. and Okoffo, E.D. (2020). Covid-19 face masks: a potential source of microplastic fibers in the environment. *The Science of the Total Environment* 737: 140279. https://doi.org/10.1016/j.scitotenv.2020.140279.

Ferronato, N. and Torretta, V. (2021). Comparison of environmental impacts related to municipal solid waste and construction and demolition waste management and recycling in a Latin American developing city. *Environmental Science and Pollution Research* https://doi.org/10.1007/s11356-021-16968-8.

Ferronato, N., Moresco, L., and Guisbert Lizarazu, G.E. (2019). Waste mismanagement in developing countries: a review of global issues. *International Journal of Environmental Research and Public Health* https://doi.org/10.3390/ijerph16061060.

Golwala, H., Zhang, X., Iskander, S.M. et al. (2021). Solid waste: an overlooked source of microplastics to the environment. *Science of the Total Environment* 769: 144581. https://doi.org/10.1016/J.SCITOTENV.2020.144581.

González-Fernández, D., Cózar, A., Hanke, G. et al. (2021). Floating macrolitter leaked from Europe into the ocean. *Nature Sustainability.* 4 (6): 474–483. https://doi.org/10.1038/s41893-021-00722-6.

Govani, J., Singh, E., Kumar, A. et al. (2021). New generation technologies for solid waste management. *Current Developments in Biotechnology and Bioengineering* 77–106. https://doi.org/10.1016/B978-0-12-821009-3.00015-4.

Grova, N., Schroeder, H., Olivier, J.-L. et al. (2019). Epigenetic and neurological impairments associated with early life exposure to persistent organic pollutants. *International Journal of Genomics* 2019: 2085496. https://doi.org/10.1155/2019/2085496.

Hantoko, D., Li, X., Pariatamby, A. et al. (2021). Challenges and practices on waste management and disposal during COVID-19 pandemic. *Journal of Environmental Management* 286: 112140. https://doi.org/10.1016/J.JENVMAN.2021.112140.

He, P., Chen, L., Shao, L. et al. (2019). Municipal solid waste (MSW) landfill: A source of microplastics? -Evidence of microplastics in landfill leachate. *Water research.* 159: 38–45. https://doi.org/10.1016/j.watres.2019.04.060.

Hosseinalizadeh, R., Izadbakhsh, H., and Shakouri, G., H. (2021). A planning model for using municipal solid waste management technologies – considering energy, economic, and environmental impacts in Tehran-Iran. *Sustainable Cities and Society* 65: 102566. https://doi.org/10.1016/J.SCS.2020.102566.

Ibrahim, M.F., Hod, R., Toha, H.R. et al. (2021). The impacts of illegal toxic waste dumping on children's health: a review and case study from Pasir Gudang, Malaysia. *International Journal of Environmental Research and Public Health* https://doi.org/10.3390/ijerph18052221.

Iqbal, A., Liu, X., and Chen, G.H. (2020). Municipal solid waste: review of best practices in application of life cycle assessment and sustainable management techniques. *Science of the Total Environment* 729: 138622. https://doi.org/10.1016/J.SCITOTENV.2020.138622.

Iqbal, J., Javed, A., and Baig, M.A. (2022). Heavy metals removal from dumpsite leachate by algae and cyanobacteria. *Bioremediation Journal* 26 (1): 31–40. https://doi.org/10.1080/10889868.2021.1884530.

Jennifer, S., Siming, Y., Christian, S. et al. (2020). 'COVID-19's unsustainable waste management. *Science* 368 (6498): 1438. https://doi.org/10.1126/science.abc7778.

Kang, K.D., Kang, H., Ilankoon, I.M.S.K. et al. (2020). Electronic waste collection systems using Internet of Things (IoT): household electronic waste management in Malaysia. *Journal of Cleaner Production* 252: 119801. https://doi.org/10.1016/J.JCLEPRO.2019.119801.

Kaza, S. Yao, L.C., Bhada-Tata, P. et al. (2018). What a waste 2.0: a global snapshot of solid waste management to 2050, Washington, DC. https://openknowledge.worldbank.org/handle/10986/30317 (accessed 3 February 2022).

Krause, S., Baranov, V., Nel, H.A. et al. (2021). Gathering at the top? Environmental controls of microplastic uptake and biomagnification in freshwater food webs. *Environmental Pollution* 268: 115750. https://doi.org/10.1016/J.ENVPOL.2020.115750.

Mohan, S. and Joseph, C.P. (2021). Potential hazards due to municipal solid waste open dumping in India. *Journal of the Indian Institute of Science* 101 (4): 523–536. https://doi.org/10.1007/s41745-021-00242-4.

Nanda, S. and Berruti, F. (2021). Municipal solid waste management and landfilling technologies: a review. *Environmental Chemistry Letters* 19 (2): 1433–1456. https://doi.org/10.1007/s10311-020-01100-y.

Ngo, H.T.T., Watchalayann, P., Nguyen, D.B. et al. (2021). Environmental health risk assessment of heavy metal exposure among children living in an informal e-waste processing village in Viet Nam. *The Science of the Total Environment* 763: 142982. https://doi.org/10.1016/j.scitotenv.2020.142982.

Njoku, P.O., Edokpayi, J.N., and Odiyo, J.O. (2019). Health and environmental risks of residents living close to a landfill: a case study of Thohoyandou landfill, Limpopo Province, South Africa. *International Journal of Environmental Research and Public Health* 16 (12): https://doi.org/10.3390/ijerph16122125.

Nzediegwu, C. and Chang, S.X. (2020). Improper solid waste management increases potential for COVID-19 spread in developing countries. *Resources, Conservation and Recycling* 161: 104947. https://doi.org/10.1016/j.resconrec.2020.104947.

Otwong, A., Jongmeewasin, S., and Phenrat, T. (2021). Legal obstacles for the circular economy in Thailand: illegal dumping of recyclable hazardous industrial waste. *Journal of Cleaner Production* 302: 126969. https://doi.org/10.1016/J.JCLEPRO.2021.126969.

Oyedotun, T.D.T., Kasim, O.F., Famewo, A. et al. (2020). Municipal waste management in the era of COVID-19: perceptions, practices, and potentials for research in developing countries. *Research in Globalization* 2: 100033. https://doi.org/10.1016/j.resglo.2020.100033.

Peter, A.E., Shiva Nagendra, S.M., and Nambi, I.M. (2019). Environmental burden by an open dumpsite in urban India. *Waste Management* 85: 151–163. https://doi.org/10.1016/j.wasman.2018.12.022.

Prata, J.C., da Costa, J.P., Lopes, I. et al. (2021). A One Health perspective of the impacts of microplastics on animal, human and environmental health. *The Science of the Total Environment* 777: 146094. https://doi.org/10.1016/j.scitotenv.2021.146094.

Rautela, R., Arya, S., Vishwakarma, S. et al. (2021). E-waste management and its effects on the environment and human health. *The Science of the Total Environment* 773: 145623. https://doi.org/10.1016/j.scitotenv.2021.145623.

Salmenperä, H., Pitkänen, K., Kautto, P. et al. (2021). Critical factors for enhancing the circular economy in waste management. *Journal of Cleaner Production* 280: 124339. https://doi.org/10.1016/J.JCLEPRO.2020.124339.

Sangkham, S. (2020). Face mask and medical waste disposal during the novel COVID-19 pandemic in Asia. *Case Studies in Chemical and Environmental Engineering* 2: 100052. https://doi.org/10.1016/j.cscee.2020.100052.

Sharma, H.B., Vanapalli, K.R., Cheela, V.S. et al. (2020). Challenges, opportunities, and innovations for effective solid waste management during and post COVID-19 pandemic. *Resouces, Conservation and Recycling* 162: 105052. https://doi.org/10.1016/J.RESCONREC.2020.105052.

Sharma, H.B., Vanapalli, K.R., Samal, B. et al. (2021). Circular economy approach in solid waste management system to achieve UN-SDGs: solutions for post-COVID recovery.

Science of the Total Environment 800: 149605. https://doi.org/10.1016/J.SCITOTENV.2021.149605.

Shukla, S. and Hait, S. (2022). Smart waste management practices in smart cities: current trends and future perspectives. *Advanced Organic Waste Management* 407–424. https://doi.org/10.1016/B978-0-323-85792-5.00011-3.

Soto-Navarro, J., Jordá, G., Compa, M. et al. (2021). Impact of the marine litter pollution on the Mediterranean biodiversity: a risk assessment study with focus on the marine protected areas. *Marine Pollution Bulletin* 165: 112169. https://doi.org/10.1016/J.MARPOLBUL.2021.112169.

Tekade, R. (2021). The impact of hazardous waste and it's impact on human health. *International Journal of Researches in Biosciences, Agriculture and Technology* 17: 567–570.

Thiounn, T. and Smith, R.C. (2020). Advances and approaches for chemical recycling of plastic waste. *Journal of Polymer Science* 58 (10): 1347–1364. https://doi.org/10.1002/pol.20190261.

United Nations Environment Programme (2020). *Waste Management During the COVID-19 Pandemic*. UNEP https://doi.org/10.18356/abfaaadd-en.

Vanapalli, K.R., Sharma, H.B., Ranjan, V.P. et al. (2021). Challenges and strategies for effective plastic waste management during and post COVID-19 pandemic. *Science of the Total Environment* 750: 141514. https://doi.org/10.1016/J.SCITOTENV.2020.141514.

Wang, W., Ge, J., Yu, X. et al. (2020). Environmental fate and impacts of microplastics in soil ecosystems: progress and perspective. *The Science of the Total Environment* 708: 134841. https://doi.org/10.1016/j.scitotenv.2019.134841.

Xie, X., Deng, T., Duan, J. et al. (2020). Exposure to polystyrene microplastics causes reproductive toxicity through oxidative stress and activation of the p38 MAPK signaling pathway. *Ecotoxicology and Environmental Safety* 190: 110133. https://doi.org/10.1016/j.ecoenv.2019.110133.

Xu, S., Ma, J., Ji, R. et al. (2020). Microplastics in aquatic environments: Occurrence, accumulation, and biological effects. *The Science of the Total Environment* 703: 134699. https://doi.org/10.1016/j.scitotenv.2019.134699.

Yousefi, M., Oskoei, V., Jonidi Jafari, A. et al. (2021). Municipal solid waste management during COVID-19 pandemic: effects and repercussions. *Environmental Science and Pollution Research* 28 (25): 32200–32209. https://doi.org/10.1007/s11356-021-14214-9.

Zhang, C., Xu, T., Feng, H. et al. (2019). Greenhouse gas emissions from landfills: a review and bibliometric analysis. *Sustainability* https://doi.org/10.3390/su11082282.

Zhang, J., Qin, Q., Li, G. et al. (2021). Sustainable municipal waste management strategies through life cycle assessment method: a review. *Journal of Environmental Management* 287: 112238. https://doi.org/10.1016/J.JENVMAN.2021.112238.

Zhao, X., Korey, M., Li, K. et al. (2022). Plastic waste upcycling toward a circular economy. *Chemical Engineering Journal* 428: 131928. https://doi.org/10.1016/J.CEJ.2021.131928.

17

One Health Approach for Eye Care

Is It a Boon or Hype?

Narayanan Janakiraman[1], *Lakshmi Badrinarayanan*[1], *Dhanashree Ratra*[2], *and Sailaja V. Elchuri*[1]

[1] *Department of Nanobiotechnology, Vision Research Foundation, Sankara Nethralaya, Chennai, India*
[2] *Shri Bhagwan Mahavir Department of Vitreo Retinal Services, Medical Research Foundation, Sankara Nethralaya, Chennai, Tamilnadu, India*

Abbreviations

AGE:	Activated glycated end products
AGM:	Antiglaucoma medication
AH:	Aqueous humor
AMD:	Age-related macular degeneration
ANTI-VEGF:	Anti-vascular endothelial growth factor
COMET:	Cultivated oral mucosa epithelial cell transplantation
DEX:	Dexamethasone/ozurdex
DM:	Diabetes mellitus
DME:	Diabetic macular edema
DR:	Diabetic retinopathy
EGF:	Epidermal growth factor
GC:	Glucocorticosteroid
HLA—B27:	Human leukocyte antigen B27
HPV:	Human papillomavirus
HPyV:	Human polyomavirus
HS:	Hypertension systemic
IRDs:	Inherited retinal disorders
LC:	Laminar cribrosa
LCA:	Leber's congenital amaurosis
LMIC:	Lower- and middle-income countries
MD:	Macular degeneration
ME:	Macular edema
NEISS:	National electronic injury surveillance system
NGS:	Next-generation sequencing
OCT:	Optical coherence tomography
OLEDs:	Organic light-emitting diodes
ONH:	Optic nerve head
POAG:	Primary open-angle glaucoma
RAAS:	Renin-angiotensin-aldosterone system
RB:	Retinoblastoma
RCD:	Rod-cone dystrophy
RGCs:	Retinal ganglion cells
RNF:	Retinal nerve fiber
RP:	Retinitis pigmentosa
RVO:	Retinal vein occlusion
SD:	Stargardt disease
SENSOR:	Sentinel event notification system for occupational risk
SIG:	Steroid-induced glaucoma
SI-OHT:	Steroid-induced ocular hypertension
TA:	Triamcinolone-acetonide
TGF:	Transforming growth factor
TM:	Trabecular meshwork
US:	Usher syndrome
UV:	Ultraviolet
WROD:	Water-related ocular disease

17.1 Introduction

One Health for ocular health approach is coined because of a tripartite agreement between the World Health Organization (WHO), World Organization for Animal Health, and the United Nations that emphasize the interaction between human, animal, and their environmental health (Mackenzie and Jeggo 2019). Now the entire world has seen several pandemics including the current COVID-19. A few examples of the earlier pandemics that affected human health and caused mortality in several people are the Great Plague of Marseille (1720–1723), Russian Plague (1770–1772), Philadelphia Yellow Fever (1793), Flu pandemic (1889–1890), American Polio Pandemic (1916), Spanish Flu (1918–1920), Asian Flu (1957–1958), H1N1 Swine flu (2009–2010), African Ebola

One Health: Human, Animal, and Environment Triad, First Edition. Edited by Meththika Vithanage and Majeti Narasimha Vara Prasad.

Pandemic (2014–2016), Zika virus pandemic (2015) conditions. Approximately 1.7 million viruses are circulating in our environment and most of them are zoonotic (Stanley et al. 1992) (Group GRS et al. 2020). The transboundary outbreaks of viral infections like Ebola, H1N1, and SARS reinforce the need to monitor the linkages between human, wildlife, and the environment (Yadav et al. 2020). Another type of infection is anthroponotic, where there is a transfection between humans to wild animals. Due to the high impact of this interaction between wildlife and the environment on human health, there is an emphasis on the concept of One Health, which is a highly interdisciplinary approach for balancing all three tiers to enhance human and animal health safety (Daszak et al. 2001).

17.2 Eye – The Visual Organ

The eye is a window to the world that helps with the general health of the people by carrying out their day-to-day tasks and maintaining their overall well-being. Human physiology is made up of different components such as cells, tissues, and organs that contribute to overall human health. The functioning of each organ is either directly or indirectly dependent on each other in one way or the other. Several factors affect human health, including genetic factors, dietary habits, and environmental factors. The ocular region is a tissue comprising different structural and functional cells, and it is highly interconnected with the nervous and brain system, which maintains its health. The parts of the eye include the cornea, iris, pupil, choroid, retina, and optic nerve. The cornea consists of the epithelial layer, stromal layer, and endothelial layer (Xuan et al. 2016). The visual processing function of the ocular system is highly dependent on the posterior components of the eye, i.e. retina (Masland 2012). It helps in processing the object's image in coordination with the brain's function (Presland 2007). Further, the ocular health homeostasis includes multifactorial perturbations such as external injury to the ocular tissue, infection by microbial population, aging, and lifestyle. However, other eye diseases are prevalent that can lead to vision loss.

17.3 Eye Diseases

The most common diseases of the eye that cause vision defects are cataract, refractive errors, diabetic retinopathy (DR), macular edema (ME), and glaucoma (Figure 17.1). Cataract – the clouding of the lens – is reported in 45% of the Indian population, which develops slowly over time, and usually, phacoemulsification surgery is done to restore

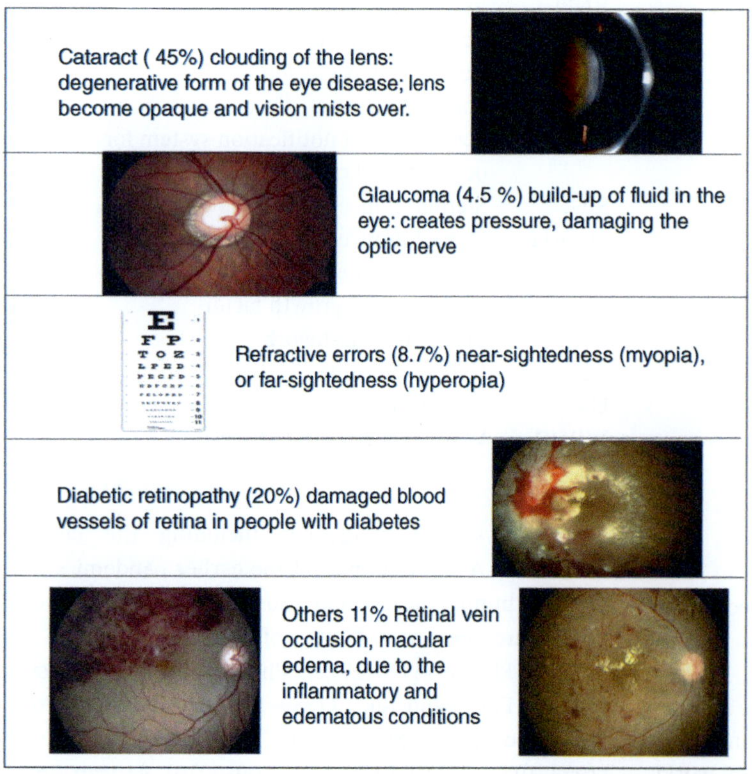

Figure 17.1 Common eye diseases in India. The percentage of common diseases are represented.

the vision. The common refractive error problems of the lens are myopia, hyperopia, astigmatism, and presbyopia, which account for 8% of vision threats in India (Sengupta et al. 2020). Glaucoma affects 4.6% of the population, which occurs due to the increased intraocular pressure of the eye (above 21 mmHg). The remaining 11% of the vision threat is contributed by posterior ocular inflammatory and edematous conditions including age-related macular degeneration (AMD), DR, and retinal vein occlusion (RVO), in which the vein that carries blood from the retina gets impaired. Keratoconus and keratitis are the few minor ailments that affect cornea accounting for 2.3% of the population.

17.4 Cornea and Its Diseases

The ocular surface comprises the epithelium of the cornea, conjunctiva, lachrymal gland, meibomian glands, and the tears, eyelashes, and eyelids with their glands. The cornea is the outermost transparent layer of the eye made up of the epithelial, stromal, and endothelial layers, respectively. The cornea receives the light from the environment and refracts it through the lens and makes it fall on the retina (Freegard 1997). The concordance of all these ocular parts performs the visual function and helps in maintaining the ocular health homeostasis. The conditions that affect corneal health include corneal injury, epithelial injury, microbial infection, and pollution (Figure 17.2).

17.4.1 Corneal Injury

The multiplayer corneal epithelial tissue prevents any microbial infections or interactions by the tight junction connections between the neighboring cells (Guttman and Finlay 2009). This filtering barrier function of epithelial tissue is being maintained by the cadherin–catenin complex (Tian et al. 2011). Corneal injuries can occur due to external injury, microbial infection, alkali or acid burn injuries, pollution, aging, and lifestyle changes (Figure 17.1), which can lead to infection susceptibility, stromal ulceration, scarring, and loss of visual acuity (Wilson et al. 2018).

17.4.2 Epithelial Injury

The nanoparticles or microparticles in the environment can bring about physical assaults (mechanical/brutal force) and/or chemical injury to the eyes inducing the damage of epithelial cells (Lasagni Vitar et al. 2019). Consequently, the architecture of corneal epithelium and stromal structures gets altered. This in turn leads to barrier dysfunction and an imbalance of the eye's homeostasis, which paves way for the microbial invasion (Augustin et al. 2011).

17.4.3 Microbial Infection

Various kinds of bacteria, viruses, and fungi can enter the eye through the cornea due to the corneal and epithelial injury, which can alter the light that falls on the retina leading to vision loss. The modus operandi of the pathogens and host ocular cells' response is completely different for each class of microbes (Vemuganti et al. 2011).

17.4.4 Gradation of the Damage

Overall, corneal injuries are classified into four grades. Wherein Grade I is confined to the corneal epithelium, Grade II includes injuries that affect the mild corneal haze, Grade III significantly causes limbus region ischemia, and Grade IV involves limbal stem cells loss. The detailed description of these grades is explained below. Several classifications do exist to describe the impact of chemical injuries on the ocular surface, guide management, and prognosis. The common factor among the various schemes

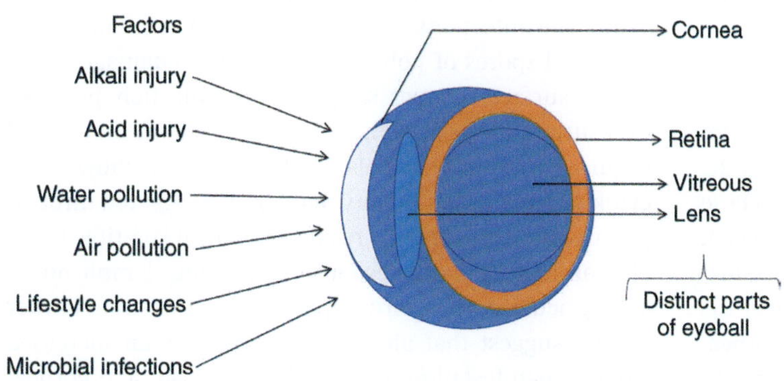

Figure 17.2 Corneal injuries due to external/environmental factors. Grade I is confined to the corneal epithelium, Grade II injuries are significant for mild corneal haze, Grade III is significant ischemia of the limbus region, and Grade IV is loss of limbal stem cells.

is a clinical presentation of the extent of conjunctival, limbal, and corneal damage at the time of initial diagnosis. The presence and degree of limbal ischemia and corneal haze are used to classify the severity. The depth of corneal involvement, including endothelial injury, may also be a prognostic marker. The Hughes classification scheme, as modified by Thoft, divides chemical injuries into four categories in order of worsening severity and prognosis.

Grade I: These injuries are confined to the corneal epithelium and there is no limbal ischemia, and the cornea is clear. These injuries carry an excellent long-term visual prognosis. **Grade II:** Injuries are significant for mild corneal haze. The presence of focal limbal ischemia and view of anterior chamber structures are the chief features. The prognosis appears to be good, but sometimes the cornea may have a focal haze and neovascularization at the site of limbal stem cell loss. **Grade III:** These injuries are characterized by significant ischemia of the limbus region and lead to the profound corneal haze that limits the view of anterior chamber structures. Due to limbal stem cell loss, patients with Grade III injuries have a limited prognosis. The corneal epithelium cannot regenerate, and the ocular surface undergoes conjunctivalization to maintain tectonic stability. This happens at the loss of visual acuity. Surgical procedure is often needed to improve the vision. **Grade IV:** This type of damage has the worst prognosis. Total loss of limbal stem cells happens. There is also damage to the proximal conjunctival epithelium. The cornea completely becomes opaque and porcelainized. This leads to melting in the acute or intermediate time frames after injury. Visual recovery may be impossible.

17.5 Types of Corneal Injuries

17.5.1 Chemical Injuries

Corneal injuries are brought about by alkali or acid, particulate components of the air and water in the environment.

17.5.1.1 Alkali Injury

Alkali injury is one of the contributors to environmental-induced vision damage. Alkali injury is caused by several chemical reagents like caustic soda, sodium hydroxide, ammonia, and calcium hydroxide (Dua et al. 2001). These chemicals are found in day-to-day use like washing powder, paint, etc. The chemical exposure happens during occupational hazards, and the affected tissues undergo necrosis (Sommer et al. 1982). Strong alkali can reach the cornea, anterior chamber of the eye including trabecular meshwork (TM), lens, and ciliary body. Direct exposure of alkali to the conjunctiva can lead to scarring, symblepharon formation, cicatricial ectropion, or entropion. If the goblet cells are damaged, it can lead to a lifetime of dry eye syndrome. Severe burns up to the limbal region can give rise to limbal stem cell deficiency. This may result in opacification and neovascularization of the cornea due to the loss of corneal epithelial progenitor cells. If the damage occurs in TM cells, it can lead to glaucoma that may, in turn, affect the retinal ganglion cells (RGCs) in the posterior segment of the eye (Dohlman et al. 2019).

17.5.1.2 Acid Injury

Acid burns are generally less destructive than the alkali counterparts and usually occur with exposure to strong acids that have a pH of less than 4 (Friedenwald et al. 1944). Hydrochloric acid (used to clean swimming pools) and sulfuric acid (found in car batteries) are some of the more common acids encountered in emergency settings. Acids tend to denature, coagulate, and precipitate the corneal proteins on contact, creating a barrier that prevents deeper penetration of the acid. This protein coagulation produces the ground-glass appearance of the cornea often seen in severe acid burns. Hydrofluoric acid (used in antirust solutions and glass etching) is an exception to the acid injuries of the cornea, as the fluoride ion can rapidly penetrate the entire thickness of the cornea through cell membranes, causing significant corneal and anterior segment destruction (Peters and Miethchen 1996). Systemic acid burns covering more than 2% of the body surface area are associated with severe hypocalcemia and can have fatal neurological, respiratory, and cardiovascular consequences.

17.5.2 Particulate Injury

17.5.2.1 Pollution

Air pollution is the biggest menace in growing cities worldwide. It hampers public health including ocular corneal surfaces. Particulate matter of different dimensions present in polluted air accumulates on the ocular surface to make a dent through which microbial infections can pervade. The infections can be immediately initiated from microbial spores of polluted air leading to damage to the ocular surface. Herpes simplex virus infection precedes exposure to air pollution, and it triggers both innate and acquired immunity imbalance. Studies have shown that cytokines and inflammatory markers are triggered through polluted air exposure that results in corneal keratitis. It can also promote a T-cell response in draining lymph nodes during acute simplex virus type 1 corneal infection. Earlier reports suggest that air pollution provokes an increased clinical manifestation of keratitis, viral load, and corneal inflammation (Sendra et al. 2021). Polluted air also promotes the recruitment of dendritic immune cells to the infection site during the early days of infection. Hence, environmental health is more important for ocular health.

17.5.2.2 Water Pollution

This pollution significantly affects the ocular surface through different mechanisms. It has been termed as "water-related ocular disease" (WROD) to express the wide spectrum of diseases associated with water pollution. The impact of water pollution on the ocular surface can be classified broadly into two types, non-infectious and infectious WROD (Ahmad 2018).

17.5.2.3 Non-Infectious Waterborne Infections

These are usually related to swimming pools, ocean swimming, or water sports that cause exposure of contaminated water to the ocular surface (https://www.cdc.gov/mmwr/preview/mmwrhtml/mm5804a3.htm). In general, chemicals added to the water in a swimming pool would bring allergic conjunctivitis to the exposed individuals. This can lead to ocular irritation with persistent eye rubbing resulting in corneal abrasions. The data sentinel event notification system for occupational risk (SENSOR) – pesticide surveillance program from National Electronic Injury Surveillance System (NEISS) data – mentioned that 33 to 42% cases of waterborne diseases were through the swimming pool (Shields et al. 2011). The pool sanitizing chemicals used are trichloramine or nitrogen trichloride, calcium/sodium hypochlorite, and chlorinated isocyanuric acid. These free chlorine chemicals after reacting with swimmers' body fluid result in the formation of trihalomethanes and chloramine that are the main reason for ocular irritation (Florentin et al. 2011). Water sports-related corneal injuries like kayaking contests or water scooters in the river or ocean can lead to a forceful splash of water onto the ocular surface, bringing about mechanical as well as chemical damage to the corneal tissue. Earlier reports on such water sports incidents mentioned the rupture of the Descemet membrane due to the chemicals present in the water and its force on the ocular surface (Mousa et al. 2018).

17.5.2.4 Infectious Waterborne Diseases

Five *Acanthamoeba* spp. cause ocular-specific waterborne infections. These are *A. polyphagia, A. castellani, A. hatchetti, A. culbertson*, and *A. rhodes*, which form keratitis when they come in contact with the ocular surface (Kilvington et al. 2004). Further, giardiasis infection is caused by protozoa named *Giardia lamblia*. The spores or cysts of the protozoans are excreted through fecal matter into the water. These spore/cysts-contaminated water can bring ocular-specific infections such as iridocyclitis, choroiditis, retinal hemorrhage, retinal vasculitis, peculiar pepper, and salt retinal degeneration.

17.5.2.5 Treatment of Corneal Injury

The treatment procedures for the alkali- and acid-damaged corneal injuries are currently in practice based on the severity and grade of the infection. If the tissue is damaged by acid/alkali, the pH would not be in the physiologic range. Hence, it needs to be irrigated to bring it to normal pH, which is the initial treatment, followed by using antibiotics based on the grade of injury. Erythromycin is a typical drug used for Grade I injury. For the remaining grades, stronger antibiotics like topical fluoroquinolone are preferred. Artificial tears are used to bring lubrication to the eyes. In some cases, clinicians also use steroids to prevent further local inflammation and corneal breakdown (Oh et al. 2008). Other treatments include the use of ascorbic acid (vitamin C) if the stromal collagen is broken during the chemical injury, which restores the collagen fibers in the corneal stroma. If any corneal tissue is necrosed on injury, it needs to be debrided as soon as possible. The delay in debridement of necrotic tissue invites inflammation and can inhibit epithelization. Amniotic membrane transplantation is another procedure to restore the conjunctival surface, limbal stem cells, and stromal cells. This procedure brings physical and biological benefits to the injured ocular surface. Additionally, it helps in reducing the biological friction between the conjunctiva and the eyelid. It also secretes transforming growth factor (TGF)-β and epidermal growth factor (EGF), which assist in the wound healing process. Another way of treating the chemical injury is through a limbal stem cell transplant, which repopulates the corneal epithelium for healthy homeostasis. Limbal stem cell transplantation helps in the speedy recovery of corneal epithelial cells and provides wound healing after a chemical injury. Cultivated oral mucosa epithelial cell transplantation (COMET) is yet another treatment method, which promotes re-epithelization upon corneal injury. The mucosal cells are isolated from the patients, grown in vitro, and transplanted to the ocular injury site to promote re-epithelialization. The advantage of COMET will be that immunosuppression is not needed for these patients.

17.6 Retina and Its Diseases

The normal retina has a shiny, healthy reflex central macula, which is the most important part of the fine vision (Figure 17.3a). A healthy optic nerve head (ONH) shows a pink appearance, which is composed of major blood vessels, the central retinal artery, and veins. ONH can be viewed with the help of non-invasive optical coherence tomography (OCT) scan, which (Figure 17.3b) helps in understanding the various diseases affecting the retina and assesses the effects of treatment such as the intravitreal

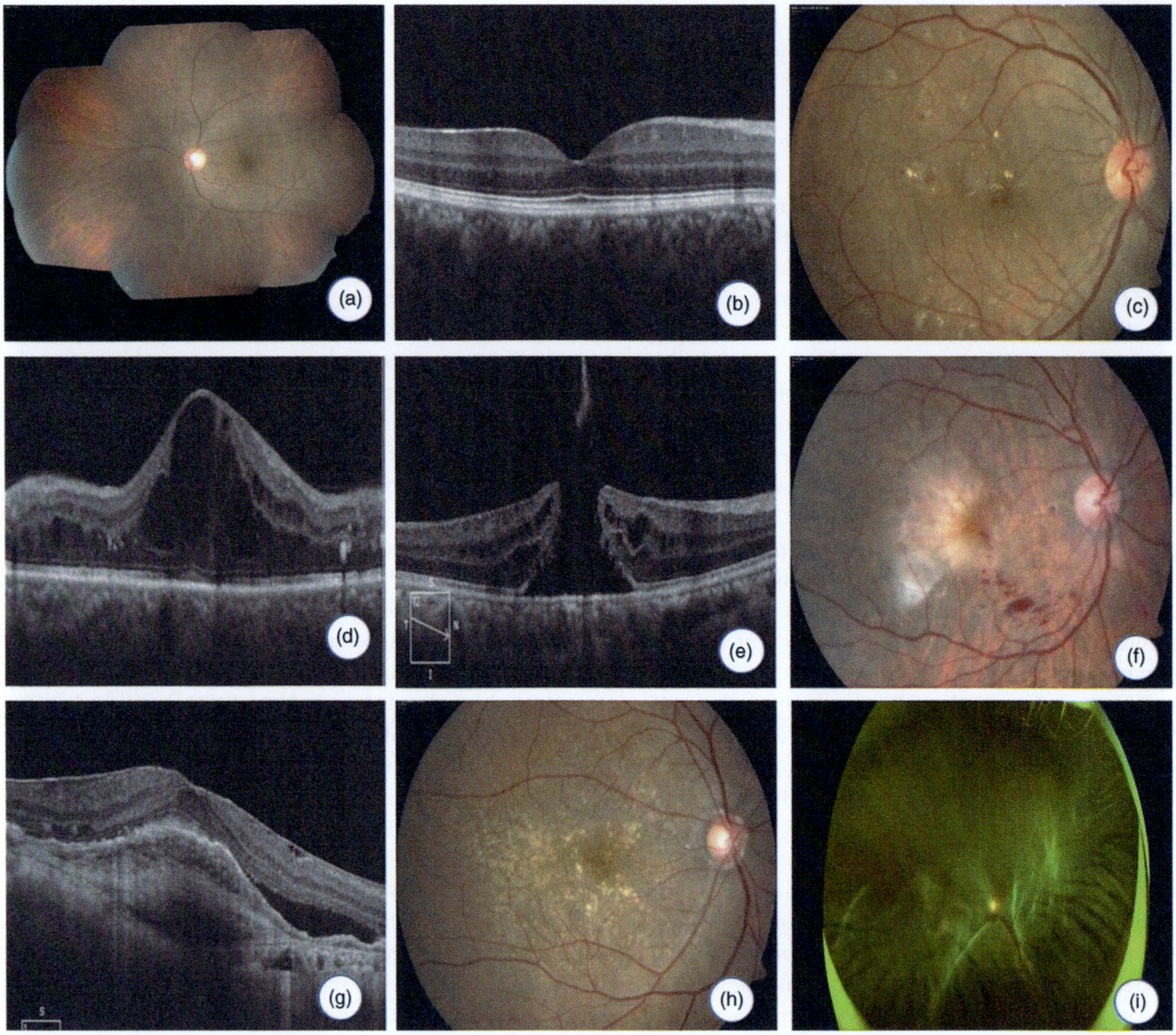

Figure 17.3 Retina and retinal diseases. (a) Shows a montage picture of a normal retina. (b) The horizontal section of an optical coherence tomography (OCT) scan of a normal retina shows the different layers of the retina, the central dip called the fovea, and a normal thickness of the retina. (c) This retinal photo shows nonproliferative diabetic retinopathy. (d) OCT scan shows thickening of the central retina known as macular edema in diabetic retinopathy (e) The OCT scan shows a break in the continuity of the retinal layer called a full-thickness macular hole. (f) Shows a grayish white subretinal choroidal neovascular membrane due to wet age-related macular degeneration. (g) This OCT scan shows a fibrovascular membrane growth under the macular area. (h) Shows dry AMD with plenty of yellow subretinal deposits called drusen. (i) A widefield photo shows partial retinal detachment.

glucocorticosteroid (GC) and anti-vascular endothelial growth factor (anti-VEGF) injections.

17.6.1 Diabetic Macular Edema (DME) and Diabetic Retinopathy (DR)

The diabetic patients predominantly possess changes in their retina due to the systemic disease. The disease is termed diabetic retinopathy (DR) (Figure 17.3c). The retinal vessels in diabetes mellitus (DM) subjects become leaky due to microvascular changes and loss of pericytes. This leads to superficial and deep hemorrhages in the retina with hard exudates and retinal thickening called macular edema (Figure 17.3d). Subjects with DM and hypertension systemic (HS) are at higher risk for DME and DR incidence. In DME, there is a disruption in the central part of the macula, due to the blood–retinal barrier (BRB) degeneration, and oxidative stress, which could increase vascular permeability. This is influenced by the renin-angiotensin-aldosterone system (RAAS) that regulates the blood pressure system. Angiotensin II is primarily involved in the vasoconstriction activity of the retinal cells that stimulates the higher secretion of VEGF in the retinal layer leading to angiogenesis (Callanan et al. 2013). Alternatively, hyperglycemic condition, oxidative stress (hypoxia), activation of proteinase kinase C, free radical synthesis, increased induction of VEGF and leukocytes adhesion molecules, endothelial cells dysfunction, and pro-inflammatory cytokines can result in the activated glycated end products (AGE) production leading to DME occurrence. Eventually, the changes observed in DME can progress to neovascularization that can proceed to the formation of fibrovascular membranes on the retina, bleeding inside the eye called vitreous hemorrhage, and retinal detachment. All these cause severe and sometimes permanent loss of vision. Periodic screening and timely treatment with intravitreal anti-VEGF and GC injections can prevent the DR progression (Figure 17.3c) and prevent vision loss. With an exponential increase in the number of diabetics in India, DR is seen to affect 18–20% of DM subjects.

17.6.2 Macular Hole

Following an injury, at times the central macular region becomes completely thick, termed as macular hole, which is generally seen in older age people (Figure 17.3e). This needs to be corrected by a vitrectomy surgery during which a mixture of an expansile gas is injected inside the eye. The patient is instructed to maintain a prone position. This maneuver gives the anticipated closure of the macular hole and improves vision.

17.6.3 Age-Related Macular Degeneration

AMD exists in two forms – dry and wet form (Figure 17.3f–h). In the wet form, there is development of a choroidal neovascular membrane and fluid accumulation under the retina in the macular area, causing membrane bleeding and leakage in the central part leading to profound central vision loss (Figure 17.3g). Dry AMD is a common cause of blindness in the elderly population and necessitates treatment with anti-VEGF usage. In dry AMD, atrophy of the central retinal tissues occurs leading to central vision loss slowly over many years (Figure 17.3h).

17.6.4 Retinal Detachment

The holes or tear in the retina causes retinal weakness and its detachment (Figure 17.3i). Treatment modality includes scleral buckle, pneumoretinopexy, or vitrectomy surgeries with appropriate head positioning.

17.6.5 Inherited Retinal Disorders

Inherited retinal disorders (IRDs) include a group of diseases that is caused due to mutations that are inherited from parents. IRDs include retinitis pigmentosa (RP), MD, rod-cone dystrophy (RCD), Usher syndrome (US), Leber's congenital amaurosis (LCA), and Stargardt disease (SD). The disease-causing mutations follow a Mendelian mode of inheritance and could be due to autosomal dominant, recessive, or X-linked inheritances (Figure 17.4a). Several other mutations are inherited via non-Mendelian fashion consisting of complex inheritance patterns including mitochondrial inheritances. However, the genetics of the disease is still evolving where the inheritance pattern is unknown in 50–70% of individuals with these ocular ailments. There are mutations in almost 300 genes (RetNet: https://sph.uth.edu/retnet; last accessed March 2022) that can cause IRDs. Some mutated genes associated with IRDs are common among various groups of diseases (Figure 17.4b). For example, two genes are common between RP and US; 12 mutated genes are common between US and retinopathy, whereas 9 genes are common between RP and LCA. Several mutated genes could be unique for each IRD group member. RP is a well-studied IRD and is known to occur in several ethnicities.

Several methods are available to date to detect these variants associated with disease progression. Next-generation sequencing (NGS) technique is one of the powerful techniques that could sequence DNA from patients at a lower cost and in a high throughput manner to get the genetic landscape of an individual affected with the disease (Audo et al. 2012; Glöckle et al. 2014; Yohe et al. 2020). Panel-based genetic testing is also reported in addition to exome sequencing in association with disease progression (Consugar et al. 2015). There is a need for understanding the inheritance pattern of the disease, and there are several studies that are published to date from different populations cohort-based studies (Table 17.1). A study of 2420 families from Israel identified RP as the most prevalent disease in autosomal recessive fashion (Sharon et al. 2020). Biswas et al. identified 35 novel variants in Indian and American IRD patients. Additionally, several patients had unclassified retinal diseases (RD), indicating that more understanding of the disease progression and clinical manifestations is still needed. The prevalence of disease was higher in Iranian families who married their close relatives (Salmaninejad et al. 2020). Usually, endogamy, geographic isolation, and marrying in relations can cause increased mutations in populations for a particular trait. If parents are related, even though they are heterozygous for a common allele that they are carrying from ancestors, there is a high chance of their children becoming homozygous for the trait and showing disease associated with the mutated gene. IRD was investigated in large families including multiple ethnicities. Clinical characterization of patients revealed RD and vision loss (de Laat et al. 2013; Ozawa et al. 2019; Pontikos et al. 2020), maternal inheritance, and mutations in mitochondrial genes associated with IRD

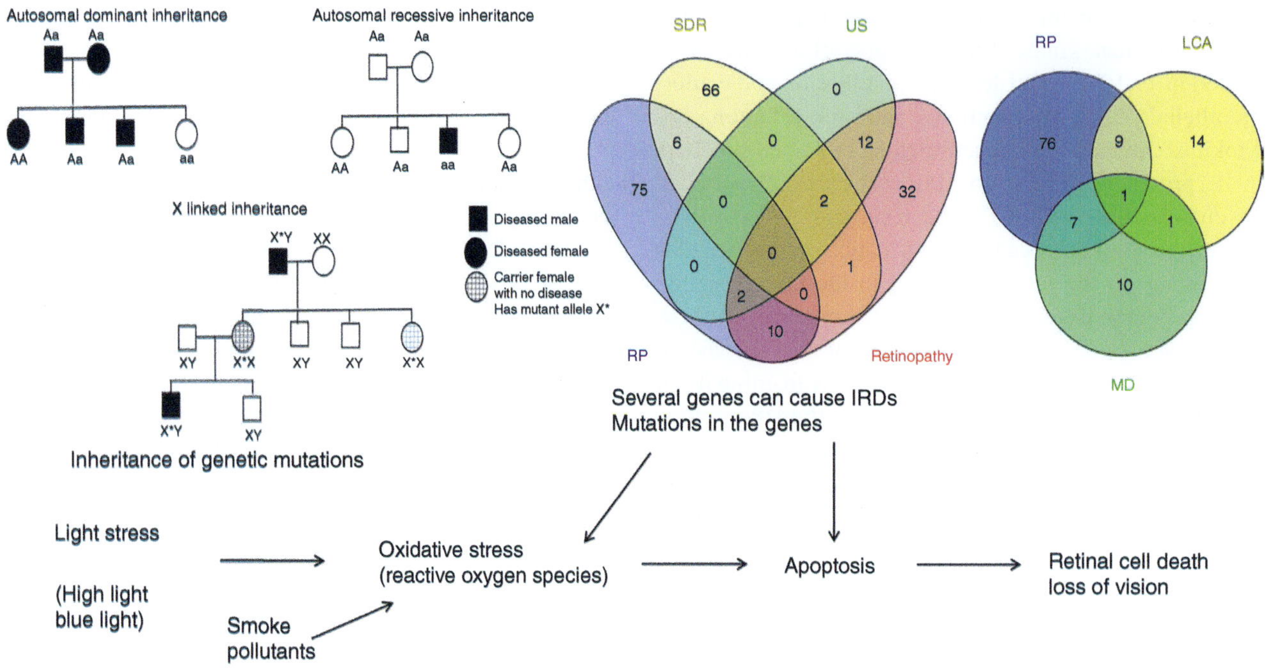

Figure 17.4 Mode of inheritance, genes causing the disease, and probable mechanisms of retinal degeneration in inherited retinal disorders. IRDs consist of several diseases that are caused by unique genes for a particular disease and common genes that can cause multiple diseases. The genes that cause diseases are downloaded from RETNET database and analyzed using Venny 2.0 (for full list check the database). Retinitis pigmentosa is a well-studied disorder with a greater number of genes identified. So this was used as a comparison to identify common genes in IRDs. A) Genes causing retinitis pigmentosa (RP) were compared to syndromic/systemic diseases with retinopathy (syndromic/systemic diseases with retinopathy [SDS]), Leber's congenital amaurosis (LCA), macular degeneration (MD), Usher syndrome (US), and other retinopathy.

progression. Mitochondrial dysfunction affects the cellular energy balance and function. The constituents of the retina including retinal pigment epithelium (RPE), rods, cones, and RGC functions are energy-demanding cells needing higher energy from mitochondrial metabolism including oxidative phosphorylation (Lock et al. 2020). The dysfunctional mitochondria caused by mutations could lead to energy imbalance and oxidative stress in IRD patients leading to RGC death (Figure 17.4c). Nonsyndromic cases included only ocular degeneration features associated with IRDs. In several cases, ocular manifestations can identify systemic complications and are termed syndromic IRD. The other affected organs could be the central nervous system, ears, musculoskeletal system, kidney, and heart (Tatour and Ben-Yosef 2020). A study of large Spanish families identified the occurrence of both syndromic and non-syndromic IRDs (Perea-Romero et al. 2021). The syndromic disease studies can counsel patients about the probability of diseases to life-threatening vital organs.

There are environmental–gene interactions for differential disease manifestations from the same gene for IRD disease progression. However, the factors governing them are not clearly understood and need further evaluation (Pierrache et al. 2016). The complex pattern of the disease is modeled recently, computationally, and the inheritance pattern is studied in six different populations worldwide (Hanany et al. 2020). In this work, researchers analyzed 276,921 variants and predicted that 10,044 could be IRD-causing variants. Additionally, it is also predicted that affected individuals could be 1 in 1380 people, which is a very high prevalence. Furthermore, about 2.7 billion people could be carriers of the disease making an enormous possibility of passing on the disease to future generations. The high carrier frequency makes it a disease of importance that should be studied and proper measures to be undertaken to educate people on the causative factors associated with the disease. There are environmental factors that could hasten the disease progression. Therefore, environmental education in addition to genetic counseling is the need of the hour.

17.6.5.1 Therapies for IRD

Genetic counseling is usually performed to discuss and understand the disease-causing alleles, probable inheritance factors passing from parents to offspring, and therapy options. Previously therapy options were limited for inherited disorders. However, the FDA approval of the gene

Country	Cohort details	Data observed			Reference
Israel	2420 families with 3413 people	Retinitis pigmentosa (RP) is the most common retinal phenotype (43%), followed by Stargardt disease (STGD), and cone/cone-rod dystrophy	ABCA4, USH2A, FAM161A, CNGA3, and EYS (603 mutations in 129 genes)	Autosomal recessive (60%), autosomal dominant (8%), and X-linked (6%)	Sharon et al. (2020)
Pakistani, Mexican, Indian, European pedigrees	409 individuals from 108 families	RP in 18, cone dystrophy in 1, macular dystrophy in 1, Leber's congenital amaurosis (LCA) in 2, Usher syndrome in 2, with the majority (Ozawa et al. 2019) having unclassified retinal degeneration	93 causative variants, 35 novel and 54 previously reported variants detected in 45 known IRD *AGBL5* and *IFT88*	9 were homozygous (in 8 pedigrees), 21 compound heterozygous (in 10 pedigrees), 2 dominant acting heterozygous (in 2 pedigrees), and 2 were X-linked variants (in 2 pedigrees)	Biswas et al. (2021)
Iranian families		Variants were found in LCA, cone-rod dystrophy, STGD, RP	9 pathogenic variants in 6IRD-associated genes (*ABCA4, MERTK, RPE65, SPATA7, TULP1*, and *USH2A*)	Autosomal recessive inheritance	Salmaninejad et al. (2020)
Affected individuals 62.2% were White, 17.9% were Asian (largely South Asian), 7.0% were Black, and 1.8% were of mixed race or ethnicity	3195 families consisting of 4236 affected individuals	Rod-cone dystrophy (49%), macular dystrophy (35%), inherited optic neuropathy (4.9%), Leber's congenital amaurosis or early onset severe retinal dystrophy (3%), rod dysfunction syndrome (3%), cone dysfunction syndrome (2%), and familial exudative vitreoretinopathy (2%)	Variants in 135 genes. Top genes with variation *ABCA4* (20.8%), *USH2A* (9.1%), *RPGR* (5.1%), *ARPH2* (4.6%), *BEST1* (3.9%), *RS1* (3.5%), *RP1* (3.3%), *RHO* (3.3%), *CHM* (2.7%), *CRB1* (2.1%), *PRPF31* (1.8%), *MY07A* (1.7%), *OPA1* (1.6), *CNGB3* (1.4%), *RPE65* (1.2%), *EYS* (1.2%), *GUCY2D* (1.2%), *PROM1* (1.2%), *CNGA3* (1.1%), *RDH12* (1.1%)	Recessive, dominant, and X-linked	Pontikos et al. (2020)
Spain	6089, 4403 unrelated families	RP (50%), 47% of the syndromic IRD cases were *USH2*, 17% *USH1* (98/577), atypical forms of Usher syndrome, ciliopathies such as *BBS* or *ALMS* (16%)	Variants in 142 different genes frequently mutated *ABCA4, USH2A, RS1, CRB1, RHO*	Sporadic (53.6%), recessive inheritance (40.2%), remaining 6.2% includes dominant (0.5%), X-linked (0.7%), mitochondrial inherited disease (0.2%), and non-classifiable cases (4.8%)	Perea-Romero et al. (2021)
Taiwan	312 families	RP (65.7%), the most macular dystrophy (12.5%), cone dystrophy/cone-rod dystrophy 6.1%), LCA (5.1%), Bietti's crystalline dystrophy (3.8%), occult macular dystrophy (1.6%), retinoschisis (RS, $n = 4$, 1.3%), choroideremia 0.6%), familial exudative vitreoretinopathy (0.6%), Alstrom syndrome (0.6%), others ($n = 6$, 1.9%)	*ABCA4* STGD, RP, CRD, *EYS, USH2A, CYP4V2, RPGR, PRPF31, RP1L1, PROM1, CEP290, BEST1, RP1*, and *GUCY2D*	64.6% autosomal recessive (AR) inheritance, whereas 26.4% autosomal dominant (AD) inheritance and 9.0% had X-linked (XL) inheritance	Chen et al. (2021)
China	800 families including 12 Consagmous families	RP (438) cone-rod dystrophy (116), Bietti crystalline corneoretinal dystrophy (Srivastava et al. 2021), LCA (Perea-Romero et al. 2021), Stargardt disease (Perea-Romero et al. 2021) individuals	*CYP4V2, BEST1, CHM, RSM, RPGR* by Sanger sequencing, *ABCA4, RPGR, USH2A* by *NGS 475* variants in 75 genes	Approximately 11.64% of 481 cases carried autosomal dominant variants, 72.97% carried AR variants, and 15.39% were found to be X-linked	Liu et al. (2021)
My Retina Tracker® – a US repository	United States (94%), 8 countries representing 75% of the international membership. Canada (14%), United Kingdom (8.9%), India (8.2%), Italy (7.1%), Mexico (6.5%), South Africa (5%), Australia (4.5%), Poland (4.2%), Germany (3.5%), Argentina (2.2%), Brazil (1.8%), France (1.7%), Netherlands (1.6%), and New Zealand (1.3%)	51% RP, including LCA, Stargardt disease, and all forms of Usher syndrome (10%), juvenile inherited macular dystrophy at 6%, 5% unknown	(6.8%) *PRPH2*, (4.8%) *RHO*, (4.7%) *EYS*, (2.6%) *BEST1*, (2.4%) *PRPF31*, (2.4%) *CRB1*, (2.3%) *RS1*, (2%) others		Fisher et al. (2016)

therapy drug, LUXTURA™, for LCA focused interest to find therapies for IRDs by pharmaceutical companies. Drugs for IRDs include gene therapy constructs mediated by adenovirus, antisense nucleic acid-based therapies, and nano-drugs. The drugs are in several phases of clinical trials registered at https://clinicaltrials.gov. The trials that are happening presently for IRD therapy are given in Table 17.2. These drugs are promising drugs for IRDs if they have successful outcomes, and they will be approved by FDA. However, environmental factors such as excessive light and pollution can enhance the degradation of photoreceptor cells and can accelerate genetically IRD progression leading to blindness.

17.6.5.2 Gene–Environmental Interactions in Inherited Retinal Diseases

AMD and RP (IRDs) cause reduction of photoreceptor cells by degradation and apoptotic cell death. The disease progression was observed to increase after the application of high light in animal models of RP, Oguchi disease, and Stargardt macular dystrophy. This observation indicates an enhanced effect of environmental factors on mutated genes (Paskowitz et al. 2006). A mouse model of RP was used to study the effect of light intensities (5, 50, and 500 Lux). In this mouse model, the phosphodiesterase 6b (Pde6b) gene had missense mutation resulting in misfolding of the protein and mimics the photoreceptor cell degradation observed in human RP disease (Wang et al. 2018). The increase in light intensity resulted in higher degradation of photoreceptors in the RP model compared to the normal mice. Furthermore, higher morphological changes, loss of synaptic connectivity, increased inflammatory cells, and oxidative stress lead to retinal degradation upon the light-induced stress (Kutsyr et al. 2020). Gut microbes were also observed to be altered in RP mice compared to normal control mice. The common bacteria such as *Rikenella* spp., *Muribaculaceace* spp., *Prevotellaceae* UGC-001 spp., and *Bacilli* spp. are present in normal mice, but *Bacteroides caecimuris* was found to be increased substantially in RP (Kutsyr et al. 2020). Interestingly, the gut microbiome was altered favoring bacteria that cause inflammation. Additionally, the fat diet administration in the same RP mouse model resulted in increased oxidative stress, photoreceptor cell degradation, and Müller glial cells loss. Hence, nutrition was indicated to play a vital role in IRD progression, in addition to high light stress (Kutsyr et al. 2020). Light-emitting diode (LED) lights are known to accelerate photoreceptor degeneration in RP patients, and photophobia is common in IRD patients. Short wavelength lights play a major role in this phenomenon (Otsuka et al. 2020). Recently, glasses that selectively filter blue and violet light are used for better vision in IRD patients (Colombo et al. 2017).

17.6.6 Glaucoma

Glaucoma is a group of chronic optic nephropathies that occur due to structural malfunctioning of two key ocular tissues, TM, and laminar cribrosa (LC) tissues (Saccà et al. 2015). TM is a web-like reticulated layer lined at the iridocorneal junction in the anterior chamber of the eye. TM's function is to maintain the eye's homeostasis by regulating aqueous humor (AH) production, circulation, and outflow. There is an impairment in the AH function that causes mechanical stress on TM and LC layers during stress conditions. Therefore, the function of the optic nerve (transmission of visual signals from the eye to the brain as neuronal signals) gets disturbed due to the distortion of LC (Weinreb et al. 2014; Wallace and O'Brien 2016). Consequently, the neuro-retinal rim layer gets thinner, leading to the loss of the central optic nerve axons with curvature-like depression referred to as a cup. These factors contribute to increased intra ocular pressures (IOP) and cup to disc ratio, loss of retinal nerve fiber (RNF) tissue, and thus RGC death (Smith et al. 2017). The burden of glaucoma in India is on a sharp rise in people of age 40–80 years, and it is estimated to reach nearly 80 million in the current decade (Ahmad et al. 2020). The factors such as genetic predisposition inflammation, ischemia, hypoxia, and oxidative stress also contribute to primary glaucoma pathogenesis (Tong et al. 2017).

17.6.6.1 External Therapeutic Drugs That Can Cause Glaucoma

There are a few instances wherein external therapeutic drugs could cause secondary glaucoma. One such adverse effect is using glucocorticoids (GC) which leads to steroid-induced glaucoma (SIG) or steroid-induced ocular hypertension (SI-OHT) in the eye. The deleterious side effect had been known for more than three decades. However, research in this field is still inconclusive. GC belongs to the family of corticosteroids that possess anti-inflammatory, anti-edematous, and antioxidant properties (Behar-Cohen 2018). Two chief functions of GCs are transactivation (anti-inflammatory cytokine expression in the nucleus) and transrepression (suppression of pro-inflammatory cytokines in the cytosol) (Patel et al. 2019). GCs are the second line of treatment paradigm for posterior ocular edematous and inflammatory conditions of RVO and ME, which are beneficial over the primary anti-VEGF usage. Different formulations of GC are available to date, which vary in their solubility, glucocorticoid receptor (GR) binding efficiency, affinity, lipophilicity, and pharmacokinetic profile, determining their therapeutic potential (Becker 2013). In the current decade, triamcinolone-acetonide (TA) and dexamethasone/ozurdex (Dex) are the

Table 17.2 Clinical trials associated with IRDs.

Number	Company	Characteristics	Phase 1
NCT05122442 2021	Novartis and SENSGENE/ Strasbourg University Hospitals (HUS)	Understand the epidemiology of IRDs, particularly the distribution of pathogenic variants in patients	Noninterventional
NCT00378742	NEI/NIH	National Ophthalmic Genotyping Network (eyeGENE)	DNA Bank
NCT03316560	Applied Genetics Technologies Corporation	This study will evaluate the safety and efficacy of a recombinant adeno-associated virus vector (rAAV2tYF-GRK1-RPGR) in patients with X-linked retinitis pigmentosa caused by RPGR mutations	Phase 1 and 2
NCT04671433	MeiraGTx UK II Ltd., Janssen Research & Development, LLC	A clinical trial of AAV5-RPGR vector for patients with X-linked retinitis pigmentosa (XLRP) biological, genetic, AAV5-RPGR, and with variants in the RPGR gene	Phase 3
NCT04611503	STZ eyetrial	Drug: subretinal injection of rAAV.hPDE6A, the goal of the *pigment* study is to develop, produce, and investigate a recombinant adeno-associated viral (AAV) gene transfer vector for the curative therapy of PDE6A-linked retinitis pigmentosa in patients	Phase 1 and 2
NCT05085964	ProQR Therapeutics	QR 421a administered via intravitreal (IVT) injection in one or both eyes, in subjects ≥18 years of age with RP due to mutations in exon 13 of the USH2A gene, retinitis pigmentosa, Usher syndrome type 2 patients (RNA: RNA antisense oligonucleotide)	Phase 2
NCT04919473	Nanoscope Therapeutics Inc.	This open-label dose-escalation study evaluated 2 dose levels in up to 11 subjects of retinitis pigmentosa (3 in low dose and 8 in high dose per dose) with active vMCO-010. Subjects with confirmed diagnosis of advanced retinitis pigmentosa (RP)	Phase 1 and 2
NCT03872479	Editas Medicine, Inc.	To evaluate the safety, tolerability, and efficacy of single escalating doses of EDIT-101 administered via subretinal injection in participants with LCA10 caused by a homozygous or compound heterozygous mutation involving c.2991+1655A>G in intron 26 of the CEP290 gene ("LCA10-IVS26"). Disease: Leber's congenital amaurosis	Phase 1 and 2
NCT04123626	ProQR Therapeutics	This study evaluates the safety, tolerability, and efficacy of QR-1123 injection in the eye, (intravitreal; IVT) injections subjects with autosomal dominant retinitis pigmentosa due to the P23H mutation in the RHO gene (AURORA)	Phase 1 and 2
NCT04855045	ProQR Therapeutics	PQ-110-005 (BRIGHTEN) is an open-label, dose escalation, and double-masked, randomized, controlled study evaluating safety and tolerability of sepofarsen administered via intravitreal (IVT) injection in pediatric subjects (<8 years of age) with LCA10 due to the c.2991+1655A>G mutation over 24 months of treatment	Phase 2 and 3
NCT03364153	IVERIC bio, Inc.	Safety and efficacy of Zimura™ (complement factor C5 inhibitor) compared to sham in subjects with autosomal recessive Stargardt disease 1 (STGD1)	Phase 2 trial

chiefly preferred GR agonists for the treatment of posterior retinal inflammatory ailments. As with the general class of steroids, the GC injection also causes considerable confounding effects such as unwarranted elevation of IOP or SI-OHT/SIG in 20–30% of Dex (Chin et al. 2017) and 30–40% of TA treatments (Maeda et al. 2019). Hence SI-OHT is of prime concern among ophthalmologists. It is predicted to be caused by genetic, environmental, and lifestyle changes. Due to the increased incidence of DM, exponential aging population, and environmental factors, intraocular diseases such as RVO and ME are projected to nearly double in number by 2040. Hence, the need for GC treatment for these ailments and subsequent SI-OHT is also expected to increase exponentially. The pathophysiology of SI-OHT is known to be remarkably similar to that of primary open-angle glaucoma (POAG) progression (Phulke et al. 2017). Administration of GC on normal human TM induces morphological changes including the crosslinking and reorganization of cytoskeletal components, which increases the TM stiffness, resulting in AH outflow resistance and IOP rise (Filla et al. 2011; Raghunathan et al. 2015; Vranka et al. 2015). The risk factors for SI-OHT include myopia, DM, HS, high cholesterol, sleep apnea, tobacco usage, or alcohol usage.

17.6.6.2 Treatment for Glaucoma

To date, IOP is the only modifiable factor for treating glaucoma with the treatment regimen involving antiglaucoma medication (AGM). AGM acts by altering AH production and outflow dynamics. In most of the glaucoma subjects (90%), the IOP rise is transient, and these patients respond well to AGM usage. On medically uncontrollable IOP with AGM, a surgical procedure termed trabeculectomy is used as an alternative therapy to drain the excess AH accumulated underneath the TM layer (Gruener et al. 2016). In this procedure, a small excision or opening is made in the TM layer or at the adjacent corneoscleral tissue. Thereby, the accumulated AH gets drained through TM.

17.7 Environmental Effect on Eye Diseases

17.7.1 Air Pollution

The harmful constituents of air are termed pollutants. Particle mass less than 2.5 μm and reduction in the ozone layer with increased ultraviolet (UV) rays' exposure are the two major constituents of air pollution that have shown severe consequences on human health, especially to heart, lung, brain, and eye-related disease. These two parameters were measured globally, and the increased risk of mortality was assessed by the global consortium. They observed that particulate matter was the fifth most important risk factor for death, and about 4.2 million people have lost their lives. Additionally, 254,000 deaths were attributed to ozone depletion (Behar-Cohen 2018). The effect of air pollution is recently studied on the damaging effects of the retina, wherein the retinal structure of 51,710 participants was examined (Chua et al. 2020). The particulate matter and increased nitrogen dioxide in the air caused alterations in retinal layers. The possible mechanism could be that particulate matter could be inhaled and gets into the blood flow and then crosses the BRB. Oxidative stress could be the main factor leading to the loss of RGC, rods, and cone cells that would affect the vision severely. The relationship between the increase in particulate matter (nitrogen dioxide, sulfur dioxide, and less than 2.5 μm particles) in the air and glaucoma and cataract progression was studied in a large Canadian cohort of 30,097adults. An increase in glaucoma risk was observed; however, the need for cataract surgeries was not affected in the cohort. Similarly, a higher risk of glaucoma and thinning of macular ganglion cell-inner plexiform layer was observed in a UK study. Particulate matter-induced pollution is associated with positive risk of heart disease and death. Hazardous effects were considerably decreased when a green environment was found in the residential neighborhoods (Gazzo et al. 2016; Son et al. 2021). Hence, the environmental interaction of humans and the environment for the well-being of humans is evident here.

17.7.2 Light Stress

The increase in artificial lighting, including LEDs, electronic devices, and television watching, has increased enormously in recent years. Light is needed for vision and is usually perceived through photoreceptors in the retina and the operation of the visual cycle through light phototransduction. However, excessive light is detrimental to the retina health by the photothermal, photochemical, and photomechanical phenomena. The excess light available to the retina after absorption can be converted to heat energy thereby increasing the temperature of the absorbing photoreceptor cells, which causes cell death. Alternatively, the excess light can be used to generate free radicles that can ultimately kill the cell. Quartz infra red heat lamps are used by people and these can cause macular damage (Zheng et al. 2017). Also, LEDs caused damage to the retina. Recently, the use of organic light-emitting diodes (OLEDs) has been suggested in place of LEDs as the latter causes higher toxicity to the retina compared to the former illuminating sources. The reason could be that OLEDs could cause lower retinal damage due to the presence of lower blue light.

17.7.3 Effect of Smoking/Tobacco Consumption on Ocular Ailments

More than one billion people smoke and use tobacco worldwide. The cigarette is composed of more than 50 harmful compounds, of which nicotine is the major harmful compound that influences the incidences of various health ailments extending from simple breathing issues to life-threatening conditions such as lung cancer, heart attack, and stroke. Even though the vision-related influence on AMD, cataract, DR, and glaucoma progression is not life threatening, cigarette usage may affect the quality of life (Kennedy et al. 2011). In the case of glaucoma, there is still a controversial debate on the relationship between smoking and glaucoma incidence, whereas the association of smoking with high IOP progression has been proven by various statistical research work (Kang et al. 2003; Lee et al. 2003; Pérez-de-Arcelus et al. 2017; Law et al. 2018). The observations of these studies cumulatively state that current smokers with high cigarette packs usage per day intend to show a high IOP rise and glaucoma incidence compared to ex-smokers and non-smokers. The nicotine compound present in the cigarette is observed to cause damage to ocular tissues such as the retina, choroid, ONH, and TM. It is mediated via reduced blood flow, ischemia, and hypoxia, resulting in collagen reorganization and increased extracellular matrix turnover that is deposited on these structures, and subsequently the AH outflow is restricted and IOP rises. Similarly, the compounds such as cadmium, copper, cyanide, and aldehyde in cigarettes mix with the bloodstream and are deposited on the lens, leading to cataract progression. The compounds may reduce the antioxidant potential of the immune system, as well as the restoration capability of the lens proteins from damage. These effects are reported to be higher when the subject has poor diet habits and alcohol consumption. Therefore, it is wiser to quit smoking and reduce alcohol consumption for better ocular health.

17.8 Microbes and Eye Diseases

The human microbiome project was undertaken by the National Institute of Health (United States) to understand the composition of microbes in various human organs. More than 100 trillion microbes live in association with humans and among themselves. The commensal microbes are known to be inherited and their composition could vary due to environmental conditions such as diet, smoking, disease, and antibiotics usage (Wang et al. 2017). The beneficial bacteria can drive away harmful disease-causing bacteria by secreting bacterial toxins and modulating the host immune system. In the eye, several microbes are identified so far by the traditional culture method. Currently, NGS techniques have sequenced ribosomal DNA (rDNA) from the microbes present on the ocular surface. The predominant microbial genera found were: *Pseudomonas*, *Propionibacterium*, *Bradyrhizobium*, *Corynebacterium*, *Acinetobacter*, *Brevundimonas*, *Staphylococcus*, *Aquabacterium*, *Sphingomonas*, *Streptococcus*, *Streptophyta*, and *Methylobacterium*, constituting about 96% of the classified microbiome (Dong et al. 2011; Lu and Liu 2016). Additionally, environmental bacteria such as *Rothia*, *Herbaspirillum*, *Leptothrichia*, and *Rhizobium* were found on the outer eye surface. *Pseudomonas* was present in healthy eyes, whereas *Bacilli* was found in dry eyes diseased condition. Further, *Staphylococci* spp. were found in people undergoing cataract surgery (Sloan et al. 2010; Lin et al. 2017).

Uveitis is caused by both microbial and eye inflammation (Forrester et al. 2018). Uveitis occurs due to the alteration in the gut microbiome composition, and it is linked to the presence of human leukocyte antigen B27 (HLA—B27) protein on the leucocyte surface (Zhou et al. 2021). Interestingly, *Helicobacter pylori* are present in the gut of glaucoma patients and the treatment of this bacteria resulted in improvement of vision due to reduction in intraocular pressures (*Kountouras* et al.). Similarly, bacterial strains of coagulase-negative *Staphylococci* (CoNS), *Pseudomonas aeruginosa*, and *Staphylococcus aureus* and fungal species such as *Aspergillus* and *Malassezia* spp. were chiefly found to be dysregulated in the gut microbe in corneal keratitis subjects. A similar pattern of varying gut microbe was observed in AMD patients and rodent DR model (Agrawal et al. 2020; Nayyar et al. 2020; Prasad et al. 2022). The possible mechanism could be alteration in the inflammatory response, oxidative stress in the intestine, which could cross the BRB and reach ocular cells, which reduce the anti-inflammatory potential of the affected subjects (Jayasudha et al. 2018). It was reported that the diet could effectively regulate microbiota and help ease the AMD symptoms (Rowan et al. 2017). Hence, the gut microbiome and ocular axis regulation by environmental factors can pave the path for novel therapeutics for ocular diseases.

17.9 Eye Cancers and Environment

Various tumors arise from different parts of the eye including the eyelid, ocular surface, retina, and melanocytes (Maheshwari and Finger 2018). One of the prominent eyelid cancers is basal cell carcinoma observed chiefly in men with immune dysfunction. Persons who are highly exposed to UV light and ionizing radiation are at a higher risk for eyelid tumors. Hence, controlling the anthropogenic UV ray's exposure and ozone layer depletion should be considered immediately by countries worldwide to reduce eyelid cancers. One of the malignant conjunctival tumors is squamous cell carcinoma, which could be caused by human immunodeficiency virus (HIV) and human papillomavirus (HPV) infection (Muchengeti et al. 2021). The E6 and E7 viral oncogenes present in these tumors affect the tumor suppressor genes, leading to cell cycle progression and tumorigenesis (Ramberg and Heegaard 2021). Uveal melanoma (in choroid, iris, and ciliary body) is the principal cause of death in adult population. These cancers affect people of different geographical regions in different ways. For example, Australia has the highest incidence, whereas Asian countries have a lower incidence of such cancers. The incidence is also dependent on the occupation of the people. Cooks and welders had a higher prevalence of such cancers. Though several chemotherapeutic treatment options such as targeted therapies, monoclonal antibodies, and gene delivery systems are available to date, the survival outcomes for uveal melanoma did not improve significantly in the last 30 years. The most common childhood cancer is retinoblastoma (RB), which is prevalent in children below five years of age. This tumor is known to occur due to the functional loss of RB tumor suppressor protein. The mode of inheritance could be either genetic or sporadic (Hill et al. 2018). Recently overexpression of Myc N was found to induce RB tumor progression. Late-stage presentation of RB and high-grade (D, E) tumors were responsible for 36% fatality in a study period of six years (Ran et al. 2014). Chemotherapy has improved the survival rate of affected children; however, the occurrence of secondary tumors and the non-availability of targeted therapies are primary concerns of these tumors. There is a disparity between higher-income countries and lower- and middle-income countries (LMIC) in cancer disease presentation. Later countries have more late age disease representation and aggressive phenotypes (Global Retinoblastoma study group 2020). The aggressiveness in LMIC is attributed to probable HPV infections in these countries. However, disease surveillance needs a global initiative to achieve 100% success rates for this cancer. A common deficiency that is associated with many eye cancers was vitamin D levels. Therefore, addressing this deficiency could improve eye tumor treatment outcomes.

17.10 Eye Diseases and COVID Infection

Coronavirus infection was first reported in Wuhan, China, in 2019 (COVID-19) and was declared as a pandemic by the WHO. The pandemic caused extensive infections (397,832,539) and loss of human life is approximately 5,752,804 to date (Accessed on 8 February 2022, https://coronavirus.jhu.edu). It has disrupted the way of modern human's life and several socioeconomic fallouts that are associated with their health. The pandemic has led to a stress on the cordial relationship between humans, the fauna around them, and the environment that houses them. The introduction of lockdowns, closure of educational institutions, and work from home patterns have increased the online device-mediated education and working system. Hence, the frequent use of electronic gadgets has increased dry eye syndrome and myopia occurrence (Alvarez-Peregrina et al. 2021; Neti et al. 2021; Saldanha et al. 2021; Wang et al. 2021). Dry eyes, even though a smaller side effect of COVID infection, were observed to be associated with mental health issues (Figure 17.5). The device-induced symptoms can be reversed by minimal usage of electronic gadgets and spending time outdoors. Another problem of COVID-19 lockdowns and home confinement is the reduction in people seeking medical assistance for their eye diseases. The numbers had drastically reduced during the pandemic (April 2020 to September 2021) in our (Sankara Nethralaya, Chennai) hospital (Figure 17.5).

The virus evolves continuously, and there is constant interaction between the host and pathogen, which is trying to evade the host immune response for its growth (Srivastava et al. 2021). Several mutants arose after the first detected COVID-19 in China. Delta variant was more virulent than the original strain leading to higher infection rate compared to the original strain. Additionally, it was associated with a surge in secondary infections such as mucormycosis (caused by fungi Mucorales), which was fatal in some individuals (Mehta and Pandey 2020). These classes of fungi are found in immunosuppressed people, especially among hematological cancer subjects. Even though the exact mechanism of mucormycosis is poorly understood, it is believed that the host immune system was weakened, and the phagocytes could not get rid of the pathogen. Factors like diabetes, excess use of steroids, high levels of circulating ferritin, and contaminated equipment were thought to contribute to mucormycosis incidence. India recorded 0.014% mucormycosis cases (Mahalaxmi et al. 2021), which was majorly treated by amphotericin B injections (Murthy et al. 2022). As tertiary eye care, our hospital has successfully treated mucormycosis-infected patients. The current omicron COVID-19 variant has substantial mutations that resulted in an upward swing in cases in the entire world. Humanity can hope for a less severe and milder strain that can coexist in humans without killing the host.

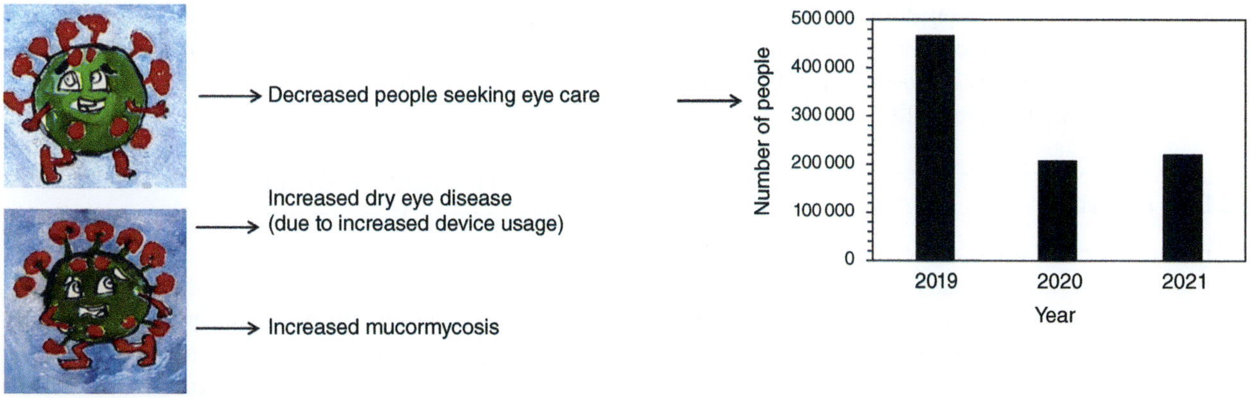

Figure 17.5 Effect of COVID-19 on eye diseases and care.

17.11 Role of Community Screening by Optometrists

India's population is at 1.39 billion as of 21 June 2021, standing second most populated country in the world. It is projected that India will overtake China to become the most populous country by reaching 1.47 billion in the year 2030. The health index of the country is also growing steadily, and life expectancy is also increasing with the population. More than 30% of the population comprises children of age less than oneyear. The neonatal and childhood diseases are addressed by health care facilities in the country leading to decreased infant mortality and childhood diseases in the country. However, in the context of eye health, there are several neonatal and newborn eye health issues like high myopia, astigmatism, anisometric amblyopia, strabismus, and premature retinopathy. There are emerging eye issues in adults as well such as AMD, DR, glaucoma, infectious keratitis, cataract, and low vision, which need attention as community health care (Figure 17.6). Lifestyle also contributes substantially to ocular morbidities.

Optometrists' role in the community is to bring awareness about the prevailing ocular diseases and their prevention methods. It is only the refractive errors and low vision aids that contribute to major functioning blindness, which can be well supported by optometrists to bring down avoidable blindness and getting the proper vision in millions of people. In a community eye care screening program, an ideal team would comprise 1 ophthalmologist, 4 optometrists, 8 eye care social workers, 8 ophthalmic assistants, and 16 ophthalmic nurses according to the LV Prasad eye institute (LVPEI) model.

17.11.1 Community Eye Care

Community eye care is the most important tool to reduce avoidable blindness in society. The community eye care system comprises ophthalmologists, optometrists, social workers, government-appointed officers, and non-governmental organizations. There are well-developed models to execute community health care by the set of people mentioned above. First, the ocular problems need to be identified by

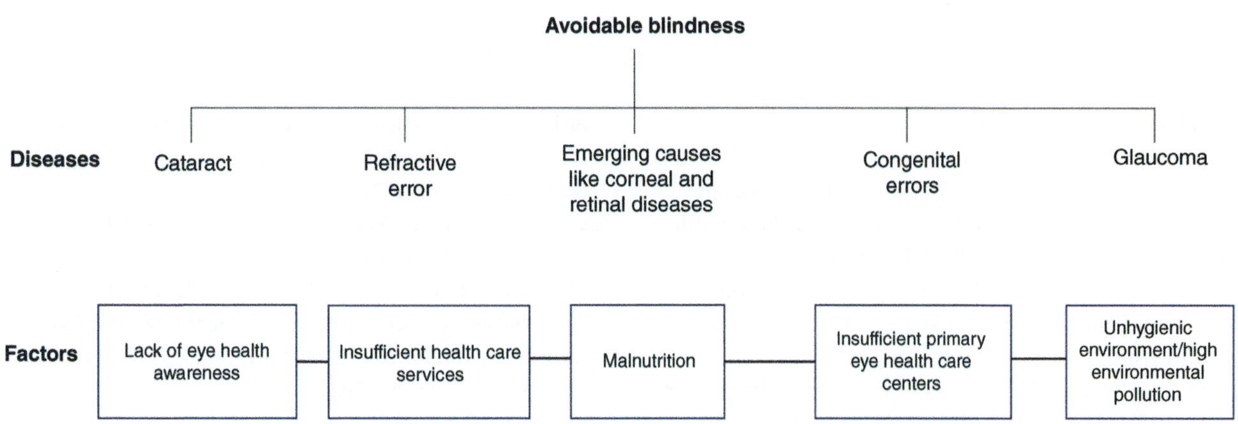

Figure 17.6 Factors that lead to eye health in a community.

the ophthalmologist and screened for 1000s of people in each area. High throughput screening of large mass disease identification and treatment protocols could be done for improving the community eye health.

17.11.2 Awareness

The modus operandi needs to be fixed by the clinician either in the top-down approach or vice versa. Once the disease pattern and the root cause of the disease are identified, then it can be shared with the common people with the help of social workers.

17.12 Role of Community Awareness Programs

Community awareness is an important tool in improving the health index of a society (Croker 2016). There are a few things that are important in creating an awareness program in a society such as information brochures, eye camps, pamphlets, and information about medical practitioners. The reason for the drop in eye care is poor awareness, insufficient infrastructure in the health care setup, and insufficient trained medical practitioners. Hence, to meet this challenge, there needs to be a proper network between primary, secondary, and tertiary health care professionals and organizations. There are several other factors including demographic, personal, socioeconomic, psychosocial, and occupational factors that need to be curbed by a governmental organization. Moreover, the program needs to be well supported by government and non-governmental organizations to sustain the activity. "Why does the community need to be made aware of eye health care?" It is an important question that gives us the absolute percentage of disease prevalence, people knowing the disease, and its treatment. Improved awareness and knowledge about eye disease in society is the only way for preventing avoidable blindness.

17.13 The Role of Green Landscapes in Eye Health

Several studies conducted on a group of children, college students, and the elderly have shown that visualizing nature and green environments have improved the well-being of people, coping with stresses, restoring attentiveness, relieving mental fatigue, and improving their mental health (Berto 2014; Amicone et al. 2018). Currently, restorativeness has become an intense area of research, and eye-tracking movements have been used that can help in urban green landscape planning for people's better health (Wu et al. 2021).

17.14 Ocular Health and One Health Approach

The perspective of One Health for ocular health approach combines environmental, animal health, and human health. This will be the perfect platform to understand the origin of diseases that causes the ecological imbalance. The vision is to develop a robust system that will survey the microbial load and its types on animal, environment, and human being's interactions. This will help us to develop a guideline to improve the health index of human beings as well as animals and the environment. It also brings a holistic collaboration of all living beings on Earth for the betterment of the ecological niche. The challenge ahead will be on developing an institutional mechanism to implement the One Health ocular health policy.

References

Agrawal, R., Testi, I., Mahajan, S. et al. (2020). The collaborative ocular tuberculosis study (COTS) consensus (CON) group meeting proceedings. *Ocular Immunology and Inflammation* 30: 1–11. https://pubmed.ncbi.nlm.nih.gov/32250731 (accessed 6 September 2021).

Ahmad, S.S. (2018). Water related ocular diseases. *Saudi Journal of Ophthalmology* 32 (3): 227–233. pmc/articles/PMC6137694/ (accessed 17 February 2022).

Ahmad, A., Ahmad, S.Z., Khalique, N. et al. (2020). Prevalence and associated risk factors of glaucoma in Aligarh, India–a population based study. *DJO* 31 (1): 36–40. www.djo.org.in/articles/31/1/Prevalence-and-Associated-Risk-Factors-of-Glaucoma-in-Aligarh-India-A-population-based-study.html (accessed 21 April 2021).

Alvarez-Peregrina, C., Martinez-Perez, C., Villa-Collar, C. et al. (2021). Impact of COVID-19 home confinement in children's refractive errors. *International Journal of Environmental Research and Public Health* 18 (10): 5347. https://www.mdpi.com/1660-4601/18/10/5347/htm (accessed 23 February 2022).

Amicone, G., Petruccelli, I., De Dominicis, S. et al. (2018). Green breaks: the restorative effect of the school environment's green areas on children's cognitive performance. *Frontiers in Psychology* 9: 1579.

Audo, I., Bujakowska, K.M., Léveillard, T. et al. (2012). Development and application of a next-generation-sequencing (NGS) approach to detect known and novel gene defects underlying retinal diseases. *Orphanet Journal of Rare Diseases* 7 (1): 8. https://www.hal.inserm.fr/inserm-00697616 (accessed 17 February 2022).

Augustin, D.K., Heimer, S.R., Tam, C. et al. (2011). Role of Defensins in corneal epithelial barrier function against *Pseudomonas aeruginosa* traversal. *Infection and Immunity* 79 (2): 595. /pmc/articles/PMC3028852/ (accessed 17 February 2022).

Becker, D.E. (2013). Basic and clinical pharmacology of glucocorticosteroids. *Anesthesia Progress* 60 (1): 25–32. https://meridian.allenpress.com/anesthesia-progress/article/60/1/25/24839/Basic-and-Clinical-Pharmacology-of (accessed 22 March 2021).

Behar-Cohen, F. (2018). Towards an optimized use of ocular corticosteroids: EURETINA award lecture 2017. *Ophthalmologica* 240 (2): 111–119. https://www.karger.com/Article/FullText/489673 (accessed 22 March 2021).

Berto, R. (2014). The role of nature in coping with psycho-physiological stress: a literature review on restorativeness. *Behavioral Science* 4 (4): 394–409. https://www.mdpi.com/2076-328X/4/4/394/htm (accessed 23 Februray 2022).

Biswas, P., Villanueva, A.L., Soto-Hermida, A. et al. (2021). Deciphering the genetic architecture and ethnographic distribution of IRD in three ethnic populations by whole genome sequence analysis. *PLoS Genetics* 17 (10): e1009848. https://doi.org/10.1371/journal.pgen.1009848.

Callanan, D.G., Gupta, S., Boyer, D.S. et al. (2013). Dexamethasone intravitreal implant in combination with laser photocoagulation for the treatment of diffuse diabetic macular edema. *Ophthalmology* 120 (9): 1843–1851. https://doi.org/10.1016/j.ophtha.2013.02.018.

Chen, T.C., Huang, D.S., Lin, C.W. et al. (2021). Genetic characteristics and epidemiology of inherited retinal degeneration in Taiwan. *NPJ Genomic Medicine* 6, 16: https://doi.org/10.1038/s41525-021-00180-1.

Chin, E.K., Almeida, D.R., Velez, G. et al. (2017). Ocular hypertension after intravitreal dexamethasone (ozurdex) sustained-release implant. *Retina (Philadelphia, Pa.)* 37 (7): 1345–1351. http://insights.ovid.com/crossref?an=00006982-201707000-00018 (6 August 2018).

Chua, S.Y.L., Khawaja, A.P., Dick, A.D. et al. (2020). Ambient air pollution associations with retinal morphology in the UK biobank. *Investigative Ophthalmology & Visual Science* 61 (5): 32–32. https://doi.org/10.1167/iovs.61.5.32 (23 February 2022).

Colombo, L., Melardi, E., Ferri, P. et al. (2017). Visual function improvement using photocromic and selective blue-violet light filtering spectacle lenses in patients affected by retinal diseases. *BMC Ophthalmology* 17 (1): 1–6. https://doi.org/10.1186/s12886-017-0545-9 https://bmcophthalmol.biomedcentral.com/articles (accessed 23 February 2022).

Consugar, M.B., Navarro-Gomez, D., Place, E.M. et al. (2015). Panel-based genetic diagnostic testing for inherited eye diseases is highly accurate and reproducible, and more sensitive for variant detection, than exome sequencing. *Genetics in Medicine: official journal of the American College of Medical Genetics* 17 (4): 253–261. https://pubmed.ncbi.nlm.nih.gov/25412400 (accessed 17 February 2022).

Croker, F. (2016). Book Reviews: Community Health And Wellness: A Socioecological Approach Anne McMurray Sydney, Mosby, 1999, Vol. 35, 2, 241–243, 408 pp. $52 95 (paperback). http://dx.doi.org/101177/144078339903500218. [Internet]. Available from: https://journals.sagepub.com/doi/10.1177/144078339903500218 (accessed 17 February 2022).

Daszak, P., Cunningham, A.A., and Hyatt, A.D. (2001). Anthropogenic environmental change and the emergence of infectious diseases in wildlife. *Acta Tropica* 78 (2): 103–116. https://pubmed.ncbi.nlm.nih.gov/11230820 (accessed 17 February 2022).

Dohlman, C.H., Zhou, C., Lei, F. et al. (2019). Glaucoma after corneal trauma or surgery – a rapid, inflammatory, IOP-independent pathway. *Cornea* 38 (12): 1589. /pmc/articles/PMC6830965/ (accessed 17 February 2022).

Dong, Q., Brulc, J.M., Iovieno, A. et al. (2011). Diversity of bacteria at healthy human conjunctiva. *Investigative Ophthalmology and Visual Science* 52 (8): 5408–5413. /pmc/articles/PMC3176057/ (accessed 23 February 2022).

Dua, H.S., King, A.J., and Joseph, A. (2001). A new classification of ocular surface burns. *The British Journal of Ophthalmology* 85 (11): 1379–1383. https://pubmed.ncbi.nlm.nih.gov/11673310 (accessed 17 February 2022).

Filla, M.S., Schwinn, M.K., Nosie, A.K. et al. (2011). Dexamethasone-associated cross-linked actin network formation in human trabecular meshwork cells involves β03 integrin signaling. *Investigative Ophthalmology & Visual Science* 52 (6): 2952–2959.

Fisher, J.K., Bromley, R.L., and Mansfield, B.C. (2016). My retina tracker™: an on-line international registry for people affected with inherited orphan retinal degenerative diseases and their genetic relatives – a new resource. *Advances in Experimental Medicine and Biology* 854: 245–251. https://doi.org/10.1007/978-3-319-17121-0_33. PMID: 26427418.

Florentin, A., Hautemanière, A., and Hartemann, P. (2011). Health effects of disinfection by-products in chlorinated swimming pools. *International Journal of Hygiene and Environmental Health* 214 (6): 461–469.

Forrester, J.V., Kuffova, L., and Dick, A.D. (2018). Autoimmunity, autoinflammation, and infection in uveitis. *American Journal of Ophthalmology* 189: 77–85. https://pubmed.ncbi.nlm.nih.gov/29505775 (accessed 23 February 2022).

Freegard, T.J. (1997). The physical basis of transparency of the normal cornea. *Eye* 11 (4): 465–471. https://www.nature.com/articles/eye1997127 (accessed 17 February 2022).

Friedenwald, J.S., Hughes, W.F., and Herrmann, H. (1944). Acid-base tolerance of the cornea. *Archives of Ophthalmology* 31 (4): 279–283. https://jamanetwork.com/journals/jamaophthalmology/fullarticle/617618 (accessed 17 February 2022).

Gazzo, A.M., Daneels, D., Cilia, E. et al. (2016). DIDA: a curated and annotated digenic diseases database. *Nucleic Acids Research* 44 (D1): D900–D907. https://academic.oup.com/nar/article/44/D1/D900/2502599 (accessed 17 February 2022).

Glöckle, N., Kohl, S., Mohr, J. et al. (2014). Panel-based next generation sequencing as a reliable and efficient technique to detect mutations in unselected patients with retinal dystrophies. *European Journal of Human Genetics* 22 (1): 99–104. https://pubmed.ncbi.nlm.nih.gov/23591405 (accessed 17 February 2022).

Group GRS, Fabian, I.D., Abdallah, E. et al. (2020). Global retinoblastoma presentation and analysis by National Income Level. *JAMA Oncology* 6 (5): 685–695. https://jamanetwork.com/journals/jamaoncology/fullarticle/2761957 (accessed 4 September 2021).

Gruener, A.M., Sharma, P., Ameen, S., and Ahmed, F. (2016). Severe corticosteroid-induced ocular hypertension requiring bilateral Trabeculectomies in a patient with Takayasu's arteritis. *Case Reports in Ophthalmological Medicine* 2016: 1–4.

Guttman, J.A. and Finlay, B.B. (2009). Tight junctions as targets of infectious agents. *Biochimica et Biophysica Acta* 1788 (4): 832–841. https://pubmed.ncbi.nlm.nih.gov/19059200 (accessed 17 February 2022).

Hanany, M., Rivolta, C., and Sharon, D. (2020). Worldwide carrier frequency and genetic prevalence of autosomal recessive inherited retinal diseases. *Proceedings of the National Academy of Sciences* 117 (5): 2710–2716. https://pubmed.ncbi.nlm.nih.gov/31964843 (accessed 17 February 2022).

Hill, J.A., Gedleh, A., Lee, S. et al. (2018). Knowledge, experiences and attitudes concerning genetics among retinoblastoma survivors and parents. *European Journal of Human Genetics* 26 (4): 505–517. https://www.nature.com/articles/s41431-017-0027-9 (accessed 23 February 2022).

Jayasudha, R., Kalyana Chakravarthy, S., Sai Prashanthi, G. et al. (2018). Alterations in gut bacterial and fungal microbiomes are associated with bacterial keratitis, an inflammatory disease of the human eye. *Journal of Biosciences* 43 (5): 835–856. https://doi.org/10.1007/s12038-018-9798-6 (accessed 23 February 2022).

Kang, J.H., Pasquale, L.R., Rosner, B.A. et al. (2003). Prospective study of cigarette smoking and the risk of primary open-angle glaucoma. *Archives of Ophthalmology* (Chicago, 1960) 121 (12): 1762–1768. https://pubmed.ncbi.nlm.nih.gov/14662597 (accessed 17 February 2022).

Kennedy, R.D., Spafford, M.M., Parkinson, C.M., and Fong, G.T. (2011). Knowledge about the relationship between smoking and blindness in Canada, the United States, the United Kingdom, and Australia: results from the International Tobacco Control Four-Country Project. *Optometry-Journal of the American Optometric Association* 82 (5): 310–317. https://pubmed.ncbi.nlm.nih.gov/21524603 (accessed 17 February 2022).

Kilvington, S., Gray, T., Dart, J. et al. (2004). Acanthamoeba keratitis: the role of domestic tap water contamination in the United Kingdom. *Investigative Ophthalmology & Visual Science* 45 (1): 165–169.

Kutsyr, O., Sánchez-Sáez, X., Martínez-Gil, N. et al. (2020). Gradual increase in environmental light intensity induces oxidative stress and inflammation and accelerates retinal neurodegeneration. *Investigative Ophthalmology & Visual Science* 61 (10): 1–1.

de Laat, P., Smeitink, J.A., Janssen, M.C. et al. (2013). Mitochondrial retinal dystrophy associated with the m.3243A > G mutation. *Ophthalmology* 120 (12): 2684–2696. https://pubmed.ncbi.nlm.nih.gov/23806424 (accessed 17 February 2022).

Lasagni Vitar, R.M., Hvozda Arana, A.G., Janezic, N.S. et al. (2019). Urban air pollution induces redox imbalance and epithelium hyperplasia in mice cornea. *Toxicology and Applied Pharmacology* 384: https://pubmed.ncbi.nlm.nih.gov/31628919 (accessed 17 February 2022).

Law, S.M., Lu, X., Yu, F. et al. (2018). Cigarette smoking and glaucoma in the United States population. *Eye* 32 (4): 716–725. https://www.nature.com/articles/eye2017292 (accessed 17 February 2022).

Lee, A.J., Rochtchina, E., Wang, J.J. et al. (2003). Does smoking affect intraocular pressure? Findings from the Blue Mountains Eye Study. *Journal of Glaucoma* 12 (3): 209–212. https://pubmed.ncbi.nlm.nih.gov/12782837 (accessed 17 February 2022).

Lin, Y.H., Kang, Y.C., Hou, C.H. et al. (2017). Antibiotic susceptibility profiles of ocular and nasal flora in patients undergoing cataract surgery in Taiwan: an observational and cross-sectional study. *BMJ Open* 7 (8): e017352.

https://bmjopen.bmj.com/content/7/8/e017352 (accessed 23 February 2022).

Liu, X., Tao, T., Zhao, L. et al. (2021). Molecular diagnosis based on comprehensive genetic testing in 800 Chinese families with non-syndromic inherited retinal dystrophies. *Clinical & Experimental Ophthalmology* 49 (1): 46–59. https://doi.org/10.1111/ceo.13875.

Lock, J., Irani, N., and Newman, N. (2020). Neuro-ophthalmic manifestations of mitochondrial disorders and their management. *Taiwan Journal of Ophthalmology* 1 (1): 39–52. https://pubmed.ncbi.nlm.nih.gov/33767954 (accessed 17 February 2022).

Lu, L.J. and Liu, J. (2016). Focus: microbiome: human microbiota and ophthalmic disease. *The Yale Journal of Biology and Medicine* 89 (3): 325. /pmc/articles/PMC5045141/ (accessed 23 February 2022).

Mackenzie, J.S. and Jeggo, M. (2019). The one health approach – why is it so important? *Tropical Medicine and Infectious Disease* 4 (2): 88. https://www.mdpi.com/2414-6366/4/2/88/htm (accessed 17 February 2022).

Maeda, Y., Ishikawa, H., Nishikawa, H. et al. (2019). Intraocular pressure elevation after subtenon triamcinolone acetonide injection; multicentre retrospective cohort study in Japan. Lewin A.S. (ed.). *PLoS One* 14 (12): e0226118. https://dx.plos.org/10.1371/journal.pone.0226118 (accessed 22 March 2021).

Mahalaxmi, I., Jayaramayya, K., Venkatesan, D. et al. (2021). Mucormycosis: an opportunistic pathogen during COVID-19. *Environmental Research* 201: 111643.

Maheshwari, A. and Finger, P.T. (2018). Cancers of the eye. *Cancer Metastasis Reviews* 37 (4): 677–690. https://pubmed.ncbi.nlm.nih.gov/30203109 (accessed 23 February 2022).

Masland, R.H. (2012). The neuronal organization of the retina. *Neuron* 76 (2): 266. /pmc/articles/PMC3714606/ (accessed 17 February 2022).

Mehta, S. and Pandey, A. (2020). Rhino-orbital mucormycosis associated with COVID-19. *Cureus* 12 (9): https://www.cureus.com/articles/40523-rhino-orbital-mucormycosis-associated-with-covid-19 (accessed 23 February 2022).

Mousa, A.M., El-Mahalaway, A.M., and El-Desoky, R.E. (2018). The protective effects of sodium hyaluronate on corneal injuries induced by chlorinated water in adult male rabbits: a histological and immunohistochemical study. *Egyptian Journal of Histology* 41 (2): 140–149. https://ejh.journals.ekb.eg/article_15895.html (accessed 17 February 2022).

Muchengeti, M., Bohlius, J., and Dhokotera, T.G. (2021). Conjunctival cancer in people living with HIV. *Current Opinion in Infectious Diseases* 34 (1): 1–7. https://pubmed.ncbi.nlm.nih.gov/33337616 (accessed 23 February 2022).

Murthy, R., Bagchi, A., Gote, Y., and Desai, S. (2022). Retrobulbar injection of amphotericin B using intravenous cannula for post-COVID-19 rhino-orbital mucormycosis. *Indian Journal of Ophthalmology* 70 (1): 302–305. https://pubmed.ncbi.nlm.nih.gov/34937263 (accessed 23 February 2022).

Nayyar, A., Gindina, S., Barron, A. et al. (2020). Do epigenetic changes caused by commensal microbiota contribute to development of ocular disease? A review of evidence. *Human Genomics* 14 (1): 1–12. https://humgenomics.biomedcentral.com/articles/10.1186/s40246-020-00257-5 (accessed 23 February 2022).

Neti, N., Prabhasawat, P., Chirapapaisan, C., and Ngowyutagon, P. (2021). Provocation of dry eye disease symptoms during COVID-19 lockdown. *Scientific Reports* 11 (1): 1–9. https://www.nature.com/articles/s41598-021-03887-4 (accessed 23 February 2022).

Oh, J.Y., Kim, M.K., Shin, M.S. et al. (2008). The anti-inflammatory and anti-angiogenic role of mesenchymal stem cells in corneal wound healing following chemical injury. *Stem Cells* 26 (4): 1047–1055. https://pubmed.ncbi.nlm.nih.gov/18192235 (accessed 17 February 2022).

Otsuka, Y., Oishi, A., Miyata, M. et al. (2020). Wavelength of light and photophobia in inherited retinal dystrophy. *Scientific Reports* 10 (1): 1–6. https://www.nature.com/articles/s41598-020-71707-2 (accessed 23 February 2022).

Ozawa, K., Mochizuki, K., Manabe, Y. et al. (2019). Retinal dystrophy associated with a single-base deletion mutation in mitochondrial DNA 3271 in patient with MELAS syndrome. *Documenta Ophthalmologica* 138 (2): 147–152. https://pubmed.ncbi.nlm.nih.gov/30701423 (accessed 17 February 2022).

Paskowitz, D.M., LaVail, M.M., and Duncan, J.L. (2006). Light and inherited retinal degeneration. *British Journal of Ophthalmology* 90 (8): 1060–1066. https://pubmed.ncbi.nlm.nih.gov/16707518 (accessed 23 February 2022).

Patel, G.C., Millar, J.C., and Clark, A.F. (2019). Glucocorticoid receptor transactivation is required for glucocorticoid-induced ocular hypertension and glaucoma. *Investigative Ophthalmology and Visual Science* 60 (6): 1967–1978. https://doi.org/10.1167%2Fiovs.18-26383 (accessed 22 March 2021).

Perea-Romero, I., Gordo, G., Iancu, I.F. et al. (2021). Genetic landscape of 6089 inherited retinal dystrophies affected cases in Spain and their therapeutic and extended epidemiological implications. *Scientific Reports* 11 (1): 1–13. https://www.nature.com/articles/s41598-021-81093-y (accessed 17 February 2022).

Pérez-de-Arcelus, M., Toledo, E., Martínez-González, M.Á. et al. (2017). Smoking and incidence of glaucoma: the SUN Cohort. *Medicine* 96 (1): e5761. https://pubmed.ncbi.nlm.nih.gov/28072720 (accessed 17 February 2022).

Peters, D. and Miethchen, R. (1996). Symptoms and treatment of hydrogen fluoride injuries. *Journal of Fluorine Chemistry* 79 (2): 161–165.

Phulke, S., Kaushik, S., Kaur, S., and Pandav, S.S. (2017). Steroid-induced glaucoma: an avoidable irreversible blindness. *Journal of Current Glaucoma Practice* 11 (2): 67–72. http://www.ncbi.nlm.nih.gov/pubmed/28924342 (accessed 6 August 2018).

Pierrache, L.H.M., Hartel, B.P., Van Wijk, E. et al. (2016). Visual prognosis in USH2A-associated retinitis pigmentosa is worse for patients with usher syndrome type IIa than for those with nonsyndromic retinitis pigmentosa. *Ophthalmology* 123 (5): 1151–1160. https://pubmed.ncbi.nlm.nih.gov/26927203 (accessed 17 February 2022).

Pontikos, N., Arno, G., Jurkute, N. et al. (2020). Genetic basis of inherited retinal disease in a molecularly characterized cohort of more than 3000 families from the United Kingdom. *Ophthalmology* 127 (10): 1384–1394. https://pubmed.ncbi.nlm.nih.gov/32423767 (accessed 17 February 2022).

Prasad, R., Asare-Bediko, B., Harbour, A. et al. (2022). Microbial signatures in the rodent eyes with retinal dysfunction and diabetic retinopathy. *Investigative Ophthalmology & Visual Science* 63 (1): 5–5. https://doi.org/10.1167/iovs.63.1.5 (accessed 23 February 2022).

Presland, A. (2007). Applied ocular physiology and anatomy. *Anaesthesia & Intensive Care Medicine.* 8 (9): 379–382.

Raghunathan, V.K., Morgan, J.T., Park, S.A. et al. (2015). Dexamethasone stiffens trabecular meshwork, trabecular meshwork cells, and matrix. *Investigative Ophthalmology and Visual Science* 56 (8): 4447–4459. /pmc/articles/PMC4509060/ (accessed 22 March 2021).

Ramberg, I. and Heegaard, S. (2021). Human papillomavirus related neoplasia of the ocular adnexa. *Viruses* 13 (8): 1522. https://www.mdpi.com/1999-4915/13/8/1522/htm (accessed 23 February 2022).

Ran, X., Cai, W.J., Huang, X.F. et al. (2014). 'RetinoGenetics': a comprehensive mutation database for genes related to inherited retinal degeneration. *Database: The Journal of Biological Databases and Curation* 2014: 47. /pmc/articles/PMC4060621/ (accessed 17 February 2022).

Rowan, S., Jiang, S., Korem, T. et al. (2017). Involvement of a gut–retina axis in protection against dietary glycemia-induced age-related macular degeneration. *Proceedings of the National Academy of Sciences* 114 (22): E4472–E4481. https://pubmed.ncbi.nlm.nih.gov/28507131 (accessed 23 February 2022).

Saccà, S.C., Pulliero, A., and Izzotti, A. (2015). The dysfunction of the trabecular meshwork during glaucoma course. *Journal of Cellular Physiology* 230 (3): 510–525. http://doi.wiley.com/10.1002/jcp.24826 (accessed 16 March 2021).

Saldanha, I.J., Petris, R., Makara, M. et al. (2021). Impact of the COVID-19 pandemic on eye strain and dry eye symptoms. *The Ocular Surface* 22: 38–46.

Salmaninejad, A., Bedoni, N., Ravesh, Z. et al. (2020). Whole exome sequencing and homozygosity mapping reveals genetic defects in consanguineous Iranian families with inherited retinal dystrophies. *Scientific Reports* 10 (1): 1–7. https://www.nature.com/articles/s41598-020-75841-9 (accessed 17 February 2022).

Sendra, V.G., Tau, J., Zapata, G. et al. (2021 Feb). Polluted air exposure compromises corneal immunity and exacerbates inflammation in acute herpes simplex keratitis. *Frontiers in Immunology* 25 (12): 163.

Sengupta, S., Honavar, S.G., Sachdev, M.S. et al. (2020). All India ophthalmological society – Indian journal of ophthalmology consensus statement on preferred practices during the COVID-19 pandemic. *Indian Journal of Ophthalmology* 68 (5): 711–724. https://pubmed.ncbi.nlm.nih.gov/32317433 (accessed 6 September 2021).

Sharon, D., Ben-Yosef, T., Goldenberg-Cohen, N. et al. (2020). A nationwide genetic analysis of inherited retinal diseases in Israel as assessed by the Israeli inherited retinal disease consortium (IIRDC). *Human Mutation* 41 (1): 140–149. https://pubmed.ncbi.nlm.nih.gov/31456290 (accessed 17 February 2022).

Shields, B.J., Wilkins, J.R. III, and Smith, G.A. (2011). Nonoccupational table saw-related injuries treated in US emergency departments, 1990–2007. *Journal of Trauma and Acute Care Surgery* 71 (6): 1902–1907. https://pubmed.ncbi.nlm.nih.gov/20065881 (accessed 17 February 2022).

Sloan, C.D., Shen, L., West, J.D. et al. (2010). Genetic pathway-based hierarchical clustering analysis of older adults with cognitive complaints and amnestic mild cognitive impairment using clinical and neuroimaging phenotypes. *American Journal of Medical Genetics Part B: Neuropsychiatric Genetics* 153 (5): 1060–1069.

Smith, C.A., Vianna, J.R., and Chauhan, B.C. (2017). Assessing retinal ganglion cell damage. *Eye* 31 (2): 209–217. http://www.nature.com/eye (accessed 22 March 2021).

Sommer, A., Green, R., and Kenyon, K.R. (1982). Clinicohistopathologic correlations in xerophthalmic ulceration and necrosis. *Archives of Ophthalmology* (Chicago, Ill: 1960) 100 (6): 953–963. https://pubmed.ncbi.nlm.nih.gov/6807264 (accessed 17 February 2022).

Son, J.Y., Sabath, M.B., Lane, K.J. et al. (2021). Long-term exposure to PM2.5 and mortality for the older population: effect modification by residential greenness. *Epidemiology (Cambridge, Mass.)* 32 (4): 477–486. https://pubmed.ncbi.nlm.nih.gov/33788795 (23 February 2022).

Srivastava, M., Hall, D., Omoru, O.B. et al. (2021). Mutational landscape and interaction of sars-cov-2 with host cellular components. *Microorganisms* 9 (9): 1794. https://www.mdpi.com/2076-2607/9/9/1794/htm (accessed 23 February 2022).

Oaks Jr, Stanley C., R. E. Shope, and J. Lederberg Emerging Infections: Microbial Threats to Health in the United States. 1992 https://pubmed.ncbi.nlm.nih.gov/25121245 (accessed 17 February 2022).

Tatour, Y. and Ben-Yosef, T. (2020). Syndromic inherited retinal diseases: genetic, clinical and diagnostic aspects. *Diagnostics* 10 (10): 779. https://pubmed.ncbi.nlm.nih.gov/33023209 (accessed 17 February 2022).

Tian, X., Liu, Z., Niu, B. et al. (2011). E-cadherin/β-catenin complex and the epithelial barrier. *Journal of Biomedicine and Biotechnology* /pmc/articles/PMC3191826/ (accessed 17 February 2022).

Tong, Y., Zhou, Y.L., Zheng, Y. et al. (2017). Analyzing cytokines as biomarkers to evaluate severity of glaucoma. *International Journal of Ophthalmology* 10 (6): 925–930. http://www.ijo.cn/gjyken/ch/reader/view_abstract.aspx?file_no=20170615&flag=1 (accessed 16 March 2021).

Vemuganti, G.K., Murthy, S.I., and Das, S. (2011). Update on pathologic diagnosis of corneal infections and inflammations. *Middle East African Journal of Ophthalmology* 18 (4): 277. /pmc/articles/PMC3249812/ (accessed 17 February 2022).

Vranka, J.A., Kelley, M.J., Acott, T.S., and Keller, K.E. (2015). Extracellular matrix in the trabecular meshwork: intraocular pressure regulation and dysregulation in glaucoma. *Experimental Eye Research* 133: 112–125. /pmc/articles/PMC4379427/ (accessed 16 March 2021).

Wallace, D.M. and O'Brien, C.J. (2016). The role of lamina cribrosa cells in optic nerve head fibrosis in glaucoma. *Experimental Eye Research* 1 (142): 102–109.

Wang, B., Yao, M., Lv, L. et al. (2017). The human microbiota in health and disease. *Engineering* 3 (1): 71–82.

Wang, T., Reingruber, J., Woodruff, M.L. et al. (2018). The PDE6 mutation in the rd10 retinal degeneration mouse model causes protein mislocalization and instability and promotes cell death through increased ion influx. *Journal of Biological Chemistry* 293 (40): 15332–15346. https://pubmed.ncbi.nlm.nih.gov/30126843 (accessed 23 February 2022).

Wang, J., Li, Y., Musch, D.C. et al. (2021). Progression of myopia in school-aged children after COVID-19 home confinement. *JAMA Ophthalmology* 139 (3): 293–300. https://jamanetwork.com/journals/jamaophthalmology/fullarticle/2774808 (accessed 23 February 2022).

Weinreb, R.N., Aung, T., and Medeiros, F.A. (2014). The pathophysiology and treatment of glaucoma: a review. *JAMA : The Journal of the American Medical Association* 311 (18): 1901–1911. /pmc/articles/PMC4523637/ (accessed 16 March 2021).

Wilson, S.E., Medeiros, C.S., and Santhiago, M.R. (2018). Pathophysiology of corneal scarring in persistent epithelial defects after PRK and other corneal injuries. *Journal of Refractive Surgery* (Thorofare, 1995) 34 (1): 59. /pmc/articles/PMC5788463/ (accessed 17 February 2022).

Wu, Y., Zhuo, Z., Liu, Q. et al. (2021). The relationships between perceived design intensity, preference, restorativeness and eye movements in designed urban Green space. *International Journal of Environmental Research and Public Health* 18 (20): 10944. https://www.mdpi.com/1660-4601/18/20/10944/htm (accessed 23 Februray 2022).

Xuan, M., Wang, S., Liu, X. et al. (2016). Proteins of the corneal stroma: importance in visual function. *Cell and Tissue Research* 364 (1): 9–16. https://link.springer.com/article/10.1007/s00441-016-2372-3 (accessed 17 February 2022).

Yadav, M.P., Singh, R.K., and Malik, Y.S. (2020). Emerging and transboundary animal viral diseases: perspectives and preparedness. *Emerging and Transboundary Animal Viruses* /pmc/articles/PMC7123659/ (accessed 17 February 2022).

Yohe, S., Sivasankar, M., Ghosh, A. et al. (2020). Prevalence of mutations in inherited retinal diseases: a comparison between the United States and India. *Molecular Genetics & Genomic Medicine* 8 (2): e1081. https://pubmed.ncbi.nlm.nih.gov/31816670 (accessed 17 February 2022).

Zheng, X., Xie, P., Hu, Z. et al. (2017). Phototoxic maculopathy induced by quartz infrared heat lamp: a clinical case report. *Medicine* 96 (3): https://pubmed.ncbi.nlm.nih.gov/28099337 (accessed 23 February 2022).

Zhou, Z., Zheng, Z., Xiong, X. et al. (2021). Gut microbiota composition and Fecal metabolic profiling in patients with diabetic retinopathy. *Frontiers in Cell and Development Biology* 9: 732204.

18

Wastes in One Health – African Perspective

R.M. Nalwanga[1], M. Kaziro[1], J. Nattabi[1], V. Kantono[2], J. Kyayesimira[3], and F. Muheirwe[4]

[1] *Department of Zoology, Entomology and Fisheries Sciences, College of Natural Sciences, Makerere University, Kampala, Uganda*
[2] *Department of Environmental Management, College of Agriculture and Environmental Sciences, Makerere University, Kampala, Uganda*
[3] *Department of Biological Sciences, Faculty of Science, Kyambogo University, Kampala, Uganda*
[4] *Department of Educational Foundation and Psychology, Faculty of Science, Mbarara University of Science and Technology, Mbarara, Uganda*

18.1 Introduction

Several countries on the African continent consider waste management independent of health, yet proper waste management is part and partial of good health. In Africa, just like other parts of the world, different forms of waste that can be biodegradable or non-biodegradable, domestic, industrial, or institutional are generated. These wastes can also be dangerous, for example sharp waste objects, body part wastes, chemical or pharmaceutical, radioactive, and cytotoxic waste. These types of waste could contribute to different health consequences. Several infectious and non-infectious diseases are associated with poor waste management. This is more evident in developing countries that make the largest part of Africa as it is highly dominated by poor waste management systems due to poor infrastructure development. Africa is often attacked by waterborne diseases that are due to poor management of wastes, for example diarrhea, cholera, and typhoid, as they are as a result of poor disposal of fecal wastes into the environment. Water-related diseases like malaria and bilharzia that are still common in developing world are also highly associated with poor and unsafe waste disposal, for example the unsafe disposal of plastics and polythene into drainage channels that lead to breakage that increases the breeding sites of mosquitoes.

The antimicrobial resistance (AMR), which is not only Africa's challenge but a global alarming issue that requires immediate actions for its control, is largely caused by improper disposal and management of wastes from hospitals, domestic, industrial, and laboratory sources. Therefore, wastes in One Health can be an appropriate approach to many of Africa's health issues. Literature from earlier studies on Africa of which some are regional specific or country specific have been used to compose this chapter. However, Africa as continent has several data gaps on waste management. Several literatures that are available on the continent are with most of data for South Africa and yet because of its economic status, it is not a proper representation of Africa as a continent. Therefore the data on South Africa has been used with precautions whenever a general picture of Africa as a continent is being sought.

18.2 Waste Categorization

Wastes are the unwanted materials that have no value in normal use (Pushpakalambiga and Jasmine 2019). These can be urban wastes, industrial wastes, agricultural wastes, biomedical wastes, and radioactive wastes. These wastes can further be classified as biodegradable and non-biodegradable (Pushpakalambiga and Jasmine 2019). Biodegradable wastes decompose easily, whereas non-biodegradable materials cannot be decomposed easily. Examples of biodegradable materials are peels of vegetables, paper, cotton, and wood while those of non-biodegradable include plastics, glasses, metal, ceramics, etc. In Africa, the category of wastes generated vary from country to country depending on the main sectors. For example, the majority of wastes generated in Egypt, Ethiopia, and Botswana are from textile industry since textile forms their main manufacturing sector while Nigeria, Senegal, and South Africa are examples that focus on food industry, and thus the majority of their wastes

One Health: Human, Animal, and Environment Triad, First Edition. Edited by Meththika Vithanage and Majeti Narasimha Vara Prasad.

are organic and biodegradable. In Uganda and Kenya, for example, the largest percentage of wastes produced (52–80%) are residential wastes comprising mainly foods with a minor portion comprising paper, plastics, and ceramics (Mwesigye et al. 2009). The different types of wastes generated in Africa include the following.

18.3 Plastics

Plastics are classified as inorganic solid waste (Awuchi et al. 2020). This is because they are non-biodegradable once disposed into the environment without proper handling. Inappropriate disposal of non-biodegradable plastic bags results in these being swept downstream resulting in blockage of drainage systems (Ziraba et al. 2016). This causes floods that not only destroy property but also have claimed lives on roads, homes, and drainage sewage systems, hence leading to widespread environmental contamination with human waste and associated risk of infection transmission. Blocked drainage systems are also breeding sites for disease transmitting vectors, for example mosquitoes, leading to the outbreak of malaria among the surrounding communities. Besides blocking water flow, a number of plastics tend to accumulate pools of water, thus acting as breeding sites for mosquitoes.

Colored plastics are harmful as their pigment contains heavy metals, for example copper, lead, chromium, cobalt, selenium, and cadmium. Increased cases of endocrine disruptors in humans, such as bisphenol A and phthalates, are associated with plastic wastes (Awuchi and Awuchi 2019a, b).

18.4 Domestic Garbage

This is commonly known as organic solid waste and it is biodegradable. It is the garbage and rubbish, which normally originates in residential households. It is also termed as municipal solid waste (MSW), and it consists of wastes of materials that people use on daily basis in their households. It involves wastes like rotten food, cloths, wood, among others. When these wastes/garbage are not properly managed from households and the community, they pose serious health hazards and lead to the spread of infectious diseases. Domestic waste lying around attracts flies, rats, and other creatures that in turn spread diseases to the surrounding communities. Organic domestic waste also poses a serious threat since they ferment, creating conditions favorable to the survival and growth of microbial pathogens. Direct handling of domestic garbage can result in various types of infectious and chronic diseases with the waste workers and the rag pickers being the most vulnerable.

Disposal site or landfills also create health hazards for the neighborhood. Thereby improperly managed and designed landfills attract all types of insects and rodents that spread diseases. There are also burns and other injuries resulting from occupational accidents at waste disposal sites or from methane gas explosion at landfill sites.

However, the group at risk from unscientific disposal of garbage include the population in areas where there is no proper waste disposal method, especially the preschool children, waste workers, and workers in facilities producing toxic and infectious materials. Other high-risk group includes population living close to a waste dump and whose water supply has become contaminated due to either waste dumping or leakages from landfill sites.

18.5 Liquid Waste

This refers to human and animal excreta, household wastewater, cooking oil, fats, and grease. Direct dumping of untreated liquid waste, i.e. wastewater in rivers, lakes, and streams, results in the accumulation of toxic substances in the food chain through plants and animals that feed on it. Hence, the two cannot be separated if we are to have a healthy community. Liquid waste can be defined as: *examples of components in liquid wastewater include fats, oils, or grease (FOG); sludges; and hazardous household liquids.* Liquid waste can also include effluents of industries, fertilizer and pesticide solutions from agricultural fields, leachate from landfills, urban runoff of untreated waste water and garbage, mining wastes, etc. The liquid waste may contain nontoxic inorganic substances or toxic organic substances.

18.6 Radioactive Waste

These are materials that contain or are contaminated with radionuclides at high concentrations. Radioactive waste is a result of many activities, including nuclear medicine, nuclear research, nuclear power generation, rare-earth mining, and nuclear weapons reprocessing. Examples of wastes that can contain radioactive radiations include wiping rags, mops, medical tubes, and laboratory animal carcasses.

Radioactive waste is considered to be hazardous because it emits radioactive particles, which if not properly managed can be a risk to human health and the environment. It is associated with physical bodily injuries such as cuts, drowning, blunt trauma, and radiation injuries like immediate skin or inhalation burns. Direct exposure to hazardous waste can also lead to diseases through chemical exposure as the release of chemical waste into the environment leads to chemical poisoning. Accident risks due to poisoning and chemical burns result from contact with small amounts of hazardous chemical wastes mixed with general waste. Waste generated from hospitals, medical laboratories, and research centers such as discarded syringe needles, bandages, swabs, plasters, and other types of infectious waste are often disposed with the regular non-infectious waste. Hence justifying waste in One Health.

18.7 Waste Electronic and Electrical Equipment (e-Waste)

Besides municipal/domestic waste, plastic waste, liquid wastes, and radioactive wastes, there are other major types of wastes that contribute to the increase in waste production in Africa, and these include end-of-life vehicles (EoLV) and electronic waste (e-waste). Africa being largely a developing continent, it mainly depends on imports of second-hand automotives/vehicles and electronics that have a short life span. These wastes can include refrigerators, computers, cell phones, circuit boards, etc. When shipped to Africa, they are dismantled for valuable metals in informal settings, resulting in significant human exposure to toxic substances. Among the common toxics released from e-wastes include lead, mercury, cadmium, beryllium, and brominated flame retardants (Awuchi et al. 2020), and these are known for being neurotoxicants. These wastes also expose humans to health risks through being breeding sites for several vectors like mosquitoes (Lebbie et al. 2021).

18.8 Drivers of Wastes Generation in Africa

The factors that influence waste generation and management vary from country to country and from city to city with a huge gap in the availability of waste data in Africa limiting the assessment of these factors. The major drivers of waste generation, collection, and disposal in Africa are population growth/increase, economic growth/income, urbanization, per capita income, level and need for industrialization, and the need for disposal (Bello et al. 2016). Majority of the African countries are experiencing rapid development with growth rate of 4% per annum (Horst and Tanya 2011). This comes with huge amounts of wastes, mainly MSW that has direct effect on human health, safety, and environment (Bello et al. 2016). Waste collection rate for African cities ranges from 20% to 80% (Achankeng 2003) and within Kampala city (64%) (Aryampa et al. 2019), Ndjamena in Chad at 15–20%, Yaoundé in Cameroon (43%) (Parrot 2019), Nairobi (30–40%) (Henry et al. 2006), and Dar es Salaam (51%) (International Solid Waste Association Report 2017). Such low collection efficiencies in African communities

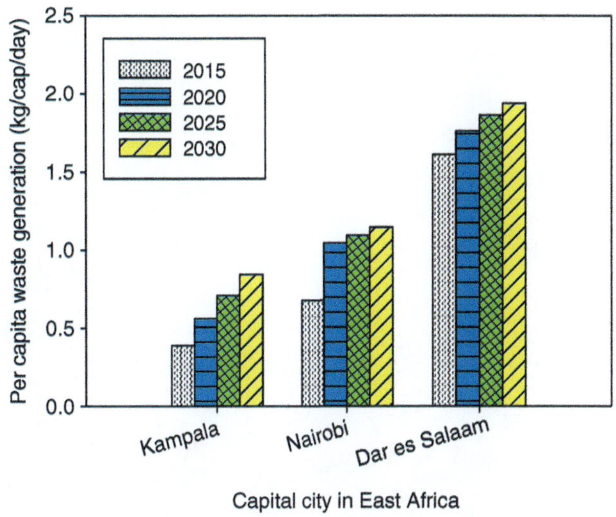

Figure 18.1 Projected waste generation rates of the three cities of East African Community (EAC). *Source:* Adapted from Aryampa et al. (2019).

clearly show that effective waste collection is a challenge to the governments and is creating environmental and human health problems for the current and future generations.

Taking examples of the capital cities in East Africa, waste generation rate in Kampala increased from 0.47 to 0.65 kg/capita/day by 2020. Projections of waste based on population indicated that waste is likely to increase by approximately 60% by 2030 in Kampala and Nairobi and by 74% in Dar es Salaam as shown in Figure 18.1.

18.9 Poor Handling Practices of Wastes

Waste continues to be a challenge in many growing urban towns in Africa (Komakech et al. 2014). Increased population means increased consumption of goods and services, and this translates into increase in the amount of waste generated (Yang et al. 2018). Research shows that over 1.3 billion tons of solid wastes is generated globally every year, and there is an increase in per capita waste generation rates, from 1.2 to 1.42 kg/person/day (Hoornweg and Bhada-Tata 2012). There are generally improper ways of disposal of wastes and insufficient funding for proper waste management (Vij 2012; Yang et al. 2018). Inappropriate waste disposal lead to environmental pollution of air, soil, and water (Yang et al. 2018) and causes health hazards of humans, animals, and environmental degradation (Vij 2012). Wastes have a complicated composition and hence require proper handling and disposal (Cao and Wang 2017). Though landfilling is the major method of disposal (Baidhe et al. 2021; Marshall and Farahbakhsh 2013; Mukama et al. 2016; Oates et al. 2019; Terazono et al. 2005), the remainder of the waste generated is indiscriminately disposed. Proper waste management involves control of

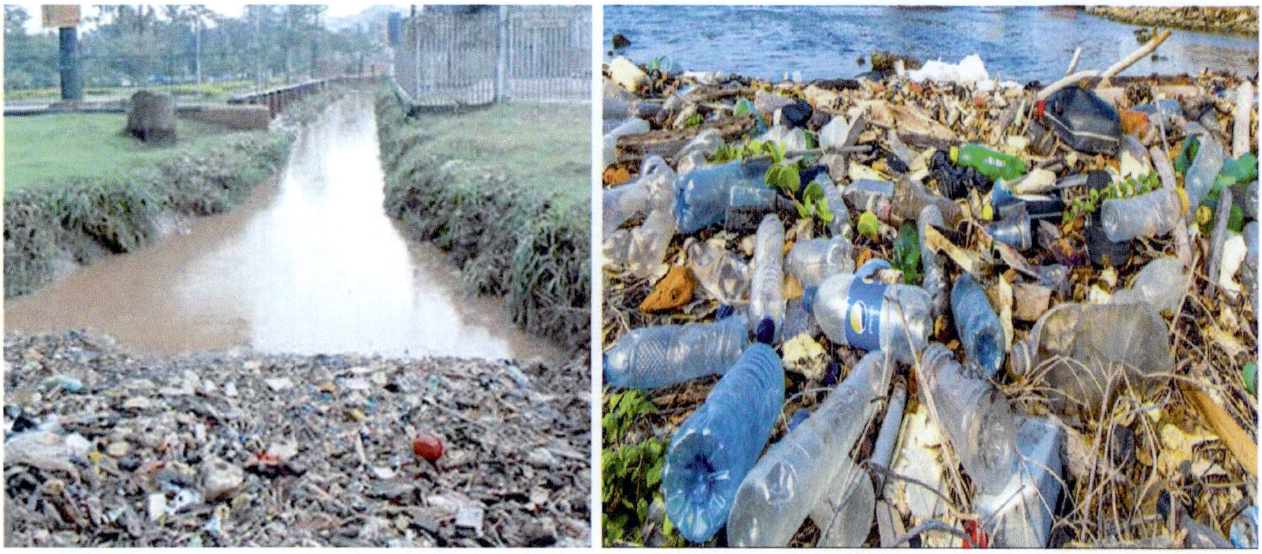

Figure 18.2 Picture of plastic wastes in water drainage channels in East Africa. *Source:* Wash Journal.

waste generation, storage, collection, transfer and transport, processing, and disposal of solid waste based on paramount practices.... that best addresses the range of public health, conservation, economic, aesthetic, engineering, and other environmental considerations. Therefore, solid waste management includes planning, administrative, financial, engineering, and legal functions. The solutions might include complex inter-disciplinary relations among fields such as public health, city and regional planning, political science, geography, sociology, economics, communication, conservation, demography, engineering, and material sciences (Ssemugabo et al. 2020). However, dumping of wastes in open areas (Figure 18.2) and roadsides or burning the biodegradable wastes and plastics (Abdel-Shafy and Mansour 2018) is a common practice in Africa both in rural and urban centres especially in slum settlements. This leads to negative effects to environment, human and animal health, as well as the aesthetic damage. For example Open burning of waste causes substantial air pollution which impacts human health and contributes to changing climates (Godfrey et al. 2019).

18.10 Knowledge, Attitudes, and Perceptions of Wastes in One Health

There is limited knowledge on proper and sustainable waste management practices in Africa (Mukama et al. 2016). Generally, there is poor public understanding of recycling of wastes (Cao and Wang 2017) and lack of knowledge on environmental effects of littering (poor waste management) (Omar et al. 2019).

Communities have still not embraced waste management hierarchy – reduce, reuse, and recycle (3R), and proper disposal (Terazono et al. 2005). The public still have an "I don't care" attitude and that the responsibility for solid waste management rests with the local government authority (WaterAid Uganda 2011). In developing countries, collection and disposal of wastes is not appropriately done (Abera 2017), and there is no sorting of wastes at household level to separate biodegradable from non-biodegradable (Hoornweg and Bhada-Tata 2012).

The poor attitudes among communities indicate lack of sufficient knowledge about good waste practices (Owojori et al. 2022) and their responsibilities in proper sustainable waste management (Mukama et al. 2016). Communities have limited skills of converting wastes into composite manure, making of briquettes for cooking, crafts, and jewelry (WaterAid Uganda 2011). Since knowledge shapes the attitude, therefore we can conclude that both knowledge and attitude are the elementary units for practice and very important in proper waste management.

18.11 Environmental Degradation of Improper Waste Disposal

Wastes in One Health if not well regulated through establishment of a waste management system could worsen environmental degradation of the communities. Illegal dumping of wastes in open fields, roadsides, and river banks and open burning (Etea et al. 2021) have been accelerated by lack of established waste management system (Henry et al. 2006) in communities, contributing to air, soil, and water pollution (Etea et al. 2021). Illegal open dumping and open incineration cause environmental degradation (Rehman et al. 2017), which causes natural resource degradation through polluting water, soil, and air (Etea et al. 2021) (Yazdani et al. 2015). Additionally, the challenge of open dumping and open air burning is that gases emitted from waste degradation process (Yazdani et al. 2015) contribute to greenhouse gases, ozone depletion, and climate change (Cogut 2016; Al-Othman and Palliam 2018; Godfrey et al. 2019). Improper waste management of wastes in One Health contaminates ground water resources, is a threat to human health and sanitation, and may contribute to environmental degradation (Ejaz et al. 2010). It is therefore important that authorities in communities establish structures for better waste management and environmental health.

18.12 Impact of Exposure to Waste on Human Health

Waste if not appropriately managed may contaminate water, soil, and the environment. This may result in releasing various pollutants in the environment (WHO 2016; Ziraba et al. 2016). Kanhai et al. (2021) report that waste could contribute to 6.5% of concentrated air pollution per annum in Ghana, while Zaman and Newman (2021) indicate that almost 79% of toxic plastics pollute the environment. This is because plastic waste releases toxic microparticles because most plastic products are made from petroleum-based fossil fuel sources. It is also noted that waste substances contribute to the release of mercury in the environment (Luz et al. 2021). Exposure to some particular types of waste especially for long time is reported to contribute to the burden of non-communicable diseases such as cancer or affect body organs (WHO 2016; Ziraba et al. 2016; Zaman and Newman 2021). The release of toxic substances in the environment emanating from waste is a health concern. The pollutants not only are destroying the environment and contributing to climate change disorders but also affect the well-being of living organisms. These pollutants may end up in the food chain or may be directly inhaled leading to multiple health consequences. For instance, Celestino et al. (2012) indicated that some chronic health issues were related to exposure to residues of agrochemicals in the environment (Celestino et al. 2012). Thus, the impact of exposure to waste on human health and other living organisms is a global concern.

Although studies exploring the relationship between exposure and health outcomes have been limited, there seems to be consensus among a few scholars that exposure to waste is associated with various health outcomes (Addo et al. 2017; Kanhai et al. 2021; Luz et al. 2021; Oyedotun et al. 2020; Ziraba et al. 2016). This is attributed to inappropriate measures for waste management in most countries, homesteads, and among waste actors especially waste pickers and recyclers (Gutberlet and Uddin 2017). Ziraba et al. (2016) endeavor to establish a framework showing the relationship between solid waste mismanagement, exposure, and poor health outcomes (see Figure 18.3). These vary from physical body injuries, acute

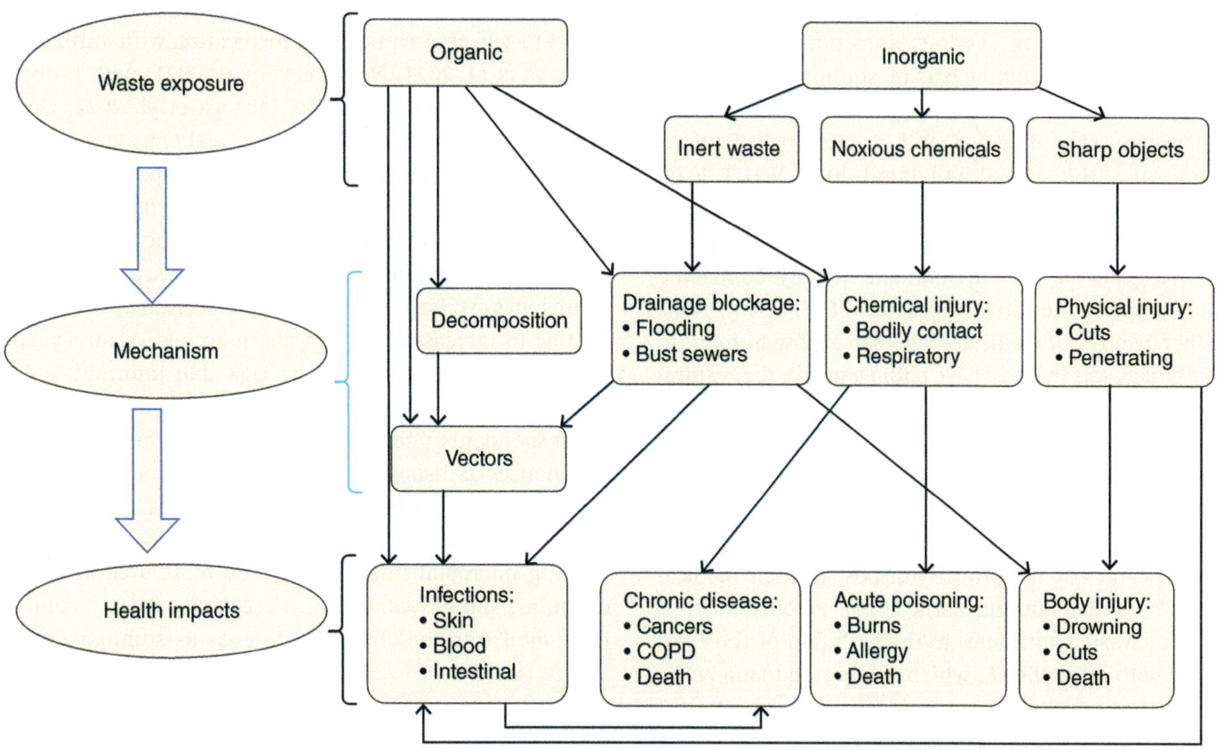

Figure 18.3 A framework for understanding the linkages between poor solid waste management and advance health outcomes. *Source:* Adopted from Ziraba et al. (2016)/Springer Nature/CC BY 4.0.

poisoning, chronic diseases and infections. Ziraba et al. (2016) caution that a person exposed to one type of waste may suffer from more than one health consequence. In this regard it should also be noted that some individuals may be exposed to more than one type of waste and are consequently likely to suffer from multiple health defects. Additionally, the health consequence of improper management of waste vary in regard to individuals vulnerable to the exposure, type of waste, and period of exposure among others (Akmal and Jamil 2021; Tsheleza et al. 2019; Ziraba et al. 2016)

The health consequences emanating from waste are double faceted. The first facet is the direct harm that waste may cause. For instance, exposure to the repugnant odor waste is not just an unsightly scene but may cause emotional stress. More so, for people that may get into direct physical contact with particular types of waste, for instance metal scraps, glass, and electronic, they may acquire injuries on their body or chemical or radiation injuries that may affect not only the skin but also the entire respiratory system and other systems since the human body is complex (Ziraba et al. 2016). It is reported that sharps from health care facilities that may contain blood contaminated with HIV can be found in many medical wastes, and puncture from the HIV-contaminated needles or blades can easily make the virus transfer to another host (Padmanabhan and Barik 2019). The second facet emanates from various waste management practices such as dumping, burning, and storage. For example, dumping of waste facilitates the breeding of disease-causing organisms such as bacteria, virus, fungus, and others, which transmit various infections as well as disease-spreading agents such as mosquitos, rodents, and flies responsible for malaria, dengue fever, gastrointestinal disorders, skin disorder, and respiratory infections (Addo et al. 2017; Akmal and Jamil 2021; WHO 2016; Ziraba et al. 2016).

With the advent of COVID-19 pandemic, poorly disposed protective gears in the environment notably contribute to the spread of the virus (Oyedotun et al. 2020). Also, improper disposal of medical wastes can expose humans to release of aerosols that can have pathogens like the respiratory syncytial virus or RSVs that can cause lung infections like pneumonia, tuberculosis, and influenza (Bates et al. 2013). Exposure of humans to hazardous materials can cause skin infections, for example anthrax can be contracted from these waste materials if laboratories that make anthrax vaccines do not properly dispose of their medical wastes (Padmanabhan and Barik 2019). Practice such as burning of waste contributes to the pollution of the environment with bisphenol-A, which is reported to affect the concentration of hormones for metabolism in human beings (Abraham et al. 2020; Chakraborty and Basu 2020). Improper disposal of waste substances contributes to the release of mercury in the environment, which could be responsible for increasing cases of emotional instabilities exhibited through high levels of anxiety, depression, and even insomnia (Luz et al. 2021). A study in Ghana that modeled waste emission to estimate its burden on health reveals that waste pollution contributes to premature deaths in Accra (Kanhai et al. 2021). It is noted that waste may be stored and not covered with lids (Addo et al. 2017) attracting flies and releasing a repugnant smell that may cause gastrointestinal disorders (Nuwematsiko et al. 2021). It is noted that improper storing, handling, and disposing of medical wastes may contain pathogens that transmit meningitis and is one of the leading diseases in Africa (Mazamay et al. 2021). Uncollected domestic garbage also increases risks of injury and infections to surrounding population. From the study it is clear that poor waste management practices contribute to the exposure to waste and its consequences on human health.

18.13 Contemporary Issues: Waste Management and Antimicrobial Resistance

Antimicrobial resistance (AMR) is threatening human and animal health as well as increasing the cost of health care. In Africa patients with limited access to health care resort to self-prescription and medication with antibiotics (Kagoya et al. 2021; Nabaweesi et al. 2021) with proportions ranging from 65 to 76% (Nayiga et al. 2022; Ocan et al. 2014). Due to the lack of an elaborate monitoring system on acquisition, use, and proper disposal of wastes containing the remaining antimicrobial drugs when self-medication is practiced, majority of the wastes and remaining drugs find their way in the environment. This causes massive horizontal transfer of resistant genes, thus leading to increased AMR in communities. A survey carried out in 2021 in one of the Ugandan informal settlements (slums) in Wakiso district, indicated that 89% of the respondents practice self-medication, thus increasing the chances of disposing the remaining medicines into the environment exposing the community and environment to health risks. Poor disposal of medical wastes used for treating microbial infections, for example used syringes, cannulas, and gloves, can also accelerate the problem of horizontal transfer of resistant genes as summarized in Figure 18.4.

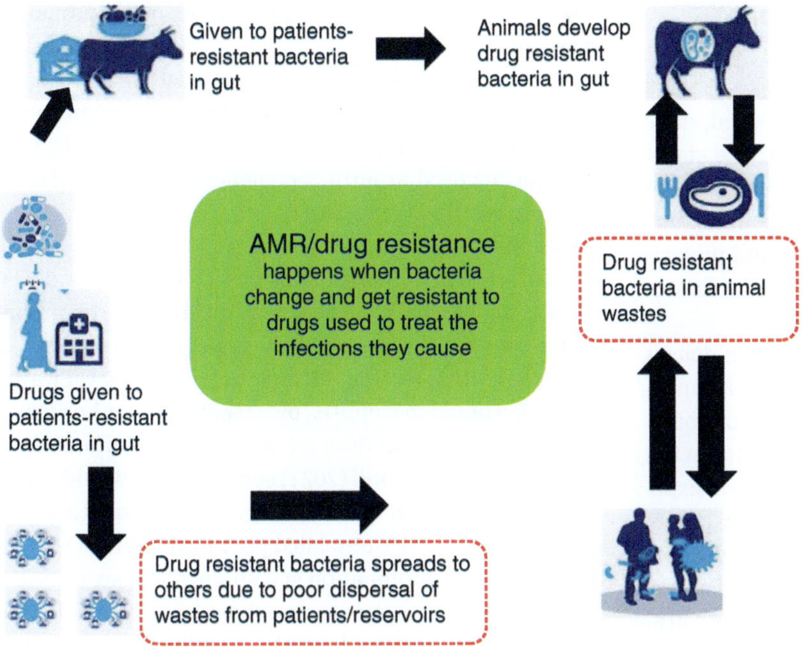

Figure 18.4 Flow of antimicrobial-resistant genes to the environment as a result of poor waste handling and disposal.

18.14 Waste Management Practices

There are several waste management practices observed at household and community level at large in most African countries. These practices include waste burning, storage of waste, waste sorting and separation, reuse and recycling, and indecent disposal of waste. Burning solid waste is one of the common practices of managing waste in Africa recorded by scholars (Lema et al. 2019; Sandra and Weghmann 2019; Tsheleza et al. 2019; Mier and Zhuo 2020; Abraham et al. 2020; Kanhai et al. 2021), which may be done in the yards of homesteads but also at dumping sites. Storage of waste is another practice that has been recorded and limited waste separation or sorting at source in terms of organic and inorganic, recyclable and unrecyclable, or toxic and nontoxic (Addo et al. 2017; Lema et al. 2019; Tsheleza et al. 2019; Zaman and Newman 2021). Nuwematsiko et al. (2021) further adds that there is a tendency of storing specific waste especially e-waste due to attachment without regard to risks of continued exposure. Reuse and recycling as well as disposal are also some of the fundamental waste management practices. Specific types of waste may be picked or sold by generators for recycling, for instance plastics and electronics (Nuwematsiko et al. 2021; Tsheleza et al. 2019; Ziraba et al. 2016). Tsheleza et al. (2019) emphasize that 89% of waste in South Africa has the potential to be recycled, reused, or composted; however, this is seldom done. Scholars (Aryampa et al. 2019; Kehinde et al. 2020; Nuwematsiko et al. 2021) concur that recycling has not been prioritized in most countries and even at household level. According to Zaman and Newman (2021) in the context of plastics, recycling initiatives have been geared toward zero-waste and not the zero-toxic concepts despite the pollution plastics have caused on land and in the marine life. Consequently, most waste that would be recycled is indecently disposed (Figure 18.4).

Dumping of waste is another rampant waste management practice. Aryampa et al. (2019) noted that recyclable waste is dumped at designated and undesignated spaces. Lema et al. (2019) concludes that improper disposal of waste such as throwing in ditches, river streams, and even in compound yards is a common practice in most poor countries. Drawing from South Africa, Tsheleza et al. (2019) reports that particularly in the informal settlements open dumping of waste is a common practice. A study by Nuwematsiko et al. (2021) reports that there were incidences of increasing illegal disposal of e-waste. The impact of waste on human health is seen in the manner in which the quality and status of the environment may be compromised though improper waste management practices and indecent disposal of waste. Conclusively, waste mismanagement contributes to the impact of exposure to waste on human health and serious action is needed to reverse the status quo (Abraham and Chakraborty 2020; Akkajit et al. 2020; Noufal et al. 2020).

18.15 Actionable Recommendations on Waste in One Health

In order to ensure that exposure to waste is reduced, there should be integrated strategies focusing on waste stakeholders right from generators, waste entrepreneurs, and policy makers. Waste management, that is proper handling and disposal, should be incorporated in all health projects to increase their effectiveness. Adding on the voices of other scholars, we recommend the following:

First, sensitization of communities about health defects arising from waste and its pollutants should be a fundamental strategy. This will ensure that generators of potentially harmful waste take responsibility to avoid harm but also to ensure that other people are not vulnerable to exposure. Sensitization has the potential to promote proper waste management practices of waste handling, collection, transportation, and disposal. Waste generators need also to understand the health risks of uncollected waste and burning waste. Sensitization campaigns should promote practices such as reuse, reduce, repair, and recycle. As Tsheleza et al. (2019) concludes, waste mismanagement can only be eliminated through sensitization and education. Recycling and reuse of wastes should also be emphasized. For example plastics can be recycled into brand new products that can be consumed by existing population, hence promoting waste in One Health.

At the household level, proper segregation of waste has to be done, and it should be ensured that all organic matter is kept aside for composting. The composted organic waste can thus be used as fertilizers, hence incorporating waste management in One Health.

Landfill sites should be located at a safe distance from all human settlement. They should be well lined and walled to ensure that there is no leakage into the nearby ground water sources. Burial in a deep geological repository is a favored solution for long-term storage of high-level waste.

There should be efforts by responsible authorities to ensure that waste services are accessible and affordable by all. As Akmal and Jamil (2021) conclude, this would reduce illegal and improper waste management practices and consequently reduce waste-related poor health outcomes.

Lastly, policy formulation and enforcement are critical to ensure that waste management practices are followed. Production of some products should be banned as has been the trend on polythene bags. We concur with Zaman and Newman (2021) that waste products whose toxicity levels have been confirmed should be banned. Incentives for waste recycles should be effective, while sanctions and punitive measures for waste dumping should be harsh enough to discourage malpractices.

References

Abdel-Shafy, H.I. and Mansour, M.S.M. (2018). Solid waste issue: sources, composition, disposal, recycling, and valorization. *Egyptian Journal of Petroleum* 27 (4): 1275–1290. https://doi.org/10.1016/j.ejpe.2018.07.003.

Abera, T. (2017). Assessment of knowledge attitude and practice towards solid and liquid waste management among Addis and Kometa Kebele Community Mizan-Aman Town, Bench – Maji Zone, Snnpr, South Waste Ethiopia, 2017. *Biomedical Journal of Scientific & Technical Research* 1 (5): 1346–1354. https://doi.org/10.26717/bjstr.2017.01.000434.

Abraham, A. and Chakraborty, P. (2020). A review on sources and health impacts of bisphenol A. *Reviews on Environmental Health* 35 (2): 201–210.

Abraham, S., Subramanian, M.V., Smitha, N.R. et al. (2020). BIOMAG-community based solid waste management through re-cycling and up- cycling in an adopted ward of corporation of Kochi, Kerala, India. *American Journal of Multidisciplinary Research & Development* 2 (12): 01–08.

Achankeng, E. (2003). Globalization, urbanization and Municipal Solid Waste Management in Africa, African Studies Association of Australasia and the Pacific. *Conference-Proceedings, African on a Global Stage.*

Addo, H.O., Dun-Dery, E.J., Afoakwa, E. et al. (2017). Correlates of domestic waste management and related health outcomes in Sunyani, Ghana: a protocol towards enhancing policy. *BMC Public Health* 17 (1): 1–10.

Akkajit, P., Romin, H., and Assawadithalerd, M. (2020). Assessment of knowledge, attitude, and practice in respect of medical waste management among healthcare workers in clinics. *Journal of Environmental and Public Health* 2020: https://doi.org/10.1155/2020/8745472.

Akmal, T. and Jamil, F. (2021). Assessing health damages from improper disposal of solid waste in metropolitan Islamabad–Rawalpindi, Pakistan. *Sustainability* 13 (5): 2717.

Al-Othman, S. and Palliam, R. (2018). *Environmental Degradation: Waste Disposal and Management in Kuwait (Issue October)*, 18. http://dx.doi.org/10.2139/ssrn.3272799 (acessed on 15 January 2023).

Aryampa, S., Maheshwari, B., Sabiiti, E. et al. (2019). Status of waste management in the East African cities: understanding the drivers of waste generation, collection and disposal and their impacts on Kampala City's sustainability. *Sustainability* 11 (19) 5523: 1–16. https://doi.org/10.3390/su11195523.

Awuchi, C.G. and Awuchi, C.G. (2019a). Physiological effects of plastic wastes on the endocrine system (bisphenol A, phthalates, bisphenol S, PBDEs, TBBPA). *International Journal of Bioinformatics and Computational Biology* 4 (2): 11–29. http://www.aascit.org/journal/archive?journalId=809.

Awuchi, C.G. and Awuchi, C.G. (2019b). Impacts of plastic pollution on the sustainability of seafood value chain and human health. *International Journal of Advanced Academic Research* 5 (11): 46–138. ISSN: 2488-9849.

Awuchi, C.G., Awuchi, C.G., Amagwula, I.O., and Igwe, V.S. (2020). Industrial and community waste management: global perspective. *American Journal of Physical Sciences* 1 (1): 1–16.

Baidhe, E., Kigozi, J., Mukisa, I. et al. (2021). Unearthing the potential of solid waste generated along the pineapple drying process line in Uganda: a review. *Environmental Challenges* 2 (November 2020): 100012. https://doi.org/10.1016/j.envc.2020.100012.

Bates, D., Zimlichman, E., Henderson, D. et al. (2013). Health care-associated infections: a meta-analysis of costs and financial impacts on the US health care system. *JAMA Internal Medicine* 2039–2046.

Bello, A.I., Ismail, N.B.M., and Kabbashi, A.N. (2016). Solid waste management in Africa: a review. *International Journal of Waste Resources* 6 (2): https://doi.org/10.4172/2252-5211.1000216.

Cao, R. and Wang, H. (2017). Research on the pollution hazard of municipal solid waste in China and its prevention and control legal countermeasures. *Nature, Environment and Pollution Technology* 16 (2): 463–469.

Celestino, J., Luz, V.B., Duarte, A.B.G., and Silva, T.F.P. (2012). Eight-cell parthenotes originated from in vitro grownb sheep preantral follicles. *Reproductive Sciences* 1219–1225.

Chakraborty, J. and Basu, P. (2020). Air quality and environmental injustice in India: connecting particulate pollution to social disadvantages. *International Journal of Environmental Research and Public Health* 2021 (18): 304. https://doi.org/10.3390/ijerph18010304.

Cogut, A. (2016). Open burning of waste: a global health disaster. R20 regions of climate action report. https://regions20.org/wp-content/uploads/2016/08/OPEN-BURNING-OF-WASTE-A-GLOBAL-HEALTH-DISASTER_R20-Research-Paper_Final_29.05.2017.pdf. (accessed 10 January 2023).

Ejaz, N., Akhtar, N., Nisar, H., and Ali Naeem, U. (2010). Environmental impacts of improper solid waste management in developing countries: a case study of Rawalpindi City. *WIT Transactions on Ecology and the Environment* 142: 379–387. https://doi.org/10.2495/SW100351.

Etea, T., Girma, E., and Mamo, K. (2021). Risk perceptions and experiences of residents living nearby municipal solid waste open dumpsite in ginchi town, Ethiopia: a qualitative study. *Risk Management and Healthcare Policy* 14: 2035–2044. https://doi.org/10.2147/RMHP.S309295.

Godfrey, L., Ahmed, T.M., Gebremedhin, G.K. et al. (2019). Solid waste management in Africa: governance failure or development opportunity?, Chapter 14. In: *Regional Development in Africa* (ed. N. Edomah). https://www.intechopen.com/chapters/68270 (accessed 20 January 2023).

Gutberlet, J. and Uddin, S.M.N. (2017). Household waste and health risks affecting waste pickers and the environment in low-and middle-income countries. *International Journal of Occupational and Environmental Health* 23 (4): 299–310.

Henry, R.K., Yongsheng, Z., and Jun, D. (2006). Municipal solid waste management challenges in developing countries – Kenyan case study. *Waste Management* 26 (1): 92–100. https://doi.org/10.1016/j.wasman.2005.03.007.

Hoornweg, D. and Bhada-Tata, P. (2012). What a waste: a global review of solid waste management. *Urban Development & Local Government Unit* https://doi.org/10.1201/9781315593173-4.

Horst and Tanya (2011). Exploring perception about the use of e-HRM tools in medium sized organisations. In: *Enterprise Information Systems: Concepts, Methodologies, Tools and Applications*, 1379–1398.

International Solid Waste Association Report (2017). International Solid Waste Association's "closing dumpsits" initiative: status of progree. *Waste Management & Research* 565–568.

Kagoya, E.K., Van Royen, K., Waako, P. et al. (2021). Experiences and views of healthcare professionals on the prescription of antibiotics in Eastern Uganda: a qualitative study. *Journal of Global Antimicrobial Resistance* 25: 66–71. https://doi.org/10.1016/j.jgar.2021.02.019.

Kanhai, G., Fobil, J.N., Nartey, B.A. et al. (2021). Urban municipal solid waste management: modeling air pollution scenarios and health impacts in the case of Accra, Ghana. *Waste Management* 123: 15–22. https://doi.org/10.1016/j.wasman.2021.01.005.

Kehinde, O., Ramonu, O.J., Babaremu, K.O., and Justin, L.D. (2020). Plastic wastes: environmental hazard and instrument for wealth creation in Nigeria. *Heliyon* 6 (10): e05131.

Komakech, A.J., Banadda, N.E., Kinobe, J.R. et al. (2014). Characterization of municipal waste in Kampala, Uganda. *Journal of the Air & Waste Management Association* 64 (3): 340–348. https://doi.org/10.1080/10962247.2013.861373.

Lebbie, T.S., Moyebi, O.D., Asante, K.A. et al. (2021). E-waste in Africa: a serious threat to the health of children. *International Journal of Environmental Research and Public Health* 18 (16): 8488.

Lema, G., Mesfun, M.G., Eshete, A., and Abdeta, G. (2019). Assessment of status of solid waste management in Asella town, Ethiopia. *BMC Public Health* 19 (1): 1–7.

Luz, D.A., Cartágenes, S.D.C., da Silveira, C.C.S.D.M. et al. (2021). Methylmercury plus ethanol exposure: how much does this combination affect emotionality? *International Journal of Molecular Sciences* 22 (23): 13131.

Marshall, R.E. and Farahbakhsh, K. (2013). Systems approaches to integrated solid waste management in developing countries. *Waste Management* 33 (4): 988–1003. https://doi.org/10.1016/j.wasman.2012.12.023.

Mazamay, S., Guégan, J.F., and Diallo, N. (2021). An overview of bacterial meningitis epidemics in Africa from 1928 to 2018 with a focus on epidemics "outside-the-belt". *BMC Infect ious Disease* 21: 1027. https://doi.org/10.1186/s12879-021-06724-1.

Mier, I.A.M. and Zhuo, L. (2020). Current status of municipal solid waste management in Juba city, South Sudan. *International Journal of Scientific and Research Publications (IJSRP)* 10 (8): 671–684. https://doi.org/10.29322/ijsrp.10.08.2020.p10485.

Mukama, T., Ndejjo, R., Musoke, D. et al. (2016). Practices, concerns, and willingness to participate in solid waste management in two urban slums in Central Uganda. *Journal of Environmental and Public Health* 2016: 7.

Mwesigye, P., Mbogoma, J., Nyakango, J. et al. (2009). Africa Review Report on Waste Management Main Report. Integrated Assessment of Present Status of Environmentally-Sound Management of Wastes in Africa. Economic and Social Council: United Nations-Economic Commission for Africa (2009-08)-main report (UN. ECA Committee on Food Security and Sustainable Development (CFSSD)/Regional Implementation Meeting (RIM) for CSD-18 (6th session: 2009, October 27–30), Addis Ababa, Ethiopia). https://hdl.handle.net/10855/3134 (accessed 10 January 2023).

Nabaweesi, I., Olum, R., Sekite, A.B. et al. (2021). Antibiotic practices, perceptions and self-medication among patients at a National Referral Hospital in Uganda. *Infection and Drug Resistance* 14: 2155–2164. doi: 10.2147/IDR.S303075. PMID: 34140783; PMCID: PMC8203198.

Nayiga, S., Denyer Willis, L., Staedke, S.G., and Chandler, C.I.R. (2022). Taking opportunities, taking medicines: antibiotic use in rural Eastern Uganda. *Medical Anthropology: Cross Cultural Studies in Health and Illness* 41 (4): 418–430. https://doi.org/10.1080/01459740.2022.2047676.

Noufal, M., Yuanyuan, L., Maalla, Z., and Adipah, S. (2020). Determinants of household solid waste generation and composition in Homs City, Syria. *Journal of Environmental and Public Health* https://doi.org/10.1155/2020/7460356.

Nuwematsiko, R., Oporia, F., Nabirye, J. et al. (2021). Knowledge, perceptions, and practices of electronic waste management among consumers in Kampala, Uganda. *Journal of Environmental and Public Health* 2021: 1–11. https://doi.org/10.1155/2021/3846428.

Oates, L., Gillard, R., Kasaija, P. et al. (2019). Supporting decent livelihoods through sustainable service provision: lessons on solid waste management from Kampala, Uganda. *Coalition for Urban Transitions* 1–20. http://newclimateeconomy.net/content/cities-working-papers(accessed 23 January 2023).

Ocan, M., Bbosa, G.S., Waako, P. et al. (2014). Factors predicting home storage of medicines in Northern Uganda. *BMC Public Health* 14: 650. https://doi.org/10.1186/1471-2458-14-650.

Omar, A.A., Hossain, M.S., and Parvin, M.M. (2019). Study on knowledge, attitude and practices towards the solid waste management in Karan District, Mogadishu Somalia. *Environmental Contaminants Reviews* 1 (2): 22–26. https://doi.org/10.26480/ecr.02.2018.22.26.

Owojori, O.M., Mulaudzi, R., and Edokpayi, J.N. (2022). Student's knowledge, attitude, and perception (KAP) to solid waste management: a survey towards a more circular economy from a rural-based tertiary institution in South Africa. *Sustainability* 14 (3): https://doi.org/10.3390/su14031310.

Oyedotun, T.D.T., Kasim, O.F., Famewo, A. et al. (2020). Municipal waste management in the era of COVID-19: perceptions, practices, and potentials for research in developing countries. *Research in Globalization* 2: 100033.

Padmanabhan, K.K. and Barik, D. (2019). Health hazards of medical waste and its disposal. *Energy from Toxic Organic Waste for Heat and Power Generation* 99–118. https://doi.org/10.1016/B978-0-08-102528-4.00008-0.

Parrot, D. (2019). 2019 full-year earnings. https://www.parrot.com/assets/s3fs-public/2020-03/Parrot_CP_FY-2019_0319_EN_DEF.pdf (accessed 1 March 2019).

Pushpakalambiga, R. and Jasmine, J. (2019). Biodegradable and Non-Biodegradable Waste Management. *Environmental Science, Journal of Community and Social Health Nursing.* 2 (1): 25–28.

Rehman, A., Saeed, S., Aslam, S.M., and Khan, W.M. (2017). Municipal solid waste management crises in the developing countries: a case study of Peshawar City. *Sarhad University International Journal of Basic and Applied Sciences* 5 (1): 23–32.

Sandra, V. N. and Weghmann, V. (2019). Municipal solid waste management services in Africa. Working Paper. PSI. France, Cedex. pp. 1–69.

Ssemugabo, C., Wafula, S.T., Lubega, G.B. et al. (2020). Status of household solid waste management and associated factors in a slum Community in Kampala, Uganda. *Journal of Environmental and Public Health* 2020: 10.1155/2020/6807630.

Terazono, A., Moriguchi, Y., Yamamoto, Y.S. et al. (2005). Waste management and recycling in Asia. *International Review for Environmental Strategies* 5 (2): 477–498.

Tsheleza, V., Nakin, M.D., Ndhleve, S. et al. (2019). Vulnerability of growing cities to solid waste-related environmental hazards: the case of Mthatha, South Africa. *Jamba: Journal of Disaster Risk Studies* 11 (1): 1–10.

Vij, D. (2012). Urbanization and solid waste management in India: present practices and future challenges. *Procedia – Social and Behavioral Sciences* 37: 437–447. https://doi.org/10.1016/j.sbspro.2012.03.309.

Water Aid Uganda. (2011). Solid waste management: study in Bwaise II parish, Kampala Division, Uganda, pp. 53. Solid-waste-management-study-in-Kawempe-Uganda-2011%20(2).pdf (accessed 7 January 2023).

WHO (2016). Environmental pollutants: genetic damage and epigenetic changes in male germ cells. *Environmental Science and Pollution* 23339–23348.

Yang, H., Ma, M., Thompson, J.R., and Flower, R.J. (2018). Waste management, informal recycling, environmental pollution and public health. *Journal of Epidemiology and Community Health* 72 (3): 237–243. https://doi.org/10.1136/jech-2016-208597.

Yazdani, M., Monavari, M., Omrani, G.A. et al. (2015). Municipal solid waste open dumping, implication for land degradation. *Solid Earth Discussions* 7 (1): 1097–1118. https://doi.org/10.5194/sed-7-1097-2015.

Zaman, A. and Newman, P. (2021). Plastics: are they part of the zero-waste agenda or the toxic-waste agenda? *Sustainable Earth* 4 (1): 1–16.

Ziraba, A.K., Haregu, T.N., and Mberu, B. (2016). A review and framework for understanding the potential impact of poor solid waste management on health in developing countries. *Archives of Public Health* 74 (1): 1–11.

19

Endocrine Disruptors and Female Reproductive Health

A Problem to Tackle with One Health Perspective

Luhan Jiang[1], *Kai-Fai Lee*[1,2], *and Suranga P. Kodithuwakku*[1,3,4]

[1] *Department of Obstetrics and Gynecology, Li Ka Shing Faculty of Medicine, The University of Hong Kong, Hong Kong SAR, China*
[2] *Shen Zhen Key Laboratory of Fertility Regulation, The University of Hong Kong-Shenzhen Hospital, Shenzhen, China*
[3] *Department of Animal Science, Faculty of Agriculture, University of Peradeniya, Peradeniya, Sri Lanka*
[4] *Institute of Veterinary Medicine and Animal Sciences, Estonian University of Life Sciences, Tartu, Estonia*

19.1 Introduction

The human population is believed to increase by 2 billion in the next 30 years reaching almost 9.7 billion mark by 2050 and by the year 2100, it is expected to reach to 11 billion mark (United Nations Population Fund 2022). Mainly Asian and African regions are expected to be the leading contributors. Therefore, the demand for basic needs like food, water, and shelter and the specific needs like transportation/mobility, health care, communication, and education will also be rapidly increased owing to the rapid economic growth of many of the Asian and African nations holding the lion's share of the total population. Interestingly, though the population increase has been seen and predicted, at the same time the fertility level around the world has seen a dramatic dip reaching the world average of 2.4 children per woman compared to 50 years back (The World Bank 2022). Interestingly, more economically developed nations have seen lower fertility rates lower than 2 where at least 2.1 children per woman are needed to maintain the society's population size (World Population Review 2022).

The increasing demands for various goods, services, lifestyle changes, and rapid industrialization paved the way for the synthesis and use of more and more chemical compounds and further expansion of the use of natural compounds from both plant and animal origins. Moreover, exposure to human beings to various chemical compounds via food webs, water, inhalation, personal care products, and personal protective equipment (PPE) due to pandemics like COVID-19 and other means also have been increased. In parallel to the increased use or presence of chemical compounds in the daily lives of humans, an increasing trend of various health issues was also observed. Therefore, scientists/clinicians started to pay more attention in figuring out relationships between the use/exposure to chemicals with various human health issues in the recent past. Interestingly, many of these daily use chemicals and their derivatives have now been identified as impacting or playing active roles in human health conditions, including reproductive health problems. Moreover, a similar trend has also been identified with animals, especially among the domesticated or farmed large animal species. This group of chemicals has now been identified as endocrine disruptors or endocrine disrupting chemicals (EDCs), and these EDCs can mimic some of the significant hormone actions and interact with the hormone receptors derailing normal homeostasis. Moreover, the impact of these EDCs can be seen at all levels in the biotic environment. Thus, most of the recent work on understanding the effects of EDCs and finding solutions for exposure of EDCs took a holistic approach based on one health principles. Traditionally one health has been restricted to zoonotic disease. However, now it has been further expanded as a trans-disciplinary approach to find answers for health issues that are common to human and animals where the environment has a direct influence. Furthermore, EDCs are becoming a one health issue given their wide range of impacts, thus, in this chapter, we will discuss the impact of selected EDCs which have significantly been studied in relation to human female reproduction functions, and highlight the need of adopting more aggressive one health and comparative medicine approaches and applications in finding solutions to prevent and mitigate the exposure to EDCs.

One Health: Human, Animal, and Environment Triad, First Edition. Edited by Meththika Vithanage and Majeti Narasimha Vara Prasad.

19.2 Endocrine Disruptors

An endocrine disruptor is an exogenous chemical or mixture of chemicals that interferes with any aspect of hormone action, including synthesis, secretion, transport, metabolism, binding action, or elimination (Sayles 2002). It was estimated that over 1000 chemicals exhibit endocrine-acting characters (Yilmaz et al. 2020). With the similar chemical structure, EDCs can easily mimic the natural hormones binding to the receptors and exert antagonist or agonist actions. They act on hormone receptors, including estrogen receptors (ERs), androgen receptors (ARs), progesterone receptors (PRs), thyroid receptors, and retinoid receptors (Diamanti-Kandarakis et al. 2009). Many known EDCs interact with ER to alter its signaling transduction via genomic and non-genomic pathways (Shanle and Xu 2011). However, they cannot fully induce the same effects and functions as natural hormones. Recently, more effects and mechanisms of EDCs on human health have been identified. EDCs can also bind to non-nuclear steroid hormone receptors, non-steroid receptors, orphan receptors, steroid biosynthesis, and metabolism pathways (Diamanti-Kandarakis et al. 2009). A wide range of EDCs can activate the aryl hydrocarbon receptor (AHR) to regulate the expression of critical enzymes for phase I and II metabolism compromising cytochrome p450-dependent monooxygenases, and UGT1A1, UGT1A6, UGT1A7, and GST-Ya (Tarnow et al. 2019). The enzyme induction mediated by AHR not only detoxify substance but also produce highly toxic metabolites (Tarnow et al. 2019). The EDCs can also affect the reproductive system or gametogenesis via epigenetic or histone modification. During early mammalian embryonic development, parental DNA methylation features are erased, and new methylation patterns are restored at a later stage (Feroe et al. 2017). The reprogrammed DNA methylation imprinting is inherited through a non-Mendelian pattern, and anything which interferes with such imprinting could alter gene expression leading to abnormal conditions (Feroe et al. 2017). Moreover, EDCs induce oxidative stress in females during first-trimester pregnancy leading to the elevation of oxidative markers expression in neonates and altered offspring gender (Puttabyatappa et al. 2020). In addition, Bisphenol A (BPA) induced oxidative response is associated with B cell cytotoxicity and impaired macrophage activation in-vivo and in-vitro (Huang et al. 2018; Jang et al. 2020). Furthermore, BPA causes and amplifies DNA damage including a double-strand break, DNA adducts, and gene mutation via impairing antioxidant enzyme pathway (Meli et al. 2020). All these modes will disrupt the genetic code leading to severe impairments of normal physiology, growth, and reproduction.

The EDCs can be divided into synthetic chemicals used in industrial products and natural chemicals found in food and feed (Diamanti-Kandarakis et al. 2009). Synthetic EDCs include Bisphenol A (BPA), phthalates, polychlorinated biphenyls (PCB), dioxins, fungicides (vinclozolin), pesticides [DDT (dichlorodiphenyltrichloroethane), methoxychlor and chlorpyrifos], phytoestrogens (genistein and coumestrol) and pharmaceutical agents [DES (diethylstilbestrol)] which are the widespread contaminants (Kawa et al. 2021). Moreover, due to industrial activities, EDCs produced by factories and processing plants would leak into the soil, seawater, or groundwater followed by accumulating in animals and can be biomagnified. In this way, EDCs have entered the food chain and reached the tail end, such as humans and carnivores, at very high doses. Lipophilic chemicals like persistent organochlorine pollutants (POPs) such as PCB can persist in the natural environment for a long time and be bioaccumulated in fatty tissue for decades (Yilmaz et al. 2020). BPA and phthalates are considered non-persistence EDCs since their half-life is 6 hours and 36 hours respectively (Encarnacao et al. 2019). Different from POPs, BPA can be excreted as BPA-glucuronide and eliminated in the urine (Encarnacao et al. 2019). Natural phytoestrogens such as genistein widely exist in soy products with low binding affinity to ERs. In recent years, the increasing usage of soybean formula has raised the discussion on the safety issue of phytoestrogens (Testa et al. 2018). Humans are exposed to EDC on daily basis mainly through diet, airway, skin absorption, maternal to the fetus and maternal to the infant. Fetus and newborn infant are the most sensitive period to EDCs (Kawa et al. 2021).

Most of the EDCs usually have a phenolic structure which can mimic the steroid hormones and bind to their receptors acting as an agonist or antagonists. The chemical structure of BPA has two hydroxyphenyl functionalities connected by two methyl groups. The analogous BPA shares a similar structure of hydroxyphenyl rings with the different connecting group. The other most common EDCs found in the environment are Phthalates and they are the esters of 1,2-di benzene dicarboxylic acid (Peijnenburg 2008). The phthalate products present various characteristics depending on the length and degree of the branching of the side chain (Encarnacao et al. 2019). The antiandrogenic effect of phthalates is largely due to reducing testosterone production (Martinez-Arguelles et al. 2011). The PCBs are derived from biphenyl with the chemical formula $C_{12}H_{10-n}Cl_n$, where n ranges from 1 to 10 (Kulkarni and Mehendale 2005). The basic structure of the dioxin molecule contains two benzene rings connected by oxygen atoms with/without chlorine or hydrogen atoms attached (Hites 2011). One of the most naturally occurring EDCs, phytoestrogens can be

Table 19.1 Summary of EDCs half-life in humans and sources.

EDCs	Half-life	Source	References
BPA	5.3 hours	Plastics	Genuis et al. (2012)
Phthalates	12 hours	Plastics and cosmetic products	Hoppin et al. (2002)
PCB	5–15 years	Dielectric fluids, heat transfer applications and plasticizers	Ritter et al. (2011), Takasuga et al. (2006)
Dioxins	7.2–15 years	Industrial by-products	Milbrath et al. (2009)
Phytoestrogens	3–10 hours	Plants and soybeans	Setchell et al. (2001)

grouped into four main subtypes including isoflavonoids, flavonoids, stilbenes and lignans (Cos et al. 2003). The general structure of isoflavonoids is consist of a 3-phenylchromen-4-one backbone, with three phenyl rings which are structural position is various from flavone (Sohn et al. 2021). Stilbenes are made up of two aromatic rings linked by an ethylene moiety (Pecyna et al. 2020). Lignans are formed by a β,β′-linkage between two phenylpropanes units (Li et al. 2018).

The EDCs can affect humans and animals via various exposure routes, at different dose levels and in various combinations. Human exposure to EDCs is mainly through dietary and other routes like inhalation and dermal absorption (Yilmaz et al. 2020). Detection of EDCs in human body fluids such as blood, urine, and breast milk confirmed human exposure to EDCs (Azzouz et al. 2016). Compared to adults, infants and children have a higher risk of exposure to EDCs mainly due to their living environmental and behavioral factors (Miller et al. 2002). With less movement ability, infants have more chances of contacting residues of cleaning reagents, dust, and pesticides on the floor, carpet, and crib (Miller et al. 2002). Furthermore, since children have more hand-to-mouth behaviors, they would uptake more EDCs via hand prehensile (Miller et al. 2002). The breathing zone of infants is closer to the floor than adults, and infants have a threefold higher breath rate than adults resulting in an increased risk of inhalation exposure to EDCs (Miller et al. 2002). In addition, the water and food consumption per unit of body weight of infants and young children is higher than adults leading to a rising intake of EDCs (Miller et al. 2002). Breast milk is one of the primary food sources for newborn babies. It was found that PCB and dioxins taken by mothers in earlier life can be concentrated in breast milk and resulted in a 50-fold higher intake per unit of body weight in the infant than in the adults (Miller et al. 2002). To manage human EDCs exposure, both the United States Environmental Protection Agency (EPA) and the European Centre for Ecotoxicology and Toxicology of Chemicals (ECETOC) performed intensive studies of various EDCs at a range of concentrations to set the lowest observed adverse effect level (LOAEL) or No Observed Adverse Effect Level (NOAEL) (Vandenberg et al. 2012; Ribeiro et al. 2017). According to the results, different from traditional toxicological concepts, EDCs show two main features: low-dose effect and non-monotonicity (Vandenberg et al. 2012). Low-dose effects indicate that a chemical exhibit a toxic effect at the lower end of the concentration spectrum (Vandenberg et al. 2012). The definition of nonmonotonicity is the dose-responsive curve changes pattern, in which the curve is U shape, at some points from positive to negative along with the concentration range or vice versa (Kohn and Melnick 2002). For example, exposure to the lower dose of DDT and Methoxychlor during mouse pregnancy would alter the litter size, the sex ratio of the litter, and the anogenital length of both male and female offspring (Palanza et al. 2001). Epidemiological studies also showed that women with intermediate PCB exposure had decreased risk of endometriosis compared to low or dose exposure (Trabert et al. 2010). With the rising consideration of the cumulative risk of EDCs, it has been well-known that humans, wildlife, and fishes have been accumulatively exposed to multiple EDCs (Table 19.1). There are three forms of the synergetic effects of EDCs, including independent action, dose addition, or interaction (De Falco and Laforgia 2021). POPs mixture is highly related to the pathogenesis of type 2 diabetes in humans, including beta-cell dysfunctions and lipid metabolisms (Zong et al. 2018). Combined EDCs treatments to seabream via dietary route would alter the lipid metabolism in the liver (Carnevali et al. 2017).

19.3 Human Female Reproductive Tract

The human female reproductive system consists of the ovary, oviduct, uterus, cervix, and vagina. The ovary is developed from germ cells, whereas the uterus, oviduct, cervix, and vagina are developed from the embryonic Mullerian tract. The ovaries are the main gametogenic and endocrine organ in the female reproductive tract. In mammalian animals, the ovarian follicle number is fixed at birth, representing the female reproductive potential (Hirshfield 1991). Follicle formation is the result of germ cell nest breakdown. Human ovary development starts from the first trimester when the germ cell migration from the genital ridge is successed and differentiated to oocyte with the formation of the primordial follicle with the somatic cell as the functional unit till the third trimester of gestation. Oocytes are arrested at the diplotene stage of late phosphate. Meiosis I meiotic division happens at puberty, and the Meiosis II division happens after fertilization. Interruptions during the oocyte development and differentiation would cause an aneuploidy embryo, premature ovarian failure (POF), and miscarriages (Diamanti-Kandarakis et al. 2009). Around the same time as germ cell formation, Mullerian ducts fuse to form the Mullerian tract, followed by further differentiation into the uterus, cervix, and upper vagina. The formation of stroma and epithelium happens at the postnatal stage and becomes functional matured during puberty with steroid hormone regulation.

The human Fallopian tube also plays a critical role in establishing successful pregnancy by providing a proper microenvironment for final gamete maturation, fertilization, early embryonic development, and finally, transporting the developing embryo to the uterus for further development subsequent implantation. The Fallopian tube also consists of epithelial and stromal cell compartments, which have active steroids, gonadotrophin, and other hormone receptors indicating the functions are under the endocrine and paracrine regulations (Maclean et al. 2020). Therefore, any EDC can quickly impart adverse effects on Fallopian tube functions through the receptors modulation.

The human uterus is the organ in the female reproductive tract that allows the embryo to implant, grow into a fetus, successfully nurse the growing fetus, and then give birth to the infant. Moreover, the endometrium can produce several hormones and factors which are essential for pregnancy and normal physiological activities of the reproductive tract. The endometrial epithelial, stromal, and smooth muscle cells in the myometrium possess hormone receptors. Depending on the stage of the menstrual cycle, these hormone receptors' expressions are varied, enabling stage-specific physiological functions (Critchley et al. 2020). Therefore, the human uterus is also a favorite target of many EDCs, and we have discussed it in detail in the following sections.

The cervix and the vagina of the female reproductive tract are also essential organs, and histologically, they share the same cell types, just like the uterus and Fallopian tube. Moreover, they also respond to the sex steroids dynamics across the menstrual cycles while expressing the receptors. Thus, EDCs have also been linked to neoplasia in the cervix and vaginal wall.

Accumulating research evidence has proven the detrimental effects of EDCs on the female reproductive system, especially on the ovary and uterus. Several critical exposure windows lead to female fertility disorders, including prenatal, postnatal, puberty, and before or during pregnancy. Moreover, few EDCs have been connected to cancer and endometriosis-like malignancies, which are becoming common in females.

19.3.1 EDCs and the Ovary

Since ovaries are the main endocrine entity in female reproduction, most of the direct impacts of EDCs can be observed in ovarian functions. In this section, we would like to highlight critical ovarian abnormalities, mainly focusing on Polycystic Ovary Syndrome (PCOS) and Premature Ovarian Failure (POF), which have been linked to EDCs exposure.

PCOS is characterized by hyperandrogenism and chronic anovulation leading to infertility (Sheehan 2004; Bachelot 2016). Half of PCOS patients also come with obesity and insulin resistance (Barber et al. 2019). In contrast to regular ovulation with one dominant follicle developed from a group of the small antral follicle, PCOS patients have multiple small antral follicles recruited at the same time leading to anovulation (Franks et al. 2000). The clinical symptoms are heterogeneous and commonly include irregular menstrual cycle, polycystic ovaries, and hirsutism (March et al. 2010). Based on the diagnostic criteria set by the Rotterdam Consensus workshop in 2003, there are three main features of PCOS patients, including ovulatory dysfunction, hyperandrogenemia, and polycystic ovaries, excluding disorders with similar clinical characteristics such as congenital adrenal hyperplasia, androgen-secreting tumors, Cushing's syndrome (Rotterdam 2004). Hypothalamic-pituitary-ovarian axis and metabolic, neuroendocrine, and other endocrine regulators are supposed to contribute to this complicated disorder (Diamanti-Kandarakis et al. 2009). However, the etiology of PCOS has not yet been identified. It is hypothesized that PCOS results from genetic and environmental co-effects (Fenichel et al. 2017). Due to the active involvement of endocrine regulation in PCOS etiology, EDCs may play a role in contributing to the pathogenesis of PCOS.

Premature ovarian failure, also known as primary ovarian insufficiency (POI), refers to the irreversible downregulation of ovarian function in advance of the typical timeline of a woman's age (Ishizuka 2021). It is a severe complication related to medical, psychological, and reproductive conditions and affects over 1% of women before 40-year-old worldwide (Jankowska 2017; Ishizuka 2021). The diagnosis criteria of POF adopted from the European Society of Human Reproduction, and Embryology (ESHRE, POI guideline development group's guidelines) are as follows, oligo/amenorrhea for at least four months and elevated FSH levels >25 mIU/ml on two occasions >four weeks apart (Ishizuka 2021). The etiology of POF is still unclear. The possible causes of POF include chromosome abnormalities, gene mutations, and autoimmunity (Ishizuka 2021). Recently, a meta-analysis pointed out the potential association between EDCs exposure and POF etiopathology. Here we would like to highlight some of the identified EDCs linked to the dysregulation of human ovarian functions. The below sections are based on the key EDCs which have been already well known to have disrupting effects on the human ovaries and their functions.

19.3.1.1 Bisphenols

Bisphenols are the most studied EDC, concerning their impacts on female reproduction. Higher BPA level was detected in women with PCOS, and they also had increased testosterone level with an inefficient BPA clearance (Takeuchi et al. 2004; Takeuchi et al. 2006). In PCOS women, urinary BPA level was negatively related to the anti-Mullerian hormone and day-3 follicular stimulating hormone levels, which indicate the ovarian reserve (Zhou et al. 2016). Recent clinical data suggest urinary BPA is associated with PCOS prevalence and irregular menstrual cycle (Hossein Rashidi et al. 2017). Furthermore, BPA may involve in insulin resistance and hyperandrogenism in PCOS patients (Hu et al. 2018). Using a rat model, it has been confirmed that BPA exposure during the neonatal stage would impair the hypothalamic-pituitary-gonadal axis of females resulting in PCOS phenotype in adulthood (Fernandez et al. 2010). Experimental evidence indicates that BPA possesses endocrine-disrupting properties by affecting steroid hormones production such as progesterone, dehydroepiandrosterone, androstenedione, estrone, testosterone, and estradiol by inhibiting the steroidogenic enzyme in mouse ovaries further impairing follicle development (Peretz et al. 2011). Moreover, BPA increases the level of testosterone production in rat ovarian theca cells via upregulating the key enzymes catalyzing androgen synthesis, including 17-hydroxylase (P450c17), cholesterol side chain cleavage enzyme (P450scc) and steroidogenic acute regulatory protein (StAR) (Zhou et al. 2008). An animal study demonstrated that Dibutyl phthalate (DBP) exposure during pregnancy resulted in reproductive system abnormalities in female offspring.

Evidence suggested that BPA exposure is related to lower oocytes survival rate, antral follicle counts, and follicle loss (Brieno-Enriquez et al. 2011; Zhou et al. 2016; Shen et al. 2020). In the rat, neonatal exposure to BPA showed a depletion of the primordial follicle and enhanced follicle recruitment which was associated with induced proliferation regulated by ER signaling pathway (Rodriguez et al. 2010). Furthermore, BPA exposure during the prepubertal period of rats also reduced follicle number and increased anti-Müllerian hormone (AMH) level indication induced primordial follicle recruitment leading to impaired ovarian reserve (Li et al. 2014). High dose and long-term BPA and its analogous exposure significantly reduced the antral follicle and corpus luteum number while enhancing oxidative stress in the post-weaning rat (Ijaz et al. 2020). However, the urinary level of BPA in premature ovarian insufficiency patients in China only marginally increased compared to the control (Li et al. 2021). A study reported that the BPA level in follicular fluid (FF) of diminished ovarian reserved patients was significantly increased and correlated with lower AMH and E2 levels in FF (Cao et al. 2018). The effect was also confirmed in the mouse model, indicating the role of BPA in the pathogenesis of DOR (Cao et al. 2018).

All these current knowledge on BPA suggests that ovaries are the most affected organ by BPA exposure in the female reproductive system. However, no exact biomarkers are available to detect the exposure, and no interventions are available to treat the exposure-related complication like in many other EDCs.

19.3.1.2 Phthalates

Platelets are also well known for their endocrine-disrupting activities, and even they have been banned from using in everyday consumables, especially in baby products. It has been intensively reported that phthalates inhibit germ cell nest breakdown, primordial follicle assembly, antral follicle growth, and oocyte saturation (Ambruosi et al. 2011; Wang et al. 2012a, b; Zhang et al. 2013, 2014). Phthalates can also induce primordial follicle recruitment and follicle atresia during the development (Hannon et al. 2014). In PCOS women, the Di(2-Ethylhexyl) phthalate (DEHP) level in follicular fluid was significantly higher than in healthy control, indicating possible involvement in the etiology of the PCOS (Jin et al. 2019). A more recent study showed that the urinary level of metabolites of phthalates such as mono-(2-ethyl-5-oxohexyl) phthalate is high in PCOS patients, again indicating the potential role of phthalates in the development of PCOS (Al-Saleh 2022). Although serum levels of DEHP and mono (2-Ethylhexyl) phthalate (MEHP) were not different between adolescents with PCOS and control, they are significantly associated with metabolic dysregulations such as insulin resistance in girls with PCOS (Akin et al. 2020). Therefore, phthalates may have a disruptive impact on ovaries through both direct and indirect pathways.

In China, a significantly increased urinary level of Mono-isobutyl phthalate was found in POF patients (Cao et al. 2020). As an indicator of ovarian function, E2/FSH ratio was negatively associated with the urinary level of phthalates metabolites suggesting phthalates impaired ovarian reserve leading to POF (Cao et al. 2020). In Korea, a cross-section study confirmed the association between urinary BPA, mono-(2-ethyl-5-hydroxyphenyl) phthalate (MEHHP), mono-(2-ethyl-5-oxohexyl) phthalate, and mono-*n*-butyl phthalate (MnBP) with increased risk of diminished ovarian reserve (Park et al. 2021). In the adult rat, the administration of 4 vinyl cyclohexene diepoxide (VCD) and phthalates mixture significantly reduced the primordial and primary follicle number and serum AMH level, indicating follicle depletion (Tran et al. 2018).

Due to many Phthalate analogs and their metabolic products in human, it is difficult to draw a complete picture of how phthalates affect ovarian function. Further animal studies and human cohort follow-ups are warranted for systematically verifying the effects of phthalates on the human female reproductive system.

19.3.1.3 Polychlorinated Biphenyls (PCB)

PCBs are also commonly found pollutants in water, air, and in food. A case-control study from China found that the serum level of PCB was nearly fourfold higher in a PCOS cohort than in a control group (Yang et al. 2015). However, another clinical study suggested no difference between PCB serum levels and PCOS prevalence (Neblett et al. 2020). PCBs are also known to modulate the steroid hormone synthesis in ovarian cells (Sechman et al. 2016), which could partly explain how they can involve in the etiology of PCOS. Moreover, a pilot study reported the antagonistic relation between the FF level of PCBs and ovarian reserve marker levels and in-vitro fertilization (IVF) outcomes (Bloom et al. 2017) and the maternal exposure to PCBs-induced ovarian follicle atresia with significantly reduced ovary weight in offspring (Shirota et al. 2006). Since the evidence of the impacts of PCBs on ovarian functional disruption is mainly from animal studies, more efforts are needed to delineate their exact impact on human ovarian functions. Methoxychlor is commonly co-occurring EDC in environmental samples with PCBs, and it could inhibit antral follicle maturation while stimulating the production of AMH in a rat model (Uzumcu et al. 2006). *In vivo* experiment showed that Methoxychlor via oral gavage significantly reduced the antral follicle number in different mouse models potentially via ERa signaling pathway (Borgeest et al. 2002; Miller et al. 2005; Tomic et al. 2006). Further in vitro study suggested that Methoxychlor partially increased the antral follicle atresia via the Bcl-2 pathway (Miller et al. 2005). However, like in PCBs, the real impact of this EDC on human ovaries is yet to be determined.

Although PCBs have been banned in commercial products in most countries since the first evidence of their harmful effect on human was published in 1968 (Keys 2002), they can still be detected in human serum nowadays (Zhang et al. 2021a). There are few investigations on stimulating the elimination of PCBs from the human body or the environment.

19.3.1.4 Genistein

Genistein is a naturally occurring phytoestrogen found in many plant-based foods, especially soy-based products. Contrary to other synthetic EDCs, genistein improved ovarian morphology and follicular distribution in the PCOS rat model mainly through the Bcl-2 signaling pathway (Chi et al. 2018). Further studies showed that Genistein could restore the estrus cycle, moderate hyperandrogenism, and reduce cystic follicles in PCOS rodent models, indicating the therapeutic potential of Genistein in the PCOS (Amanat et al. 2021; Luo et al. 2021) Genistein supplement could improve antioxidant response by increasing superoxide dismutase enzyme activity and the ovarian secretion functions in PCOS rodents dependent on ER signaling (Amanat et al. 2021; Luo et al. 2021). Furthermore, genistein administration decreased circulating low-density lipoprotein and pro-inflammatory cytokines such as tumor necrosis factor-alpha in rats with PCOS (Amanat et al. 2021). In human, a three-month genistein regiment for PCOS women showed a decreasing level of serum LH, triglyceride, LDL cholesterol, and testosterone which are usually increased in PCOS patients (Khani et al. 2011). The benefit of genistein or soy isoflavone to PCOS patients also includes reducing BMI, insulin resistance, glycemic control, circulating testosterone, and lipid profiles, significantly increasing circulating nitric oxide and glutathione (Jamilian and Asemi 2016; Karamali et al. 2018). Though genistein showed the above positive outcomes, it is also well known to disrupt ovarian development at the neonate stage in mice (Wu et al. 2019). There are various records of the disruptive endocrine effects of Genistein in animal models (Jefferson and Williams 2011), and very few human studies are available. In human cell culture study, Genistein directly inhibits 17 β-hydroxysteroid dehydrogenase activity, which is a critical enzyme in steroids production in the human ovary (Whitehead et al. 2002) and also disrupts aromatase activities as well (Rice et al. 2006). Thus, given the phytoestrogen in nature, it is worth further investigating the endocrine disruptive impact of Genistein. It would be better to be cautious when using soy products, especially the females with known other ovary-related reproductive problems.

Genistein also exhibits therapeutic potential to POF, like PCOS. In the gamma radiation-treated rat model, the administration of genistein would reverse the primordial follicle depletion, activate follicle number, and reduce follicle atresia (Haddad et al. 2020). Genistein can also prevent follicle granulosa cell apoptosis by reducing the Bax/Bcl-2 ratio followed by reduction of cytochrome c and caspase three expression (Haddad et al. 2020). Genistein upregulated the expression of C-X-C chemokine ligand 12 (CXCL12) and early growth response gene-1 (EGR-1), which would prevent POF in both young and aging rat (Zhang et al. 2021b). However, in the neonatal mouse ovary, genistein inhibited the oocyte nest breakdown and primordial follicle formation leading to multiple oocyte follicle (Chen et al. 2007). The adult female mice exposed to genistein during the neonatal stage exhibited a decreased corpora lutea formation with cystic follicle (Wu et al. 2019). Furthermore, none of the mice treated with genistein during the neonatal stage achieved successful pregnancy after mating with a fertile male for two months (Wu et al. 2019). Genistein also induced IGF-1 and IGFBP-1 expression in rat ovaries suggesting its role in preventing ovary reserve depletion via the insulin-like growth factor signaling pathway (Chi et al. 2019).

In summary, PCOS and POF are two significant complications related to reduce female fertility affecting more than 1–20% of women during reproductive age, causing pregnancy failure and stress (Jankowska 2017; Deswal et al. 2020). Etiological studies clearly showed that EDCs levels in human body fluid are related to the prevalence of PCOS and POF. Therefore, various EDCs overexposure has been proven to be one of the etiological factors. However, rodent models were commonly used to identify the molecular mechanisms of EDCs during folliculogenesis and reproductive system development, while more direct human evidence is needed. Animal studies reported the transgenerational germline inheritance of the epimutation induced by EDCs which may be one of the reasons leading to ovarian development defects. In contrast, further studies are needed to prove the mechanisms.

19.3.2 EDCs and the Endometrium

The endometrium is the innermost lining of the uterus, and it consists of epithelium, glands, and stromal cells together with a complex vascular, neural, and lymphatic network. The endometrium is the lining mainly interacts with the embryo during the implantation process and subsequently lets the implanted embryo grow through placentation. Moreover, the endometrium produces various hormones, including steroids, which are critical in normal and pregnant endometrial physiology. Endometrium shows cyclical changes in anatomy and functions along with the menstrual cycle phase responding to the hormones and expressing the hormone receptors. Thus, any exogenous entity that can mimic hormonal activities like EDCs can directly or indirectly impair the normal physiology and functions of the human endometrium, resulting in various abnormalities leading to subfertility and infertility. Moreover, some abnormalities could also lead to benign or malignant cancer conditions. In the below section, we discuss a few necessary abnormal conditions in the human endometrium where the etiologies have been linked to EDCs.

Endometriosis is an estrogen-dependent disease found only in human and a few high-order primates; which are defined as ectopic growth of endometrial-like tissue (glands and stroma) resulting in the chronic inflammatory response and lesions on the peritoneum and ovary (Parasar et al. 2017; Lagana et al. 2018). It causes chronic pelvic pain, dysmenorrhea, dyspareunia, irregular uterine bleeding, and infertility (Lagana et al. 2018). It affects 5–10% of women of reproductive age, causing severe influence on patients' physical well-being and life quality (Vitale et al. 2017). According to the American Society for Reproductive Medicine guidelines, the classification of Endometriosis should be based on the morphology and percentage of involvement in the peritoneal and pelvic lesion (Canis et al. 1997; Parasar et al. 2017). For diagnosing endometriosis, the number, size, and location of endometrial implants, plaques, endometriomas, and adhesions should be carefully inspected (Canis et al. 1997). Endometriosis can be sub-grouped into peritoneal superficial lesions, ovarian cysts (endometriomas), and deep infiltrating endometriosis. It can be scored into four stages minimal, mild, moderate, and severe, based on the revised American Fertility Society classification (Dunselman et al. 2014). With little knowledge of the etiology of endometriosis, animal models have been established, including rodents, rabbits, and non-human primates, for understanding the molecular mechanisms of endometriosis and developing new diagnostic and therapeutic methods (Lagana et al. 2018). Many EDCs have been indicated in the pathophysiology of endometriosis, and most of the information comes from animal models. However, there is some limited interesting evidence in human as well.

Repeated implantation failure (RIF) is referred to as failure to implant causing pregnancy loss after transferring good-quality embryos in three consecutive in-vitro fertilization attempts (Simon and Laufer 2012; Polanski et al. 2014). However, the exact diagnostic criteria remain controversial (Coughlan et al. 2014; Somigliana et al. 2018). Implantation failure can be affected by maternal age, embryo quality, and uterus factors. The parental chromosomal abnormities can also cause various pregnancy complications, and the couples with balanced chromosomal translocation had a higher chance of implantation failure than the control group (Stern et al. 1999). Moreover, most RIF patients have abnormal endometrial immune profiles compared to control patients (Ledee et al. 2016). Uterine factors leading to recurrent implantation failure include congenital uterine abnormities, acquired intracavity pathologies such as submucous fibroids, endometrial polyps, intrauterine adhesions, and adenomyosis (Coughlan et al. 2014). Apart from the intracavity structural complications, the endometrium's immune response also plays a part in regulating the optimal endometrial receptivity (Kwak-Kim et al. 2005). A recent study illustrated a higher prevalence of chronic endometritis in RIF patients with an increasing level of CD138+ cells, a marker of inflammation in the endometrium, than in the control (Saxtorph et al. 2020). Thus, any external entity, including chemicals that modulate the immune system, could contribute to the etiology and progression of RIF. Lifestyle factors such as smoking and obesity also contribute to the pathogenesis of the RIF (Practice Committee of the American Society for Reproductive Medicine. Electronic address and Practice Committee of the American Society for Reproductive 2012, 2021).

19.3.2.1 Bisphenol A

The association between EDCs and endometriosis morbidity has been well-identified in recent years. An example regarding urinary BPA level and the prevalence of endometriosis has been conducted in different cohort studies. Upson and co-workers conducted a population-based case-control study and reported a positive association between the increased urinary BPA level and raised risk of non-ovarian pelvic endometriosis in US women (Upson et al. 2014). Wen and co-workers showed that the creatinine-adjusted urinary BPA concentrations are associated with serum MMP2 and MMP9 levels, a risk factor for peritoneal endometriosis (Wen et al. 2020). Iranian women also observed a similar phenomenon (Rashidi et al. 2017). However, a case-control study found no significant relationship between Bisphenol F and S and the risk of endometriosis (Peinado et al. 2020). Interestingly, Simonelie and co-workers found that the prevalence of endometriosis is not relevant to patients with a high risk of BPA exposure. However, they still proved that urinary BPA level is associated with endometriosis (Simonelli et al. 2017). Most of the clinical studies used the urinary BPA level to represent the exposure, Simonelie and co-workers attempted to collect pelvic fluid to measure the BPA level by using gas chromatography-tandem mass spectrometry (GC/MSMS). However, the statistical analysis did not result in significant outcomes owing to the limited sample number (Simonelli et al. 2017). The possible mechanism of BPA causing endometriosis can be due to an induced inflammatory response, hyperestrogenic environment, embryogenetic pathogenesis, development of progesterone resistance, and early onset of puberty (Signorile et al. 2010; Wen et al. 2020; Stephens et al. 2021). An *in vitro* study further reported that the environmental dosage of BPA would enhance the invasion ability of endometrial stromal cells by upregulating the MMP2 and MMP9 expression (Wen et al. 2020). Furthermore, BPA can induce oxidative stress and inflammatory response in human endometrial stromal cells through ER signaling (Cho et al. 2018). Using a mouse model, Signorile and co-workers demonstrated that prenatal exposure to BPA would cause an endometriosis phenotype in female offspring (Signorile et al. 2010). Since BPA can contaminate many environmental components, it is worth performing continuous monitoring and environmental assessment to prevent unintentional exposure. Moreover, females experiencing fertility issues due to endometriosis would ideally be aware of the sources of different BPs and should be advised to avoid the exposures as much as possible.

19.3.2.2 Phthalates

It is confirmed that the exposure of both Phthalate esters and their metabolites is related to the morbidity of endometriosis (Sirohi et al. 2021). A matched population and operative cohort study proved that sixteen types of phthalates could be detected in women's urine. Six of them are positively related to twofold higher odds of an endometriosis diagnosis in the population group (Buck Louis et al. 2013). The urinary level of monooctyl phthalate is related to visualized and histological endometriosis in the operative population (Buck Louis et al. 2013). However, a case-control study performed in the US found an inverse association between the fourth and fifth-quartile urinary mono-(2-ethyl-5-hexyl) phthalate (MEHP), which is a metabolite of DEHP, concentration, and endometriosis risk (Upson et al. 2013). The result of the work from Upson and co-workers also showed that an increased endometriosis risk is associated with urinary mono-benzyl phthalate (MBzP) and mono-ethyl phthalate (MEP) levels; however, it is not statistically significant (Upson et al. 2013). Measurement of urinary phthalates and their derivatives is quite tricky and method sensitive. Thus, it is essential to use the most appropriate method based on the sample type with proper storage and handling of samples. The association between phthalates and endometriosis has been confirmed in different regions worldwide, indicating a broad exposure to them and a rising risk leading to endometriosis in women. Both Rozati and Reddy, with their co-workers, have reported an association between increased serum levels of phthalates and endometriosis in Indian women (Reddy et al. 2006; Rozati et al. 2008). Kim and co-workers also found that the plasma level of monoethylhexyl phthalate and DEHP was significantly higher in an advanced-stage endometriosis patient cohort (Kim et al. 2011). In Taiwan, two studies showed a significant association between endometriosis and Phthalate metabolites, including mono-*n*-butyl phthalate (MnBP) and MEHP (Huang et al. 2010; Chou et al. 2020). A recent meta-analysis summarized eight studies and found that only MEHHP out of the other five phthalates metabolites was potentially associated with endometriosis in Asia but not in USA (Cai et al. 2019). Moreover, an investigation using a rodent model demonstrated that chronic exposure to *n*-Butyl benzyl phthalate (BBP) would increase the surgically induced endometriotic lesion survival rate via enhancing CD44 on plasmacytoid dendritic cells (Sharma et al. 2021). Like in bisphenols, phthalates are also commonly found in many environmental sources and food/feed due to the commonly used plastic-based materials. Therefore, getting more insights through animals and other environment-related research would be edificial under one health concept.

19.3.2.3 Polychlorinated Biphenyls

Persistent organic pollutants (PoPs) have also become common in many environmental components, including air and water. Both PCBs and dioxins belong to POPs. There are non-dioxin-like PCBs (NDL-PCBs) and dioxin-like PCBs (DL-PCBs) (Porpora et al. 2009). The concern about the effect of PCB on endometriosis morbidity and progression was never ended. Based on the quoted thirteen recent pieces of research, the association between PCB and endometriosis has remained controversial (Lebel et al. 1998; Pauwels et al. 2001; De Felip et al. 2004; Heilier et al. 2005; Louis et al. 2005; Porpora et al. 2006, 2009; Niskar et al. 2009; Cai et al. 2011; Buck Louis et al. 2012; Martinez-Zamora et al. 2015; Trabert et al. 2015; Ploteau et al. 2017). Most of the published data reported a significant association between endometriosis body fluid levels of PCBs, including PCB-105, PCB-114, and DL-PCB-118, DL-PBC-156, DL-PCB-167, NDL-PCB-101, NDL-PCB-138, NDL-PCB-153, NDL-PCB-170, NDL-PCB-180 in France, Italy or US (Louis et al. 2005; Porpora et al. 2009; Ploteau et al. 2017). Especially, Plateau and co-workers reported that significant correlation between the adipose level of PCB and dioxin with a deep infiltrated endometriosis (Ploteau et al. 2017). However, Fierens and colleagues found no association between the increased serum level of NDL-PCBs or dioxins and endometriosis in a Belgium women cohort (Fierens et al. 2003). Moreover, Louis, Trabet, and their co-workers found an inverse association between PCB-74, DL-PCB-156, NDL-PCB-170, PCB-196, and PCB-201with endometriosis (Buck Louis et al. 2012; Trabert et al. 2015). Dioxin includes 2,3,7,8-tetrachlorodibenzo-*p*-dioxin (TCDD), polychlorinated-dibenzo-*p*-dioxin (PCDD), and polycholarinated-dibenzo-furans (PCDF) (Sirohi et al. 2021). By comparing 29 dioxins levels in serum and peritoneal fluid, Cai and colleagues found that a higher level of PCDD and PCDF in the peritoneal fluid was associated with an increased risk of endometriosis (Cai et al. 2011). However, a pilot case-control study reported that dioxin-like compounds exposure is not relevant to endometriosis. At the same time, the serum level of dioxins in Belgian women was significantly higher in Italian women at reproductive age (De Felip et al. 2004). Since PoPs are co-founded in endometriosis and are also known as biomagnified through the food chains, females are at increased risk of exposure to PoPs, just like other EDCs. The interactions or combined effects of different PoPs in animal and human systems have limited information available in the literature since many studies focus only on a single or couple of EDCs simultaneously. Thus, it would be time to use one health approach to investigate the combined effects of already identified main EDCs on endometriosis and other female endometrium-related disorders.

19.3.2.4 Genistein

Under the impact of EDCs on human endometrium, we have highlighted the possible disruptive effects of phytoestrogens, including Genistein, along with the reported positive effects on specific ovarian abnormalities. Usually, estrogen is known to increase ectopic endometrial cell proliferation and promote endometriotic lesions. However, Genistein was found to elicit a potentially therapeutic potential against endometriosis. A recent clinical study reported no association between urinary level of phytoestrogen and the risk of endometriosis in premenopausal women (Mumford et al. 2017). In a rat model, three weeks of genistein treatment caused a reduction of the endometriotic implants (Yavuz et al. 2007). Genistein could inhibit the inflammatory response and angiogenesis in the peritoneal endometriosis mouse model by reducing the expression of ERα, VEGF, and HIF-1a while increasing the ERβ level in the endometrium (Sutrisno et al. 2018). Treating the stromal cell isolated from ovarian endometrioma with daidzein-rich isoflavone aglycones such as daidzein and genistein inhibited the cell proliferation, suggesting a potential therapeutic role of these phytoestrogens (Takaoka et al. 2018). The potent anti-inflammatory of genistein was found previously by inhibiting NF-κB, prostaglandins, and pro-inflammatory cytokines, including IL-1β, IL-6, and TNF-α as well as Nitric Oxide signaling (Goh et al. 2022).

Many clinical studies have been performed to evaluate the EDCs exposure and pregnancy outcomes or implantation rate of women after IVF treatment. It was reported in a clinical cohort study that high levels of urinary PCB metabolites, including MEHP, MEHHP, MEOHP, MECPP, ∑DEHP (MEHP + MEHHP + MEOHP + MECPP), and MCNP, were related to poor outcomes of the oocyte yield and matured oocyte retrieved (Hauser et al. 2016). Further, in the highest urinary ∑DEHP level, women showed a decreased proportion of cycles leading to a living birth (Hauser et al. 2016). In the Saudi population, urinary MEP and MEHP level is positively related to the risk of failed clinical pregnancy and decreased live birth rate of women who undergo IVF (Al-Saleh et al. 2019). Both clinical studies and *in vivo* mouse models suggested that BPA exposure is associated with implantation failure. The urinary BPA level is positively related to the implantation failure rate in women undergoing IVF (Ehrlich et al. 2012). A case-control study demonstrated that environmental exposure to bisphenol analogs such as bisphenol AP (BPAP), bisphenol AF (BPAF), and BPA are associated with unexplained recurrent miscarriage in Chinese women over 30-year-old (Ao et al. 2022). Yuan et al. demonstrated that preimplantation exposure to BPA would potentially decrease implantation site number in mouse models via progesterone receptor (PGR) and ERs signaling (Yuan et al. 2015). In contrast to the positive effect of genistein in POF and endometriosis, rat model showed that genistein and daidzein reduced endometrium receptivity (Toktay et al. 2020).

Endometrium plays vital functions in female reproduction and the continuation of humankind. Due to the periodic regulation of hormones, the endometrium is vulnerable to exogenous hormones such as EDCs. The altered hormone signaling pathway would cause dysfunction of the endometrium leading to implantation failure and miscarriage. Further, EDCs would induce oxidative stress and aberrant immune response, resulting in reproductive diseases such as endometriosis. However, only some studies focused on the relationship between RIF and EDCs exposure. It is possibly due to the unclear and complex pathogenesis of RIF. More detailed clinical and molecular studies are still needed to understand further the role of EDCs in mediating female reproductive functions.

19.3.3 EDCs and Transgenerational and Multigenerational Effect

It is well known that EDCs cause multigenerational and transgenerational effects in the male and female reproductive systems. If the pregnant female (F0) is exposed to EDCs, offspring in the F1 generation are directly exposed to EDCs in the uterus since most EDCs bypass the placental barrier (Brehm and Flaws 2019). Multigenerational effects of EDCs have been considered that the offspring is exposed to EDCs during development in the uterus (F1) or as germ cell (F2) (Brehm and Flaws 2019). The offspring (F3) of F2 are not directly exposed to EDCs; the effects observed on F3 are defined as transgenerational (Brehm and Flaws 2019). EDCs-induced transgenerational epigenetic inheritance effects range from reproductive and behavioral changes to obesity (Skinner 2014). The germ line epigenetic mutations include DNA methylation, histone modifications, non-coding RNA, and chromosomal structural alteration (Skinner 2016). The inheritance of PCOS and POI has been proven to be related to epigenome and transcriptome alteration induced by ancestral EDCs exposure (Nilsson et al. 2018). Ancestral exposure to vinclozolin and DDT caused changes in differentially methylated regions, long noncoding, and small non-coding RNA expression in the ovarian granulosa cells of the F3 generation rats (Nilsson et al. 2018). Similar ovarian diseases, such as primordial follicle loss and PCOS, were also observed in F3 generation rats that had been ancestrally exposed to EDCs derived from plastics, including BPA, DEHP, and DBP at lower dose (Manikkam et al. 2013). Pesticides such as Methoxychlor exposure to pregnant rats induced the incidence of polycystic ovary disease in the F3 generation without affecting the E2 and testosterone level (Manikkam et al. 2014). PCB affected the hormone, neurotransmission, and neuropeptides-related gene expression in the F1–F3 generation female hypothalamus (Gore et al. 2021). Aroclor 1221, which is a chlorinated mixture PCB with weak estrogenic characteristics, reported that its effect on reproductive and social sexual behaviors could persist through subsequent three generations of female rats after ancestral exposure indicating the effect might be epigenetic germline transmitted (Kermath et al. 2022). The F2 and F3 offspring of female Wistar rats which had been exposed to a mixture of 13 EDCs including di-*n*-butyl phthalate (DnBP), DEHP, BPA, vinclozolin, prochloraz, procymidone, linuron, epoxynaxole, dichlorodiphenyldichloroethylene, octyl methoxynimmate, 4-methyl benzylidene camphor (4-MBC), butylparaben, and acetaminophen showed delayed onset of puberty, altered estrus cycle and folliculogenesis defects with an increasing of atretic and cystic follicle number (Lopez-Rodriguez et al. 2021). The study further proved that hypothalamic genes such as Kiss1, Esr1, and Oxt regulating puberty and ovulation were altered in a transgenerational epigenetic mechanism via maternal germline lineage (Lopez-Rodriguez et al. 2021). In the hamster, gestational exposure to TCDD would severely alter the reproductive function of F1 and F2 female offspring leading to increased implantation failure and reduced litter size (Wolf et al. 1999). Although it has been shown that EDCs can modulate the germline epigenetic patterns, which can further affect female folliculogenesis, hormone production, and reproductive behaviors, most evidence are not comprehensive enough. Thus, further mechanical studies on the epi-mutation germ line inheritance are warranted.

19.4 Mitigating the Exposure/Impact of EDCs and Future Research Through the "One Health" Approach

Female reproductive health and well-being are fundamental for the successful reproduction process for the continuation of eutherian mammals, including humans. As we have highlighted in the above sections, our work and many others have indicated the impact of various endocrine disruptors in different functions of female reproduction, which ultimately leads to reproductive tract complications and subsequent fertility issues plus possible cancer incidences as well (Karwacka et al. 2019). Due to the seriousness of EDCs exposure, many countries, including the USA, the European Union, China, and Canada, have given prominent attention to preventing and mitigating EDC exposure by targeting both reproductive health and the human and animal environment. Holistically considering whole living entities in answering issues related to health is the crucial concept of one health approach and comparative biomedicine, i.e. use of the same models to understand both human and animal disease etiology and treatment options. Most of the EDCs in the environment could be biomagnified through food chains and can be concentrated in the animal and human bodies via the food chain. Thus, higher-order animals like human are at high risk of being exposed to very high doses, specifically in the case of many persistent pollutants. Therefore, the preventive and mitigation measures for EDCs must encompass all these aspects, and one health principle could play a pivotal role (Frazzoli and Mantovani 2018). Traditionally one health has been only limited to talking about zoonotic diseases. However, recently it has been redefined to encompass many other aspects including the environmental health (PÈrez and Pierce Wise Sr. 2018) and WHO has already recognized the impact of one health in reducing the exposure to EDCs and adaptation of mitigation measures through one health approach as well (EHI 2021). The impact of ECDs on outcomes of human-assisted reproduction is also well documented (Xu and Yang 2021). In recent years, even some of the chemicals and consumables in artificially assisted reproduction came under scrutiny due to known EDCs like bisphenols. Thus, there may still be some minor avenues we must find with proper auditing to prevent accidental and unintentional exposures.

Given the broader scope of the one health concept and recent other similar approaches like planetary health, it would be time to appreciate and adopt such to minimize, prevent and mitigate the undesirables effects of EDCs on human female reproductive health. Therefore, to reduce the release of EDCs to the environment and mitigate animal and human exposures, we need to improve; the education of all segments that could potentially produce & release such into the environment, enhance testing facilities to identify the EDCs, strengthen the research with the novel *in vitro* 3D models and approaches like exosomes-based biomarkers to recognize the new and exact mode of actions of many EDCs and their derivatives could be identified as priority areas. Furthermore, much comprehensive collaboration between various disciplines is needed. To check the levels of different EDCs and distribution of EDCs, various biomonitoring can be employed using different animal types, including vertebrates, non-vertebrates, and microorganisms. Moreover, with the recent COVID-19 pandemic, the use of PPE has increased alarmingly, and discarding such will release many EDCs to the environment, including micro and nano-plastics, and there is no collective agreement in different countries as to how to manage these to avoid any environmental damage. Thus, one health approach would be an ideal platform to find solutions with multidisciplinary research and educate all sectors collectively.

19.5 Concluding Remarks

All the existing evidence suggests that EDCs directly impact female reproductive health, which will heavily impact many parts of the world where already negative birth rates are being experienced. Moreover, the number of couples seeking assisted reproductive therapies like embryo transfer is also increasing. With the advancement of societal requirements, there is a high risk of exposure to EDCs daily with the population expansion with further escalation of repercussions concerning female reproductive health. We have discussed a few key EDCs and their known impact on female reproduction and disease conditions; however, a lot needs to be further explored and known. Since bioaccumulation via food webs and other environmental factors like air and water are the primary sources of exposure to EDCs, a wholistic approach encompassing ecological health, one health, and comparative biomedicine must be employed to identify the exact roles of different EDCs on female reproduction, and to design preventive and mitigation including targeted therapy to alleviate the exposure aftermath. Thus, adopting and practicing one health approach would be a way to find answers for often complex female reproduction issues. More priority must be given to research and development using one health principle.

References

(EHI), E.H.I.A (2021). *Identification of Risks from Exposure to Endocrine-Disrupting Chemicals at the Country Level.* World Health Organization.

Akin, L., Kendirci, M., Narin, F. et al. (2020). Endocrine disruptors and polycystic ovary syndrome: phthalates. *J. Clin. Res. Pediatr. Endocrinol.* 12: 393–400.

Al-Saleh, I. (2022). The relationship between urinary phthalate metabolites and polycystic ovary syndrome in women undergoing in vitro fertilization: nested case-control study. *Chemosphere* 286: 131495.

Al-Saleh, I., Coskun, S., Al-Doush, I. et al. (2019). Couples exposure to phthalates and its influence on in vitro fertilization outcomes. *Chemosphere* 226: 597–606.

Amanat, S., Ashkar, F., Eftekhari, M.H. et al. (2021). The effect of genistein on insulin resistance, inflammatory factors, lipid profile, and histopathologic indices in rats with polycystic ovary syndrome. *Clin. Exp. Reprod. Med.* 48: 236–244.

Ambruosi, B., Uranio, M.F., Sardanelli, A.M. et al. (2011). in vitro acute exposure to DEHP affects oocyte meiotic maturation, energy and oxidative stress parameters in a large animal model. *PLoS One* 6: e27452.

Ao, J., Huo, X., Zhang, J. et al. (2022). Environmental exposure to bisphenol analogues and unexplained recurrent miscarriage: a case-control study. *Environ. Res.* 204: 112293.

Azzouz, A., Rascon, A.J., and Ballesteros, E. (2016). Simultaneous determination of parabens, alkylphenols, phenylphenols, bisphenol A and triclosan in human urine, blood and breast milk by continuous solid-phase extraction and gas chromatography-mass spectrometry. *J. Pharm. Biomed. Anal.* 119: 16–26.

Bachelot, A. (2016). Polycystic ovarian syndrome: clinical and biological diagnosis. *Ann. Biol. Clin. (Paris)* 74: 661–667.

Barber, T.M., Hanson, P., Weickert, M.O., and Franks, S. (2019). Obesity and polycystic ovary syndrome: implications for pathogenesis and novel management strategies. *Clin. Med. Insights. Reprod. Health* 13: 1179558119874042.

Bloom, M.S., Fujimoto, V.Y., Storm, R. et al. (2017). Persistent organic pollutants (POPs) in human follicular fluid and in vitro fertilization outcomes, a pilot study. *Reprod. Toxicol.* 67: 165–173.

Borgeest, C., Symonds, D., Mayer, L.P. et al. (2002). Methoxychlor may cause ovarian follicular atresia and proliferation of the ovarian epithelium in the mouse. *Toxicol. Sci.* 68: 473–478.

Brehm, E. and Flaws, J.A. (2019). Transgenerational effects of endocrine-disrupting chemicals on male and female reproduction. *Endocrinology* 160: 1421–1435.

Brieno-Enriquez, M.A., Robles, P., Camats-Tarruella, N. et al. (2011). Human meiotic progression and recombination are affected by bisphenol A exposure during in vitro human oocyte development. *Hum. Reprod.* 26: 2807–2818.

Buck Louis, G.M., Chen, Z., Peterson, C.M. et al. (2012). Persistent lipophilic environmental chemicals and endometriosis: the ENDO study. *Environ. Health Perspect.* 120: 811–816.

Buck Louis, G.M., Peterson, C.M., Chen, Z. et al. (2013). Bisphenol A and phthalates and endometriosis: the endometriosis: natural history, diagnosis and outcomes study. *Fertil. Steril.* 100 (162–9): e1–e2.

Cai, L.Y., Izumi, S., Suzuki, T. et al. (2011). Dioxins in ascites and serum of women with endometriosis: a pilot study. *Hum. Reprod.* 26: 117–126.

Cai, W., Yang, J., Liu, Y. et al. (2019). Association between phthalate metabolites and risk of endometriosis: a meta-analysis. *Int. J. Environ. Res. Public Health* 16: 1–11.

Canis, M., Donnez, J.G., Guzick, D.S. et al. (1997). Revised american society for reproductive medicine classification of endometriosis: 1996. *Fertil. Steril.* 67: 817–821.

Cao, Y., Qu, X., Ming, Z. et al. (2018). The correlation between exposure to BPA and the decrease of the ovarian reserve. *Int. J. Clin. Exp. Pathol.* 11: 3375–3382.

Cao, M., Pan, W., Shen, X. et al. (2020). Urinary levels of phthalate metabolites in women associated with risk of premature ovarian failure and reproductive hormones. *Chemosphere* 242: 125206.

Carnevali, O., Notarstefano, V., Olivotto, I. et al. (2017). Dietary administration of EDC mixtures: a focus on fish lipid metabolism. *Aquat. Toxicol.* 185: 95–104.

Chen, Y., Jefferson, W.N., Newbold, R.R. et al. (2007). Estradiol, progesterone, and genistein inhibit oocyte nest breakdown and primordial follicle assembly in the neonatal mouse ovary in vitro and in vivo. *Endocrinology* 148: 3580–3590.

Chi, X.X., Zhang, T., Chu, X.L. et al. (2018). The regulatory effect of Genistein on granulosa cell in ovary of rat with PCOS through Bcl-2 and Bax signaling pathways. *J. Vet. Med. Sci.* 80: 1348–1355.

Chi, X.X., Zhang, T., and Chu, X.L. (2019). Effect of genistein on IGF-1 and IGFBP-1 in young and aged female rat ovary. *J. Anim. Physiol. Anim. Nutr. (Berl)* 103: 1594–1601.

Cho, Y.J., Park, S.B., Park, J.W. et al. (2018). Bisphenol A modulates inflammation and proliferation pathway in human endometrial stromal cells by inducing oxidative stress. *Reprod. Toxicol.* 81: 41–49.

Chou, Y.C., Chen, Y.C., Chen, M.J. et al. (2020). Exposure to mono-*n*-butyl phthalate in women with endometriosis and its association with the biological effects on human granulosa cells. *Int. J. Mol. Sci.* 21: 1–16.

Cos, P., De Bruyne, T., Apers, S. et al. (2003). Phytoestrogens: recent developments. *Planta Med.* 69: 589–599.

Coughlan, C., Ledger, W., Wang, Q. et al. (2014). Recurrent implantation failure: definition and management. *Reprod. BioMed. Online* 28: 14–38.

Critchley, H.O.D., Maybin, J.A., Armstrong, G.M., and Williams, A.R.W. (2020). Physiology of the endometrium and regulation of menstruation. *Physiol. Rev.* 100: 1149–1179.

De Falco, M. and Laforgia, V. (2021). Combined effects of different endocrine-disrupting chemicals (EDCs) on prostate gland. *Int. J. Environ. Res. Public Health* 18: 9772.

De Felip, E., Porpora, M.G., Di Domenico, A. et al. (2004). Dioxin-like compounds and endometriosis: a study on Italian and Belgian women of reproductive age. *Toxicol. Lett.* 150: 203–209.

Deswal, R., Narwal, V., Dang, A., and Pundir, C.S. (2020). The prevalence of polycystic ovary syndrome: a brief systematic review. *J. Hum. Reprod. Sci.* 13: 261–271.

Diamanti-Kandarakis, E., Bourguignon, J.P., Giudice, L.C. et al. (2009). Endocrine-disrupting chemicals: an Endocrine society scientific statement. *Endocr. Rev.* 30: 293–342.

Dunselman, G.A.J., Vermeulen, N., Becker, C. et al. (2014). ESHRE guideline: management of women with endometriosis. *Hum. Reprod.* 29: 400–412.

Ehrlich, S., Williams, P.L., Missmer, S.A. et al. (2012). Urinary bisphenol A concentrations and implantation failure among women undergoing in vitro fertilization. *Environ. Health Perspect.* 120: 978–983.

Encarnação, T., Pais, A.A., Campos, M.G., and Burrows, H.D. (2019). Endocrine disrupting chemicals: Impact on human health, wildlife and the environment. *Sci. Prog.* 102: 3–42.

Fenichel, P., Rougier, C., Hieronimus, S., and Chevalier, N. (2017). Which origin for polycystic ovaries syndrome: genetic, environmental or both? *Ann. Endocrinol. (Paris)* 78: 176–185.

Fernández, M., Bourguignon, N., Lux-Lantos, V., and Libertun, C. (2010). Neonatal exposure to bisphenol a and reproductive and endocrine alterations resembling the polycystic ovarian syndrome in adult rats. *Environ. Health Perspect.* 118: 1217–1222.

Feroe, A., Broene, R., Albuquerque, D., and Ruiz, P. (2017). Endocrine disrupting chemicals, transgenerational epigenetics and metabolic diseases. *EC Endocrinol. Metab. Res.* 21: 31–51.

Fierens, S., Mairesse, H., Heilier, J.F.O. et al. (2003). Dioxin/polychlorinated biphenyl body burden, diabetes and endometriosis: findings in a population-based study in Belgium. *Biomarkers* 8: 529–534.

Franks, S., Mason, H., and Willis, D. (2000). Follicular dynamics in the polycystic ovary syndrome. *Mol. Cell. Endocrinol.* 163: 49–52.

Frazzoli, C. and Mantovani, A. (2018). Editorial: the environment-animal-human web: a "one health" view of toxicological risk analysis. *Front. Public Health* 6: 353.

Genuis, S.J., Beesoon, S., Birkholz, D., and Lobo, R.A. (2012). Human excretion of bisphenol A: blood, urine, and sweat (BUS) study. *J. Environ. Public Health* 2012: 185731.

Goh, Y.X., Jalil, J., Lam, K.W. et al. (2022). Genistein: a review on its anti-inflammatory properties. *Front. Pharmacol.* 13: 820969.

Gore, A.C., Thompson, L.M., Bell, M., and Mennigen, J.A. (2021). Transgenerational effects of polychlorinated biphenyls: 2. Hypothalamic gene expression in ratsdagger. *Biol. Reprod.* 105: 690–704.

Haddad, Y.H., Said, R.S., Kamel, R. et al. (2020). Phytoestrogen genistein hinders ovarian oxidative damage and apoptotic cell death-induced by ionizing radiation: co-operative role of ER-beta, TGF-beta, and FOXL-2. *Sci. Rep.* 10: 13551.

Hannon, P.R., Peretz, J., and Flaws, J.A. (2014). Daily exposure to Di(2-ethylhexyl) phthalate alters estrous cyclicity and accelerates primordial follicle recruitment potentially via dysregulation of the phosphatidylinositol 3-kinase signaling pathway in adult mice. *Biol. Reprod.* 90: 136.

Hauser, R., Gaskins, A.J., Souter, I. et al. (2016). Urinary phthalate metabolite concentrations and reproductive outcomes among women undergoing in vitro fertilization: results from the EARTH study. *Environ. Health Perspect.* 124: 831–839.

Heilier, J.F., Nackers, F., Verougstraete, V. et al. (2005). Increased dioxin-like compounds in the serum of women with peritoneal endometriosis and deep endometriotic (adenomyotic) nodules. *Fertil. Steril.* 84: 305–312.

Hirshfield, A.N. (1991). Development of follicles in the mammalian ovary. *Int. Rev. Cytol.* 124: 43–101.

Hites, R.A. (2011). Dioxins: an overview and history. *Environ. Sci. Technol.* 45: 16–20.

Hoppin, J.A., Brock, J.W., Davis, B.J., and Baird, D.D. (2002). Reproducibility of urinary phthalate metabolites in first morning urine samples. *Environ. Health Perspect.* 110: 515–518.

Hossein Rashidi, B., Amanlou, M., Lak, T.B. et al. (2017). The association between bisphenol A and polycystic ovarian syndrome: a case-control study. *Acta Med. Iran.* 55: 759–764.

Hu, Y., Wen, S., Yuan, D. et al. (2018). The association between the environmental endocrine disruptor bisphenol A and polycystic ovary syndrome: a systematic review and meta-analysis. *Gynecol. Endocrinol.* 34: 370–377.

Huang, P.C., Tsai, E.M., Li, W.F. et al. (2010). Association between phthalate exposure and glutathione S-transferase M1 polymorphism in adenomyosis, leiomyoma and endometriosis. *Hum. Reprod.* 25: 986–994.

Huang, F.M., Chang, Y.C., Lee, S.S. et al. (2018). Bisphenol A exhibits cytotoxic or genotoxic potential via oxidative stress-associated mitochondrial apoptotic pathway in murine macrophages. *Food Chem. Toxicol.* 122: 215–224.

Ijaz, S., Ullah, A., Shaheen, G., and Jahan, S. (2020). Exposure of BPA and its alternatives like BPB, BPF, and BPS impair subsequent reproductive potentials in adult female Sprague Dawley rats. *Toxicol. Mech. Methods* 30: 60–72.

Ishizuka, B. (2021). Current understanding of the etiology, symptomatology, and treatment options in premature ovarian insufficiency (POI). *Front. Endocrinol. (Lausanne)* 12: 626924.

Jamilian, M. and Asemi, Z. (2016). The effects of soy isoflavones on metabolic status of patients with polycystic ovary syndrome. *J. Clin. Endocrinol. Metab.* 101: 3386–3394.

Jang, J.W., Lee, J.W., Yoon, Y.D. et al. (2020). Bisphenol A and its substitutes regulate human B cell survival via Nrf2 expression. *Environ. Pollut.* 259: 113907.

Jankowska, K. (2017). Premature ovarian failure. *Prz. Menopauzalny* 16: 51–56.

Jefferson, W.N. and Williams, C.J. (2011). Circulating levels of genistein in the neonate, apart from dose and route, predict future adverse female reproductive outcomes. *Reprod. Toxicol.* 31: 272–279.

Jin, Y., Zhang, Q., Pan, J.X. et al. (2019). The effects of di(2-ethylhexyl) phthalate exposure in women with polycystic ovary syndrome undergoing in vitro fertilization. *J. Int. Med. Res.* 47: 6278–6293.

Karamali, M., Kashanian, M., Alaeinasab, S., and Asemi, Z. (2018). The effect of dietary soy intake on weight loss, glycaemic control, lipid profiles and biomarkers of inflammation and oxidative stress in women with polycystic ovary syndrome: a randomised clinical trial. *J. Hum. Nutr. Diet.* 31: 533–543.

Karwacka, A., Zamkowska, D., Radwan, M., and Jurewicz, J. (2019). Exposure to modern, widespread environmental endocrine disrupting chemicals and their effect on the reproductive potential of women: an overview of current epidemiological evidence. *Hum. Fertil. (Camb)* 22: 2–25.

Kawa, I.A., Akbar, M., Fatima, Q. et al. (2021). Endocrine disrupting chemical bisphenol A and its potential effects on female health. *Diabetes Metab. Syndr.* 15: 803–811.

Kermath, B.A., Thompson, L.M., Jefferson, J.R. et al. (2022). Transgenerational effects of prenatal endocrine disruption on reproductive and sociosexual behaviors in Sprague Dawley male and female rats. *Toxics* 10: 47.

KEYS, J.G.K.A.J. (2002). PCBs and the precautionary principle. *Environmental Issue report* 22: 64–75.

Khani, B., Mehrabian, F., Khalesi, E., and Eshraghi, A. (2011). Effect of soy phytoestrogen on metabolic and hormonal disturbance of women with polycystic ovary syndrome. *J. Res. Med. Sci.* 16: 297–302.

Kim, S.H., Chun, S., Jang, J.Y. et al. (2011). Increased plasma levels of phthalate esters in women with advanced-stage endometriosis: a prospective case-control study. *Fertil. Steril.* 95: 357–359.

Kohn, M.C. and Melnick, R.L. (2002). Biochemical origins of the non-monotonic receptor-mediated dose-response. *J. Mol. Endocrinol.* 29: 113–123.

Kulkarni, S.G. and Mehendale, H.M. (2005). Polychlorinated biphenyls (PCBs). In: *Encyclopedia of Toxicology*, 2e (ed. P. Wexler), 509–511. New York: Elsevier.

Kwak-Kim, J.Y., Gilman-Sachs, A., and Kim, C.E. (2005). T helper 1 and 2 immune responses in relationship to pregnancy, nonpregnancy, recurrent spontaneous abortions and infertility of repeated implantation failures. *Chem. Immunol. Allergy* 88: 64–79.

Laganà, A.S., Garzon, S., Franchi, M. et al. (2018). Translational animal models for endometriosis research: a long and windy road. *Ann. Transl. Med.* 6: 431.

Lebel, G., Dodin, S., Ayotte, P. et al. (1998). Organochlorine exposure and the risk of endometriosis. *Fertil. Steril.* 69: 221–228.

Lédée, N., Petitbarat, M., Chevrier, L. et al. (2016). The uterine immune profile may help women with repeated unexplained embryo implantation failure after in vitro fertilization. *Am. J. Reprod. Immunol.* 75: 388–401.

Li, Y., Zhang, W., Liu, J. et al. (2014). Prepubertal bisphenol A exposure interferes with ovarian follicle development and its relevant gene expression. *Reprod. Toxicol.* 44: 33–40.

Li, Y., Xie, S., Ying, J. et al. (2018). Chemical structures of lignans and neolignans isolated from Lauraceae. *Molecules* 23: 1–18.

Li, C., Cao, M., Qi, T. et al. (2021). The association of bisphenol A exposure with premature ovarian insufficiency: a case-control study. *Climacteric* 24: 95–100.

López-Rodríguez, D., Aylwin, C.F., Delli, V. et al. (2021). Multi- and transgenerational outcomes of an exposure to a mixture of endocrine-disrupting chemicals (EDCs) on puberty and maternal behavior in the female rat. *Environ. Health Perspect.* 129: 87003.

Louis, G.M., Weiner, J.M., Whitcomb, B.W. et al. (2005). Environmental PCB exposure and risk of endometriosis. *Hum. Reprod.* 20: 279–285.

Luo, M., Zheng, L.W., Wang, Y.S. et al. (2021). Genistein exhibits therapeutic potential for PCOS mice via the ER-Nrf2-Foxo1-ROS pathway. *Food Funct.* 12: 8800–8811.

Maclean, A., Bunni, E., Makrydima, S. et al. (2020). Fallopian tube epithelial cells express androgen receptor and have a distinct hormonal responsiveness when compared with endometrial epithelium. *Hum. Reprod.* 35: 2097–2106.

Manikkam, M., Tracey, R., Guerrero-Bosagna, C., and Skinner, M.K. (2013). Plastics derived endocrine disruptors (BPA, DEHP and DBP) induce epigenetic transgenerational inheritance of obesity, reproductive disease and sperm epimutations. *PLoS One* 8: e55387.

Manikkam, M., Haque, M.M., Guerrero-Bosagna, C. et al. (2014). Pesticide methoxychlor promotes the epigenetic transgenerational inheritance of adult-onset disease through the female germline. *PLoS One* 9: e102091.

March, W.A., Moore, V.M., Willson, K.J. et al. (2010). The prevalence of polycystic ovary syndrome in a community sample assessed under contrasting diagnostic criteria. *Hum. Reprod.* 25: 544–551.

Martinez-Arguelles, D.B., Guichard, T., Culty, M. et al. (2011). In utero exposure to the antiandrogen di-(2-ethylhexyl) phthalate decreases adrenal aldosterone production in the adult rat. *Biol. Reprod.* 85: 51–61.

Martinez-Zamora, M.A., Mattioli, L., Parera, J. et al. (2015). Increased levels of dioxin-like substances in adipose tissue in patients with deep infiltrating endometriosis. *Hum. Reprod.* 30: 1059–1068.

Meli, R., Monnolo, A., Annunziata, C. et al. (2020). Oxidative stress and bpa toxicity: an antioxidant approach for male and female reproductive dysfunction. *Antioxidants (Basel)* 9: 1–24.

Milbrath, M.O.G., Wenger, Y., Chang, C.W. et al. (2009). Apparent half-lives of dioxins, furans, and polychlorinated biphenyls as a function of age, body fat, smoking status, and breast-feeding. *Environ. Health Perspect.* 117: 417–425.

Miller, M.D., Marty, M.A., Arcus, A. et al. (2002). Differences between children and adults: implications for risk assessment at California EPA. *Int. J. Toxicol.* 21: 403–418.

Miller, K.P., Gupta, R.K., Greenfeld, C.R. et al. (2005). Methoxychlor directly affects ovarian antral follicle growth and atresia through Bcl-2- and Bax-mediated pathways. *Toxicol. Sci.* 88: 213–221.

Mumford, S.L., Weck, J., Kannan, K., and Buck Louis, G.M. (2017). Urinary phytoestrogen concentrations are not associated with incident endometriosis in premenopausal women. *J. Nutr.* 147: 227–234.

Neblett, M.F., Curtis, S.W., Gerkowicz, S.A. et al. (2020). Examining reproductive health outcomes in females exposed to polychlorinated biphenyl and polybrominated biphenyl. *Sci. Rep.* 10: 3314.

Nilsson, E., Klukovich, R., Sadler-Riggleman, I. et al. (2018). Environmental toxicant induced epigenetic transgenerational inheritance of ovarian pathology and granulosa cell epigenome and transcriptome alterations: ancestral origins of polycystic ovarian syndrome and primary ovarian insufiency. *Epigenetics* 13: 875–895.

Niskar, A.S., Needham, L.L., Rubin, C. et al. (2009). Serum dioxins, polychlorinated biphenyls, and endometriosis: a case-control study in Atlanta. *Chemosphere* 74: 944–949.

Palanza, P., Parmigiani, S., and Vom Saal, F.S. (2001). Effects of prenatal exposure to low doses of diethylstilbestrol, o,p'DDT, and methoxychlor on postnatal growth and neurobehavioral development in male and female mice. *Horm. Behav.* 40: 252–265.

Parasar, P., Ozcan, P., and Terry, K.L. (2017). Endometriosis: epidemiology, diagnosis and clinical management. *Curr. Obstet. Gynecol. Rep.* 6: 34–41.

Park, S.Y., Jeon, J.H., Jeong, K. et al. (2021). The association of ovarian reserve with exposure to bisphenol A and phthalate in reproductive-aged women. *J. Korean Med. Sci.* 36: e1.

Pauwels, A., Schepens, P.J.C., D'Hooghe, T. et al. (2001). The risk of endometriosis and exposure to dioxins and polychlorinated biphenyls: a case-control study of infertile women. *Hum. Reprod.* 16: 2050–2055.

Pecyna, P., Wargula, J., Murias, M., and Kucinska, M. (2020). More than resveratrol: new insights into stilbene-based compounds. *Biomolecules* 10: 1–40.

Peijnenburg, W.J.G.M. (2008). Phthalates. In: *Encyclopedia of Ecology* (ed. S.E. Jørgensen and B.D. Fath), 2733–2738. Oxford: Academic Press.

Peinado, F.M., Lendínez, I., Sotelo, R. et al. (2020). Association of urinary levels of bisphenols A, F, and S with endometriosis risk: preliminary results of the EndEA study. *Int. J. Environ. Res. Public Health* 17: 1–13.

Peretz, J., Gupta, R.K., Singh, J. et al. (2011). Bisphenol A impairs follicle growth, inhibits steroidogenesis, and downregulates rate-limiting enzymes in the estradiol biosynthesis pathway. *Toxicol. Sci.* 119: 209–217.

Pèrez, A. and Pierce Wise, J. Sr. (2018). One Environmental Health: an emerging perspective in toxicology [version 1; peer review: 2 approved]. *F1000Research* 7: 10.

Ploteau, S., Cano-Sancho, G., Volteau, C. et al. (2017). Associations between internal exposure levels of persistent organic pollutants in adipose tissue and deep infiltrating endometriosis with or without concurrent ovarian endometrioma. *Environ. Int.* 108: 195–203.

Polanski, L.T., Baumgarten, M.N., Quenby, S. et al. (2014). What exactly do we mean by 'recurrent implantation failure'? A systematic review and opinion. *Reprod. BioMed. Online* 28: 409–423.

Porpora, M.G., Ingelido, A.M., Di Domenico, A. et al. (2006). Increased levels of polychlorobiphenyls in Italian women with endometriosis. *Chemosphere* 63: 1361–1367.

Porpora, M.G., Medda, E., Abballe, A. et al. (2009). Endometriosis and organochlorinated environmental pollutants: a case-control study on Italian women of reproductive age. *Environ. Health Perspect.* 117: 1070–1075.

Practice Committee of the American Society For Reproductive Medicine (2012). Smoking and infertility: a committee opinion. *Fertil. Steril.* 98: 1400–1406.

Practice Committee of the American Society for Reproductive Medicine (2021). Electronic address, a. a. o. & practice Committee of the American Society for reproductive, medicine, obesity and reproduction: a committee opinion. *Fertil. Steril.* 116: 1266–1285.

Puttabyatappa, M., Banker, M., Zeng, L. et al. (2020). Maternal exposure to environmental disruptors and sexually dimorphic changes in maternal and neonatal oxidative stress. *J. Clin. Endocrinol. Metab.* 105: 492–505.

Rashidi, B.H., Amanlou, M., Lak, T.B. et al. (2017). A case-control study of bisphenol A and endometrioma among subgroup of Iranian women. *J. Res. Med. Sci.* 22 (7): 1–5.

Reddy, B.S., Rozati, R., Reddy, B.V., and Raman, N.V. (2006). Association of phthalate esters with endometriosis in Indian women. *BJOG* 113: 515–520.

Ribeiro, E., Ladeira, C., and Viegas, S. (2017). EDCs mixtures: a stealthy hazard for human health? *Toxics* 5: 1–17.

Rice, S., Mason, H.D., and Whitehead, S.A. (2006). Phytoestrogens and their low dose combinations inhibit mRNA expression and activity of aromatase in human granulosa-luteal cells. *J. Steroid Biochem. Mol. Biol.* 101: 216–225.

Ritter, R., Scheringer, M., MacLeod, M. et al. (2011). Intrinsic human elimination half-lives of polychlorinated biphenyls derived from the temporal evolution of cross-sectional biomonitoring data from the United Kingdom. *Environ. Health Perspect.* 119: 225–231.

Rodríguez, H.A., Santambrosio, N., Santamaría, C.G. et al. (2010). Neonatal exposure to bisphenol A reduces the pool of primordial follicles in the rat ovary. *Reprod. Toxicol.* 30: 550–557.

Rotterdam, E.A.-S.P.C.W.G. (2004). Revised 2003 consensus on diagnostic criteria and long-term health risks related to polycystic ovary syndrome. *Fertil. Steril.* 81: 19–25.

Rozati, R., Simha, B., Bendi, N., and Sekhar, C. (2008). Evaluation of the phthalate esters in South Indian women with endometriosis. *Int. J. Fertil. Steril.* 1: 165–170.

Saxtorph, M.H., Hallager, T., Persson, G. et al. (2020). Assessing endometrial receptivity after recurrent implantation failure: a prospective controlled cohort study. *Reprod. BioMed. Online* 41: 998–1006.

Sayles, G.D. (2002). Environmental engineering and endocrine disrupting chemicals Arnold, R.G. (ed.). *J. Environ. Eng.* 128: 1–2.

Sechman, A., Batoryna, M., Antos, P.A., and Hrabia, A. (2016). Effects of PCB 126 and PCB 153 on secretion of steroid hormones and mRNA expression of steroidogenic genes (STAR, HSD3B, CYP19A1) and estrogen receptors (ERalpha, ERbeta) in prehierarchical chicken ovarian follicles. *Toxicol. Lett.* 264: 29–37.

Setchell, K.D., Brown, N.M., Desai, P. et al. (2001). Bioavailability of pure isoflavones in healthy humans and analysis of commercial soy isoflavone supplements. *J. Nutr.* 131: 1362S–1375S.

Shanle, E.K. and Xu, W. (2011). Endocrine disrupting chemicals targeting estrogen receptor signaling: identification and mechanisms of action. *Chem. Res. Toxicol.* 24: 6–19.

Sharma, P., Lee, J.Y.L., Tsai, E.M. et al. (2021). n-Butyl benzyl phthalate exposure promotes lesion survival in a murine endometriosis model. *Int. J. Environ. Res. Public Health* 18: 1–13.

Sheehan, M.T. (2004). Polycystic ovarian syndrome: diagnosis and management. *Clin. Med. Res.* 2: 13–27.

Shen, J., Kang, Q., Mao, Y. et al. (2020). Urinary bisphenol A concentration is correlated with poorer oocyte retrieval and embryo implantation outcomes in patients with tubal factor infertility undergoing in vitro fertilisation. *Ecotoxicol. Environ. Saf.* 187: 109816.

Shirota, M., Mukai, M., Sakurada, Y. et al. (2006). Effects of vertically transferred 3,3',4,4',5-pentachlorobiphenyl (PCB-126) on the reproductive development of female rats. *J. Reprod. Dev.* 52: 751–761.

Signorile, P.G., Spugnini, E.P., Mita, L. et al. (2010). Pre-natal exposure of mice to bisphenol A elicits an endometriosis-like phenotype in female offspring. *Gen. Comp. Endocrinol.* 168: 318–325.

Simon, A. and Laufer, N. (2012). Repeated implantation failure: clinical approach. *Fertil. Steril.* 97: 1039–1043.

Simonelli, A., Guadagni, R., De Franciscis, P. et al. (2017). Environmental and occupational exposure to bisphenol A and endometriosis: urinary and peritoneal fluid concentration levels. *Int. Arch. Occup. Environ. Health* 90: 49–61.

Sirohi, D., Al Ramadhani, R., and Knibbs, L.D. (2021). Environmental exposures to endocrine disrupting chemicals (EDCs) and their role in endometriosis: a systematic literature review. *Rev. Environ. Health* 36: 101–115.

Skinner, M.K. (2014). Endocrine disruptor induction of epigenetic transgenerational inheritance of disease. *Mol. Cell. Endocrinol.* 398: 4–12.

Skinner, M.K. (2016). Endocrine disruptors in 2015: epigenetic transgenerational inheritance. *Nat. Rev. Endocrinol.* 12: 68–70.

Sohn, S.I., Pandian, S., Oh, Y.J. et al. (2021). Metabolic engineering of isoflavones: an updated overview. *Front. Plant Sci.* 12: 670103.

Somigliana, E., Vigano, P., Busnelli, A. et al. (2018). Repeated implantation failure at the crossroad between statistics, clinics and over-diagnosis. *Reprod. BioMed. Online* 36: 32–38.

Stephens, V.R., Rumph, J.T., Ameli, S. et al. (2021). The potential relationship between environmental endocrine disruptor exposure and the development of endometriosis and adenomyosis. *Front. Physiol.* 12: 807685.

Stern, C., Pertile, M., Norris, H. et al. (1999). Chromosome translocations in couples with in-vitro fertilization implantation failure. *Hum. Reprod.* 14: 2097–2101.

Sutrisno, S., Aprina, H., Simanungkalit, H.M. et al. (2018). Genistein modulates the estrogen receptor and suppresses angiogenesis and inflammation in the murine model of peritoneal endometriosis. *J. Tradit. Complement. Med.* 8: 278–281.

Takaoka, O., Mori, T., Ito, F. et al. (2018). Daidzein-rich isoflavone aglycones inhibit cell growth and inflammation in endometriosis. *J. Steroid Biochem. Mol. Biol.* 181: 125–132.

Takasuga, T., Senthilkumar, K., Matsumura, T. et al. (2006). Isotope dilution analysis of polychlorinated biphenyls (PCBs) in transformer oil and global commercial PCB formulations by high resolution gas chromatography-high resolution mass spectrometry. *Chemosphere* 62: 469–484.

Takeuchi, T., Tsutsumi, O., Ikezuki, Y. et al. (2004). Positive relationship between androgen and the endocrine disruptor, bisphenol A, in normal women and women with ovarian dysfunction. *Endocr. J.* 51: 165–169.

Takeuchi, T., Tsutsumi, O., Ikezuki, Y. et al. (2006). Elevated serum bisphenol A levels under hyperandrogenic conditions may be caused by decreased UDP-glucuronosyltransferase activity. *Endocr. J.* 53: 485–491.

Tarnow, P., Tralau, T., and Luch, A. (2019). Chemical activation of estrogen and aryl hydrocarbon receptor signaling pathways and their interaction in toxicology and metabolism. *Expert Opin. Drug Metab. Toxicol.* 15: 219–229.

Testa, I., Salvatori, C., Di Cara, G. et al. (2018). Soy-based infant formula: are phyto-oestrogens still in doubt? *Front. Nutr.* 5: 110.

The World Bank (2022). Fertility rate, total (births per woman). The World Bank. https://data.worldbank.org/indicator/SP.DYN.TFRT.IN (accessed 17 June 2022).

Toktay, E., Selli, J., Gurbuz, M.A. et al. (2020). Effects of soy isoflavonoids (genistein and daidzein) on endometrial receptivity. *Iran. J. Basic Med. Sci.* 23: 1603–1609.

Tomic, D., Frech, M.S., Babus, J.K. et al. (2006). Methoxychlor induces atresia of antral follicles in ERalpha-overexpressing mice. *Toxicol. Sci.* 93: 196–204.

Trabert, B., De Roos, A.J., Schwartz, S.M. et al. (2010). Non-dioxin-like polychlorinated biphenyls and risk of endometriosis. *Environ. Health Perspect.* 118: 1280–1285.

Trabert, B., Chen, Z., Kannan, K. et al. (2015). Persistent organic pollutants (POPs) and fibroids: results from the ENDO study. *J. Expo. Sci. Environ. Epidemiol.* 25: 278–285.

Tran, D.N., Jung, E.M., Yoo, Y.M. et al. (2018). Depletion of follicles accelerated by combined exposure to phthalates and 4-vinylcyclohexene diepoxide, leading to premature ovarian failure in rats. *Reprod. Toxicol.* 80: 60–67.

United Nations Population Fund (2022). World population dashboard. https://www.unfpa.org/data/world-population-dashboard (accessed 23 June 2022).

Upson, K., Sathyanarayana, S., De Roos, A.J. et al. (2013). Phthalates and risk of endometriosis. *Environ. Res.* 126: 91–97.

Upson, K., Sathyanarayana, S., De Roos, A.J. et al. (2014). A population-based case-control study of urinary bisphenol A concentrations and risk of endometriosis. *Hum. Reprod.* 29: 2457–2464.

Uzumcu, M., Kuhn, P.E., Marano, J.E. et al. (2006). Early postnatal methoxychlor exposure inhibits folliculogenesis and stimulates anti-Mullerian hormone production in the rat ovary. *J. Endocrinol.* 191: 549–558.

Vandenberg, L.N., Colborn, T., Hayes, T.B. et al. (2012). Hormones and endocrine-disrupting chemicals: low-dose effects and nonmonotonic dose responses. *Endocr. Rev.* 33: 378–455.

Vitale, S.G., La Rosa, V.L., Rapisarda, A.M.C., and Lagana, A.S. (2017). Impact of endometriosis on quality of life and psychological well-being. *J. Psychosom. Obstet. Gynaecol.* 38: 317–319.

Wang, W., Craig, Z.R., Basavarajappa, M.S. et al. (2012a). Di (2-ethylhexyl) phthalate inhibits growth of mouse ovarian antral follicles through an oxidative stress pathway. *Toxicol. Appl. Pharmacol.* 258: 288–295.

Wang, W., Craig, Z.R., Basavarajappa, M.S. et al. (2012b). Mono-(2-ethylhexyl) phthalate induces oxidative stress and inhibits growth of mouse ovarian antral follicles. *Biol. Reprod.* 87: 152.

Wen, X., Xiong, Y., Jin, L. et al. (2020). Bisphenol a exposure enhances endometrial stromal cell invasion and has a positive association with peritoneal endometriosis. *Reprod. Sci.* 27: 704–712.

Whitehead, S.A., Cross, J.E., Burden, C., and Lacey, M. (2002). Acute and chronic effects of genistein, tyrphostin and lavendustin A on steroid synthesis in luteinized human granulosa cells. *Hum. Reprod.* 17: 589–594.

Wolf, C.J., Ostby, J.S., Gray, L.E., and JR. (1999). Gestational exposure to 2,3,7,8-tetrachlorodibenzo-p-dioxin (TCDD) severely alters reproductive function of female hamster offspring. *Toxicol. Sci.* 51: 259–264.

World Population Review (2022). 2022 World population by country. World Population Review. https://worldpopulationreview.com/ (accessed 30 June 2022).

Wu, G., Wei, Q., Yu, D., and Shi, F. (2019). Neonatal genistein exposure disrupts ovarian and uterine development in the mouse by inhibiting cellular proliferation. *J. Reprod. Dev.* 65: 7–17.

Xu, X. and Yang, M. (2021). Effects of environmental EDCs on oocyte quality, embryo development, and the outcome in human IVF process. *Adv. Exp. Med. Biol.* 1300: 181–202.

Yang, Q., Zhao, Y., Qiu, X. et al. (2015). Association of serum levels of typical organic pollutants with polycystic ovary syndrome (PCOS): a case-control study. *Hum. Reprod.* 30: 1964–1973.

Yavuz, E., Oktem, M., Esinler, I. et al. (2007). Genistein causes regression of endometriotic implants in the rat model. *Fertil. Steril.* 88: 1129–1134.

Yilmaz, B., Terekeci, H., Sandal, S., and Kelestimur, F. (2020). Endocrine disrupting chemicals: exposure, effects on human health, mechanism of action, models for testing and strategies for prevention. *Rev. Endocr. Metab. Disord.* 21: 127–147.

Yuan, M., Bai, M.Z., Huang, X.F. et al. (2015). Preimplantation exposure to Bisphenol A and triclosan may lead to implantation failure in humans. *Biomed. Res. Int.* 2015: 184845.

Zhang, X.F., Zhang, L.J., Li, L. et al. (2013). Diethylhexyl phthalate exposure impairs follicular development and affects oocyte maturation in the mouse. *Environ. Mol. Mutagen.* 54: 354–361.

Zhang, T., Li, L., Qin, X.S. et al. (2014). Di-(2-ethylhexyl) phthalate and bisphenol A exposure impairs mouse primordial follicle assembly in vitro. *Environ. Mol. Mutagen.* 55: 343–353.

Zhang, D., Saktrakulkla, P., Tuttle, K. et al. (2021a). Detection and quantification of polychlorinated biphenyl sulfates in human serum. *Environ. Sci. Technol.* 55: 2473–2481.

Zhang, T., Chi, X.X., Kong, F.X., and Chu, X.L. (2021b). Effect of genistein on the gene and protein expressions of CXCL-12 and EGR-1 in the rat ovary. *J. Anim. Physiol. Anim. Nutr. (Berl)* 105: 191–197.

Zhou, W., Liu, J., Liao, L. et al. (2008). Effect of bisphenol A on steroid hormone production in rat ovarian theca-interstitial and granulosa cells. *Mol. Cell. Endocrinol.* 283: 12–18.

Zhou, W., Fang, F., Zhu, W. et al. (2016). Bisphenol A and ovarian reserve among infertile women with polycystic ovarian syndrome. *Int. J. Environ. Res. Public Health* 14 (1): 7.

Zong, G., Valvi, D., Coull, B. et al. (2018). Persistent organic pollutants and risk of type 2 diabetes: a prospective investigation among middle-aged women in nurses' health study II. *Environ. Int.* 114: 334–342.

20

Emerging and Re-emerging Zoonoses in South Asia

Challenges of One Health

T.M.A.H. Tennakoon[1] *and K.K. Wijesundera*[2]

[1] *Department of Pathology, Faculty of Medicine, University of Peradeniya, Peradeniya, Sri Lanka*
[2] *Department of Veterinary Pathobiology, Faculty of Veterinary Medicine and Animal Science, University of Peradeniya, Peradeniya, Sri Lanka*

Emerging and re-emerging zoonoses have become a serious public health concern recently. Forty percent (600 million people) of the poor in developing countries are living in the South Asian region. In addition, almost all known zoonoses have been recorded in this area. The emergence of leishmaniasis, trypanosomiasis, Nipah virus, and SARS-CoV infections and the re-emergence of rabies, leptospirosis, anthrax, influenza, helminth, and fungal zoonoses have created a significant public health burden and socio-economic impact in South Asian countries. One Health approach, the concept of combining human, animal, and environmental components to address global health challenges like zoonoses, is advantageous. This chapter will discuss the common zoonoses and the challenges in the implementation of One Health concept in the South Asian region.

> Between animal and human medicine there is no dividing line – nor should there be. The object is different but the experience obtained constitutes the basis of all medicine.
>
> *Rudolph Virchow*

20.1 One Health Concept

Diseases of variable origin affect the well-being and welfare of humans and animals, equally. The outcomes of diseases were observed for a long time by humankind and the concept of One Health paradigm has been invented (Evans and Leighton 2014). Historically, the pathologic convergence between domestic species and humans was most clearly described by Jenner, a well-known physician for his acclaimed work, long before the time of Virchow and Osler. Jenner could generate immunity and thereby prevent infection with smallpox virus in humans after intended inoculation with cowpox virus (later believed as horsepox virus) (Sundberg and Schofield 2009). Yet another major milestone was the discovery of Smith and Kilborne regarding the spread of diseases by ticks (Smith and Kilborne 1893). As the knowledge and understanding of causative agents, specific genetic, and environmental effects associated with each disease become more broadened, the general mechanisms of disease among animals and humans become more obvious (Sundberg and Schofield 2009).

Historically, the notion of One Health can be found in the writings of Hippocrates as early as 300 BC (460–367 BCE) (Evans and Leighton 2014). In addition, studies by Aristotle (384–322 BCE) on common characteristics among human and other mammalian diseases brought up the concept of comparative medicine (Dunlop and Williams 1996). Later, a German physician and a pathologist named Rudolf Virchow (1821–1902) coined the term "zoonosis" and is quoted as saying; "between animal and human medicines there are no dividing lines – nor should there be." Furthermore, it is described that object is different between human and animal medicine, but the experience obtained constitutes the basis of all medicine (Greek 2012). Sir William Osler (1849–1919), the father of modern medicine, who studied under Virchow, promoted the concepts of comparative medicine and comparative biology and the integration of human and animal health (Monath et al. 2010).

The concept of One Health has been in the South Asian culture from the ancient time. In the recent past, the concept of One Health in the South Asian region was encouraged and nurtured with the support of funding and advice from international aid agencies. However, it is observed that the progress of One Health policies is slow due to poor

One Health: Human, Animal, and Environment Triad, First Edition. Edited by Meththika Vithanage and Majeti Narasimha Vara Prasad.

institutionalization, economic, and political restrictions (Thresia 2018). Technically, the One Health paradigm promotes the integration of human and animal health with the environment through communication and collaboration among medical professionals, veterinarians, wildlife professionals, environmental and public health experts, chemists, agriculturists, educationists, economists, policymakers, and other interested parties (Monath et al. 2010). Tracing human diseases for their origin plays a pivotal role in epidemiology. Veterinarian Calvin W. Schwabe (1927–2006) was a noted epidemiologist and a parasitologist who pioneered the application of human disease-tracking techniques in the study of animal diseases. In fact, in 1984, Schwabe in his textbook named *Veterinary Medicine and Human Health* proposes a unified human and veterinary approach to zoonotic diseases and paved the pathway to the modern concept of one health (Monath et al. 2010). Interestingly, the collaborative efforts of Frederick A. Murphy, a veterinarian, and Karl M. Johnson, a physician, helped to unravel the hidden facts behind the initial outbreak of Ebola hemorrhagic fever in Africa (Notable "One Health" endorsements-One health Initiative 2022). In fact, the recent accomplishments of the One Health paradigm would be the investigation of crossing of species barrier by the SARS-CoV-2 virus (Yesudhas et al. 2021).

Accelerated deforestation for agriculture and livestock, poaching, increasing human density, and transboundary human movements during the past two decades have triggered the emergence and re-emergence of zoonoses in the South Asian region. These emerging and re-emerging zoonoses highlight the importance and active implementation of One Health in the region than any other time in the history.

20.2 Zoonoses

Zoonoses account for about 60% of emerging infectious diseases and about 70% has a wildlife origin (Jones et al. 2008). According to the World Health Organization (WHO) expert committee "any disease or infection that is naturally transmissible between vertebrate animals and humans" is known as a zoonosis ("JOINT WHO/FAO expert committee on zoonoses" 1959) (Figure 20.1). The term "zoonosis" is derived from two Greek words "zoon" and "nosos" meaning animal and illness, respectively. However, the definition of zoonosis should include the word "infestations" to cover parasitic diseases as well. Essentially, zoonoses are limited to microbial agents that can replicate in the animal host. Therefore, it does not include pathological conditions caused by envenomation of reptile or fish origin, toxicities, or by allergies in vertebrates. It also excludes diseases mechanically transmitted by animals or food of animal origin. Furthermore, the transmissibility of zoonoses should occur naturally and all

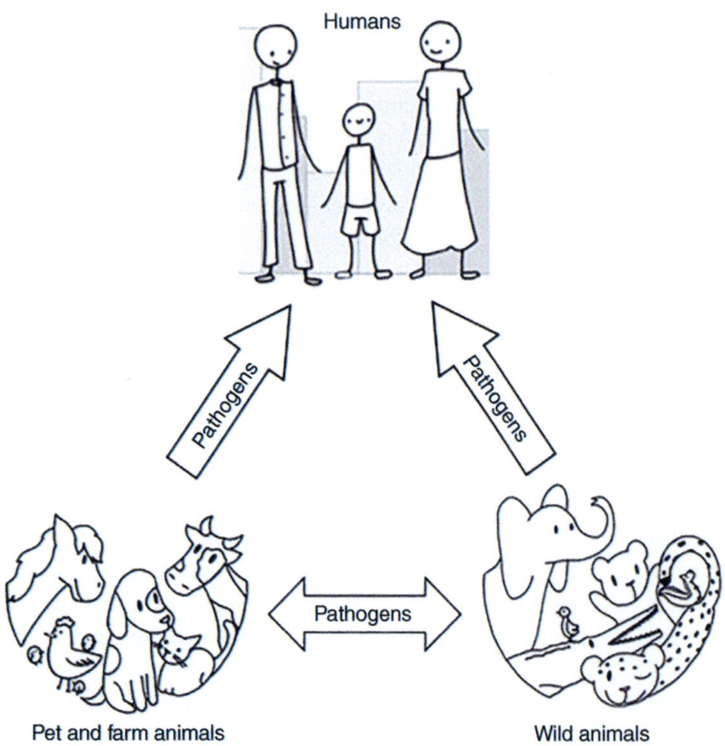

Figure 20.1 The zoonotic cycle. Humans acquired disease causing pathogens from pet, farm, and wild animals.

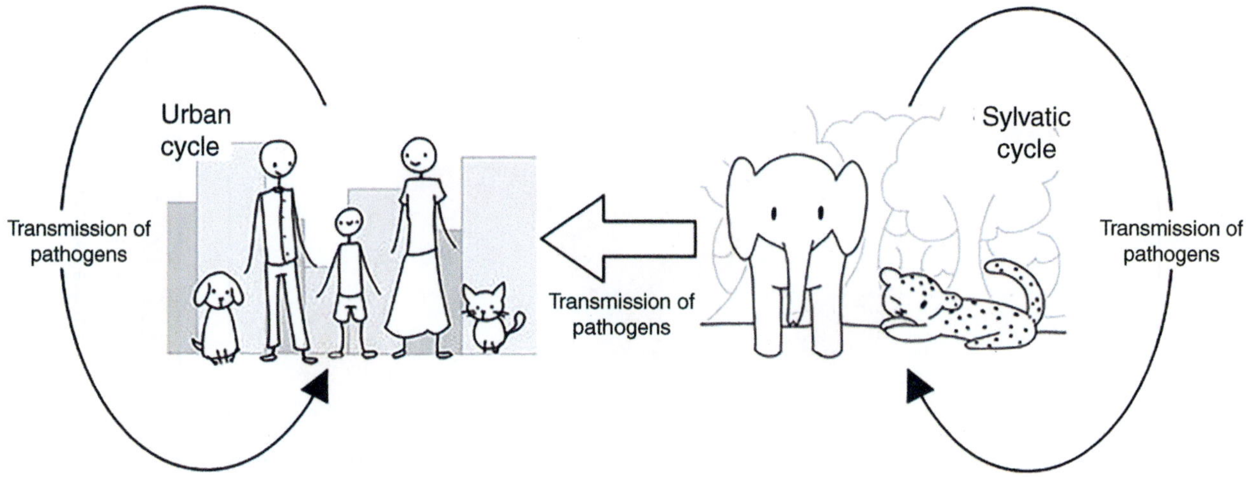

Figure 20.2 The urban and sylvatic cycles of zoonotic spread.

experimental infections of human pathogens to non-human vertebrates should be excluded.

Almost all zoonoses have a sylvatic cycle and an urban cycle (Figure 20.2). In the sylvatic cycle the causative agents are transmitted between wild animals and humans, whereas the urban cycle occurs between humans and domestic animals such as dogs, cats, livestock, and feral animals. However, in almost all zoonotic diseases the sylvatic and the urban cycles have crossed their pathways at least once. The livestock industry in majority of South Asian countries relies on the traditional pastoral system, where there would be increased contact of wildlife, domestic animals, and humans.

Zoonoses can be classified based on etiology such as bacterial zoonoses (e.g. anthrax, salmonellosis, tuberculosis, Lyme disease, brucellosis, and plague), viral zoonoses (e.g. rabies, Ebola, coronavirus including SARS-CoV, and avian influenza), parasitic zoonoses (e.g. trichinosis, toxoplasmosis, leishmaniasis, giardiasis, and echinococcosis), fungal zoonoses (e.g. ringworm, rhinosporidium), rickettsial zoonoses (e.g. Q-fever), chlamydial zoonoses (e.g. psittacosis), and diseases caused by acellular non-viral pathogenic agents (e.g. transmissible spongiform encephalopathies). Another categorization describes zoonoses as emerging, re-emerging, and neglected. Epidemiologically zoonoses are classified as follows: (i) endemic zoonoses that are present in many places and affect many people and animals, (ii) epidemic zoonoses that are sporadic in temporal and spatial distribution, and (iii) emerging and re-emerging zoonoses that are newly appearing in a population or have existed previously but are rapidly increasing in incidence or geographical range. In addition, a neglected zoonotic disease is a zoonosis that is commonly associated with poverty and impacts the lives and livelihoods of people in underdeveloped countries including South Asia.

20.3 Emerging and Re-emerging Zoonoses in South Asia

South Asia comprises the countries of Afghanistan, Bangladesh, Bhutan, India, Maldives, Nepal, Pakistan, and Sri Lanka. This area inhabits the most densely populated subregion in the world, having a total area of 5,134,641 km^2 with a density of 362.3 people/km^2 (Acharya et al. 2021). However, according to the World Bank report in 2019, the per capita GDP of this region (US$1779) remains much lower than the rest of the middle- and low-income countries in the world, which are US$10,636 and US$4497, respectively. Most of the people in the South Asian region make their livelihood by agriculture, livestock farming, or by fisheries. Furthermore, most of the countries belonging to South Asian region show rapid economic development. These economic developments are generally seen in the areas of industry, international trade, and tourism, which at the same time imposes a global threat in spreading of zoonoses and creating pandemics as happened in 1955 with plague. The region has been identified as a hot spot for emerging and re-emerging zoonotic diseases (Figure 20.3) (Grace et al. 2012; Laxminarayan et al. 2017). South Asia accounts for approximately one-quarter of the world's soil-transmitted helminth infections, one-third or more of the global deaths from rabies, and one-half or more of the global burden of lymphatic filariasis and visceral leishmaniasis (Lobo et al. 2011). The following few paragraphs will discuss the most common emerging and re-emerging zoonoses that threaten the well-being of South Asian ecosystems.

20.3.1 Rabies

Rabies is considered a re-emerging and a neglected zoonosis (Fooks et al. 2017). It is caused by infection with

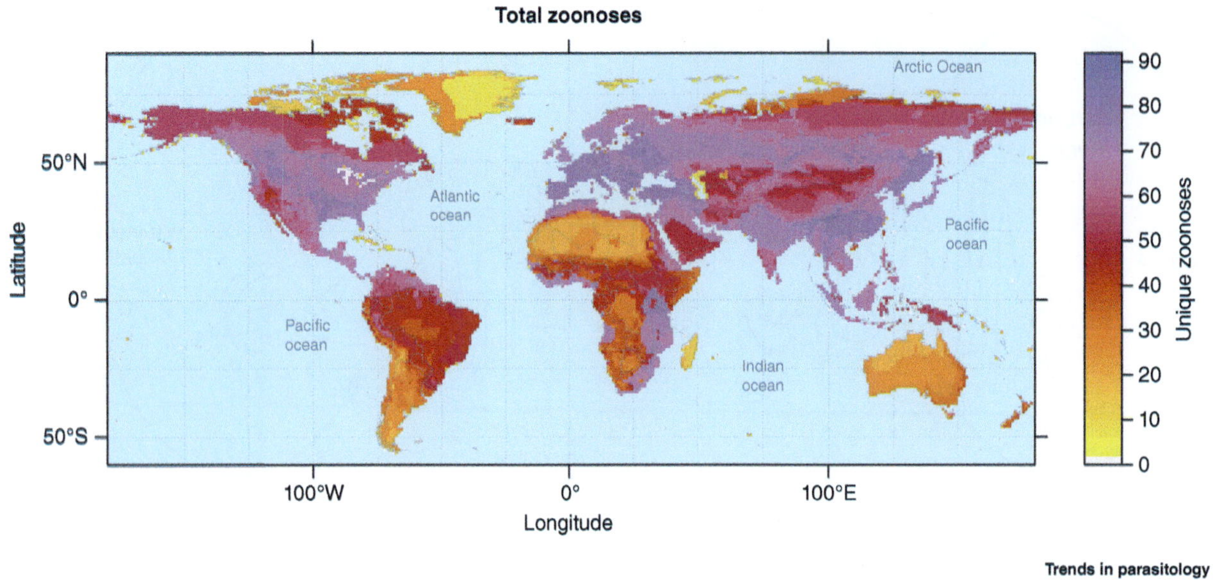

Figure 20.3 Geographic distribution of zoonoses carried by 27 orders of wild terrestrial mammals. South Asian region lies on the top of the zoonotic prevalence. *Source:* Adapted from Han et al. (2016).

viruses of the Lyssa virus genus. Rabies is transmitted primarily by the bite of an infected host and less frequently by the deposition of saliva containing viral particles on wounds or mucous membranes (Radhakrishnan et al. 2020). The main transmission pathway involves the contact between infected saliva and neuromuscular junctions. The dog is considered the causative agent of up to 99% of rabies transmission to humans in most rabies-endemic countries including the countries in South Asia (Figure 20.4). In addition, cats, monkeys, mongoose, civet cats, jackals, and occasionally bats have been identified as reservoirs of rabies in the South Asian countries (Sudarshan and Ashwath Narayana 2019). Rabies is a 100% fatal disease. Three South Asian countries namely India, Pakistan, and Bangladesh are considered as the top five rabies endemic countries of the world. Around 55,000 people die of rabies every year globally and 45% of them belong to South and Southeast Asia (Chowdhury et al. 2015). In fact, 22,000–28,000 deaths due to rabies are recorded annually, in the South Asian region (Chowdhury et al. 2015). About 35% of the global dog-mediated rabies deaths occur in India. These figures show the significance of rabies as a zoonosis in the region. Depending on the number of cases rabies-endemic countries in South Asia can be categorized into three groups: high (India, Pakistan, and Bangladesh), medium (Bhutan, Nepal, and Sri Lanka), and low (Afghanistan). Both animal and human rabies are preventable through immunization. Despite this burden, only two countries (Bhutan and Sri Lanka) have coordinated rabies control activities at their national level. Interestingly, Maldives is completely free of rabies (Gongal and Wright 2011). This would probably be due to the low wildlife population and the geography of Maldives by being an archipelago. In contrast, the other South Asian countries have a rich wildlife population coupled with poor rabies vaccination programs, which facilitates the urban and sylvatic cycle of rabies. Therefore, control of rabies among domestic animals is the most practical solution to preventing rabies-related deaths. It has been suggested that 70% or more of dogs in a population should be vaccinated to prevent epidemics and to eliminate endemic rabies (Franka et al. 2013). However, the high cost of modern rabies vaccines and the lack of education and awareness about rabies especially among the South Asian rural populations limit the use of immunization for rabies.

Despite the joint call for action to eliminate rabies by 2030, by the WHO, the epidemiological control of rabies in the South Asian region is constrained by the lack of political commitment and mired rabies control activities (*Prevention and Control of Rabies in SAARC Countries: Report of the Workshop Colombo, Sri Lanka, 11–13 August 2015* 2016).

20.3.2 Leishmaniasis

Leishmaniasis is a disease caused by an intracellular protozoan parasite, Leishmania. This parasite is transmitted by the sand flies (*Phlebotomus* and *Lutzomyia*), and clinically manifested as skin lesions (cutaneous leishmaniasis) to fatal visceral infections (visceral leishmaniasis, also known as kala-azar) (Karunaweera et al. 2021). The latter

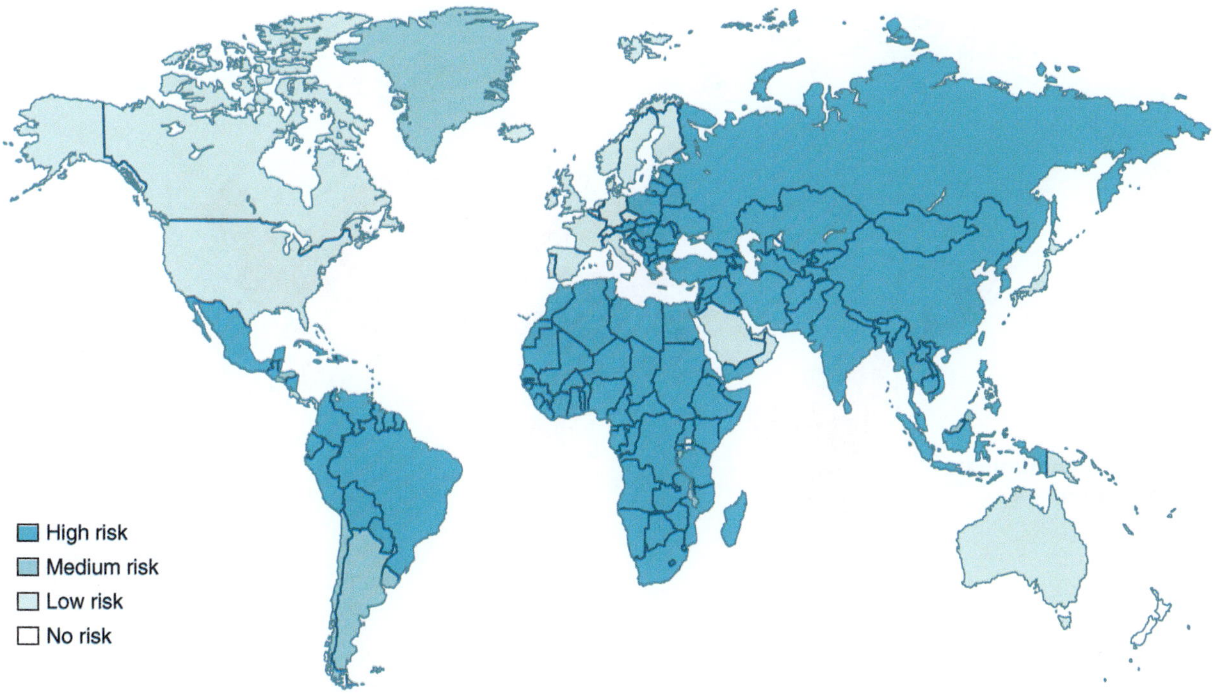

Figure 20.4 Map of rabies-endemic areas. South Asian region is endemic for rabies. *Source:* Adapted from Crowcroft and Thampi (2015).

is a clinical form seen in India, Bangladesh, and Nepal. Leishmaniasis is considered as one of the seven most important tropical diseases that can have a fatal outcome (Andrade-Narváez et al. 2001). About 70 animal species, including humans, have been found as natural reservoir hosts of *Leishmania* parasites (Esteva et al. 2017). Visceral leishmaniasis has been recorded on the Indian subcontinent since the early nineteenth century and the three most affected countries in South Asia at present are India, Bangladesh, and Nepal (Rijal et al. 2019). Interestingly, these South Asian countries account for more than 50% of the global visceral leishmaniasis burden. In addition, a significant number of cutaneous leishmaniasis cases were recorded in Pakistan and Afghanistan (WHO 2016). Sporadic cases have been reported in Bhutan, and leishmaniasis appears as an emerging zoonosis in Sri Lanka in contrast to the declining trend in the rest of South Asia (Karunaweera et al. 2021). Leishmaniasis is a disease very commonly seen in human habitats near forests. In 2005, the governments of Bangladesh, India, and Nepal with the lead of the WHO jointly established a regional alliance to eliminate visceral leishmaniasis (kala-azar) (Hirve et al. 2017) and set a target to reduce the public health burden by 2015. However, according to the epidemiological studies done in the region (Figure 20.5), it is revealed that leishmaniasis still prevails significantly in non-immunized populations (Rijal et al. 2019).

20.3.3 Trypanosomiasis

Trypanosomiasis is caused by the unicellular flagellar protozoan belonging to the family of Trypanosomatidae and the genus *Trypanosoma* (Sobhy et al. 2017). Diseases caused by trypanosomes have been identified in humans, domestic animals, and wild animals specially in sub-Saharan Africa, South Asia, and South America (Sánchez et al. 2015). African Trypanosomiasis (African human trypanosomiasis or African sleeping sickness) is a disease caused by the parasite *Trypanosoma brucei gambiense* or *Trypanosoma brucei rhodesiense* and transmitted by the tsetse fly (Franco et al. 2022). Chagas disease, which is also known as American trypanosomiasis and is caused by *Trypanosoma cruzi* and transmitted by the Reduuvid bugs (Hemmige et al. 2012).

Trypanosoma evansi is the causative agent of trypanosomiasis (surra) in bovids, camelids, and equids (Aregawi et al. 2019). This parasite has been in the domestic and wild animals in the South Asian region for a long time. However, the first human case of trypanosomiasis was reported in 2005, in the Indian subcontinent. Furthermore, this was the first confirmed infection of a human by *T. evansi* (Joshi et al. 2005). Later, a similar case of human infection was reported in 2015 in Mumbai (Wabale et al. 2015), indicating the possibility of the emergence of surra as a human zoonosis. Recent evidence of infections of *T. evansi* in domestic dogs in Sri Lanka and Afghanistan (Aref

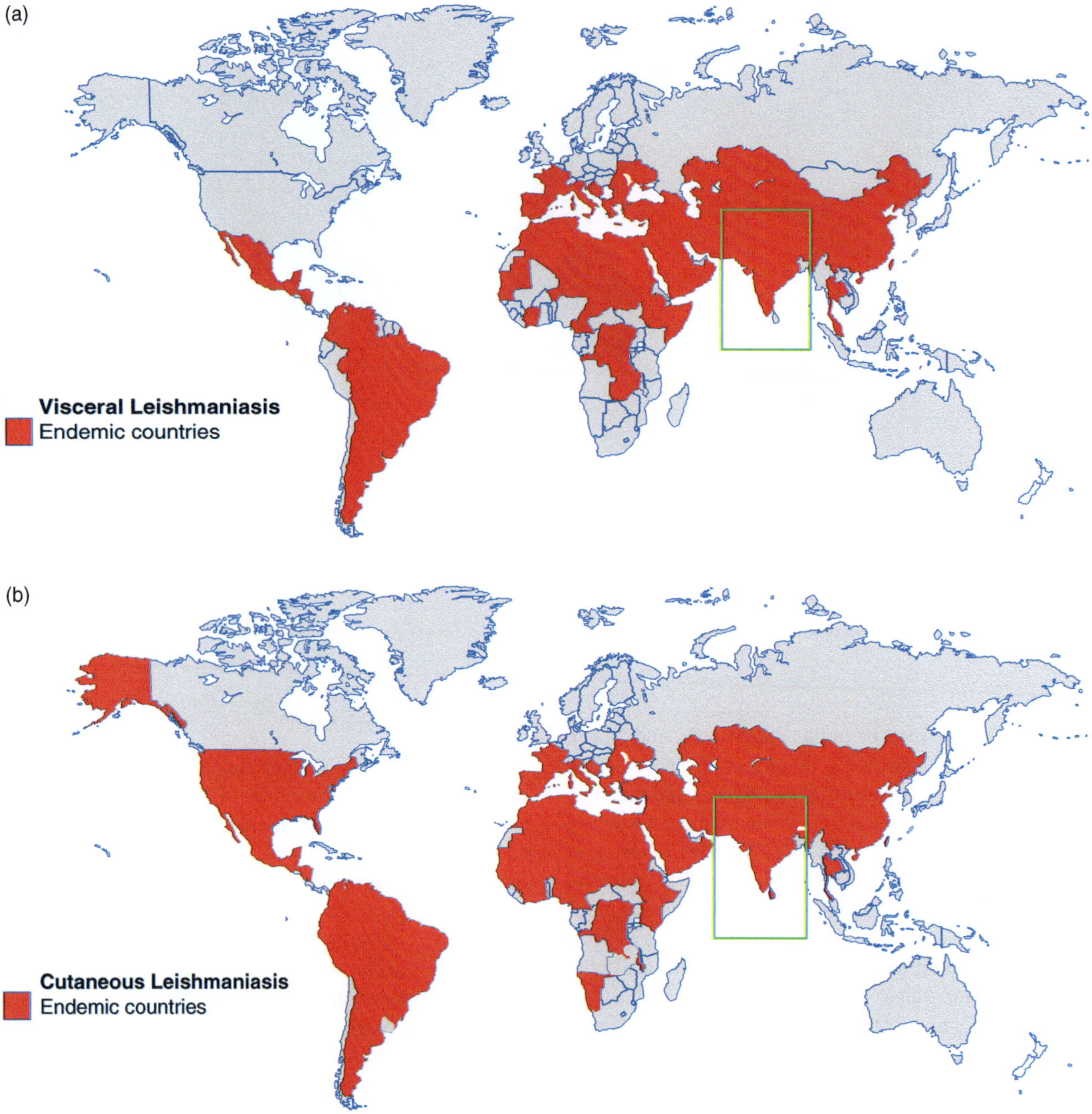

Figure 20.5 Status of the leishmaniasis in the world. Both visceral leishmaniasis (a) cutaneous leishmaniasis (b) are endemic in the South Asian region. *Source:* Adapted from Sasidharan and Saudagar (2021).

et al. 2013; Dangolla et al. 2020) shows the ability to overcome the species barrier by the protozoan, which will impose a heavy zoonotic potential in the coming years in the region.

20.3.4 Nipah Virus

Nipah is one of the emerging deadly zoonotic diseases and is caused by the viruses of the order Mononegavirales. The other deadly virus in this order includes Hendra, Ebola, and Marburg. Nipah can cause encephalitis and severe acute respiratory failure and result in mortality (Soman Pillai et al. 2020). Considering the high mortality rate of the Nipah virus, it is identified as a biological safety level 4 (BSL 4) pathogen (Devnath and Masud 2021). Pteropus fruit bats (flying foxes) have been identified as the natural reservoir of the Nipah virus (Halpin et al. 2011), and pigs act as the intermediate (amplifying) hosts through the consumption of bat-eaten fruits (Luby 2013). Nipah-infected bats are symptomless carriers, and they shed the viruses in their saliva, urine, semen, and feces (Luby 2013). The first human case of Nipah virus was first identified in Sungai Nipah village in Malaysia in 1998. Furthermore, it was thought to be transmitted from pigs that served as the intermediate host (Hauser et al. 2021). Interestingly, all identified cases of Nipah virus in humans after 2001 have occurred in India and Bangladesh (Luby et al. 2009). Bangladesh and India represent 42 and 15%, respectively, of the total incident cases worldwide (Soman Pillai et al. 2020). Nipah virus is identified as a potential pandemic agent since it can infect a broad range of mammals and is capable of person-to-person transmission (Luby 2013). In Bangladesh drinking raw date palm sap that is contaminated with bat saliva is the most common form of transmission from bats to humans (Luby 2013). In addition, in Bangladesh and India, person-to-person transmission has been found to be an important mode of transmission (Aditi and Shariff 2019).

20.3.5 Coronavirus (SARS, MERS, CoV) Infections

Severe acute respiratory syndrome (SARS-CoV-1), Middle East respiratory syndrome (MERS-CoV), and coronavirus disease 2019 (COVID-19/SARS-CoV-2) are all caused by coronaviruses. MERS-CoV was first reported in Saudi Arabia in September 2012 and has since spread to 27 countries, but no human cases were reported in South Asia (Al-Tawfiq et al. 2021). SARS-CoV-1 is the first major novel infectious disease to hit the global community, particularly in Asia, in the twenty-first century (Lam et al. 2003). During the 2002–2004 SARS-CoV-1 outbreak, three cases were reported from India, and none were reported from other South Asian countries (Lee and McKibbin 2004). Research evidence suggests that both SARS-CoV-1 and MERS-CoV originated in bats. Then, SARS-CoV spread to humans from infected civets, while MERS-CoV spread from infected dromedary to people (Zhu et al. 2020). Coronavirus disease 2019 (COVID-19 caused by SARS-CoV-2) invaded the world unexpectedly in 2019 (Niu et al. 2021), and 21% of the reported total number of cases and 11% of COVID-19 deaths worldwide were reported in South Asia (Babu et al. 2021). There is growing evidence that the SARS-CoV-2 has an animal origin (Yesudhas et al. 2021). Interestingly, the first wave of SARS-CoV-2 infections remained relatively low in South Asian countries even without vaccination coverage. However, the second wave of infections attained a much higher level, likely due to invasion of the Delta strain and possibly relaxing of control measures (Song et al. 2021).

The COVID-19 pandemic has exposed the vulnerabilities of the South Asian region. Despite poor pandemic preparedness, South Asian countries mounted a reasonably good response against the COVID-19 crisis (Babu et al. 2021).

20.3.6 Leptospirosis

Leptospirosis is caused by 11 pathogenic and 5 intermediate species of Leptospira from the genus *Leptospira* of the family Leptospiraceae. South Asia accounts for the third commonest region of global outbreaks (Munoz-Zanzi et al. 2020). It is endemic in India and Sri Lanka. Humans are accidental hosts and the primary reservoir hosts are infected animals such as rodents, dogs, cattle, and pigs. These primary reservoir hosts shed the Leptospira with their urine. Humans acquire the infection through direct or indirect contact with water or soil contaminated by the urine of infected animals (Holla et al. 2018). Leptospirosis is one of the zoonoses that have a large geographical distribution due to a large number of reservoir hosts and wider environmental conditions. Sri Lanka and India have experienced several outbreaks during the last decade (Agampodi et al. 2009). However, most leptospirosis cases in both South Asian countries remain unreported due to poor surveillance (Warnasekara and Agampodi 2017). In India and Malaysia, it has been found that floods heighten the possibility of leptospirosis outbreaks because the close contact of humans and rodents on higher ground facilitates the spread of the pathogen (Watson et al. 2007). Therefore, tropical climate with seasonal storms that frequently result in flooding makes India and Sri Lanka more vulnerable to leptospirosis. Leptospirosis outbreaks in these countries will be more frequent with climatic changes.

20.3.7 Anthrax

Anthrax is a bacterial infection caused by *Bacillus anthracis*, an aerobic, Gram-positive spore-forming bacterium, and occurs primarily as a cutaneous, pulmonary, or gastrointestinal infection, and humans commonly get infected directly or indirectly through contact with infected animals and their products (Sushma et al. 2021). Anthrax outbreaks occur during the hot and humid transition period between the dry and wet seasons, and human case rates are highest in Africa, Central Asia, and South Asia ("Anthrax in humans and animals Fourth edition Food and Agriculture Organization of the United Nations World Organisation for Animal Health" 2008). Animal anthrax is endemic in Afghanistan, India, and Bangladesh causing frequent human outbreaks of the disease and in Bhutan, sporadic anthrax outbreaks occur annually among animals, posing health risks to persons who come into contact with the infected animals (Bhattacharya et al. 2021). Furthermore, bioterrorism-related anthrax has been reported in Pakistan (Tin et al. 2022).

20.3.8 Avian Influenza

Avian influenza is caused by influenza A viruses that are RNA viruses of the family Orthomyxoviridae. Furthermore, influenza viruses are classified into different subtypes based on the antigenic variation of their surface glycoproteins, hemagglutinin (HA), and neuraminidase (NA). Currently, there are 16 HA and 9 NA subtypes (Webster et al. 1992). The main natural host of the avian influenza virus is aquatic birds (Webster et al. 1992). However, the avian influenza virus has been found in other birds and mammals including humans (Webster et al. 1992; Alexander and Brown 2000). Generally, influenza A viruses are host specific and are not capable of transmitting from one species to another. However, due to environmental, viral, and host factors, the influenza viruses can transmit from one host to another (Chen et al. 2012).

Highly pathogenic avian influenza (HPAI), H5N1, has caused many outbreaks in poultry in Asia, Europe, and Africa (OIE 2019). Poultry, especially chicken, are susceptible to HPAI (H5N1), with high morbidity and a case fatality rate as high as 100% (Alexander 2006). Furthermore, in South Asia, people live very close to poultry farms and have poor knowledge about the risk of avian influenza. HPAI, which was introduced to the subcontinent in 2005 through wild birds, has since become endemic across large parts of Northeast India and Bangladesh (Laxminarayan et al. 2017). Since 2006, HPAI outbreaks were reported in six South Asian countries, namely, Afghanistan, Bangladesh, Bhutan, India, Nepal, and Pakistan. In addition, human cases of HPAI were reported in Bangladesh and Pakistan, since 2007 (WHO 2019). Interestingly, Maldives and Sri Lanka did not report any HPAI outbreaks in poultry or in humans probably due to their geographic location (OIE 2019; WHO 2019).

20.3.9 Other Zoonoses

In addition to aforementioned major zoonoses, there are records of some other emerging and re-emerging zoonoses in the South Asian region during the past two decades. Most of these zoonoses are caused by different etiological agents such as bacteria (brucellosis, shigellosis), fungi (rhinosporidiosis, basidobolomycosis), helminths (schistosomiasis, *Orientobilharzia* infections, toxocariasis), rickettsia, and protozoans (toxoplasmosis, cryptosporidiosis). Outbreaks of such diseases occur sporadically in the South Asian region and would impose a huge public health threat in the coming years. Arthropod-borne zoonoses impose a huge threat on human lives in the tropics. The major arthropod-borne diseases that cause severe morbidity and mortality are Japanese B encephalitis, dengue, Zika, and Chikungunya. Japanese B encephalitis is one of the epidemic encephalitis that is reported in all countries of South Asia except Afghanistan (Partridge et al. 2007; Turtle and Solomon 2018). The viral etiological agent of the Japanese B encephalitis belongs to the family Flaviviridae. Pigs and birds act as the natural reservoir of the Japanese B encephalitis virus, and the transmission between animals and humans occurs due to Culex mosquitoes (Filgueira and Lannes 2019). Dengue is another arthropod-borne disease that is caused by the viruses of the family Flaviviridae, which threatens the lifestyles of people in the tropics including South Asia. Recent climatic changes have increased the number of dengue cases in the region probably due to favorable environments for mosquito breeding (Udayanga et al. 2020). Furthermore, even though it is underestimated, the emergence and re-emergence of dengue outbreaks in the region could be attributed to a sylvatic cycle where non-human primates would be playing a significant role (Aliaga-Samanez et al. 2021). Chikungunya is another arthropod-borne human disease that can be related to non-human mammalian involvement (Darwish et al. 1983). During the period of 2005–2017, Chikungunya outbreaks have been reported in several South Asian countries, namely, India, Sri Lanka, Bangladesh, Bhutan, Nepal, and Pakistan (Ng and Hapuarachchi 2010; Rahman et al. 2019). Most of the above diseases are undervalued or the connection to the animal host has not yet been confirmed.

20.4 Challenges of Implementing One Health in South Asia

Most of the South Asian countries are geographically located in and around the equator. Therefore, most of the Indian subcontinent, Bangladesh, Pakistan, Sri Lanka, and Maldives has a tropical climate throughout the years that favors transmission of most zoonotic pathogens. Furthermore, the South Asian region comprises one of the most vivid areas of biodiversity in the world (Chowdhury et al. 2022). Being the most populated region in the world, there is continuous and constant competition between humans, domestic animals, and wildlife for space and food. This competition for basic needs along with other socioeconomic factors such as poverty, low education, political instability, and lack of rules and regulations lead to increased outbreaks of zoonoses and their transboundary propagation. This section will encompass some of the main socioeconomic factors that increase the zoonotic burden and constraint the effective application of the One Health paradigm in South Asian countries.

20.4.1 Poverty and Overpopulation

South Asia is the most populated region followed by Southeast Asia (Figure 20.6). Currently, there is a population of nearly two billion living in an area of 5.2 million km^2. Therefore, the population density in the region is

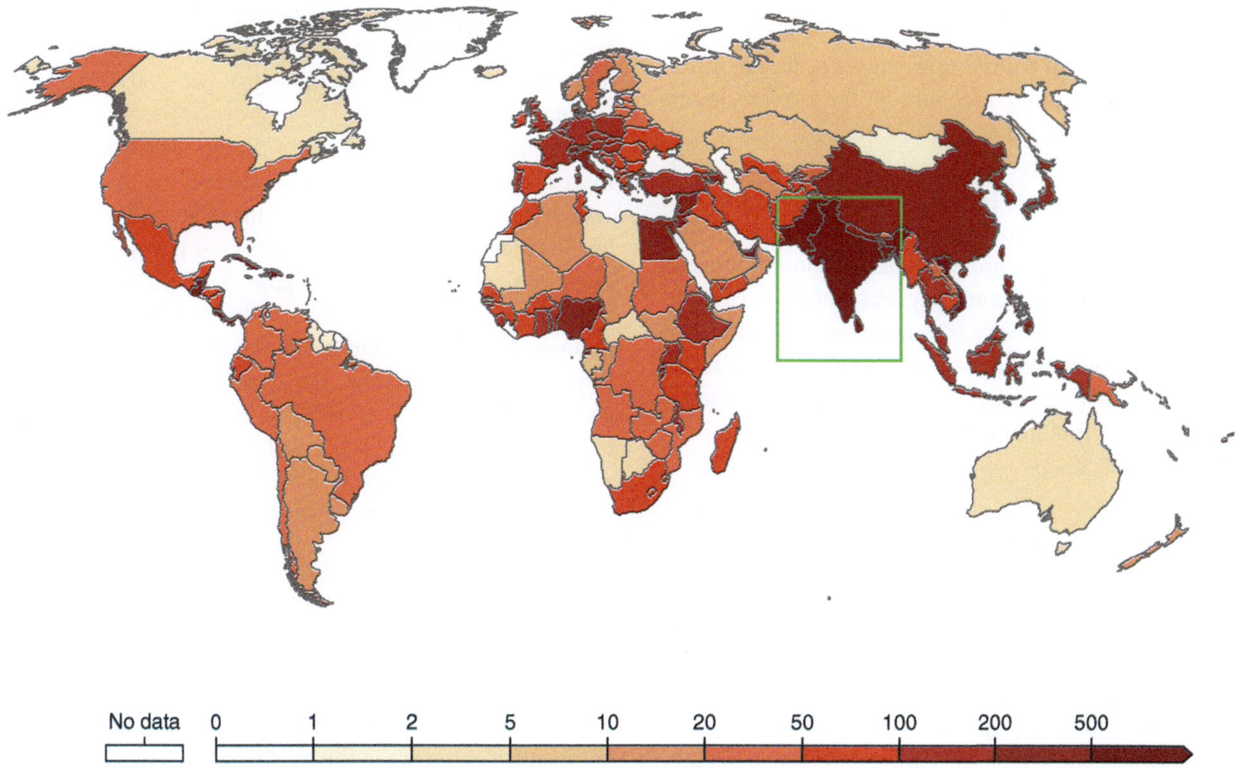

Figure 20.6 World population density map. The South Asian region is the most populated region in the world. *Source:* World Bank (2021).

approximately $400/km^2$. This number is far high in reality due to urbanization and geographical differences in the land. Furthermore, most of the countries in South Asia are underdeveloped and people are living with very minimum necessities. In fact, the world's most poor people live in South Asia next to sub-Saharan Africa (Islam et al. 2021). An insufficient level of safe drinking water, food, clothes, and shelter is termed "poverty," which is used as a benchmark for a society in terms of lack of opportunities to learn, better employment, quality of life, and societal admiration (Karim 2013; Keeley 2015).

These people have very limited access to nutritional food, potable water, education, health, and sanitary facilities (Deen et al. 2020). Furthermore, most of these people share their habitats with farm animals or in certain situations with wild or feral animals. This is more commonly seen in livestock farmers and pastoral livestock herders (Grace et al. 2017). Factors that are coupled with poverty and overcrowding such as poor sanitation, lack of medical facilities, and under education make the population fall into a disease burden, especially to zoonotic diseases (Leonardo et al. 2019).

20.4.2 Identification of Zoonoses in Animals

In most zoonotic diseases the reservoir hosts remain asymptomatic. This is more commonly seen in zoonoses such as leptospirosis, toxoplasmosis, and brucellosis. Certain zoonoses such as tuberculosis are transmitted with animal products and make it difficult to diagnose under a farm or without laboratory facilities (Almeria et al. 2021). In the South Asian region, the veterinary and food safety systems are at a suboptimum level, especially in the rural and remote areas (Bruschi 2012). In addition, most of the people in the region live close to wildlife habitats and there are no proper mechanisms to investigate wildlife deaths, which would most of the time be due to a zoonotic important disease. Therefore, failure in diagnosing zoonotic threats in advance will lead to major outbreaks in the region.

20.4.3 Poor Collaboration Between Different Parties Involved in Zoonosis Control

Effective implementation of the One Health paradigm needs communication between different parties, mainly medical and veterinary professionals. However, severe compartmentalization is seen in different institutes among each country of the region specially during the implementation of One Health project (Rubin et al. 2014). Working in isolation by different entities needed to control zoonoses and promote One Health impedes the early detection and control measures.

20.4.4 Lack of Awareness

Lack of awareness in control of zoonoses occurs in different stages. At the ground level, most of the farmers, herdsmen, pet owners, and other people who work closely with animals or animal products have no proper awareness about zoonotic diseases (Hundal et al. 2016). In fact, the majority of people are not aware of the existence of zoonoses. In addition, health professionals are more interested in treating human patients and pay less attention to the origin of diseases. This is very commonly seen in rural and remote areas where people have very limited health facilities. Besides, in these areas there are limited diagnostic facilities, and symptomatic treatment is given a priority (Kamineni et al. 2012).

20.4.5 Political Instability

Political instability in the South Asian countries has severely impeded the upgrading of life standards and poverty alleviation of the people. Most South Asian countries have party policies and their attitudes on agriculture, livestock, health, and education vary with the political party in power. This is seen since the post-colonial era and invariably affected the control of zoonotic diseases. In addition, political conflicts in the region in the forms of insurgencies, counterinsurgencies, civil fighting, terrorism, and communal riots have been occurring continuously and sporadically. Furthermore, these conflicts result in displacement, cross border migration, and human trafficking that will result in a population of people who are unable to access health care, livelihood, and public health aspects (Babu et al. 2021). In addition, these conflicts drain a large amount of national income on military expenses and inhibit spending on vaccination, health care, and other zoonotic containment measures (Bhutta et al. 2021). Besides, most South Asian nations do not have robust national plans, guidelines, or laws that account for surveillance and control of zoonotic diseases, concerns of public health, and antibiotic resistance. It has been noted that all South Asian countries are short of health workers and have less than one field epidemiologist per 200,000 people (Haidar 2020).

In addition to the five main factors described above, there are some other socioeconomic reasons that load the zoonotic potential in the region. One of such factors would be globalization where the migration of people will introduce new zoonoses to the region. Second, South Asian countries have a huge cultural diversity. This brings about different food habits and public health concerns such as resistance to vaccination based on religious and other beliefs (Rozier 2017). Furthermore, these beliefs make people resistant to lifestyle changes that are needed for zoonotic control.

20.5 Conclusion

South Asia plays a huge role in the global economy and political scenario. Besides, this region inhabits 25% of the world's population along with livestock and wildlife. Most of the major zoonoses in the world are still prevalent in the region. One Health paradigm that is an effective and economical method of controlling zoonoses is still novel to the region and progressing at a slow phase due to certain constraints that are indigenous to the region. Zoonotic outbreaks in the South Asian region would impose health threats to the whole world. Therefore, more regional and global partnerships are expected to overcome such constraints and implement the One Health paradigm in the South Asian region.

Acknowledgments

The authors like to extend their acknowledgment to Dihini Wijesundera for artwork.

References

Acharya, K.P., Subedi, D., and Wilson, R.T. (2021). Rabies control in South Asia requires a one health approach. *One Health* 12: 100215.

Aditi and Shariff, M. (2019). Nipah virus infection: a review. *Epidemiology and Infection*. https://doi.org/10.1017/S0950268819000086 147.

Agampodi, S., Peacock, S., and Thevanesam, V. (2009). The potential emergence of leptospirosis in Sri Lanka. *The Lancet Infectious Diseases* 9 (9): 524–526.

Alexander, D.J. (2006). Avian influenza viruses and human health. *Developments in Biologicals* 2006 (124): 77–84.

Alexander, D. and Brown, I. (2000). Recent zoonoses caused by influenza A viruses. *Revue Scientifique et Technique de l'OIE* 19 (1): 197–225.

Aliaga-Samanez, A., Cobos-Mayo, M., Real, R. et al. (2021). Worldwide dynamic biogeography of zoonotic and anthroponotic dengue. *PLoS Neglected Tropical Diseases* 15 (6): e0009496.

Almeria, S., Robertson, L., and Santin, M. (2021). Why foodborne and waterborne parasites are important for veterinarians. *Research in Veterinary Science* 136: 198–199.

Al-Tawfiq, J., Azhar, E., Memish, Z., and Zumla, A. (2021). Middle East respiratory syndrome coronavirus. *Seminars in Respiratory and Critical Care Medicine* 42 (06): 828–838.

Andrade-Narváez, F., Vargas-González, A., Canto-Lara, S., and Damián-Centeno, A. (2001). Clinical picture of cutaneous leishmaniases due to *Leishmania* (*Leishmania*) Mexicana in the Yucatan peninsula, Mexico. *Memórias do Instituto Oswaldo Cruz* 96 (2): 163–167.

Aref, M., Yasin, S.M., Bahear, W. et al. (2013). Canine *Trypanosoma evansi* infection in Afghanistan. *Veterinary Parasitology* 197 (3–4): 638–641.

Aregawi, W.G., Agga, G.E., Abdi, R.D., and Büscher, P. (2019). Systematic review and meta-analysis on the global distribution, host range, and prevalence of *Trypanosoma evansi*. *Parasites & Vectors* 12 (1): 67.

Babu, G., Khetrapal, S., John, D. et al. (2021). Pandemic preparedness and response to COVID-19 in south Asian countries. *International Journal of Infectious Diseases* 104: 169–174.

Bhattacharya, D., Kshatri, J., Choudhary, H. et al. (2021). One Health approach for elimination of human anthrax in a tribal district of Odisha: study protocol. *PLoS One* 16 (5): e0251041.

Bhutta, Z.A., Mitra, A., Salman, A. et al. (2021). Conflict, extremism, resilience and peace in South Asia; can covid-19 provide a bridge for peace and rapprochement? *BMJ* 15 (375): e067384.

Bruschi, F. (2012). Trichinellosis in developing countries: is it neglected? *Journal of Infection in Developing Countries* 6 (3): 216–222.

Chen, W., Zhong, Y., Qin, Y. et al. (2012). The evolutionary pattern of glycosylation sites in influenza virus (H5N1) hemagglutinin and neuraminidase. *PLoS One* 7 (11): e49224.

Chowdhury, F., Basher, A., Amin, M. et al. (2015). Rabies in South Asia: fighting for elimination. *Recent Patents on Anti-Infective Drug Discovery* 10 (1): 30–34.

Chowdhury, S., Alam, S., Labi, M.M. et al. (2022). Protected areas in South Asia: status and prospects. *The Science of the Total Environment* 811: 152316.

Crowcroft, N.S. and Thampi, N. (2015). The prevention and management of rabies. *BMJ* 350: g7827. doi: 10.1136/bmj.g7827. Erratum in: BMJ. 2015;350:h581. PMID: 25589091.

Dangolla, A., Wijesundara, D., Blair, D. et al. (2020). Canine trypanosomosis in Sri Lanka: an emerging problem reported from three distinct geographic locations. *Parasitology International* 77: 102129.

Darwish, M., Hoogstraal, H., Roberts, T. et al. (1983). A sero-epidemiological survey for certain arboviruses (Togaviridae) in Pakistan. *Transactions of the Royal Society of Tropical Medicine and Hygiene* 77 (4): 442–445.

Deen, J., Mengel, M.A., and Clemens, J.D. (2020). Epidemiology of cholera. *Vaccine* 38 (Suppl 1): A31–A40.

Devnath, P. and Masud, H.M.A.A. (2021). Nipah virus: a potential pandemic agent in the context of the current severe acute respiratory syndrome coronavirus 2 pandemic. *New Microbes and New Infections* 41: 100873.

Dunlop, R.H. and Williams, D.J. (1996). *Veterinary Medicine: An Illustrated History*. St. Louis: Mosby-Year Book.

Esteva, L., Vargas, C., and Vargas de León, C. (2017). The role of asymptomatics and dogs on leishmaniasis propagation. *Mathematical Biosciences*. United States 293: 46–55.

Evans, B. and Leighton, F. (2014). A history of One Health. *Revue Scientifique et Technique de l'OIE* 33 (2): 413–420.

Filgueira, L. and Lannes, N. (2019). Review of emerging Japanese encephalitis virus: new aspects and concepts about entry into the brain and inter-cellular spreading. *Pathogens* 8 (3): 111.

Fooks, A., Cliquet, F., Finke, S. et al. (2017). Rabies. *Nature Reviews. Disease Primers* 3 (1).

Franco, J., Cecchi, G., Paone, M. et al. (2022). The elimination of human African trypanosomiasis: achievements in relation to WHO road map targets for 2020. *PLoS Neglected Tropical Diseases* 16 (1): e0010047.

Franka, R., Smith, T., Dyer, J. et al. (2013). Current and future tools for global canine rabies elimination. *Antiviral Research* 100 (1): 220–225.

Gongal, G. and Wright, A. (2011). Human rabies in the WHO Southeast Asia region: forward steps for elimination. *Advances in Preventive Medicine* 2011: 1–5.

Grace, D., Mutua, F., Ochungo, P., et al. (2012). Mapping of poverty and likely zoonoses hotspots. Zoonoses Project 4. Report to the UK Department for International Development. Nairobi, Kenya: ILRI.

Grace, D., Lindahl, J., Wanyoike, F. et al. (2017). Poor livestock keepers: ecosystem-poverty-health interactions. *Philosophical Transactions of The Royal Society B Biological Sciences* 372 (1725): 20160166.

Greek, R. (2012). Zoobiquity: what animals can teach us about health and the science of healing. *Animals: An Open Access Journal from MDPI* 2 (4): 559–563.

Haidar, S. (2020). Coronavirus|South Asia remains an outlier in infections. *The Hindu*. http://www.thehindu.com/news/national/coronavirus-south-asia-remains-an-outlier-in-infections/article31378180.ece (accessed 23 February 2022)

Halpin, K., Daszak, P., Field, H. et al. (2011). Pteropid bats are confirmed as the reservoir hosts of Henipaviruses: a comprehensive experimental study of virus transmission. *The American Journal of Tropical Medicine and Hygiene* 85 (5): 946–951.

Han, B.A., Kramer, A.M., and Drake, J.M. (2016 Jul). Global patterns of zoonotic disease in mammals. *Trends in Parasitology* 32 (7): 565–577. https://doi.org/10.1016/j.pt.2016.04.007. Epub 2016 Jun 14. PMID: 27316904; PMCID: PMC4921293.

Hauser, N., Gushiken, A., Narayanan, S. et al. (2021). Evolution of Nipah virus infection: past, present, and future considerations. *Tropical Medicine and Infectious Disease* 6 (1): 24.

Hemmige, V., Tanowitz, H., and Sethi, A. (2012). *Trypanosoma cruzi* infection: a review with emphasis on cutaneous manifestations. *International Journal of Dermatology* 51 (5): 501–508.

Hirve, S., Kroeger, A., Matlashewski, G. et al. (2017). Towards elimination of visceral leishmaniasis in the Indian subcontinent – translating research to practice to public health. *PLoS Neglected Tropical Diseases* 11 (10): e0005889.

Holla, R., Darshan, B., Pandey, L. et al. (2018). Leptospirosis in Coastal South India: a facility based study. *BioMed Research International* 2018: 1–5.

Hundal, J.S., Sodhi, S.S., Gupta, A. et al. (2016). Awareness, knowledge, and risks of zoonotic diseases among livestock farmers in Punjab. *Veterinary World* 9 (2): 186–191.

Islam, T.T., Newhouse, D., and Yanez-Pagans, M. (2021). International comparisons of poverty in South Asia. *Asian Development Review* 38: 142–175.

JOINT WHO/FAO Expert Committee on Zoonoses (1959). *World Health Organization Technical Report Series.* Switzerland, 58 (169), pp. 1–84.

Jones, K., Patel, N., Levy, M. et al. (2008). Global trends in emerging infectious diseases. *Nature* 451 (7181): 990–993.

Joshi, P., Truc, P., Salkar, H. et al. (2005). Human trypanosomiasis caused by *Trypanosoma evansi* in India: the first case report. *The American Journal of Tropical Medicine and Hygiene* 73 (3): 491–495.

Kamineni, V.V., Wilson, N., Das, A. et al. (2012). Addressing poverty through disease control programmes: examples from tuberculosis control in India. *International Journal for Equity in Health* 26 (11): 17.

Karim, M.M. (2013). Socio-economic and political development of South Asian countries: in Bangladesh perspective. *International Journal of Humanities and Social Science Invention* 2 (2): 29–43.

Karunaweera, N., Senanayake, S., Ginige, S. et al. (2021). Spatiotemporal distribution of cutaneous leishmaniasis in Sri Lanka and future case burden estimates. *PLoS Neglected Tropical Diseases* 15 (4): e0009346.

Keeley, B. (2015). *Income Inequality: The Gap between Rich and Poor.* OECD Insights, OECD Publishing https://doi.org/10.1787/9789264246010-en.

Lam, W.K., Zhong, N.S., and Tan, W.C. (2003). Overview on SARS in Asia and the world. *Respirology* 8 (s1): S2–S5.

Laxminarayan, R., Kakkar, M., Horby, P. et al. (2017). Emerging and re-emerging infectious disease threats in South Asia: status, vulnerability, preparedness, and outlook. *BMJ* 357: j1447.

Lee, J. and McKibbin, W. (2004). Globalization and disease: the case of SARS. *Asian Economic Papers* 3 (1): 113–131.

Leonardo, L., Bergquist, R., Utzinger, J. et al. (2019). Challenges and way forward. *Advances in Parasitology* 105: 125–132.

Lobo, D., Velayudhan, R., Chatterjee, P. et al. (2011). The neglected tropical diseases of India and South Asia: review of their prevalence, distribution, and control or elimination. *PLoS Neglected Tropical Diseases* 5 (10): e1222.

Luby, S. (2013). The pandemic potential of Nipah virus. *Antiviral Research* 100 (1): 38–43.

Luby, S.P., Gurley, E.S., and Hossain, M.J. (2009). Transmission of human infection with Nipah virus. *Clinical Infectious Diseases* 49 (11): 1743–1748.

Monath, T.P., Kahn, L.H., and Kaplan, B. (2010). Introduction: One Health perspective. *ILAR Journal* 51 (3): 193–198.

Munoz-Zanzi, C., Groene, E., Morawski, B. et al. (2020). A systematic literature review of leptospirosis outbreaks worldwide, 1970–2012. *Revista Panamericana de Salud Pública* 44: 1.

Ng, L. and Hapuarachchi, H. (2010). Tracing the path of chikungunya virus – evolution and adaptation. *Infection, Genetics and Evolution* 10 (7): 876–885.

Niu, Y., Rui, J., Wang, Q. et al. (2021). Containing the transmission of COVID-19: a modeling study in 160 countries. *Frontiers in Medicine* 8: 701836.

OIE (2019). Update on Avian Influenza in animals (types H5 and H7). http://www.oie.int/animal-health-in-the-world/update-on-avian-influenza (accessed on 15 September 2019).

One Health Initiative (2022). *Notable "one health" endorsements – One Health Initiative.* http://onehealthinitiative.com/notable-one-health-endorsements (accessed 23 February 2022).

Partridge, J., Bista, M., Ghimire, P. et al. (2007). Endemic Japanese encephalitis in the Kathmandu Valley, Nepal. *The American Journal of Tropical Medicine and Hygiene* 77 (6): 1146–1149.

Radhakrishnan, S., Vanak, A., Nouvellet, P., and Donnelly, C. (2020). Rabies as a public health concern in India – a historical perspective. *Tropical Medicine and Infectious Disease* 5 (4): 162.

Rahman, M., Yamagishi, J., Rahim, R. et al. (2019). East/Central/South African genotype in a chikungunya outbreak, Dhaka, Bangladesh, 2017. *Emerging Infectious Diseases* 25 (2): 370–372.

Regional Office for South-East Asia, World Health Organization (2016). Prevention and control of rabies in SAARC countries: report of the workshop Colombo, Sri Lanka (11–13 August 2015). New Delhi, India: WHO Regional Office for South-East Asia.

Rijal, S., Sundar, S., Mondal, D. et al. (2019). Eliminating visceral leishmaniasis in South Asia: the road ahead. *BMJ* 364: k5224.

Rozier, M. (2017). Religion and public health: moral tradition as both problem and solution. *Journal of Religion and Health* 56 (3): 1052–1063.

Rubin, C., Dunham, B., and Sleeman, J. (2014). Making One Health a reality–crossing bureaucratic boundaries. *Microbiology Spectrum* 2 (1): OH-0016-2012.

Sánchez, E., Perrone, T., Recchimuzzi, G. et al. (2015). Molecular characterization and classification of *Trypanosoma* spp. Venezuelan isolates based on microsatellite markers and kinetoplast maxicircle genes. *Parasites & Vectors* 8 (1): 566.

Sasidharan, Santanu, and Prakash Saudagar. "Leishmaniasis: where are we and where are we heading?" Parasitology Research, vol. 120, no. 5, May 2021, pp. 1541+. Gale Academic OneFile, link.gale.com/apps/doc/A660213797/AONE?u=anon~5032d589&sid=googleScholar&xid=799691de (accessed 2 January 2023).

Smith, T. and Kilborne, F.L. (1893). *Investigations Into the Nature, Causation, and Prevention of Texas or Southern Cattle Fever*. Washington: US Department of Agriculture, Bureau of Animal Industry.

Sobhy, H.M., Barghash, S.M., Behour, T.S., and Razin, E.A. (2017). Seasonal fluctuation of trypanosomiasis in camels in North-West Egypt and effect of age, sex, location, health status and vector abundance on the prevalence. *Beni-Suef University Journal of Basic and Applied Sciences* 6: 64–68.

Soman Pillai, V., Krishna, G., and Valiya Veettil, M. (2020). Nipah virus: past outbreaks and future containment. *Viruses* 12 (4): 465.

Song, H., Fan, G., Liu, Y. et al. (2021). The second wave of COVID-19 in South and Southeast Asia and the effects of vaccination. *Frontiers in Medicine* 8: 773110.

Sudarshan, M.K. and Ashwath Narayana, D.H. (2019). Providing evidence for effective prevention and control of rabies in India. *Indian Journal of Public Health* 63 (Suppl 1): S1.

Sundberg, J. and Schofield, P. (2009). One medicine, one pathology, and the One Health concept. *Journal of the American Veterinary Medical Association* 234 (12): 1530–1531.

Sushma, B., Shedole, S., Suresh, K. et al. (2021). An estimate of global anthrax prevalence in livestock: a meta-analysis. *Veterinary World* 1263–1271.

Thresia, C. (2018). Health inequalities in South Asia at the launch of sustainable development goals: exclusions in health in Kerala, India need political interventions. *International Journal of Health Services* 48 (1): 57–80.

Tin, D., Sabeti, P., and Ciottone, G.R. (2022). Bioterrorism: an analysis of biological agents used in terrorist events. *The American Journal of Emergency Medicine* 54: 117–121.

Turtle, L. and Solomon, T. (2018). Japanese encephalitis – the prospects for new treatments. *Nature Reviews. Neurology* 14: 298–313. https://doi.org/10.1038/nrneurol.2018.30.

Udayanga, L., Gunathilaka, N., Iqbal, M.C.M., and Abeyewickreme, W. (2020). Climate change induced vulnerability and adaption for dengue incidence in Colombo and Kandy districts: the detailed investigation in Sri Lanka. *Infectious Diseases of Poverty* 9 (1): 102.

Wabale, V., Nalage, P., Joshi, A. et al. (2015). Human Asian Trypanosomiasis due to *Trypanosoma evansi*: a rare case. *The Journal of Advances in Parasitology* 3 (3): 65–68.

Warnasekara, J. and Agampodi, S. (2017). Leptospirosis in Sri Lanka. *Sri Lankan Journal of Infectious Diseases* 7 (2): 67.

Watson, J.T., Gayer, M., and Connolly, M.A. (2007). Epidemics after natural disasters. *Emergeging Infectious Diseases* 13: 1–5.

Webster, R., Bean, W., Gorman, O. et al. (1992). Evolution and ecology of influenza A viruses. *Microbiological Reviews* 56 (1): 152–179.

WHO (2019). WHO cumulative number of confirmed human cases of Avian Influenza A (H5N1) reported to WHO. https: //http://www.who.int/influenza/human_animal_interface/2019_09_27_tableH5N1.pdf? ua=1.%202019 (accessed 10 October 2019).

World Bank (2021). Food and Agriculture Organization of the United Nations via World Bank (2021); Gapminder (v6); HYDE (v3.2); UN (2022).

World Health Organization, Food and Agriculture Organization of the United Nations & World Organisation for Animal Health (2008). *Anthrax in humans and animals*, 4e. World Health Organization https://apps.who.int/iris/handle/10665/97503.

Yesudhas, D., Srivastava, A., and Gromiha, M.M. (2021). COVID-19 outbreak: history, mechanism, transmission, structural studies and therapeutics. *Infection* 49 (2): 199–213.

Zhu, Z., Lian, X., Su, X. et al. (2020). From SARS and MERS to COVID-19: a brief summary and comparison of severe acute respiratory infections caused by three highly pathogenic human coronaviruses. *Respiratory Research* 21 (1): 224.

21

Impacts of Crop Protection Practices on Human Infectious Diseases

Agroecology as the Preferred Strategy to Integrate Crop Plant Health Within the Extended "One Health" Framework

Alain Ratnadass[1,2], Peninna Deberdt[3,4], Thibaud Martin[3,4], Mathilde Sester[2,5], and Jean-Philippe Deguine[6]

[1] *CIRAD, UPR Aïda, Réunion, France*
[2] *CIRAD, Aïda, Univ Montpellier, Montpellier, France*
[3] *CIRAD, UPR HortSys, Montpellier, France*
[4] *CIRAD, HortSys, Univ Montpellier, Montpellier, France*
[5] *CIRAD, UPR Aïda, Institut Technologique du Cambodge, Phnom Penh, Cambodia*
[6] *CIRAD, UMR PVBMT, Can Tho University, Can Tho City, Vietnam*

21.1 Introduction

Recent viral zoonotic epidemics have been ascribed to the negative impact of human activities, including agricultural practices (Morand et al. 2019). Authors have stressed the relevance of a "One Health" approach to tackle these problems (FAO, CIRAD, CIFOR, WCS 2020). However, plant health was never fully part of the concept, which mainly encompasses the health of humans and domestic animals, with a recent extension to environmental health, namely mainly the health of wild animals as potential or confirmed reservoirs of zoonotic diseases, in natural ecosystems (Destoumieux-Garzón et al. 2018).

Wild plants are considered as parts of these natural ecosystems, while cultivated plants (or crops) within agroecosystems are largely ignored (Van Bruggen et al. 2019). Some organizational efforts have, however, been made to bring plant and animal health together in the One Health framework, e.g. Plant Clinics promoted by the Centre for Agricultural Biosciences International (CABI) (Boa et al. 2015; Danielsen 2013; Rushton et al. 2018), or shared methodological approaches, e.g. the impact of biodiversity on human and animal health and plant health (Keesing et al. 2006; Ratnadass et al. 2012; Van Bruggen and Finckh 2016).

In view of the better integration of crop plant health to the One Health concept, we conducted a series of literature reviews on the interactions between crop protection (CP) practices and human infectious diseases, which had never been done before, although CP stands at the interface between crop plant and ecosystem health (specifically via biodiversity and soil health), and human health. Then, not all agricultural practices were considered in these reviews, but only those that explicitly aim at a better plant health via alleviation of crop pest and pathogen aggressions.

These reviews pertained, respectively, to viral zoonotic diseases (Ratnadass and Deguine 2021), bacterial infectious diseases (Ratnadass and Deberdt 2021), human parasitic diseases (Ratnadass and Martin 2022), and human fungal diseases (Ratnadass and Sester 2023) (Table 21.1). In this book chapter, we will highlight the main conclusions of these reviews, whether generic or specific.

21.2 Limits of the Study

Many agricultural practices not aiming at crop pest or disease control per se may affect plant health by indirectly affecting pests or pathogens or their natural enemies. For instance, in Argentina, deforestation for agricultural purposes resulted in the occupation of corn plots by *Calomys musculinus* and *Calomys laucha*, and occupation of soybean and alfalfa plots by *Akodon azarae*, and *Necromys obscurus*, all pest rodent species originating from the natural environment, also reservoirs of the Junin virus (Mammarenavirus, Arenaviridae), and involved in its transmission to rural workers, causing Argentine viral hemorrhagic fever outbreaks (Tapia-Ramírez et al. 2022).

In addition, many studies highlighted the impacts of non-CP agricultural practices on parasitic diseases, particularly crop irrigation systems and regimes regarding malaria and bilharzia [e.g. (De Clercq et al. 2000; Haileselassie et al. 2021)] or use of wastewater regarding protozoan or helminthic intestinal diseases (Kouamé et al. 2017). On another note, some crop health problems

One Health: Human, Animal, and Environment Triad, First Edition. Edited by Meththika Vithanage and Majeti Narasimha Vara Prasad.

Table 21.1 Examples of human infectious diseases addressed in the series of literature reviews supporting this book chapter.

Main disease groups and corresponding review articles		Examples	Causative agents
Viral diseases (Ratnadass and Deguine 2021)		West Nile fever (WNF)	WN virus (Flaviviridae)
		Japanese encephalitis (JE)	JE virus (Flaviviridae)
		Hemorrhagic fever with renal syndrome	Hantaviruses (Bunyaviridae)
		Lassa fever	Lassa virus (Arenaviridae)
		Nipah virus infection	Nipah virus (Paramyxoviridae)
		Crimean–Congo hemorrhagic fever	CCHF Orthonairovirus (Bunyaviridae)
		Avian flu	H5N1 Alphainfluenzavirus (Orthomyxoviridae)
		Ebola hemorrhagic fever	Ebola virus (Filoviridae)
Bacterial diseases (Ratnadass and Deberdt 2021)		Plague	*Yersinia pestis* (Enterobacteriaceae)
		Murine typhus	*Rickettsia typhi* (Rickettsiaceae)
		Leptospirosis	*Leptospira* (Leptospiraceae)
		Colibacillosis	*Escherichia coli* (Enterobacteriaceae)
		Salmonellosis	*Salmonella* spp. (Enterobacteriaceae)
		Burkholderia infection	*Burkholderia* spp. (Burkholderiaceae)
		Pseudomonas infection	*Pseudomonas* spp. (Pseudomonadaceae)
Parasitic diseases (Ratnadass and Martin 2022)	Protozoan	Malaria	*Plasmodium* spp. (Plasmodiidae)
		Chagas disease	*Trypanosoma cruzi* (Trypanosomatidae)
		African sleeping sickness	*Trypanosoma brucei* (Trypanosomatidae)
		Giardiasis	*Giardia duodenalis* (Hexamitidae)
		Cryptosporidiosis	*Cryptosporidium* spp. (Cryptosporidiidae)
	Helminthic	Lymphatic filariasis	*Wuchereria bancrofti* (Onchocercidae)
		Bilharzia (Schistosomiasis)	*Schistosoma* spp. (Schistosomatidae)
Fungal diseases (Ratnadass and Sester 2023)		Pulmonary aspergillosis	*Aspergillus fumigatus* (Trichocomaceae)
		Candidiasis	*Candida* spp. (Saccharomycetaceae)
		Cryptococcosis	*Cryptococcus* spp. (Tremeliaceae)
		Histoplasmosis	*Histoplasma capsulatum* (Ajellomycetaceae)
		Chronic rhino facial zygomycosis	*Conidiobolus coronatus* (Ancylistaceae)

involving pests or plant pathogens have also been associated with increased human infectious disease risk, without reference to CP practices though. This is the case of the Lethal Yellowing Disease, caused by a phytoplasma, which from the 1990s onward swept the coconut plantations of the Garifuna community along the coast of Honduras, forcing a significant part of male population to migrate abroad. This forced migration is thought to be a major driver of HIV/AIDS epidemic among the community (Stansbury and Sierra 2004).

Other agricultural practices affect plant health although they do not target pests or diseases, but because they have an effect on plant physiology, directly or via what is referred to as "soil health" (Husson 2013; Husson et al. 2021). None of these practices were covered in our literature reviews.

Our reviews did not encompass the effect of CP practices on non-infectious diseases, e.g. intoxications/poisoning by mycotoxins produced by plant pathogenic or entomopathogenic fungi, or by pesticides, with acute or chronic effects in terms of food and fodder safety and on ecosystem health. Our reviews did not address either the effects of CP measures on the immune responses of humans and animals to infectious diseases, as they were geared toward population-level interactions, not individual interactions between pathogens and hosts as affected by pesticides for instance. Our reviews did not encompass either the damage caused by pests and pathogens to food crops that has a major negative impact on human and animal health via reduced food and fodder security (and indeed food and fodder safety in the case of mycotoxins: see above).

21.3 A Conceptual Framework to Position Crop Protection Practices

CP practices are "classically" classified according to the type of "pest" (*sensu lato*) targeted (invertebrate or vertebrate pest; fungal/oomycete, bacterial, or viral pathogen; or weed or parasitic plant) or to the type of management practice (chemical, genetic, biological, cultural, etc.). However, in order to justify the necessary transition of agricultural practices toward sustainability, we chose to review interactions between CP practices and human infectious diseases, using the E-S-R conceptual framework, proposed by Hill and MacRae in 1996 (Hill and Mac Rae 1996), and broadly used since [e.g. (Wezel et al. 2014)].

Applied to CP, this framework covers, respectively: (i) improving the Efficiency (E) of conventional CP practices (which are mostly agrochemical); (ii) Substitution (S) of these practices (mainly by genetic, physical/mechanical, or bioprotection methods); and (iii) agroecosystem Redesign (R) to improve resilience to pests, notably with recourse to conservation biological control (CBC) through habitat conservation and management or agroecological systems (Figure 21.1).

21.3.1 Examples of Conventional Crop Protection Practices or Those Aiming at Improving the Efficiency of the Same (=E-Based)

Instances of evidence of impacts of conventional and Efficiency-based CP practices on infectious disease risks are provided in Table 21.2.

21.3.1.1 Synthetic Insecticides

Initially, insecticide treatments applied in irrigated rice fields could reduce populations of mosquito vectors of infectious diseases. For instance, the application of the pyrethroid lambda cyhalothrin against the aquatic rice weevil *Lissorhoptrus oryzophilus* in the United States had a beneficial impact in terms of mosquito population reduction, particularly *Culex* spp. (notably *Culex pipiens*) (Lenzi et al. 2021), which are potentially vectors of viral zoonoses [VZs, particularly the one caused by the West Nile virus: WNV (flavivirus)]. Similarly, relatively low survivorship of immature stages of *Anopheles arabiensis* (a malaria vector) in irrigated rice fields in Kenya was ascribed to exposure to insecticides, particularly Sumithion (Muturi et al. 2013). However, insecticides have also a negative impact on predators of mosquito vectors, ultimately favoring mosquitoes (Roger et al. 1994; Service 1977).

Many studies highlight the role of insecticide applications in agriculture, on the emergence of mosquito vectors of VZs [e.g. Japanese encephalitis (flavivirus) and WNV fever] that are resistant to insecticides of the same families as those used in public health. This is the case for pyrethroids used in rice cultivation in China [e.g. (Wang et al. 2020)] and in the United States (Lawler et al. 2007). This is also the case for malaria vector *Anopheles* mosquitoes in Africa, particularly vis-à-vis pyrethroids [e.g. (Gnankiné et al. 2013)] applied on cotton and vegetable crops (Yadouleton et al. 2009, 2011). This also applies to *Culex quinquefasciatus*, mosquito vector of *Wuchereria bancrofti*, the nematode causing lymphatic filariasis (Kibuthu et al. 2016). A similar relationship is suspected in assassin bugs (*Rhodnius* spp.), vectors of the trypanosome *Trypanosoma cruzi* causing Chagas disease in Latin America, following insecticide treatments on oil palm plantations against the palm weevil *Rhynchophorus palmarum*, with the same pyrethroids used for indoor bedbug treatments (Calderón et al. 2020).

The effect of synthetic agricultural insecticides is thus negative overall, in terms of human vectored disease risk. True there are some instances when their application reduces disease incidence via vector suppression, but it generally results in increased disease risk either by suppression of natural enemies of vectors, or, more importantly, by the emergence of vector populations that are resistant to synthetic agricultural insecticides, particularly pyrethroids that are also used in public health. This, of course, has a tremendous negative impact on human health.

21.3.1.2 Synthetic Rodenticides

Apodemus agrarius is a major rodent crop pest and a reservoir of hantaviruses transmissible to humans via inhalation of aerosols from excreta of infected rodents, provoking hemorrhagic fevers with renal syndrome, in both continental China and Taiwan. A study highlighted the susceptibility of this rodent to the anticoagulant rodenticide diphacinone in continental China (Zhi and Cheng-Xin 1984), translating to a drastic reduction in the incidence of hemorrhagic fever. The effectiveness of another anticoagulant rodenticide (flocoumafen) was also demonstrated in Taiwan (Lu 1990). In contrast, a study showed that in Indonesian oil palm plantations, the application of anticoagulant rodenticides (coumatetralyl) against *Rattus tanezumi*, rodent pest and reservoir of hantaviruses, rather resulted in the emergence of rodenticide-resistant rodent populations (Andru et al. 2013).

Similarly, regarding bacterial infections, rodenticides (particularly anticoagulants) used to control rodent pests of crops grown in the fields or stored after harvest, first proved efficient in reducing populations of these bacterial disease reservoirs, e.g. *Rattus* spp. for the plague bacterium (Rahelinirina et al. 2021), the murine typhus rickettsia (Rakotonanahary et al. 2017) in Madagascar, or the

ESR positioning	Process	Examples
Efficiency (E)	Intensive use of synthetic inputs (particularly pesticides) and move for a more rational use of the same to improve "efficiency"	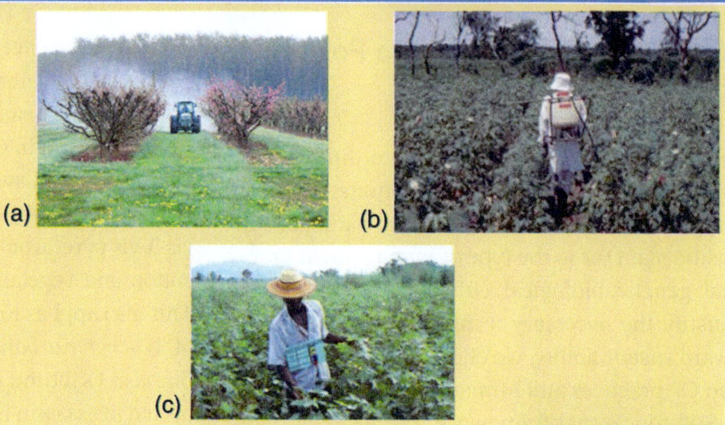
Substitution (S)	Substitution of synthetic pesticides by non-synthetic ones, or other levers (e.g. mechanical) used exactly in the same way and for the same purpose	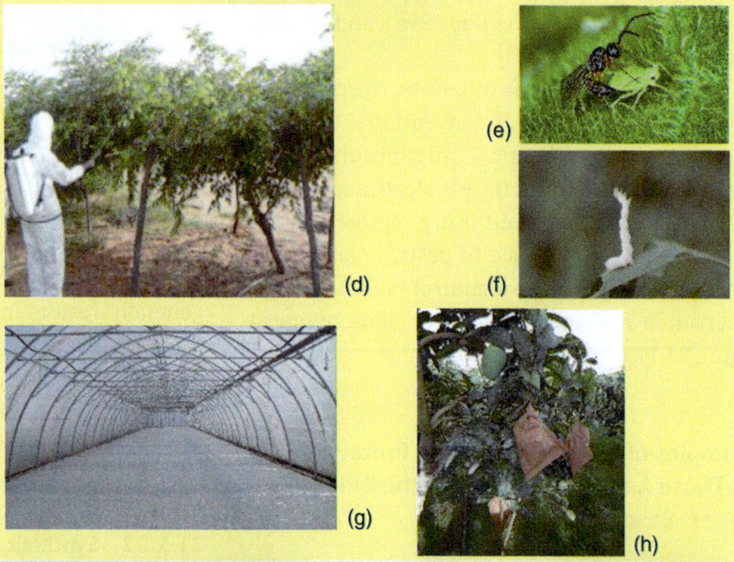
Redesign (R)	Redesign of the entire system as an agro ecosystem based on ecological processes rather than external inputs	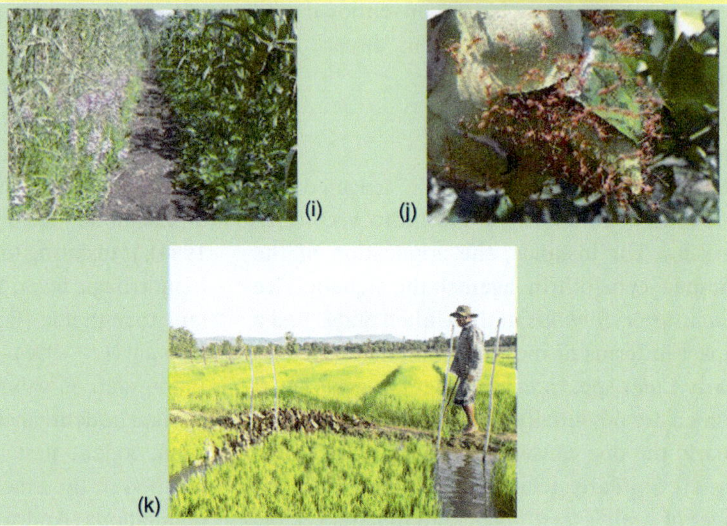

Figure 21.1 Examples of Efficiency-based, Substitution-based and Redesign-based crop protection practices (Hill and MacRae 1996): (a) Mechanized spraying of a pesticide in an orchard (*Source:* © MAITRE Christophe/ INRAE). (b) Manual spraying of insecticide in a cotton field (*Source:* © P. Silvie – IRD-CIRAD). (c) Using pegboard to scout cotton pests prior to threshold-based control (*Source:* © P. Silvie – IRD-CIRAD). (d) Spot spraying with food attractant mixed with biological insecticide for fruit fly control (*Source:* © A. Ratnadass – CIRAD). (e) Augmentative biological control with parasitoid (*Source:* © A. Franck – CIRAD). (f) Augmentative biological control with entomopathogenic fungus (*Source:* © P. Silvie – IRD-CIRAD). (g) Solarization as a substitute to fumigation for nematode control (*Source:* © JEANNEQUIN Benoît – INRAE). (h) Mango bagging as a physical barrier against fruit flies (*Source:* © A. Ratnadass – CIRAD). (i) Push-pull system for stemborer and Striga control on maize (*Source:* © J. van den Berg – NWU). (j) Conservation biological control with weaver ants in an orchard (*Source:* © J.-P. Deguine – CIRAD). (k) Integrated rice-duck farming for weed, pest and disease control (*Source:* © R. Sry – GDA Cambodia).

Table 21.2 Instances of evidence of impacts of conventional and Efficiency-based crop protection practices on infectious disease risks.

Type of causative pathogen	Virus		Bacterium		Parasite		Fungus
Impact[a]	+	–	+	–	+	–	–
Synthetic insecticides	West Nile Fever (Lawler et al. 2007)	WNF (Lawler et al. 2007) Japanese encephalitis (Liu et al. 2019; Shi et al. 2019; Wang et al. 2020)			Sleeping sickness (Rutto et al. 2013)	Malaria (Akogbeto et al. 2006; Chouaibou et al. 2008; Corbel et al. 2007; Darriet et al. 2012; Diabate et al. 2002; Haileselassie et al. 2021; Mouhamadou et al. 2019; Orondo et al. 2021; Reid and McKenzie 2016; Yadouleton et al. 2009, 2011) Lymphatic filariasis (Kibuthu et al. 2016) Chagas disease (Calderón et al. 2020) Bilharzia (Becker et al. 2020; Hoover et al. 2020)	
Synthetic rodenticides	Hemorrhagic fever with renal syndrome (Lu 1990; Zhi and Cheng-Xin 1984)	HFRS (Andru et al. 2013)	Plague (Ratovonjato et al. 2003)	Leptospirosis (Marquez et al. 2019)			
Synthetic herbicides				Colibacillosis and Salmonellosis (Kurenbach et al. 2018)	Bilharzia (Ibrahim et al. 2019)	Bilharzia (Hoover et al. 2020)	
Synthetic fungicides							Aspergillosis (Alvarez-Moreno et al. 2019; Barber et al. 2020; Bromley et al. 2014; Cao et al. 2021; Gómez Londoño et al. 2019; Kano et al. 2015; Prigitano et al. 2014; Ren et al. 2017; Rocchi et al. 2014, 2018; Schoustra et al. 2019; Shi et al. 2019) Candidiosis (Brilhante et al. 2019; Chen et al. 2019; Faria-Ramos et al. 2014; Lo et al. 2017; Muller et al. 2007; Potocki et al. 2020; Rocha et al. 2016; Yang et al. 2012) Cryptococcosis (Bastos et al. 2018, 2019; Carneiro et al. 2020)

For supporting references, see reference list.
[a] +, positive impact (reduced disease risk); –, negative impact (increased disease risk).

leptospirosis spirochetes in the French West Indies island of Martinique (Marquez et al. 2019). But resistances to these rodenticides then appear. For leptospirosis, European and French law therefore restricts the use of anticoagulant rodenticides to the fields alone and to only two sugarcane growing periods in a year in the French Indian Ocean island of Réunion (Mansuy and Fontaine 2014).

In the case of synthetic rodenticides, there are thus more instances than in the case of synthetic insecticides, of a positive effect in terms of human infectious disease risk alleviation. However, there are also many instances when their excessive use results in the emergence of rodent reservoir populations that are resistant to these (particularly anticoagulant) rodenticides. However, efforts are being made to regulate their use and therefore reduce the emergence of resistances and consequently alleviate adverse impact on human health.

21.3.1.3 Synthetic Herbicides

Regarding bacterial infections, convincing evidence was provided of the contribution of herbicides, particularly glyphosate (whose use pertains to conventional, agrochemical-based practices), to resistance to antibiotics (Kurenbach et al. 2018). This is notably due to shifts in microbial community compositions in soil, rhizosphere, and animal guts (Van Bruggen et al. 2021).

On another note, water pollution from agricultural herbicides has rather mixed effects as far as bilharzia is concerned. Atrazine promotes the growth of the freshwater planorbid snail *Biomphalaria alexandrina* and its infection by *Schistosoma* spp. by stimulating some algae and thus the quantity of algae ingested (bottom-up effect) [e.g. (Halstead et al. 2018)], whereas a certain dose of atrazine has a direct toxic effect on the survival and reproduction of gastropods, as does glyphosate (Barky et al. 2012). Of note, glyphosate may equally stimulate the development of some algae.

Although direct effects of herbicides on animals and humans are considered as limited, major concerns have thus arisen about their indirect harmful side effects. In particular, glyphosate appears to contribute to antimicrobial resistance (AMR) by interacting with the microbiome of soil, plants, and animals and thus also humans, as harmful microorganisms are often more tolerant to it than beneficial organisms.

21.3.1.4 Synthetic Bactericides and Fungicides

There is no documented case when the application of antibiotics for CP purposes against phytopathogenic bacteria would be conducive to AMR in public health and/or veterinary health. However, it is precisely the extent of the crisis due to generalized AMR in humans that restricts the use of antibiotics in CP to high-value horticultural crops (McManus et al. 2002). Antibiotic injections in fruit tree trunks, are thus not likely to significantly contribute to AMR of bacteria of medical or veterinary importance to these antibiotics (notably streptomycin). In contrast, large-scale foliar spraying of antibiotics to combat citrus Greening (Huanglongbing), caused par *Candidatus Liberibacter* sp., as recently used in Florida (McKenna 2019), or the inconsiderate application of medical antibiotics with the same objective, like in Thailand (Chanvatik et al. 2019), are a cause of concern.

Concerning pulmonary aspergillosis, the agricultural azole fungicides have been demonstrated in the laboratory as inducers of cross-resistance to medical triazoles (Snelders et al. 2012). The higher incidence of azole resistance in agricultural environments was demonstrated particularly in Denmark (Mortensen et al. 2010), Germany (Barber et al. 2020), India (Chowdhary et al. 2012), the Netherlands (Schoustra et al. 2019), and the United Kingdom (Bromley et al. 2014) and was attributed to different horticultural and grain crops. The presence of resistant isolates in patients with no previous exposition to triazole is also considered as an evidence of the environmental origin of these resistant strains (Beer et al. 2018; Sharma et al. 2015). Some studies however found a very low number of azole-resistant isolates in cereal crops treated by fungicides, either in Europe (Fraaije et al. 2020) or in Japan (Toyotome et al. 2016) and ornamental crops were pointed rather (Godeau et al. 2020; Hagiwara 2020).

The same phenomenon was reported with other pathogenic fungi and other types of fungicides, because of the proximity of the molecules used in agriculture and in medical treatments inducing the same resistance mechanisms. Cross-resistance reported in pathogenic yeasts *Candida* spp. and with *Cryptococcus* spp. was ascribed to fungicide treatments on various crops (Brilhante et al. 2019; Carneiro et al. 2020).

AMR, which is a major public health concern, and particularly relevant to the One Health concept, thus pertains much more to the use of agricultural fungicides than to the use of agricultural antibiotics. This however does not preclude the contribution of the use of antibiotics in agriculture, but it is mainly for veterinary not CP purposes.

21.3.2 Examples of Substitution (S)-Based Crop Protection Practices

Instances of evidence of impacts of Substitution-based CP practices on infectious disease risks are provided in Table 21.3.

21.3.2.1 Crop Plant Resistance

Since crop plant varieties resistant to specific pests or pathogens are alternatives to replace some inefficient

Table 21.3 Instances of evidence of impacts of Substitution-based crop protection practices on infectious disease risks.

Type of causative pathogen	Virus		Bacterium		Parasite	Fungus
Impact[a]	+	–	+	–	–	–
Crop plant resistance			Leptospirosis (Quénéhervé et al. 2005) Enterobacteria infection (Lenzi et al. 2021)			
Trapping, hunting, and culling of vertebrate pests	Bolivian hemorrhagic fever (Mills 1999) Argentine hemorrhagic fever (Mills 1999) Lassa fever (Mari Saez et al. 2018)	Ebola, Nipah, Hendra virus infection (Andru et al. 2013; Leroy et al. 2009)				
Physical barriers	Lassa fever (Orondo et al. 2021) Nipah virus encephalitis (Calisher et al. 2006; Nahar et al. 2010, 2012, 2014; Smith and Wang 2013)					
Mineral, botanical, or organic pesticides			Enterobacteria infection (Lenzi et al. 2021) *P. aeruginosa* infection (Rasamiravaka et al. 2018)	Enterobacteria infection (Xie et al. 2018; Yoshizawa et al. 2020)	Malaria (Talom et al. 2020)	Histoplasmosis (Jayasvati and Jayasvati 2018) Cryptococcidiosis (Dongmo et al. 2016)
Biological control				Burkholderia infection (Eberl and Vandamme 2016) Enterobacteria infection (Damasceno et al. 2019) *P. aeruginosa* infection (Bodey et al. 1983)		*M. anisopliae* infection (Dorin et al. 2015) *B. bassiana* infection (Tucker et al. 2004) Entomophthoromycosis (El-Shabrawi et al. 2014)
Soil solarization			Enterobacteria infection (Lenzi et al. 2021)	Enterobacteria infection (Lenzi et al. 2021)		

[a] +, positive impact (reduced disease risk); –, negative impact (increased disease risk).

components of a cropping system, their deployment may be considered as being part of an "S" approach. For instance, for sugarcane, which is particularly subject to rodent attacks, it is the case of cultivars with hard bark and erected stalk like B 82.333 in Martinique (Quénéhervé et al. 2005) or R 570 (resistant to the stemborer *Chilo sacchariphagus*) in Réunion (Nibouche and Tibère 2010). These are less damaged by rodents than cultivar R 59.92. Reduced damage translates into reduced risk of on-field infection with leptospirosis.

There are also varietal differences in the capacity of vegetable crops to shelter human-pathogenic enterobacteria (Lenzi et al. 2021). Growing vegetable varieties resistant to phytopathogenic fungi and bacteria that facilitate vegetable colonization by enterobacteria reduces the risk of human bacterial infections. This is the case of cucumber cultivar Marketmore 97 or tomato cultivars "Sun Gold" and "Snow White" vis-à-vis *Salmonella enterica* (Lenzi et al. 2021).

Beyond the reduction of pesticide use allowed by the cultivation of such varieties, and the associated reduced risk of emergence of insecticide resistance in vectors, and of AMR in bacteria and fungi of medical importance (cf. above section), there are thus specific pathways through which crop plant resistance to pests or diseases may alleviate infectious disease risks.

21.3.2.2 Trapping, Hunting, and Culling of Vertebrate Pests

Trapping of rodent pests of crop and stored product is a means of reducing their populations and associated damages. Such trapping also contributes to the control of hemorrhagic fever transmitted by commensal rodents (Mari Saez et al. 2018). However, although they are generally not consumed, these trapped rodents may be handled manually, dead or alive, hence the need to follow strict procedures to avoid disease transmission (Soarimalala et al. 2019). Disease transmission risk is particularly high in the case of plague and murine typhus (as compared to VZs and leptospirosis), since it is related to fleas, which when leaving dead rodents are actively seeking new mammal hosts, e.g. humans (Miarinjara et al. 2019).

Although its effectiveness has not yet been established, government-backed trapping and culling of fruit bats such as *Pteropus* spp. is sometimes employed to reduce losses incurred in orchards. These practices may, however, increase VZ risk if live or dead captured bats are handled manually or eaten as bushmeat without prior knowledge of their reservoir status (Nahar et al. 2020).

Beyond the ethical aspects raised, trapping, hunting, and culling of vertebrate pests are thus a double-edged sword. On the one hand, like in the case of synthetic rodenticides, they have a positive effect in terms of human infectious disease alleviation via the reduction of the populations of disease reservoirs. On the other hand, even though they cannot result in the emergence of "resistant" pest/reservoir populations, they may more directly increase the risk of infectious disease transmission to humans, unless strict procedures to avoid the same are taken.

21.3.2.3 Physical Barriers

Some devices that reduce food loss by preventing pest rodents from accessing crops (notably perennial fruit crops) and stored products may also contribute to alleviate infectious disease risks. For instance, placing metal sleeves (or "rat guards") on the posts supporting the platform of elevated granaries (Ratnadass et al. 1991) excluded pest rodents from products stored therein but also resulted in reduced incidence of Lassa fever (Arenavirus), of which the multi-mammate rat *Mastomys natalensis* is the reservoir in Sierra Leone (Olugasa et al. 2014).

In orchards, physical barriers against vertebrate and arthropod fruit pests reduce damage, both direct (fruit consumption) and indirect (contamination of fruits and other perennial crop products). These barriers are, however, not always cost-effective, which affects uptake by farmers: e.g. fruit bat netting in Australia (Aziz et al. 2016). On the other hand, the use of "bamboo skirts," although seldom adopted traditionally to prevent date-palm sap losses in Malaysia, was successfully extended to specifically reduce transmission of the Nipah virus (Nahar et al. 2014).

On another note, nets may prevent beneficial bat species from reaching crops, e.g. pollinators of fruit crops such as durian (Chaiyarat et al. 2020) or as predators of insect pests. Also, insect nets that are widely used to protect high-value crops, notably fruit orchards against insect pests in Europe (Alaphilippe et al. 2016), may actually increase pest rodent numbers (and associated infectious disease risks) because they hamper predation of the latter by birds of prey (Baumgartner et al. 2019).

On the basis of documented cases, most physical barriers aiming at CP, particularly against vertebrate pests (either rodents or fruit bats) thus seem to generally alleviate disease transmission risks, rather than increase them. However, some may hamper some ecosystem services and increase some infectious disease risks.

21.3.2.4 Mineral, Botanical, or Organic Pesticides

On tomato, foliar sprays of copper against fungal diseases reduce populations of enterobacteria, e.g. *Salmonella* and *Paenibacillus* (Lenzi et al. 2021). It should however be noted that the use of copper-based fungicides/bactericides in market gardening is suspected to favor the cross-resistance to insecticides of malaria-vector *Anopheles* mosquitoes (Talom et al. 2020). Conversely, various plant extracts have a bacteriostatic effect both on *Ralstonia solanacearum*, which causes bacterial wilt in Solanaceae and on *Pseudomonas aeruginosa*, a potential human pathogen (see below) (Rasamiravaka et al. 2018).

On the other hand, feces of frugivorous and insectivorous bats (=bat guano) are commonly used, particularly in organic agriculture, mainly for their fertilizing effect, but also for their antimicrobial and anti-nematode effect against crop pathogens (Keleher 1996; Zuhair et al. 2022). Bat guano manipulation may, however, expose users to VZs, including one caused by a coronavirus (Wacharapluesadee et al. 2013). Guano has also been reported as a potential source of many human diseases including pathogenic fungi, e.g. *Cryptococcus* spp. (Dongmo et al. 2016) The risk is even worse concerning the health hazard due to inhalation of fungal spores from *Histoplasma capsulatum*, causing life-threatening histoplasmosis in humans (Jayasvati and Jayasvati 2018). However, the risk may be reduced with adequate composting process (Gómez Londoño et al. 2019).

Depending on their type or origin, the so-called bioproduction products, while reducing crop pest or disease damage, may thus either decrease or increase populations of human-pathogenic organisms or their vectors, via various pathways.

21.3.2.5 Augmentative Biological Control

Many strains of *Burkholderia*, registered as active on phytopathogenic soil fungi, have seen their agreement withdrawn because they caused human diseases (Eberl and Vandamme 2016). Similarly, many bacteria with proven effectiveness against banana anthracnose (e.g. *Enterobactercloacae*, *Serratia marcescens*, and *Stenotrophomonas maltophilia*) are pathogenic for humans, particularly immunodepressed persons (Damasceno et al. 2019).

Also, while *Pseudomonas fluorescens* is extensively mentioned in the literature as bioprotection agent, the close species *P. aeruginosa*, which also shows a CP effect, particularly against *Botrytis cinerea* on tomato, presents a real infectious risk for humans during processes of isolation, purification, and multiplication to elaborate bioprotection products. As a typical example of nosocomial opportunistic bacterium, *P. aeruginosa* is little or not virulent in a healthy person, but may prove dreadful for immunodepressed persons (Bodey et al. 1983).

Similarly, some fungi used in CP as entomopathogens for biological insect pest control have been reported as potentially causing health problems for humans. This is notably the case for the hyphomycetes *Metarhizium* spp. (Nourrisson et al. 2017) and the entomophthorale *Conidiobolus coronatus* (Vilela and Mendoza 2018).

Augmentative biological control using either bacteria or fungi to control phytopathogenic fungi or insect pests of crops may thus also result in human infection by the same, particularly in the case of immunodepressed persons.

21.3.2.6 Soil Solarization

As a substitute to fumigation, soil solarization using plastic mulches controls nematodes and other soilborne plant pathogenic organisms. It also decontaminates the soil from enterobacteria (*Escherichia coli* and *Salmonella*) (Lenzi et al. 2021), and is also used to control weeds in market gardening. In addition, by preventing direct contact between plant aerial parts and the soil, it reduces the incidence of some plant diseases and contamination with enterobacteria.

Conversely, as opposed to bare soil, it favors the persistence of enterobacteria within the soil and their dispersal by splash due to rain or irrigation. On the other hand, pathogenic *E. coli* populations were shown to be better sustained in mulch-grown (either with plastic, biodegradable, or vegetal mulch) lettuce than in bare ground-grown lettuce (Lenzi et al. 2021).

Soil solarization using plastic mulches, which is an effective substitute to fumigation for the control of soilborne pathogenic organisms, has thus a mixed effect in terms of human enterobacterial contamination risk.

21.3.3 Examples of Redesign (R)-Based Crop Protection Practices

Instances of evidence of impacts of Redesign-based CP practices on infectious disease risks are provided in Table 21.4.

21.3.3.1 Sanitizing Rotations

Beyond microbes beneficial to plant growth and plant pathogenic organisms, opportunistic bacteria pathogenic to humans can be found in the microbiome of the plant rhizosphere (belonging to genera *Burkholderia, Enterobacter, Herbaspirillum, Ochrobactrum, Pseudomonas, Ralstonia, Staphylococcus,* and *Stenotrophomonas*) (Mendes et al. 2013). These are facilitated if "service" plants that shelter them in their rhizosphere are grown in rotation with the main crop. For instance, growing some wheat cultivars as previous crops make soils suppressive toward *Rhizoctonia solani*, a fungus that negatively affects the growth of young apple seedlings (Gu and Mazzola 2003). This suppressive effect is, however, due to competition with *Pseudomonas putida*, which is potentially a human pathogen (Fernández et al. 2015).

Table 21.4 Instances of evidence of impacts of Redesign-based crop protection practices on infectious disease risks.

Type of causative pathogen	Virus			Bacterium		Parasite		Fungus
Impact[a]	+	+/−	−	+/−	−	+	−	+
Sanitizing rotations					*Pseudomonas* infection (Fernández et al. 2015)			
Crop-livestock integration	Avian flu H5N1 (Suh 2014) Japanese encephalitis (Zhao and Xue 2021)	Crimean–Congo hemorrhagic fever (Sekercioglu 2013)	Nipah virus infection (Singh et al. 2019)		Bacterial gastroenteritis (Pires et al. 2019; Theofel et al. 2020)	Malaria (Zhao and Xue 2021) Bilharzia (Kloos et al. 2001)	Cryptosporidiosis (Robertson et al. 2020)	
CBC with arthropod natural enemies	Ebola hemorrhagic fever, Nipah virus infection, and other VZs (Lokkers 1990; Peach et al. 2019; Van Mele et al. 2009)			Bacterial gastroenteritis (Sellers et al. 2018)	Plague (Rahelinirina et al. 2010) Tularemia (Rodríguez-Pastor et al. 2017)			
CBC with vertebrate natural enemies	Hantavirus pulmonary syndrome (Muñoz-Pedreros et al. 2016)					Malaria (Howard 1920)		
Conversion to organic agriculture								Aspergillosis (Rocchi et al. 2021; Schoustra et al. 2019)

[a] +, positive impact (reduced disease risk); +/−, mixed impact or no impact; −, negative impact (increased disease risk).

21.3.3.2 Push-Pull

This technique involves trap plant borders, of which some are bushy, and repellent plants, of which many have a high covering capacity, intercropped with cereals (Khan et al. 2011). These border crops and intercrops may serve as habitats to rodent pests that are also potential reservoirs of infectious bacteria. For instance, hedges of vetiver grass (*Vetiveria zizanoides*), which serve as a trap crop for cereal stem borers (van den Berg 2006), are considered by some as shelters for rodents, while others consider they are repellent for both rodents and snakes (Grimshaw and Faiz 1995).

21.3.3.3 Crop-Livestock Integration

This integration may take two main forms: either domestic animals are introduced into the cropping system for a CP purpose, or manure from animals raised as part of the farming system is applied onto crop fields with (at least partly) a CP objective.

21.3.3.3.1 Introduction of Domestic Animals into Cultivated Plots Examples of introduction of livestock into fields or orchards to control weeds, pathogens, or pests are many (Ratnadass and Deguine 2021). For instance, the introduction of ducks into rice fields has been extensively studied (Furuno 2001). In integrated rice-duck farming (IRDF), ducklings are released into paddy fields during the rice growing period, primarily with a weed and pest control objective, targeting particularly weeds such as the cockspur grass, the Brown Plant Hopper, *Nilaparvata lugens (*Men et al. 2002*)*, and Golden Apple Snails (*Pomacea canaliculata*) (Liang et al. 2014) and second, to control plant pathogenic fungus *R. solani*, which causes rice sheath blight disease (Su et al. 2012). This ancient Chinese practice has recently been extended to other Asian countries (Suh 2014) and to Camargue in southern France (Mouret and Falconnier 2018).

A distinction should be made between traditional rice-duck farming focusing on fattening ducks and IRDF, where ducks are released for the purpose of increasing rice yield, particularly via weeding and pest and disease control. In the IRDF system, ducks are introduced to paddy fields during the rice growing period, when there are few migratory birds, whereas in traditional rice-duck farming, they are released to graze post-harvest. In these latter situations, they may come into proximity to wild birds (particularly Anatidae). This might result in transmission and epidemics of avian flu including H5N1, Alphainfluenzavirus, and Orthomyxoviridae (Gilbert et al. 2007; Henning et al. 2016). In addition, ducks being fond of golden apple snails, they also contribute to the control of planorbid freshwater snails, intermediate hosts of *Schistosoma* trematode worms (Kloos et al. 2001).

Fish (namely, common carp, African catfish, and Nile tilapia) were also found to play a vital role in the integrated management of pests, including golden apple snails, and weeds in rice-fish cropping systems (Frei et al. 2007; Sin 2006). Fish predation on mosquito larvae could also dramatically reduce the incidence of malaria and Japanese encephalitis (Zhao and Xue 2021).

On another note, feeding pigs with insect-infested fruits (e.g. fruit flies: Diptera, Tephritidae) may facilitate the transmission of Nipah virus if these fruits are also contaminated with fruit bat excreta. Such cross-contamination was observed in Asia with *Pteropus* spp. bats and pigsties in the vicinity of orchards (Singh et al. 2019). The introduction of poultry in orchards may also aggravate the risk of enterobacteria transmission (Theofel et al. 2020).

The introduction of domestic animals into cultivated plots for CP purposes may therefore alleviate some infectious disease risks, while aggravating some others. Regarding the latter case, the example of duck-rice integration shows that if adequately managed, the sanitary risk may be minimized. For instance, although contacts with migratory birds may be responsible for the transmission of zoonotic diseases to domestic ducks, the risk of disease outbreak is lower when ducks are outside in paddy fields, than when confined in sheds.

21.3.3.3.2 Application of Farm-Produced Animal Manure to Crop Fields Agricultural manure can be used on cultivated crops, partly due to its role in reducing plant parasitic nematode populations, although its effect in this respect is less pronounced than that of plant compost. Conversely, agricultural manure can transmit human pathogens, in particular AMR bacteria (Yoshizawa et al. 2020) and parasites (Squire et al. 2017). The risk of zoonotic contamination by the latter (namely, *Giardia* and *Cryptosporidium*) is, however, reduced if manures are composted at sufficiently high temperatures (e.g. >55 °C for a period of 15 days) before application (Van Herk et al. 2004).

21.3.3.4 Conservation Biological Control with Arthropod Natural Enemies

The enhancement of weaver ant (*Oecophylla* spp.) populations in tropical orchards is a CBC practice that helps control fruit flies and other insect pests (Thurman et al. 2019). Weaver ant establishment may be facilitated by manipulating plant species in orchards, particularly with respect to hemipteran trophobionts and antagonistic ants (Vayssières et al. 2016). CBC generally has also a positive impact on VZ regulation, since weaver ants repel fruit bats (Van Mele et al. 2009), which may be reservoirs of Ebola (Ebolavirus, Filoviridae), Nipah virus, or other VZs (Aziz et al. 2016). In addition, they do not hamper insectivorous vertebrates that hunt flying prey.

Conversely, several studies suggest that flowering plants, part of the spontaneous vegetation cover of cultivated areas or of flower strips, which are used in CBC with arthropodan predators and parasitoids, can promote mosquito vectors of infectious diseases, e.g. *Anopheles* spp., malaria vectors; yellow fever mosquito *Aedes aegypti*; and *Culex* spp., potential vectors of VZs and of lymphatic filariasis (Peach et al. 2019; Peach and Gries 2019; Stone et al. 2018).

In addition, just like trap plant borders, flowering plants in the spontaneous weed cover of cropped fields or in hedges, used in CBC, may serve as habitats for many rodent species, some of which are reservoirs of infectious diseases, e.g. plague (Rahelinirina et al. 2010), or tularemia caused by the bacterium *Francisella tularensis (*Rodríguez-Pastor et al. 2017*)*, or leptospirosis.

Plant species diversity enhancement, notably as part of ecological infrastructures for habitat management in view of CBC with arthropod natural enemies, may thus alleviate some infectious disease risks, while aggravating some others. This particularly pertains to diseases with arthropod vectors and/or vertebrate reservoirs.

21.3.3.5 Conservation Biological Control with Vertebrate Natural Enemies

21.3.3.5.1 Enhancement of Insectivorous Bats

Provision of nest boxes or artificial shelters for insectivorous bats results in a reduction of insect pest populations and their damage to crops (Russo et al. 2018). This type of control may result in either positive or negative effects on infectious disease transmission. Insectivorous bats may thus reduce populations of VZ- and malaria-vector mosquitoes (Gonsalves et al. 2013; Howard 1920).

On the other hand, in oases, where Acacia trees are critical as habitats for insectivorous bats, flowering *Acacia raddiana* provides to adult *Anopheles sergentii*, the desert malaria vector (Gu et al. 2011), primary sugar sources whose availability in the local environment is considered a major determinant regulating the dynamics of mosquito populations and their vector potential.

The enhancement of insectivorous bats has thus an overall positive impact in terms of insect pest control, but its impact may be negative in terms of infectious disease risk alleviation, due to the mixed impact of some enhancement measures on vector mosquitoes.

21.3.3.5.2 Enhancement of Insectivorous Birds Insectivorous birds, as recognized predators of arthropod pests of crops [e.g. (Sow et al. 2020)], are considered less of a problem for VZ transmission than insectivorous bats. However, they may themselves serve as reservoirs as well (Nabi et al. 2021) and are often blamed for the predation of natural enemies of crop pests (Grass et al. 2017) or as pests themselves (Elser et al. 2019). Insectivorous birds are also recognized as predators of arthropods such as mosquitoes, and ticks, which may potentially be vectors of infectious diseases (Medlock and Snow 2008; Samish and Rehacek 1999). On another note, American crows acted as sentinels for human health, in 1999–2000 in the United States with WNV (Brugère-Picoux and Le Floc'h Soye 2014), which they do not transmit to man. In addition, the light collateral damage to crops these crows cause (Elser et al. 2019) is largely compensated for by the insect pest regulatory service they provide.

21.3.3.5.3 Enhancement of Predators of Rodent Pests Poles or nest boxes that are provided to increase raptor numbers (particularly barn owls) in cultivated plots contribute to the reduction of rodent pest populations (*Rattus* spp.) and the damage they cause to crops, as highlighted in Indonesia and in Malaysia (Bessou et al. 2017; Verwilghen 2015). The same is true for arrangements in agroforestry landscapes that may increase populations of small mammal carnivore species predating on rodent pests (Jennings et al. 2015; Verwilghen 2015).

These devices or spatial arrangements may thus have either positive or negative effects in terms of pest rodent control and associated infectious disease (notably VZ) regulation. On the one hand, enhanced rodent control by barn owls reduces potential reservoirs of such diseases. On the other hand, while populations of small carnivore species enhanced by new landscape arrangements also facilitate control of rodents (as crop pests and disease reservoirs), notably of these species (e.g. civets), they may themselves act as reservoirs of VZs (Guan et al. 2003).

One should note that unlike the IRDF system, which is truly R-based since it is exclusive of pesticide use (as ducks replace pesticides, which in turn would result in high duck mortality), the facilitation of barn owl predation is not necessarily exclusive of rodenticide use. Actually, some on the contrary think that implementation of both is necessary to warrant satisfactory control. This stand is supported by the fact that results on the extent of the adverse effect of rodenticides (mainly via food chains) on raptors, particularly barn owls, are contradictory. In any case, research is still needed to establish whether combined effect of barn owls and small mammal carnivores, via truly agroecological spatial arrangements, may allow a full waiver of rodenticide use.

21.3.3.6 Organic Agriculture

Organic agriculture is often given as an example of redesign, especially when it relies on "Alternative on-farm inputs" as proposed by Dupré et al. (Dupré et al. 2017) in their framework adapted from Hill and MacRae (1996). To us, this category is rather encompassed by the "Redesign" category of Hill and MacRae, rather than the "Alternative off-farm inputs," which falls indeed within the "Substitution" category of Hill and MacRae.

Besides studies on specific agroecological sets of practices (see above), comparisons have also been done between organic and non-organic agriculture, specifically to confirm the increase of resistant pathogenic populations of fungi in environments with repeated use of agricultural fungicides. Actually, breaking with the use of azole as practiced in organic farms appears to be the best way to decrease the pressure of selection and hence the level of azole-resistant strains in the environment (Rocchi et al. 2021).

21.4 Discussion and Conclusion

21.4.1 Irrelevance of Conventional Crop Protection Practices or Those Aiming at Improving the Efficiency of the Same (="E"-Based)

Regarding conventional and E-based CP practices, there are much more instances of them aggravating the risk of infectious disease, than alleviating it. This is particularly due to: i) the importance of the buildup of public health insecticide resistance in mosquito vectors of malaria (and to a lesser extent of VZs), following their exposition to agricultural insecticides; and ii) the importance of clinical azole-resistance buildup in populations suffering from pulmonary aspergillosis or candidiasis (and to a lesser extent crypto-coccidiosis) following their exposition to agricultural fungicides, particularly triazoles.

21.4.2 Relevance of Some Substitution (S)-Based and Most Redesign (R)-Based Crop Protection Practices

Regarding S-based CP practices, there were broadly equally as many instances of them alleviating the infectious disease risk than worsening it. For the former, it was particularly due to the case of physical barriers against fruit bats reducing the risk of Nipah virus transmission. Regarding R-based CP practices, there were some cases of "mixed impacts" for viral, bacterial, and parasitic infections and an overall positive impact (reduced disease risk) for viral, parasitic, and fungal disease risks, while the impact was generally negative for bacterial diseases.

21.4.3 Agroecology as the Preferred Strategy to Integrate Crop Plant Health Within the Extended "One Health" Framework

All these effects are summarized in Figure 21.2. Overall, Redesign-based CP practices, which are mostly agroecological practices, are the ones that generally result in alleviation of the risk of infectious diseases, as compared to Efficiency-based and even Substitution-based CP practices. Agroecological crop protection (ACP) that is the declension of agroecology to CP (Deguine et al. 2023) is therefore the most relevant strategy for integrating crop plant health within the extended "One Health" concept.

In addition, our literature reviews also highlighted a negative impact of climate change on infectious diseases (namely, an increased disease risk), notably via the northward extension of the distribution area of arthropodan disease vectors or the potential re-emergence of zoonotic viruses (e.g. Spanish flu) or bacteria (e.g. anthrax) frozen

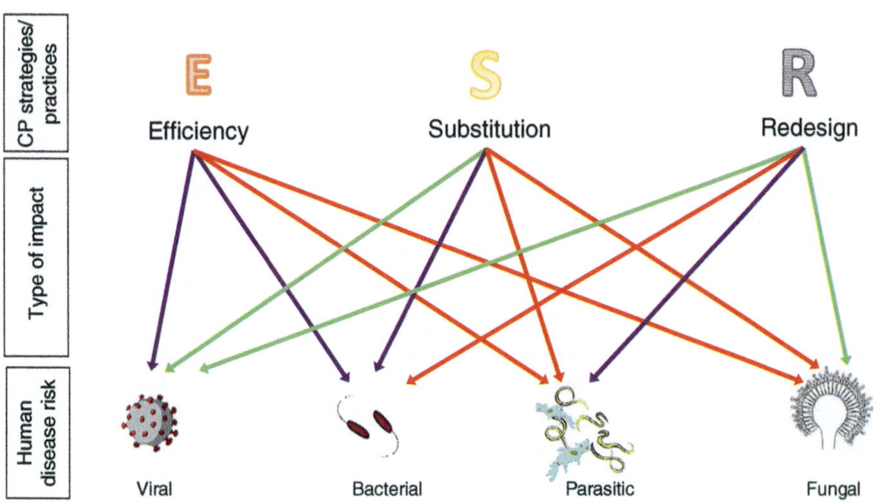

Figure 21.2 Impacts of crop protection (CP) practices according to the Efficiency-Substitution-Redesign framework (Hill and Mac Rae 1996), i.e. whether conventional (Efficiency improvement-based), bioprotection/Substitution-based, or agroecological (Redesign-based), on human (including zoonotic) disease risks. Green arrow: positive impact (reduced disease risk); red arrow: negative impact (increased disease risk); purple arrow: mixed impact. *Source:* Artwork © S. Ratnadass – ILOI.

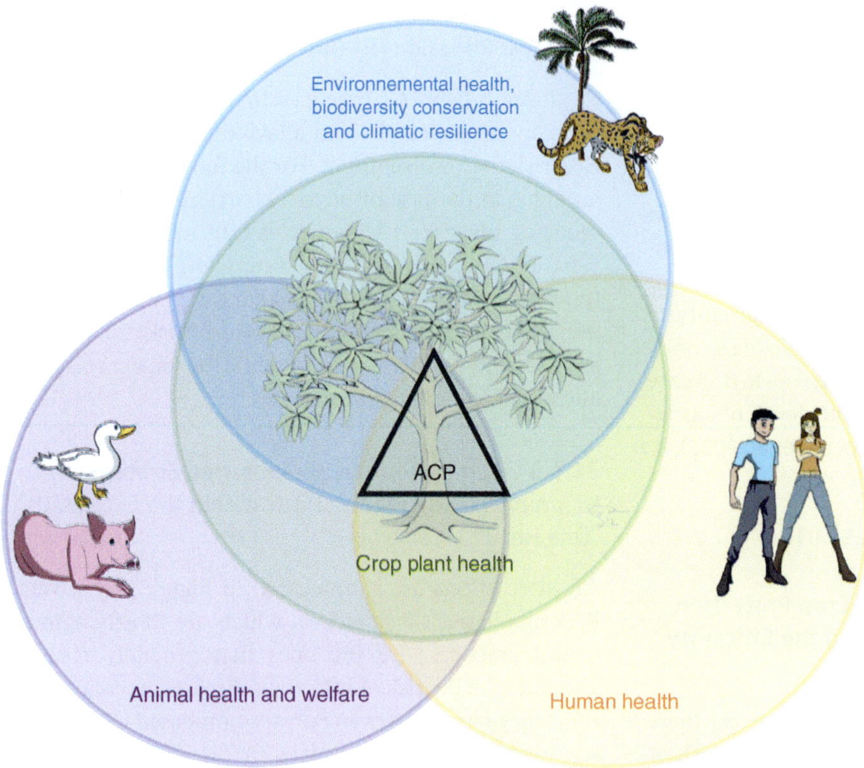

Figure 21.3 Agroecological crop protection (ACP) (central black triangle): contribution to the One Health concept extended to the four health types (circles), including global challenges of climatic resilience, biodiversity conservation, and animal welfare. *Source:* Adapted from Ratnadass and Deguine (2021).

in permafrost, due to global warming (Houwenhuyse et al. 2017). ACP, as a climate-smart approach, both in terms of adaptation and mitigation (Lamichhane et al. 2015) is also thwarting this trend. Similarly, ACP contributes to the conservation of biodiversity in agroecosystems, in natural ecosystems, and in many cases (e.g. livestock-cropping integration with poultry raised in the open air rather than confined in intensive rearing units) to animal welfare (Keeling et al. 2019). These virtuous contributions are depicted in Figure 21.3.

References

Akogbeto, M.C., Djouaka, R.F., and Kinde-Gazard, D.A. (2006). Screening of pesticide residues in soil and water samples from agricultural settings. *Malar. J.* 5: 22. https://doi.org/10.1186/1475-2875-5-22.

Alaphilippe, A., Capowiez, Y., Severac, G. et al. (2016). Codling moth exclusion netting: an overview of French and Italian experiences. *IOBC-WPRS Bull* 112: 31–35.

Alvarez-Moreno, C., Lavergne, R.A., Hagen, F. et al. (2019). Fungicide-driven alterations in azole-resistant *Aspergillus fumigatus* are related to vegetable crops in Colombia, South America. *Mycologia* 111: 217–224. https://doi.org/10.1080/00275514.2018.1557796.

Andru, J., Cosson, J.F., Caliman, J.P., and Benoit, E. (2013). Coumatetralyl resistance of *Rattus tanezumi* infesting oil palm plantations in Indonesia. *Ecotoxicology* 22: 377–396. https://doi.org/10.1007/s10646-012-1032-y.

Aziz, S.A., Olival, K.J., Bumrungsri, S. et al. (2016). The conflict between pteropodid bats and fruit growers: species, legislation and mitigation. In: *Bats in the Anthropocene: Conservation of Bats in a Changing World* (ed. C.C. Voigt and T. Kingston), 377–426. New York: Springer International Publishing https://doi.org/10.1007/978-3-319-25220-913.

Barber, A.E., Riedel, J., Sae-Ong, T. et al. (2020). Effects of agricultural fungicide use on *Aspergillus fumigatus* abundance, antifungal susceptibility, and population structure. *MBio* 11: e02213–e02220. https://doi.org/10.1128/mBio.02213-20.

Barky, F.A., Abdelsalam, H.A., Mahmoud, M.A., and Hamdi, S.A.H. (2012). Influence of atrazine and roundup pesticides on biochemical and molecular aspects of *Biomphalaria alexandrina* snails. *Pestic. Biochem. Physiol.* 104: 9–18. https://doi.org/10.1016/j.pestbp.2012.05.012.

Bastos, R.W., Carneiro, H.C.S., Oliveira, L.V.N. et al. (2018). Environmental triazole induces cross-resistance to clinical drugs and affects morphophysiology and virulence of *Cryptococcus gattii* and *C. neoformans*. *Antimicrob. Agents Chemother.* 62: e01179–e01117. https://doi.org/10.1128/AAC.01179-17.

Bastos, R.W., Freitas, G.J.C., Carneiro, H.C.S. et al. (2019). From the environment to the host: how non-azole agrochemical exposure affects the antifungal susceptibility and virulence of *Cryptococcus gattii*. *Sci. Total Environ.* 681: 516–523. https://doi.org/10.1016/j.scitotenv.2019.05.094.

Baumgartner, J.A., Kross, S., Heath, S., and Connor, S. (2019). *Supporting Beneficial Birds and Managing Pest Birds*. Watsonville: Wild Farm Alliance.

Becker, J.M., Ganatra, A.A., Kandie, F. et al. (2020). Pesticide pollution in freshwater paves the way for schistosomiasis transmission. *Sci. Rep.* 10: 3650. https://doi.org/10.1038/s41598-020-60654-7.

Beer, K.D., Farnon, E.C., Jain, S. et al. (2018). Multidrug-resistant *Aspergillus fumigatus* carrying mutations linked to environmental fungicide exposure – three states, 2010–2017. *Morb. Mortal. Wkly Rep.* 67: 1064.

Bessou, C., Verwilghen, A., Beaudoin-Ollivier, L. et al. (2017). Agroecological practices in oil palm plantations: examples from the field. *OCL* 24: D305. https://doi.org/10.1051/ocl/2017024.

Boa, E., Danielsen, S., and Haesen, S. (2015). Better together: identifying the benefits of a closer integration between plant health, agriculture and one health. In: *One Health: The Theory and Practice of Integrated Health Approaches* (ed. J. Zinsstag, E. Schelling, D. Waltner-Toews, et al.), 258–271. UK: CABI Publishing.

Bodey, G.P., Bolivar, R., Fainstein, V., and Jadeja, L. (1983). Infections caused by *Pseudomonas aeruginosa*. *Rev. Infect. Dis.* 5: 279–313. https://doi.org/10.1093/clinids/5.2.279.

Brilhante, R.S.N., de Alencar, L.P., Bandeira, S.P. et al. (2019). Exposure of *Candida parapsilosis* complex to agricultural azoles: an overview of the role of environmental determinants for the development of resistance. *Sci. Total Environ.* 650: 1231–1238. https://doi.org/10.1016/j.scitotenv.2018.09.096.

Bromley, M.J., Van Muijlwijk, G., Fraczek, M.G. et al. (2014). Occurrence of azole-resistant species of Aspergillus in the UK environment. *J. Glob. Antimicrob. Resist.* 2: 276–279. https://doi.org/10.1016/j.jgar.2014.05.004.

Brugère-Picoux, J. and Le Floc'h Soye Y. (2014). Importance de l'implication de la faune sauvage dans les zoonoses émergentes ou résurgentes. *B. Acad. Nat. Med. Paris* 198: 1411–1422. https://doi.org/10.1016/S0001-4079(19)31237-3.

Calderón, J.M., Fuya, P., Santacoloma, L., and González, C. (2020). Deltamethrin resistance in Chagas disease vectors colonizing oil palm plantations: implications for vector control strategies in a public health-agriculture interface. *Parasit. Vectors* 13: 163. https://doi.org/10.1186/s13071-020-04048-8.

Calisher, C.H., Childs, J.E., Field, H.E. et al. (2006). Bats: important reservoir hosts of emerging viruses. *Clin. Microbiol. Rev.* 19: 531–545. https://doi.org/10.1128/CMR.00017-06.

Cao, D., Wang, F., Yu, S. et al. (2021). Prevalence of azole-resistant *Aspergillus fumigatus* is highly associated with azole fungicide residues in the fields. *Environ. Sci. Technol.* 55: 3041–3049. https://doi.org/10.1021/acs.est.0c03958?ref=pdf.

Carneiro, H.C.S., Bastos, R.W., Ribeiro, N.Q. et al. (2020). Hypervirulence and cross-resistance to a clinical antifungal are induced by an environmental fungicide in *Cryptococcus gattii*. *Sci. Total Environ.* 740: 140135. https://doi.org/10.1016/j.scitotenv.2020.140135.

Chaiyarat, R., Boonma, W., and Koedrith, P. (2020). The role of pteropodid bats in pollination of durian (*Durio zibethinus*) in managed orchards in suburban habitat of Thailand. *Urban Ecosyst.* 23: 97–106. https://doi.org/10.1007/s11252-019-00919-w.

Chanvatik, S., Donnua, S., Lekagul, A. et al. (2019). Antibiotic use in mandarin production (*Citrus reticulata* Blanco) in major mandarin-producing areas in Thailand: a survey assessment. *PLoS One* 14: e0225172. https://doi.org/10.1371/journal.pone.0225172.

Chen, P.Y., Chuang, Y.C., Wu, U.I. et al. (2019). Clonality of fluconazole-nonsusceptible *Candida tropicalis* in bloodstream infections, Taiwan, 2011–2017. *Emerg. Infect. Dis.* 25: 1668. https://doi.org/10.3201/eid2509.190520.

Chouaibou, M., Etang, J., Brevault, T. et al. (2008). Dynamics of insecticide resistance in the malaria vector *Anopheles gambiae s. l.* from an area of extensive cotton cultivation in Northern Cameroon. *Tropical Med. Int. Health* 13: 476–486. https://doi.org/10.1111/j.1365-3156.2008.02025.x.

Chowdhary, A., Kathuria, S., Randhawa, H.S. et al. (2012). Isolation of multiple-triazole-resistant *Aspergillus fumigatus* strains carrying the TR/L98H mutations in the cyp51A gene in India. *J. Antimicrob. Chemother.* 67: 362–366. https://doi.org/10.1093/jac/dkr443.

Corbel, V., N'Guessan, R., Brengues, C. et al. (2007). Multiple insecticide resistance mechanisms in *Anopheles gambiae* and *Culex quinquefasciatus* from Benin. *West Africa. Acta Trop.* 101: 207–216. https://doi.org/10.1016/j.actatropica.2007.01.005.

Damasceno, C.L., Duarte, E.A.A., dos Santos, L.B.P.R. et al. (2019). Postharvest biocontrol of anthracnose in bananas by endophytic and soil rhizosphere bacteria associated with sisal (*Agave sisalana*) in Brazil. *Biol. Control* 137: 104016. https://doi.org/10.1016/j.biocontrol.2019.104016.

Danielsen, S. (2013). Including plant health in the "one health" concept – in theory and in Uganda. In: *A Success Story in Danish Development Aid-DBL (1964–2012)* (ed. A. Olsen, N. Ørnbjerg and K. Winkel), 107–113. Copenhagen: DBL.

Darriet, F., Rossignol, M., and Chandre, F. (2012). The combination of NPK fertilizer and deltamethrin insecticide favors the proliferation of pyrethroid-resistant *Anopheles gambiae* (Diptera: Culicidae). *Parasite* 19: 159–164. https://doi.org/10.1051/parasite/2012192159.

De Clercq, D., Vercruysse, J., Sène, M. et al. (2000). The effects of irrigated agriculture on the transmission of urinary schistosomiasis in the middle and upper valleys of the Senegal River basin. *Ann. Trop. Med. Parasitol.* 94: 581–590.

Deguine, J.-P., Aubertot, J.-N., Bellon, S. et al. (2023). Agroecological crop protection for sustainable agriculture. *Adv. Agron.* 178. https://doi.org/10.1016/bs.agron.2022.11.002.

Destoumieux-Garzón, D., Mavingui, P., Boetsch, G. et al. (2018). The one health concept: 10 years old and a long road ahead. *Front. Vet. Sci.* 5: 14. https://doi.org/10.3389/fvets.2018.00014.

Diabate, A., Baldet, T., Chandre, F. et al. (2002). The role of agricultural use of insecticides in resistance to pyrethroids in *Anopheles gambiae s. l.* in Burkina Faso. *Am. J. Trop. Med. Hyg.* 67: 617–622. https://doi.org/10.4269/ajtmh.2002.67.617.

Dongmo, W., Kechia, F., Tchuenguem, R. et al. (2016). in vitro antifungal susceptibility of environmental isolates of *Cryptococcus* spp. from the west region of Cameroon. *Ethiop. J. Health Sci.* 26: 555–560. https://doi.org/10.4314/ejhs.v26i6.2.

Dorin, J., Debourgogne, A., Zaïdi, M. et al. (2015). First unusual case of keratitis in Europe due to the rare fungus *Metarhizium anisopliae*. *Int. J. Med. Microbiol.* 305: 408–412. https://doi.org/10.1016/j.ijmm.2015.03.004.

Dupré, M., Michels, T., and Le Gal, P.Y. (2017). Diverse dynamics in agroecological transitions on fruit tree farms. *Eur. J. Agron.* 90: 23–33. https://doi.org/10.1016/j.eja.2017.07.002.

Eberl, L. and Vandamme, P. (2016). Members of the genus Burkholderia: good and bad guys. *F1000Research* 5: 1007. https://doi.org/10.12688/f1000research.8221.1.

Elser, J.L., Lindell, C.A., Steensma, K.M.M. et al. (2019). Measuring bird damage to three fruit crops: a comparison of grower and field estimates. *Crop Prot.* 123: 1–4. https://doi.org/10.1016/j.cropro.2019.05.010.

El-Shabrawi, M.H., Arnaout, H., Madkour, L., and Kamal, N.M. (2014). Entomophthoromycosis: a challenging emerging disease. *Mycoses* 57: 132–137. https://doi.org/10.1111/myc.12248.

FAO, CIRAD, CIFOR, WCS (2020). *White Paper: Build Back Better in a Post-COVID-19 World – Reducing Future Wildlife-Borne Spillover of Disease to Humans: Sustainable Wildlife Management (SWM) Programme*. Rome: FAO https://doi.org/10.4060/cb1503en.

Faria-Ramos, I., Tavares, P.R., Farinha, S. et al. (2014). Environmental azole fungicide, prochloraz, can induce cross-resistance to medical triazoles in *Candida glabrata*. *FEMS Yeast Res.* 14: 1119–1123. https://doi.org/10.1111/1567-1364.12193.

Fernández, M., Porcel, M., de la Torre, J. et al. (2015). Analysis of the pathogenic potential of nosocomial pseudomonas putida strains. *Front. Microbiol.* 6: 871. https://doi.org/10.3389/fmicb.2015.00871.

Fraaije, B., Atkins, S., Hanley, S. et al. (2020). The multi-fungicide resistance status of *Aspergillus fumigatus* populations in arable soils and the wider European environment. *Front. Microbiol.* 11: 599233. https://doi.org/10.3389/fmicb.2020.599233.

Frei, M., Khan, M.A.M., Razzak, M.A. et al. (2007). Effects of a mixed culture of common carp, *Cyprinus carpio* L., and Nile tilapia, *Oreochromis niloticus* (L.), on terrestrial arthropod population, benthic fauna, and weed biomass in rice fields in Bangladesh. *Biol. Control* 41: 207–213. https://doi.org/10.1016/j.biocontrol.2007.02.001.

Furuno, T. (2001). *The Power of Duck*. Tasmania: Tagari Publications.

Gilbert, M., Xiao, X., Chaitaweesub, P. et al. (2007). Avian influenza, domestic ducks and rice agriculture in Thailand. *Agric. Ecosyst. Environ.* 119: 409–415. https://doi.org/10.1016/j.agee.2006.09.001.

Gnankiné, O., Bassolé, I.H.N., Chandre, F. et al. (2013). A review: insecticide resistance in *Bemisia tabaci* Gennadius (Homoptera: *Aleyrodidae*) and *Anopheles gambiae* Giles (Diptera: *Culicidae*) could compromise the sustainability of malaria vector control strategies in West Africa. *Acta Trop.* 6: 7–17. https://doi.org/10.1016/j.actatropica.2013.06.004.

Godeau, C., Reboux, G., Scherer, E. et al. (2020). Azole-resistant *Aspergillus fumigatus* in the hospital: surveillance from flower beds to corridors. *Am. J. Infect. Control* 48: 702–704. https://doi.org/10.1016/j.ajic.2019.10.003.

Gómez Londoño, L.F., Pérez León, L.C., McEwen Ochoa, J.G. et al. (2019). Capacity of *Histoplasma capsulatum* to survive the composting process. *Appl. Environ. Soil Sci.* 2019: https://doi.org/10.1155/2019/5038153.

Gonsalves, L., Bicknell, B., Law, B. et al. (2013). Mosquito consumption by insectivorous bats: does size matter? *PLoS One* 8: e77183. https://doi.org/10.1371/journal.pone.0077183.

Grass, I., Lehmann, K., Thies, C., and Tscharntke, T. (2017). Insectivorous birds disrupt biological control of cereal aphids. *Ecology* 98: 1583–1590. https://doi.org/10.1002/ecy.1814.

Grimshaw, R.G. and Faiz. A. (1995). Vetiver grass: application for stabilization of structures. *Proceedings of the Sixth International Conference on Low-Volume Roads*, Minneapolis, MN (25–29 June 1995). pp. 74–81. National Academy Press, Washington, DC

Gu, Y.-H. and Mazzola, M. (2003). Modification of fluorescent pseudomonad community and control of apple replant disease induced in a wheat cultivar-specific manner. *Appl. Soil Ecol.* 24: 57–72. https://doi.org/10.1016/S0929-1393(03)00066-0.

Gu, W., Müller, G., Schlein, Y. et al. (2011). Natural plant sugar sources of anopheles mosquitoes strongly impact malaria transmission potential. *PLoS One* 6: e15996. https://doi.org/10.1371/journal.pone.0015996.

Guan, Y., Zheng, B.J., He, Y.Q. et al. (2003). Isolation and characterization of viruses related to the SARS coronavirus from animals in Southern China. *Science* 302: 276–278. https://doi.org/10.1126/science.1087139.

Hagiwara, D. (2020). Isolation of azole-resistant *Aspergillus fumigatus* from imported plant bulbs in Japan and the effect of fungicide treatment. *J. Pestic. Sci.* 45: 147–150. https://doi.org/10.1584/jpestics.D20-017.

Haileselassie, W., Zemene, E., Lee, M.C. et al. (2021). The effect of irrigation on malaria vector bionomics and transmission intensity in Western Ethiopia. *Parasit. Vectors* 14: 1–11. https://doi.org/10.1186/s13071-021-04993-y.

Halstead, N.T., Hoover, C.M., Arakala, A. et al. (2018). Agrochemicals increase risk of human schistosomiasis by supporting higher densities of intermediate hosts. *Nat. Commun.* 9: 837. https://doi.org/10.1038/s41467-018-03189-w.

Henning, J., Pfeiffer, D.U., Stevenson, M. et al. (2016). Who is spreading avian influenza in the moving duck flock farming network of Indonesia? *PLoS One* 11: e0152123. https://doi.org/10.1371/journal.pone.0152123.

Hill, S.B. and MacRae, R.J. (1996). Conceptual framework for the transition from conventional to sustainable agriculture. *J. Sustain. Agric.* 7: 81–87. https://doi.org/10.1300/J064v07n01_07.

Hoover, C.M., Rumschlag, S.L., Strgar, L. et al. (2020). Effects of agrochemical pollution on schistosomiasis transmission: a systematic review and modelling analysis. *Lancet Planet. Health* 4: e280–e291. https://doi.org/10.1016/S2542-5196(20)30105-4.

Houwenhuyse, S., Macke, E., Reyserhove, L. et al. (2017). Back to the future in a petri dish: origin and impact of resurrected microbes in natural populations. *Evol. Appl.* 11: 29–41. https://doi.org/10.1111/eva.12538.

Howard, L.O. (1920). Mosquitoes and bats. *Public Health Rep.* (1896–1970) 35: 1789.

Husson, O. (2013). Redox potential (Eh) and pH as drivers of soil/plant/microorganism systems: a transdisciplinary overview pointing to integrative opportunities for agronomy. *Plant Soil* 362: 389–417. https://doi.org/10.1007/s11104-012-1429-7.

Husson, O., Sarthou, J.P., Bousset, L. et al. (2021). Soil and plant health in relation to dynamic sustainment of Eh and pH homeostasis: a review. *Plant Soil* 466: 391–447. https://doi.org/10.1007/s11104-021-05047-z.

Ibrahim, A.M., Ahmed, A.K., Bakry, F.A. et al. (2019). Toxicological impact of butralin, glyphosate-isopropylammonium and pendimethalin herbicides on physiological parameters of *Biomphalaria alexandrina* snails. *Molluscan Res.* 39: 224–233. https://doi.org/10.1080/13235818.2019.1592296.

Jayasvati, I. and Jayasvati, M. (2018). Bat guano as the component of fertilizer or the health hazard? SE Asian. *J. Trop. Med.* 49: 331–339.

Jennings, A.P., Naim, M., Advento, A.D. et al. (2015). Diversity and occupancy of small carnivores within oil palm plantations in Central Sumatra, Indonesia. *Mamm. Res.* 60: 181–188. https://doi.org/10.1007/s13364-015-0217-1.

Kano, R., Kohata, E., Tateishi, A. et al. (2015). Does farm fungicide use induce azole resistance in *Aspergillus fumigatus*? *Med. Mycol.* 53: 174–177. https://doi.org/10.1093/mmy/myu076.

Keeling, L., Tunón, H., Olmos Antillón, G. et al. (2019). Animal welfare and the United Nations sustainable development goals. *Front. Vet. Sci.* 6: 336. https://doi.org/10.3389/fvets.2019.00336.

Keesing, F., Holt, R.D., and Ostfeld, R.S. (2006). Effects of species diversity on disease risk. *Ecol. Lett.* 9: 485–498. https://doi.org/10.1111/j.1461-0248.2006.00885.x.

Keleher, S. (1996). Guano: bats gift to gardeners. *Bats* 14: 15–17.

Khan, Z.R., Midega, C.A.O., Pittchar, J. et al. (2011). Push–pull technology: a conservation agriculture approach for integrated management of insect pests, weeds and soil health in Africa. *Int. J. Agric. Sustain.* 9: 162–170. https://doi.org/10.3763/ijas.2010.0558.

Kibuthu, T.W., Njenga, S.M., Mbugua, A.K., and Muturi, E.J. (2016). Agricultural chemicals: life changer for mosquito vectors in agricultural landscapes? *Parasit. Vectors* 9: 500, 27624456.

Kloos, H., De Souza, C., Gazzinelli, A. et al. (2001). The distribution of *Biomphalaria* spp. in different habitats in relation to physical, biological, water contact, and cognitive factors in a rural area in Minas Gerais, Brazil. *Mem. Inst. Oswaldo Cruz* 96: 57–66.

Kouamé, P.K., Nguyen-Viet, H., Dongo, K. et al. (2017). Microbiological risk infection assessment using QMRA in agriculture systems in Côte d'Ivoire, West Africa. *Environ.*

Monit. Assess. 189: 1–11. https://doi.org/10.1007/s10661-017-6279-6.

Kurenbach, B., Hill, A.M., Godsoe, W. et al. (2018). Agrichemicals and antibiotics in combination increase antibiotic resistance evolution. *Peer J* 6: e 5801. https://doi.org/10.7717/peerj.5801.

Lamichhane, J.R., Barzman, M., Booij, K. et al. (2015). Robust cropping systems to tackle pests under climate change. A review. *Agron. Sustain. Dev.* 35: 443–459. https://doi.org/10.1007/s13593-014-0275-9.

Lawler, S.P., Dritz, D.A., Christiansen, J.A., and Cornel, A.J. (2007). Effects of lambda-cyhalothrin on mosquito larvae and predatory aquatic insects. *Pest Manag. Sci.* 63: 234–240. https://doi.org/10.1002/ps.1279.

Lenzi, A., Marvasi, M., and Baldi, A. (2021). Agronomic practices to limit pre-and post-harvest contamination and proliferation of human pathogenic *Enterobacteriaceae* in vegetable produce. *Food Control* 119: 107486. https://doi.org/10.1016/j.foodcont.2020.107486.

Leroy, E.M., Epelboin, A., Mondonge, V. et al. (2009). Human Ebola outbreak resulting from direct exposure to fruit bats in Luebo, Democratic Republic of Congo. *Vector-Borne Zoonot.* 9: 723–728.

Liang, K., Zhang, J., Song, C. et al. (2014). Integrated management to control golden apple snails (Pomacea canaliculata) in direct seeding rice fields: an approach combining water management and rice-duck farming. *Agroecol. Sust. Food* 38: 264–282. https://doi.org/10.1080/21683565.2013.809562.

Liu, H., Xie, L., Cheng, P. et al. (2019). Trends in insecticide resistance in *Culex pipiens* pallens over 20 years in Shandong, China. *Parasites Vectors* 12: 167. https://doi.org/10.1186/s13071-019-3416-9.

Lo, H.J., Tsai, S.H., Chu, W.L. et al. (2017). Fruits as the vehicle of drug resistant pathogenic yeasts. *J. Inf. Secur.* 75: 254–262. https://doi.org/10.1016/j.jinf.2017.06.005.

Lokkers C. (1990). Colony dynamics of the green tree ant (Oecophylla smaragdina Fab.) in a seasonal tropical climate. PhD thesis. James Cook University, Australia.

Lu, K. (1990). The susceptibility of *Apodemus agrarius* and *Rattus losea* to the anticoagulant ro-denticide, flocoumafen. *Int. Biodeterior.* 26: 69–74.

Mansuy, A. and Fontaine, R. (2014). Fiche phytosanitaire canne à sucre – rats. Ecophytopic. http://www.bsv-reunion.fr/wp-content/uploads/2015/02/Fiche-phyto-rats.pdf (accessed 10 March 2021)

Mari Saez, A., Cherif Haidara, M., Camara, A. et al. (2018). Rodent control to fight Lassa fever: evaluation and lessons learned from a 4-year study in upper Guinea. *PLoS Negl. Trop. Dis.* 12: e0006829. https://doi.org/10.1371/journal.pntd.0006829.

Marquez, A., Khalil, R.A., Fourel, I. et al. (2019). Resistance to anticoagulant rodenticides in Martinique could lead to inefficient rodent control in a context of endemic leptospirosis. *Sci. Rep.* 9: 13491. https://doi.org/10.1038/s41598-019-49661-5.

McKenna, M. (2019). Antibiotics set to flood Florida's troubled orange orchards. *Nature* 567: 302–303.

McManus, P.S., Stockwell, V.O., Sundin, G.W., and Jones, A.L. (2002). Antibiotic use in plant agriculture. *Annu. Rev. Phytopathol.* 40: 443–465. https://doi.org/10.1146/annurev.phyto.40.120301.093927.

Medlock, J.M. and Snow, K.R. (2008). Natural predators and parasites of British mosquitoes – a review. *Eur. Mosq. Bull.* 25: 1–11.

Men, B.X., Ogle, R.B., and Lindberg, J.E. (2002). Studies on integrated duck-rice systems in the Mekong Delta of Vietnam. *J. Sustain. Agric.* 20: 27–40. https://doi.org/10.1300/J064v20n01_05.

Mendes, R., Garbeva, P., and Raaijmakers, J.M. (2013). The rhizosphere microbiome: significance of plant beneficial plant pathogenic and human pathogenic microorganisms. *FEMS Microbiol. Rev.* 37: 634–663. https://doi.org/10.1111/1574-6976.12028.

Miarinjara, A., Rahelinirina, S., Razafimahatratra, N.L. et al. (2019). Field assessment of insecticide dusting and bait station treatment impact against rodent flea and house flea species in the Madagascar plague context. *PLoS Negl. Trop. Dis.* 13: e0007604. https://doi.org/10.1371/journal.pntd.0007604.

Mills, J.N. (1999). The role of rodents in emerging human disease: examples from the hantaviruses and arenaviruses. In: *Ecologically-Based Rodent Management* (ed. G.R. Singleton, L.A. Hinds, H. Leirs and Z. Zhang), 134–160. Canberra: ACIAR.

Morand, S., Blasdell, K., Bordes, F. et al. (2019). Changing landscapes of Southeast Asia and rodent-borne diseases: decreased diversity but increased transmission risks. *Ecol. Appl.* 29: e01886. https://doi.org/10.1002/eap.1886.

Mortensen, K.L., Mellado, E., Lass-Flörl, C. et al. (2010). Environmental study of azole-resistant *Aspergillus fumigatus* and other aspergilli in Austria, Denmark, and Spain. *Antimicrob. Agents Chemother.* 54: 4545–4549. https://doi.org/10.1128/AAC.00692-10.

Mouhamadou, C.S., de Souza, S.S., Fodjo, B.K. et al. (2019). Evidence of insecticide resistance selection in wild *Anopheles coluzzii* mosquitoes due to agricultural pesticide use. *Infect. Dis. Poverty* 8: 64. https://doi.org/10.1186/s40249-019-0572-2.

Mouret, J.C. and Falconnier, G.N. (2018). La gestion des adventices en riziculture biologique. In: *Le riz et la Camargue: vers des agroécosystèmes durables* (ed. J.C. Mouret and B. Leclerc), 437–150. Dijon: Educagri-Cardère.

Muller, F.M.C., Staudigel, A., Salvenmoser, S. et al. (2007). Cross-resistance to medical and agricultural azole drugs in yeasts from the oropharynx of human immunodeficiency virus patients and from environmental Bavarian vine grapes. *Antimicrob. Agents Chemother.* 51: 3014–3016. https://doi.org/10.1128/AAC.00459-07.

Muñoz-Pedreros, A., Gil, C., Yáñez, J. et al. (2016). Trophic ecology of two raptors, barn owl (*Tyto alba*) and white-tailed kite (*Elanus leucurus*), and possible implications for biological control of hantavirus reservoir in Chile. *Wilson J. Ornithol.* 128: 391–403. https://doi.org/10.1676/wils-128-02-391-403.1.

Muturi, E.J., Mwangangi, J.M., Beier, J.C. et al. (2013). Ecology and behavior of *Anopheles arabiensis* in relation to agricultural practices in Central Kenya. *J. Am. Mosq. Control Assoc.* 29: 222–230. https://doi.org/10.2987/13-6328R.1.

Nabi, G., Wang, Y., Lü, L. et al. (2021). Bats and birds as viral reservoirs: a physiological and ecological perspective. *Sci. Total Environ.* 754: 142372. https://doi.org/10.1016/j.scitotenv.2020.142372.

Nahar, N., Sultana, R., Gurley, E.S. et al. (2010). Date palm sap collection: exploring opportunities to prevent Nipah transmission. *Ecosyst. Health* 7: 196–203. https://doi.org/10.1007/s10393-010-0320-3.

Nahar, N., Mondal, U.K., Sultana, R. et al. (2012). Piloting the use of indigenous methods to prevent Nipah virus infection by interrupting bats' access to date palm sap in Bangladesh. *Health Promot. Int.* 28: 378–386. https://doi.org/10.1093/heapro/das020.

Nahar, N., Mondal, U.K., Hossain, M.J. et al. (2014). Piloting the promotion of bamboo skirt barriers to prevent Nipah virus transmission through date palm sap in Bangladesh. *Glob. Health Promot.* 21: 7–15. https://doi.org/10.1177/1757975914528249.

Nahar, N., Asaduzzaman, M., Mandal, U.K. et al. (2020). Hunting bats for human consumption in Bangladesh. *Ecosyst. Health* 17: 139–151. https://doi.org/10.1007/s10393-020-01468-x.

Nibouche, S. and Tibère, R. (2010). Mechanism of resistance to the spotted stalk borer, *Chilo sacchariphagus*, in the sugar cane cultivar R570. *Entomol. Exp. Applic.* 135: 308–314. https://doi.org/10.1111/j.1570-7458.2010.00996.x.

Nourrisson, C., Dupont, D., Lavergne, R.A. et al. (2017). Species of *Metarhizium anisopliae* complex implicated in human infections: retrospective sequencing study. *Clin. Microbiol. Infect.* 23: 994–999. https://doi.org/10.1016/j.cmi.2017.05.001.

Olugasa, B.O., Dogba, J.B., Nykoi, J.D. et al. (2014). The rubber plantation environment and Lassa fever epidemics in Liberia, 2008-2012: a spatial regression. *Spat. Spatio-Temporal Epidemiol.* 11: 163–174. https://doi.org/10.1016/j.sste.2014.04.005.

Orondo, P., Nyanjom, S., Atieli, H. et al. (2021). Insecticide resistance status of *Anopheles arabiensis* in irrigated and non-irrigated areas in Western Kenya. *Parasit. Vectors* 14: 335. https://doi.org/10.1186/s13071-021-04833-z.

Peach, D.A.H. and Gries, G. (2019). Mosquito phytophagy – sources exploited, ecological function, and evolutionary transition to haematophagy. *Entomol. Exp. Appl.* 168: 120–136.

Peach, D.A., Gries, R., Zhai, H. et al. (2019). Multimodal floral cues guide mosquitoes to tansy inflorescences. *Sci. Rep.* 9: 3908. https://doi.org/10.1038/s41598-019-39748-4.

Pires, A.F.A., Patterson, L., Kukielka, E.A. et al. (2019). Prevalence and risk factors associated with *Campylobacter* spp. and *Salmonella enterica* in livestock raised on diversified small-scale farms in California. *Epidemiol. Infect.* 147: e321. https://doi.org/10.1017/S095026881900205X.

Potocki, L., Baran, A., Oklejewicz, B. et al. (2020). Synthetic pesticides used in agricultural production promote genetic instability and metabolic variability in Candida spp. *Gen. Dent.* 11: 848. https://doi.org/10.3390/genes11080848.

Prigitano A, Venier V, Cogliati M, De Lorenzis G, Esposto MC, Tortorano AM. 2014. Azole-resistant *Aspergillus fumigatus* in the environment of northern Italy, May 2011 to June 2012. *Euro Surveill.* 19: 20747. http: //http://www.eurosurveillance.org/View Article. aspx? Article Id=20747 (accessed 13 October 2021)

Quénéhervé, P., Dao, J.-C., Ducelier, D. et al. (2005). Faisabilité technique de l'agriculture biologique en Martinique: productions. In: *Agriculture biologique en Martinique* (ed. M. François, R. Moreau and B. Sylvander), 149–233. Montpellier: IRD éditions.

Rahelinirina, S., Duplantier, J.-M., Ratovonjato, J. et al. (2010). Study on the movement of *Rattus rattus* and evaluation of the plague dispersion in Madagascar. *Vector-Borne Zoonotic Dis.* 10: 77–84. https://doi.org/10.1089/vbz.2009.0019.

Rahelinirina, S., Scobie, K., Ramasindrazana, B. et al. (2021). Rodent control to fight plague: field assessment of methods based on rat density reduction. *Integr. Zool.* 0: 1–18. https://doi.org/10.1111/1749-4877.12529.

Rakotonanahary, R.J.L., Harrison, A., Maina, A.N. et al. (2017). Molecular and serological evidence of flea-associated typhus group and spotted fever group rickettsial infections in Madagascar. *Parasit. Vectors* 10: 125. https://doi.org/10.1186/s13071-017-2061-4.

Rasamiravaka, T., Raveloson, P.A., Rajaonarivelo, P.J. et al. (2018). Malagasy traditional treatments of infectious plant diseases exert anti-virulence activities against *Pseudomonas aeruginosa* and *Ralstonia solanacearum*. *J. Microbiol. Biotechnol. Food Sci.* 7: 377–382.

Ratnadass, A. and Deberdt, P. (2021). Pratiques de protection des cultures en agroécosystèmes tropicaux et risques de maladies humaines et animales d'origine bactérienne. *Cah. Agric.* 30: 42. https://doi.org/10.1051/cagri/2021028.

Ratnadass, A. and Deguine, J.-P. (2021). Crop protection practices and viral zoonotic risks within a one health framework. *Sci. Total Environ.* 774: 145172. https://doi.org/10.1016/j.scitotenv.2021.145172.

Ratnadass, A. and Martin, T. (2022). Crop protection practices and risks associated with infectious tropical parasitic diseases. *Sci. Total Environ.* 823: 153633. https://doi.org/10.1016/j.scitotenv.2022.153633.

Ratnadass, A. and Sester (2023). Crop protection practices and risks associated with human fungal diseases: a one health perspective. *Cah. Agric.* 32: 7. https://doi.org/10.1051/cagri/2022036.

Ratnadass, A., Evans, D.C., Way, B.S. et al. (1991). Amélioration des techniques de stockage des vivriers en vue de la réduction des pertes post-récolte occasionnées par les rongeurs au niveau de village de la République Centrafricaine. In: *Proceedings International Working Conference on Stored-Product Protection*, vol. 5 (ed. F. Fleurat-Lessard and P. Ducom), 1507–1516.

Ratnadass, A., Fernandes, P., Avelino, J., and Habib, R. (2012). Plant species diversity for sustainable management of crop pests and diseases in agroecosystems: a review. *Agron. Sustain. Dev.* 32: 273–303. https://doi.org/10.1007/s13593-011-0022-4.

Ratovonjato, J., Duchemin, J.B., Duplantier, J.M. et al. (2003). Lutte contre la peste à Madagascar: évaluation de l'efficacité des boîtes de Kartman en milieu urbain. *Arch. Inst. Pasteur Madagascar* 69: 41–45.

Reid, M.C. and McKenzie, F.E. (2016). The contribution of agricultural insecticide use to increasing insecticide resistance in African malaria vectors. *Malar. J.* 15: 107. https://doi.org/10.1186/s12936-016-1162-4.

Ren, J., Jin, X., Zhang, Q. et al. (2017). Fungicides induced triazole-resistance in *Aspergillus fumigatus* associated with mutations of TR46/Y121F/T289A and its appearance in agricultural fields. *J. Hazard. Mater.* 326: 54–60. https://doi.org/10.1016/j.jhazmat.2016.12.013.

Robertson, L.J., Johansen, Ø.H., Kifleyohannes, T. et al. (2020). Cryptosporidium infections in Africa – how important is zoonotic transmission? A review of the evidence. *Front. Vet. Sci.* 7: 575881. https://doi.org/10.3389/fvets.2020.575881.

Rocchi, S., Daguindau, E., Grenouillet, F. et al. (2014). Azole-resistant *Aspergillus fumigatus* isolate with the TR34/L98H mutation in both a fungicide-sprayed field and the lung of a hematopoietic stem cell transplant recipient with invasive aspergillosis. *J. Clin. Microbiol.* 52: 1724–1726. https://doi.org/10.1128/JCM.03182-13.

Rocchi, S., Ponçot, M., Morin-Crini, N. et al. (2018). Determination of azole fungal residues in soils and detection of *Aspergillus fumigatus*-resistant strains in market gardens of eastern France. *Environ. Sci. Pollut. Res.* 25: 32015–32023. https://doi.org/10.1007/s11356-018-3177-6.

Rocchi, S., Godeau, C., Scherer, E. et al. (2021). One year later: the effect of changing azole-treated bulbs for organic tulips bulbs in hospital environment on the azole-resistant *Aspergillus fumigatus* rate. *Med. Mycol.* 59: 741–743. https://doi.org/10.1093/mmy/myab007.

Rocha, M.F.G., Alencar, L.P.D., Paiva, M.A.N. et al. (2016). Cross-resistance to fluconazole induced by exposure to the agricultural azole tetraconazole: an environmental resistance school? *Mycoses* 59: 281–290. https://doi.org/10.1111/myc.12457.

Rodríguez-Pastor, R., Escudero, R., Vidal, D. et al. (2017). Density-dependent prevalence of *Francisella tularensis* in fluctuating vole populations, Northwestern Spain. *Emerg. Infect. Dis.* 23: 1377–1379. https://doi.org/10.1016/j.agee.2016.06.041.

Roger, P.A., Simpson, I., Oficial, R. et al. (1994). Effects of pesticides on soil and water microflora and mesofauna in wetland ricefields: a summary of current knowledge and extrapolation to temperate environments. *Aust. J. Exp. Agric.* 34: 1057–1068.

Rushton, J., Nielsen, L.R., Cornelsen, L. et al. (2018). Evaluation of integrated approaches to health with a focus on one health. In: *Integrated Approaches to Health: A Handbook for the Evaluation of One Health* (ed. S. Rüegg, B. Häsler and J. Zinsstag), 14–21. Wageningen: Wageningen Academic Publishers https://doi.org/10.3920/978-90-8686-875-9.

Russo, D., Bosso, L., and Ancillotto, L. (2018). Novel perspectives on bat insectivory highlight the value of this ecosystem service in farmland: research frontiers and management implications. *Agric. Ecosyst. Environ.* 266: 31–38. https://doi.org/10.1016/j.agee.2018.07.024.

Rutto, J.J., Osano, O., Thuranira, E.G. et al. (2013). Socio-economic and cultural determinants of human African trypanosomiasis at the Kenya–Uganda transboundary. *PLoS Negl. Trop. Dis.* 7: e 2186. https://doi.org/10.1371/journal.pntd.0002186.

Samish, M. and Rehacek, J. (1999). Pathogens and predators of ticks and their potential in biological control. *Annu. Rev. Entomol.* 44: 159–182. https://doi.org/10.1146/annurev.ento.44.1.159.

Schoustra, S.E., Debets, A.J., Rijs, A.J. et al. (2019). Environmental hotspots for azole resistance selection of *Aspergillus fumigatus*, the Netherlands. *Emerg. Infect. Dis.* 25: 1347–1353. https://doi.org/10.3201/eid2507.181625.

Sekercioglu, C.H. (2013). Guineafowl, ticks and Crimean-Congo hemorrhagic fever in Turkey: the perfect storm? *Trends Parasitol.* 29: 1–2. https://doi.org/10.1016/j.pt.2012.10.001.

Sellers, L.A., Long, R.F., Jay-Russell, M.T. et al. (2018). Impact of field-edge habitat on mammalian wildlife abundance, distribution, and vectored foodborne pathogens in adjacent crops. *Crop Prot.* 108: 1–11. https://doi.org/10.1016/j.cropro.2018.02.005.

Service, M.W. (1977). Mortalities of the immature stages of species B of the *Anopheles gambiae* complex in Kenya: comparison between rice fields and temporary pools, identification of predators, and effects of insecticidal spraying. *J. Med. Entomol.* 13: 535–545. https://doi.org/10.1093/jmedent/13.4-5.535.

Sharma, C., Hagen, F., Moroti, R. et al. (2015). Triazole-resistant *Aspergillus fumigatus* harbouring G54 mutation: is it de novo or environmentally acquired? *J. Glob. Antimicrob. Resist.* 3: 69–74. https://doi.org/10.1016/j.jgar.2015.01.005.

Shi, Q., Song, X., Lv, Y. et al. (2019). Potential risks associated with Japanese encephalitis prevalence in Shandong Province, China. *Vector-Borne Zoonot.* 19: 640–645. https://doi.org/10.1089/vbz.2018.2416.

Sin, T.S. (2006). Evaluation of different species of fish for biological control of golden apple snail *Pomacea canaliculata* (Lamarck) in rice. *Crop Prot.* 25: 1004–1012. https://doi.org/10.1016/j.cropro.2006.01.012.

Singh, R.K., Dhama, K., Chakraborty, S. et al. (2019). Nipah virus: epidemiology, pathology, immunobiology and advances in diagnosis, vaccine designing and control strategies – a comprehensive review. *Vet. Q.* 39: 26–55. https://doi.org/10.1080/01652176.2019.1580827.

Smith, I. and Wang, L.F. (2013). Bats and their virome: an important source of emerging viruses capable of infecting humans. *Curr. Opin. Virol.* 3: 84–91. https://doi.org/10.1016/j.coviro.2012.11.006.

Snelders, E., Camps, S.M.T., Karawajczyk, A. et al. (2012). Triazole fungicides can induce cross-resistance to medical triazoles in *Aspergillus fumigatus*. *PLoS One* 7: e31801. https://doi.org/10.1371/journal.pone.0031801.

Soarimalala, V., Jean, P., and Rakotovao, F. (2019). Les rats dans le monde rural du centre-est et du centre-sud de Madagascar: Dommages causés et systèmes de contrôle. *Malagasy Nature* 13: 125–151.

Sow, A., Seye, D., Faye, E. et al. (2020). Birds and bats contribute to natural regulation of the millet head miner in tree-crop agroforestry systems. *Crop Prot.* 132: 105127. https://doi.org/10.1016/j.cropro.2020.105127.

Squire, S.A., Yang, R., Robertson, I. et al. (2017). Molecular characterization of cryptosporidium and giardia in farmers and their ruminant livestock from the coastal Savannah zone of Ghana. *Infect. Genet. Evol.* 55: 236–243. https://doi.org/10.1016/j.meegid.2017.09.025.

Stansbury, J.P. and Sierra, M. (2004). Risks, stigma and Honduran Garífuna conceptions of HIV/AIDS. *Soc. Sci. Med.* 59: 457–471. https://doi.org/10.1016/j.socscimed.2003.11.013.

Stone, C.M., Witt, A.B., Walsh, G.C. et al. (2018). Would the control of invasive alien plants reduce malaria transmission? A review. *Parasite. Vector.* 11: 76. https://doi.org/10.1186/s13071-018-2644-8.

Su, P., Liao, X.L., Zhang, Y., and Huang, H. (2012). Influencing factors on rice sheath blight epidemics in integrated rice-duck system. *J. Integr. Agric.* 11: 1462–1473. https://doi.org/10.1016/S2095-3119(12)60146-4.

Suh, J. (2014). Theory and reality of integrated rice–duck farming in Asian developing countries: a systematic review and SWOT analysis. *Agric. Syst.* 125: 74–81. http://doi.org/10.1016/j.agsy.2013.11.003.

Talom, A.D., Essoung, M.A., Gbankoto, A. et al. (2020). A preliminary analysis on the effect of copper on *Anopheles coluzzii* insecticide resistance in vegetable farms in Benin. *Sci. Rep.* 10: 6392. https://doi.org/10.1038/s41598-020-63086-5.

Tapia-Ramírez, G., Lorenzo, C., Navarrete, D. et al. (2022). A review of mammarenaviruses and rodent reservoirs in the Americas. *Ecosyst. Health* 1-18: https://doi.org/10.1007/s10393-022-01580-0.

Theofel, C.G., Williams, T.R., Gutierrez, E. et al. (2020). Microorganisms move a short distance into an almond orchard from an adjacent upwind poultry operation. *Appl. Environ. Microbiol.* 86: e00573–e00520. https://doi.org/10.1128/AEM.00573-20.

Thurman, J.H., Northfield, T.D., and Snyder, W.E. (2019). Weaver ants provide ecosystem services to tropical tree crops. *Front. Ecol. Evol.* 7: 120. https://doi.org/10.3389/fevo.2019.00120.

Toyotome, T., Fujiwara, T., Kida, H. et al. (2016). Azole susceptibility in clinical and environmental isolates of *Aspergillus fumigatus* from Eastern Hokkaido, Japan. *J. Infect. Chemother.* 22: 648–650. https://doi.org/10.1016/j.jiac.2016.03.002.

Tucker, D.L., Beresford, C.H., Sigler, L., and Rogers, K. (2004). Disseminated *Beauveria bassiana* infection in a patient with acute lymphoblastic leukemia. *J. Clin. Microbiol.* 42: 5412–5414. https://doi.org/10.1128/JCM.42.11.5412-5414.2004.

Van Bruggen, A.H.C. and Finckh, M. (2016). Plant diseases and management approaches in organic farming systems. *Annu. Rev. Phytopathol.* 54: 25–54. https://doi.org/10.1146/annurev-phyto-080615-100123.

Van Bruggen, A.H.C., Goss, E.M., Havelaar, A. et al. (2019). One health-cycling of diverse microbial communities as a connecting force for soil, plant, animal, human and ecosystem health. *Sci. Total Environ.* 664: 927–937. https://doi.org/10.1016/j.scitotenv.2019.02.091.

Van Bruggen, A.H.C., Finckh, M.R., He, M. et al. (2021). Indirect effects of the herbicide glyphosate on plant, animal and human health through its effects on microbial communities. *Front. Environ. Sci.* 9: 763917. https://doi.org/10.3389/fenvs.2021.763917.

Van den Berg, J. (2006). Vetiver grass (*Vetiveria zizanioides* (L.) Nash) as trap plant for *Chilo partellus* (Swinhoe) (Lepidoptera: Pyralidae) and *Busseola fusca* (Fuller) (Lepidoptera: Noctuidae). *Ann. Soc. Entomol. Fr.* 42: 449–454. https://doi.org/10.1080/00379271.2006.10697478.

Van Herk, F.H., McAllister, T.A., Cockwill, C.L. et al. (2004). Inactivation of giardia cysts and cryptosporidium oocysts in beef feedlot manure by thermophilic windrow composting. *Compost Sci. Util.* 12: 235–241. https://doi.org/10.1080/1065657X.2004.10702188.

Van Mele, P., Camara, K., and Vayssieres, J.-F. (2009). Thieves, bats and fruit flies: local ecological knowledge on the weaver ant *Oecophylla longinoda* in relation to three 'invisible' intruders in orchards in Guinea. *Int. J. Pest Manage.* 55: 57–61. https://doi.org/10.1080/09670870802450276.

Vayssières, J.-F., Offenberg, J., Sinzogan, A. et al. (2016). The use of weaver ants in the management of fruit flies in Africa. In: *Fruit Fly Research and Development in Africa* (ed. S. Ekesi, S.A. Mohamed and M. De Meyer), 389–422. Basel: Springer International Publishing.

Verwilghen, A. (2015). Rodent pest management and predator communities in oil palm plantations in Indonesia: a comparison of two contrasting systems. PhD thesis. Université de Franche-Comté, Besançon, France.

Vilela, R. and Mendoza, L. (2018). Human pathogenic *Entomophthorales*. *Clin. Microbiol. Rev.* 31: e00014–e00018. https://doi.org/10.1128/CMR.00014-18.

Wacharapluesadee, S., Sintunawa, C., Kaewpom, T. et al. (2013). Group C betacoronavirus in bat guano fertilizer, Thailand. *Emerg. Infect. Dis.* 19: 1349–1351. https://doi.org/10.3201/eid1908.130119.

Wang, Y., Cheng, P., Jiao, B. et al. (2020). Investigation of mosquito larval habitats and insecticide resistance in an area with a high incidence of mosquito-borne diseases in Jining, Shandong Province. *PLoS One* 15: e0229764. https://doi.org/10.1371/journal.pone.0229764.

Wezel, A., Casagrande, M., Celette, F. et al. (2014). Agroecological practices for sustainable agriculture. A review. *Agron. Sustain. Dev.* 34: 1–20. https://doi.org/10.1007/s13593-013-0180-7.

Xie, W.Y., Shen, Q.R., and Zhao, F.J. (2018). Antibiotics and antibiotic–resistance from animal manures to soil: a review. *Eur. J. Soil Sci.* 69: 181–195. https://doi.org/10.1111/ejss.12494.

Yadouleton, A.W.M., Asidi, A., Djouaka, R.F. et al. (2009). Development of vegetable farming: a cause of the emergence of insecticide resistance in populations of *Anopheles gambiae* in urban areas of Benin. *Malar. J.* 8: 103. https://doi.org/10.1186/1475-2875-8-103.

Yadouleton, A., Martin, T., Padonou, G. et al. (2011). Cotton pest management practices and the selection of pyrethroid resistance in *Anopheles gambiae* population in Northern Benin. *Parasit. Vectors* 4: 60. https://doi.org/10.1186/1756-3305-4-60.

Yang, Y.-L., Lin, C.-C., Chang, T.-P. et al. (2012). Comparison of human and soil *Candida tropicalis* isolates with reduced susceptibility to fluconazole. *PLoS One* 7: e34609. https://doi.org/10.1371/journal.pone.0034609.

Yoshizawa, N., Usui, M., Fukuda, A. et al. (2020). Manure compost is a potential source of tetracycline-resistant *Escherichia coli* and tetracycline resistance genes in Japanese farms. *Antibiotics* 9: 76. https://doi.org/10.3390/antibiotics9020076.

Zhao, T.Y. and Xue, R.D. (2021). Integrated mosquito management in rice field in China. *Wetl. Ecol. Manag.* 1-11: https://doi.org/10.1007/s11273-021-09840-6.

Zhi, D. and Cheng-Xin, W. (1984). Rodent control in China. In: *Proceedings of the Vertebrate Pest Conference 1984* (ed. D.O. Clark), 47–53. Sacramento.

Zuhair, R.M., Al-Assiuty, A.N.I., Khalil, M.A., and Salama, W.M. (2022). Efficacy of vermicompost amended and bacterial diversity on plant growth and pathogen control. *Int. J. Recycl. Org. Waste Agric.* 11: 131–141. https://doi.org/10.30486/IJROWA.2021.1919606.1176.

22

Tackling Antimicrobial Resistance Needs One Health Approach

Yasodhara Gunasekara[1], Sanda Kottawatta[1], Thilini Nisansala[2], Ayona Silva-Fletcher[3], and Ruwani Kalupahana[1]

[1] Department of Veterinary Public Health and Pharmacology, Faculty of Veterinary Medicine and Animal Science, University of Peradeniya, Peradeniya, Sri Lanka
[2] Faculty of Veterinary Medicine, Universiti Malaysia Kelantan, Kota Bharu, Kelantan, Malaysia
[3] Department of Veterinary Clinical Sciences, The Royal Veterinary College, University of London, United Kingdom

22.1 Antimicrobial Resistance (AMR): A Brief Overview

Antimicrobials are broader categories of chemicals that act against bacteria, viruses, fungi, and parasites and are named as antibacterials, antivirals, antifungals, and antiparasitics, respectively. Any substance with the ability of inhibiting or killing the microorganism with no or less damage to the host is termed as an antimicrobial (Purssell 2020). These could have an origin that could be natural, semisynthetic, or synthetic. Antibacterials are the commonly used and mostly studied class of antimicrobials. Therefore "antibacterials" are often used interchangeably with the term "antimicrobials" and antibiotics (Scott et al. 2019).

These antimicrobials are used to prevent and treat bacterial, viral, fungal, and parasitic infections in humans, animals, and plants. When bacteria, viruses, fungi, and parasites change over time and no longer respond to respective medicines, it is called antimicrobial resistance (AMR). As a result of drug resistance, antimicrobials become ineffective and infections become harder or impossible to treat. The resulting consequences are increased number of days of hospital stays and health care costs, disease spread, and high mortality rates. Further, these drug-resistant organisms are transmitted between humans and animals or vice versa with the involvement of environment. Current perceptions are that AMR could result in the loss of millions of lives of humans and animals per year in this century damaging the health care and agriculture industries. Therefore, the World Health Organization (WHO) and Centers for Disease Control and Prevention (CDC) have declared AMR as one of the urgent threats to global public health and development (WHO 2015b; CDC 2019). The World Organization for Animal Health (OIE) states that "Antimicrobial resistance (AMR) is a serious global threat to human health, animal health and welfare, plant health, food security, and also impacts to the environment throughout the world and cannot be successfully tackled without multi-sectoral cooperation" (OIE 2022). In this book chapter on "tackling AMR under One Health concept," the focus will be on bacterial resistance to antibiotics, so antibacterial resistance will be discussed under the term "antimicrobial resistance" (AMR).

22.2 AMR: Antimicrobials, Their Origin, and Development of Resistance

A Nobel Prize-winning German physician, Paul Ehrlich (1854–1915), theorized the perception of antibiotics first and termed his imaginary agent as a "magic bullet." He comprehended that magic bullet could target specific microbes, which cause diseases in the body without harming the body itself. Alexander Fleming in 1928 discovered the world's first antibiotic penicillin, and this instigated the era of antibiotics that subsequently led to the discovery and development of extensive range of diverse antimicrobials. Majority of antimicrobials that we use today were discovered and introduced during the period of 1950–1960, which is known as the golden era of antibiotic discovery (Hutchings et al. 2019). Unfortunately, in recent years there have been very limited discovery and introduction of novel antimicrobial agents. This discovery rate is not sufficient to cope with the wide antimicrobial usage globally. Antimicrobials that are used today either are derived from natural resources like fungi and bacteria or are chemically synthesized. Details of antimicrobials that are currently in use are summarized in Table 22.1.

One Health: Human, Animal, and Environment Triad, First Edition. Edited by Meththika Vithanage and Majeti Narasimha Vara Prasad.

Table 22.1 Antibiotic classification, common examples, and their mode of action.

Classes of antibiotics	Common examples	Mode of action
Penicillins (β-lactam antibiotics)	Ampicillin Amoxicillin Penicillin G Oxacillin	Bactericidal: prevents bacteria from forming cell wall via competitive inhibition of the transpeptidase enzyme
Cephalosporins (β-lactam antibiotics)	Cephalexin Cefuroxime Ceftriaxone Ceftazidime	Bactericidal: prevents bacteria from forming cell wall via competitive inhibition of the transpeptidase enzyme
Aminoglycosides	Gentamicin Neomycin Amikacin Streptomycin	Bactericidal: prevents bacteria from producing proteins that they need to grow and multiply by irreversibly binding to 30S
Carbapenems (β-lactam antibiotics)	Doripenem Ertapenem Imipenem Meropenem	Bactericidal: prevents bacteria from forming cell wall
Fluoroquinolones	Nalidixic acid Ciprofloxacin Gatifloxacin Moxifloxacin	Bactericidal: inhibits DNA synthesis by interfering with the activity of DNA gyrase enzyme
Glycopeptides and lipoglycopeptides	Vancomycin Oritavancin Teicoplanin Telavancin	Bactericidal: prevents Gram-positive bacteria from forming cell wall
Macrolides	Azithromycin Clarithromycin Erythromycin Fidaxomicin	Bacteriostatic: prevents bacteria from producing proteins that they need to grow and multiply by reversibly binding to 50S
Oxazolidinones	Linezolid Tedizolid	Prevents bacteria from producing proteins that they need to grow and multiply by binding to 50S
Polypeptides	Bacitracin Colistin Polymyxin B	Prevents bacteria from forming cell wall and/or disrupting the cell membrane underlying the cell wall
Rifamycins	Rifabutin Rifampin Rifapentine Rifaximin	Bactericidal: inhibits RNA transcription by inhibiting RNA polymerase
Sulfonamides	Sulfadiazine Sulfadoxine Sulfamethizole Sulfamethoxazole	Bacteriostatic: inhibits production of folic acid that bacteria need to grow and multiply
Isoniazid	Isoniazidz	Bacteriostatic: inhibits production of mycolic acid that bacteria need to grow and multiply
Tetracyclines	Doxycycline Minocycline Tetracycline	Bacteriostatic: prevents bacteria from producing proteins that they need to grow and multiply by blocking tRNA

Unfortunately, in 1940s shortly after the discovery of penicillin, Abraham and Chain discovered and reported an *Escherichia coli* strain that produces penicillinase against penicillin (Abraham and Chain 1940). This was the first alarming news of AMR. When bacteria are exposed to antimicrobials, susceptible organisms are either killed or inhibited but under the selective pressure of the antimicrobials, resistant bacteria will escape, survive, and multiply. There are a number of reasons for the wide development and spread of AMR worldwide. Some explanations include ease of accessibility, higher intake of antimicrobials without proper prescriptions and treatment guidelines, wide usage of antimicrobials in animal husbandry and agricultural sectors, poor hygienic practices, dissemination by wildlife, poor sewage removal systems, and lack of public awareness (Ayukekbong et al. 2017).

22.3 AMR: Types and Mechanisms

Resistance of microorganisms against antimicrobials can be "natural" or "acquired" (Peterson and Kaur 2018). As most of antimicrobial agents are natural products, surrounding coresident organisms have developed mechanisms to survive by escaping the activity of naturally occurring antimicrobials. Therefore, natural resistance is considered to be "intrinsic," which can be observable within the species or "induced" where these bacteria harbor relevant genes that are expressed only after exposure to a particular antimicrobial agent. An example of intrinsic resistance is penicillin G resistance in Gram-negative bacteria but not in Gram-positive bacteria.

Development and expression of resistance to an antimicrobial agent that was susceptible to an antibiotic previously is known as acquired resistance. Mechanisms involved in acquired resistance are result of (i) either the gene mutations responsible for regular biological processes and cellular structures under selective pressure (ii) or the acquisition of resistance genes from other cells (vertical or horizontal) or by both mechanisms (Vikesland et al. 2019). Unlike the natural resistance where that particular trait is shared universally within a bacterial species, acquired resistance can be observable only in some strains or subpopulations of a bacterial species.

Bacteria that possess resistance toward antimicrobials have developed different mechanisms to attack the action of antimicrobials, mainly (i) modification or degradation of antimicrobials, (ii) decreased antimicrobial permeability and efflux, and (iii) receptor modification (Pandra et al. 2010).

Modification or degradation of antimicrobial drug by microbes is one of the most common biological mechanisms that have been reported. This occurs when bacteria are able to produce enzymes that chemically degrade or modify the antibiotic making them inactive against the bacteria. Production of β-lactamase enzymes against β-lactamase antibiotics is a classic example for this (Bush and Bradford 2016). Decreased antimicrobial permeability and efflux is another mechanism that is commonly found in Gram-negative bacteria. With this trait bacteria are able to prevent the antibiotics penetrating into its intracellular or periplasmic target, thus resulting in a concentration below that is required for antibacterial activity. Activity of vancomycin against Gram-negative bacteria is a well-known example for the decreased antimicrobial permeability because of the presence of natural barrier in outer membrane (Antonoplis et al. 2019). Receptor modification is one of the most successful bacterial strategies to avoid the action of the antimicrobial by interfering with their target site. This character is fulfilled either by target protection or by modification, which results in lack of binding and consequently the lack of antibacterial effect. Some of the classic and best-studied examples for the modifications in the structural conformation is penicillin-binding proteins observed in certain types of penicillin resistance; ribosomal alterations that can render aminoglycosides, macrolides, or tetracyclines inactive; and DNA-gyrase modifications resulting in resistance to fluoroquinolones (Hooper and Jacoby 2015) (Figure 22.1). Methicillin-resistant *Staphylococcus aureus* (MRSA) and extended spectrum β-lactamase (ESBL) producers are leading bacterial pathogens that cause AMR infections throughout the world (Sah and Hemalatha 2015; Vestergaard et al. 2019).

22.4 AMR: No Boundaries for Transmission

As discussed above bacteria display resistance either naturally (intrinsic resistance) or via the mechanisms displayed through resistant genes, which are the key genes that were mutated during replication. The resistant genes are then transferred to next generations of bacteria via either vertical transmission or horizontal gene transfer. In vertical transmission resistant genes are transmitted to their daughter cells during replication. Transmission of antimicrobial-resistant genetic materials between organisms can happen through different mechanisms that involve horizontal gene transfer by conjugation, transformation, and transduction (Lerminiaux and Cameron 2019) (Figure 22.2). Among three horizontal gene transfer methods, conjugation is the most common and is a significant mechanism of transmission of resistance among bacteria. During the conjugation, mobilization of plasmid from a donor bacterium to a

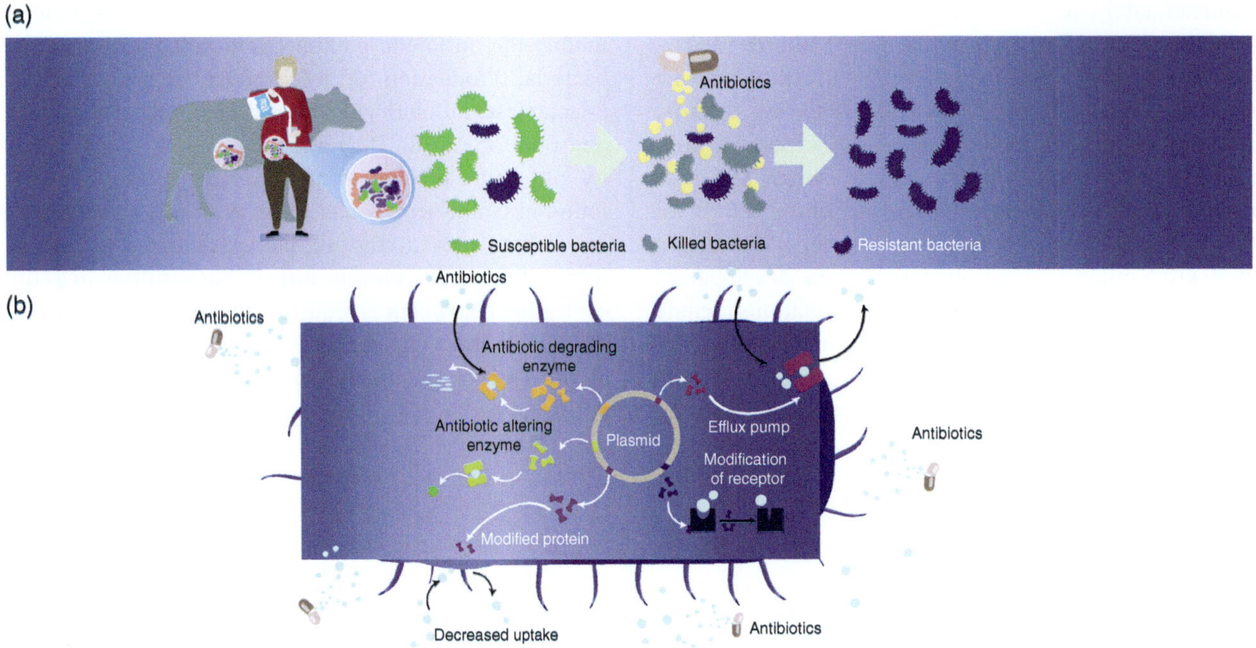

Figure 22.1 Main mechanisms by which microorganisms exhibit resistance to antimicrobials a substantial majority of bacteria that are found in the human and animal microbiome are susceptible to antimicrobials, and only a few of them are resistant to antibiotics, which can be acquired or natural. Antibiotics only kill bacteria that are susceptible to the antibiotics that are being used, and the bacteria that are resistant to those antibiotics take over and proliferate (a). Bacteria have developed a variety of methods that make them impotent against antimicrobial agents, and these mechanisms in bacteria can be classified into categories, namely modification or degradation of antimicrobial drug, decreased antimicrobial permeability, and efflux and receptor modification (b).

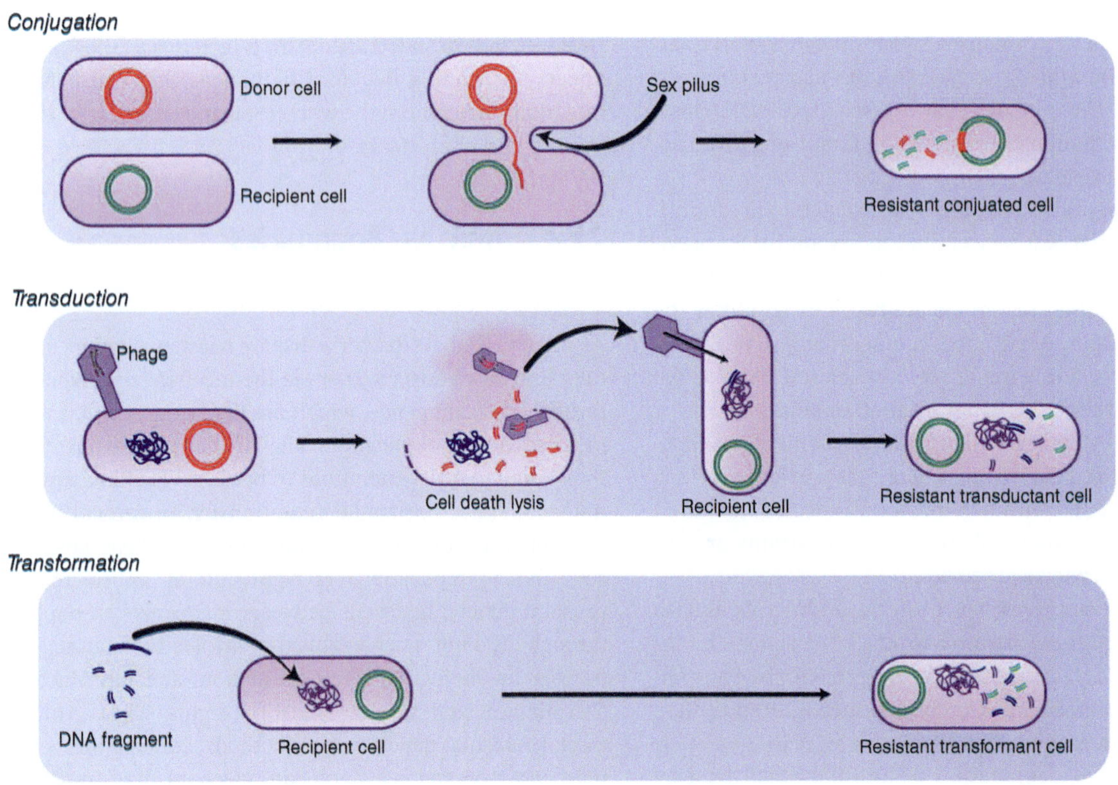

Figure 22.2 Horizontal gene transformation. Conjugation is the mechanism by which one bacterium transfers genetic material to another through direct contact. Transduction is the process by which a virus transfers genetic material from one bacterium to another. Transformation is the process of horizontal gene transfer by which some bacteria take up foreign genetic material (naked DNA) from the environment.

recipient bacterium occurs through a pilus that forms between the two bacteria when they are next to each other (Virolle et al. 2020). Transformation occurs when there is direct uptake of naked DNA by a competent bacterium that is released by a dead bacterium nearby (Seitz and Blokesch 2013). The recipient bacterium incorporates naked DNA into its own genetic material after receiving into its cytoplasm. Transduction is the genetic transfer of the resistant genes from one bacterial cell to another via vector or bacteriophage (Fillol-Salom et al. 2019). These vectors and bacteriophages are most often viruses. Most importantly, in horizontal transmission of resistant genes any bacteria can transfer resistance genes and elements to any other bacterial species, even to taxonomically and genetically distant ones. This poses a serious global threat as the resistant bacteria can transfer the AMR genes among humans, animals, and the environment leading to rapid dissemination of AMR everywhere (Von Wintersdorff et al. 2016).

22.5 AMR: Current Status

22.5.1 Burden of AMR in Human Health

In the ancient world before the discovery of antimicrobials, infectious diseases like cholera, tuberculosis, and typhoid fever were highly prevalent, and such bacterial illnesses were the major cause of highest morbidity and mortality among human populations. The discovery of antibiotics and subsequent treatment of people for bacterial infections helped to save millions of lives by reducing associated morbidity and mortality. Further, antimicrobials continue as the key treatment option not only in potentially significant bacterial infections like tuberculosis, sepsis, pneumonia, and urinary tract infection but also in preventing infections in several fields of modern medicine such as chemotherapy for cancer treatment, organ transplantation, hip replacement surgery, and intensive care for preterm newborns. But the rapid development of AMR is threatening all these benefits of the antibiotics and can be catastrophic (Huemer et al. 2020).

CDC has assessed AMR threats according to several factors and classified bacterial pathogens as urgent, serious, and concerning threats. *Clostridium difficile*, carbapenem-resistant Enterobacteriaceae, and drug-resistant *Neisseria gonorrhoeae* are the three bacterial species that are classified under urgent threats (CDC 2019). There are several pathogenic bacteria listed under serious threats, and some common examples found under this category are multidrug-resistant Acinetobacter, ESBL-producing Enterobacteriaceae, MRSA, and drug-resistant tuber-culosis. Classical examples under concerning threats are vancomycin-resistant *S. aureus* (VRSA), erythromycin-resistant Group A *Streptococcus*, and clindamycin-resistant Group B *Streptococcus* (Ventola 2015).

The burden of AMR is substantial among human populations resulting in 700,000 deaths annually worldwide (Allcock et al. 2017). The threat of AMR affects all countries, but the burden is disproportionately aggravated in low-income and middle-income countries. Deaths attributed to AMR in 2019 was highest in western sub-Saharan Africa, at 27.3 deaths per 100,000 and lowest in Australasia, at 6.5 deaths (4.3–9.4) per 100,000 (Stanaway et al. 2019). The main causes behind this are irrational use of antimicrobials and poverty-related issues in developing countries as discussed in detail in following paragraph.

One of the top factors explained in this scenario is poor utilization of antimicrobial agents by people. Both misuse and overuse of antimicrobials due to purchase of antimicrobials over the counter without a prescription, irrational usage of antimicrobials without proper medical guidelines or self-medication, stop taking antimicrobials before completing the full course are responsible in the development of drug-resistant pathogens (Michael et al. 2014). In some instances, lack of proper strategies for prevention and control of infectious diseases in health care facilities and global pandemics like COVID-19 that might cause massive use of antimicrobial drugs can exacerbate the problem of AMR (Chibabhai et al. 2020). In addition, empirical antimicrobial treatments in resource-poor settings are hampered by lack of point of care diagnostic assays, which can distinguish bacterial from viral infections. The start of empirical antimicrobial treatments whiles waiting for the results of microbiological tests that can be delayed due to lack of resources further aggravates AMR development. Antimicrobials are also prescribed or administered for viral infections such as cold and flu, which do not necessitate antimicrobials at all but as preventive medicines of secondary bacterial infection. Sometimes unnecessary prescription of broad-spectrum antibiotics for the illnesses that could be treated with narrow-spectrum antibiotics also worsen the situation of bacterial resistance. Paucity-driven factors like sharing of medicines, use of leftovers or expired medicines, and use of low-quality antimicrobials also contribute to the occurrence of AMR. Lack of proper and cautious guidelines for antimicrobial usage and national action plans to combat this emerging AMR in most parts of the world has also contributed to the development of bacterial resistance (Ayukekbong et al. 2017).

Even though there are existing rules and regulations on antimicrobial usage in some countries, there may be a gap of proper implementation of them. Not only these factors but the low number of new antimicrobial drugs that are in the development and manufacturing processes result in minimal options of treatment strategies and worsen AMR development (Michael et al. 2014). There is evidence that general public and some health care workers lack knowledge regarding AMR development and spread (Prestinaci et al. 2015).

22.5.2 Burden of AMR in Animal Sector

Similar to human medicine, veterinary medicine requires antimicrobials for treatment of bacterial infections in companion and food producing animals, wild animals, and aquaculture (Ibrahim et al. 2020). Antimicrobials are broadly used in animals to treat infectious diseases ranging from simple topical infections to severe systemic illnesses (septicemias, respiratory infections, and mastitis), as prophylactic agents in disease prevention and as growth promoters in subtherapeutic levels in healthy animals.

Widespread antimicrobial usage in food producing animals and excessive and misuse in humans are considered to be the major drivers identified for AMR. Majority of livestock are reared under intensive management systems where animals are kept in high densities, making them susceptible to infectious diseases. Lack of proper biosecurity measures such as vaccination and hygienic practices in such scenario further aggravate the situation and increase the prevalence of infectious diseases leading to usage of antimicrobials and the development of AMR. Livestock are managed at herd or flock level and not at individual animal level (Davies and Wales 2019). When one or few animals become ill, all the animals in the herd/flock are treated with antimicrobials at therapeutic level as it is difficult to distinguish or treat animals at individual level. This procedure works as both treatment for sick animals and as a preventive strategy against infection in those animals who are healthy but risk of becoming infected. This unnecessary approach of antimicrobial usage is a factor in the development of AMR. Further oral antimicrobials are administered through mixing with feed or water in large herds/flocks (poultry and swine). This can result in overdosing or underdosing due to various reasons such as chemical or heat destruction of antimicrobials during mixing and low/high intake of mixed feed/water by animals leading to variations of exposure and the evolution of resistance (Chattopadhyay 2014). Moreover, usage of antimicrobials through several routes of administration (oral and systemic) in some farm systems like swine is a common practice that results in selection pressure among bacteria. Sometimes farmers might use antimicrobials without proper advices or guidance from veterinarians. Such repeated and continued use of antimicrobials to treat recurrent infectious diseases increases the risk of emergence of resistance. Lack of diagnostic facilities in resource-poor setting that results in the use of antimicrobials unnecessarily, administration of antimicrobials for viral infections rather than for bacterial infections, and the use of broad-spectrum antimicrobials without performing antimicrobial susceptibility testing are all contributing to AMR development. Again, antimicrobials are unreasonably given to animals at subtherapeutic levels as growth promotors in many countries. Antimicrobial growth promoters that are used as feed additives are administered via drinking water or feed for prolonged periods to improve growth rates of farm animals. Prolonged exposure of gut microbiota to subtherapeutic concentrations of antimicrobials leads to the emergence of AMR. Biocide (substances that hinder the activity of broad-spectrum bacteria) usage in livestock industry as animal feed preservatives and disinfectants and antiseptics could lead to the development of resistance mechanisms against biocides and thus might express resistance against antimicrobials also through non-specific mechanisms (Capita et al. 2019). In developing countries where antimicrobial production and storage chains are insufficient, antimicrobial agents may degrade resulting in low concentration and bactericidal activity. When using such antimicrobials, it allows survival of exposed microorganisms and emergence of AMR (Ayukekbong et al. 2017).

The data on the extent and significance of AMR in companion animals (dogs and cats) remains scarce due to limited surveillance systems. There is a critical threat of emergence of AMR in companion animals, because of the proximity of them with humans. Again, the most important contributing factor in resistance development is extensive use of antimicrobials among companion animals. Lack of proper diagnostic facilities and over-prescription without laboratory-based diagnosis (antimicrobial susceptibility testing), over the counter purchase of antimicrobials without guidance of registered veterinarians, preference for leftover antimicrobials used for human diseases due to easy availability, errors in required dosage calculations that result in underdosing, and not continuing the prescribed proper duration are some common reasons mentioned in literature for responsible reasons of emergence of AMR in companion animals (Galarce et al. 2021).

Antimicrobial agents are extensively used in aquaculture for therapeutic as well as prophylactic treatment and presence of AMR is largely reported, evidences from Sri Lanka are presented in Text Box 22.1 (Dhanapala et al. 2021). AMR observed in aquatic animals may be due to direct exposure to antimicrobials that are used as group therapy but also due to animal and human excreta containing resistant bacteria, resistance genes, and antimicrobial residues. Further, antimicrobials are used as metaphylactic in aquatic animals as individual treatment is impossible that exposes the non-target animals to such treatment.

Text Box 22.1 Research data from our ongoing research study on identifying the extent of AMR/ABR among animals, humans, and environment in selected three ecosystems of Sri Lanka

Published data:

1) This study was conducted to identify the distribution of AMR among wild animals, urban wild animals, and livestock in and around a selected wildlife region in Sri Lanka. We found that 52.7%, 20%, and 52% of *E. coli* from wild animals, urban wild animals, and livestock were resistant to at least one antimicrobial among the 12 antimicrobials tested. Further, multidrug-resistant *E. coli* was also found from all three groups (Bamunusinghage et al. 2022).
2) This study was conducted to identify the distribution of AMR among ornamental fish and their farming environments using selected set of ornamental fish farms in Sri Lanka. *Aeromonas* spp. was isolated from ornamental freshwater fish farming environment; apparently healthy and diseased fish were tested to see their AMR patterns for 13 antimicrobials and found resistance frequencies as amoxicillin (92.5%), enrofloxacin (67.1%), nalidixic acid (63.4%), erythromycin (26.1%), tetracycline (23.6%), imipenem (18%), trimethoprim-sulfamethoxazole (16.8%), and gentamicin (16.8%). Multidrug resistance (MDR) was also widespread (Dhanapala et al. 2021).

Though wildlife animals are hardly treated with antimicrobials, presence of AMR genes in microorganisms of wildlife animals has been reported in several countries including Sri Lanka and stated in Text Box 22.1 (Bamunusinghage et al. 2022). This might be as a result of indirect exposure to antimicrobial residues that are present in the environment and resistant bacteria in human and animal excreta due to the overlap between habitats. Therefore, many studies suggest that wildlife species act as reservoirs that disperse AMR across several niches (Vittecoq et al. 2016).

In high-income countries, trends in AMR in animals are monitored via systematic surveillance by organizations such as the European Food Safety Authority (EFSA) in Europe (Authority et al. 2021), the National Antimicrobial Resistance Monitoring System for Enteric Bacteria (NARMS) in the United States, or the Canadian Integrated Program for Antimicrobial Resistance Surveillance (CIPARS) in Canada (Karp et al. 2017). However, in low- and middle-income countries (LMICs), where demand for meat (and antimicrobials) is rising, rapid systematic surveillance systems remain largely absent.

22.5.3 AMR in the Environment

The environment (soil and water) has been concerned as a reservoir of AMR and is suggested to play a main role in the spreading of AMR bacteria and genes between humans and animals across different ecosystems (Holmes et al. 2016). There are millions of non-pathogenic microorganisms that live in soil and water, and there is no direct application of antimicrobials on them. However, incidental exposure of antimicrobials that contaminate environment such as elimination of leftover antimicrobials, removal of feed or water with antimicrobials that are used in livestock, antimicrobial application to aquatic environments and agricultural fields result in the emergence of AMR among environmental residing bacteria (Thanner et al. 2016; Dhanapala et al. 2021). There are variations in the efficiency of antimicrobial processing within the gut: antimicrobial agent itself, animal species, route of administration, and duration since administration; thus, these factors determine the volume of residue excreted and duration of the bioavailability of these excreted residues in the environment. Around 90% of antimicrobials administered in livestock animals and fish are excreted out into environment in unmetabolized form due to poor metabolization and gut absorption, thus resulting in high concentration of antimicrobial residues in the environment. This is a critical hazard that influences the emergence of AMR in said environments. Further, there may be resistant gut microflora that contaminates the environment through animal excreta (dung/feces and urine). These resistant organisms might exchange genetic materials responsible for AMR to other residing environmental bacteria (Fletcher 2015).

22.6 AMR: Inter and Intra Transmission Among Humans, Animals, and Environment

The hosts for bacteria are not limited to one species. Therefore, AMR in one animal has the potential to extend to another animal, while the environment acts as a reservoir for resistance. Humans can be exposed to animal-originated AMR mainly through animal-based food products and contaminated water, while animals might be exposed to AMR via humans through environmental contamination (Figure 22.3). AMR transmission can be occurred within intra-species and between inter-species.

Consumption and handling of animal-originated foods such as milk, meat, fish, and egg act as one of the main pathways by which humans are exposed directly to AMR organisms via ingestion of them. Foodborne pathogens, *E. coli*, *Salmonella*, *Campylobacter*, and *Shigella* can be transmitted widely (Founou et al. 2016). AMR bacteria might be present in milk from dairy cows treated for example for mastitis during lactation or drying-off. Inadequate environmental hygiene and inappropriate milk storage can also cause AMR bacterial contamination in milk. Raw milk and milk products have a higher potential to carry AMR bacteria (Al-Harbi et al. 2021). Several studies have reported the presence of AMR bacteria in commonly available meat types, namely beef, pork, and chicken that can act as a reservoir for AMR bacteria. Meat can be contaminated by AMR bacteria throughout the processing chain and at the retail level (Mateus et al. 2016). Consumption of raw and undercooked meat had shown a higher potential of transmission of AMR bacteria to humans compared to properly cooked meat (James et al. 2021). Further, AMR bacteria were detected in processed meat items such as sausages, ham, and bacon (Jans et al. 2018; Monger et al. 2021).

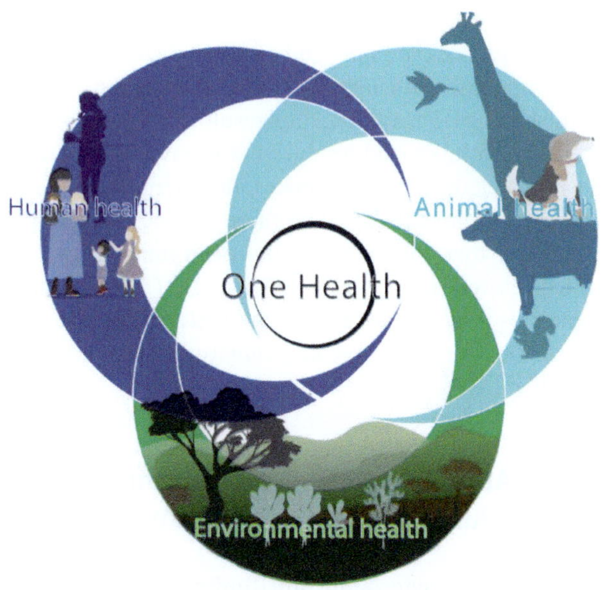

Figure 22.3 Interconnection between human health, animal health, and environmental health in One Health concept (because antimicrobials used to treat various infectious diseases in animals may be the same or comparable to those used in people, and environment can link human and animals, addressing the emerging issue of AMR requires a One Health approach).

Drinking water was identified as a reservoir and transmission route of AMR bacteria to human beings (Alawi et al. 2022). Not only by drinking water and animal-originated foods, but AMR organisms can also be carried by contaminated fruits and vegetables (Thanner et al. 2016). For example, ESBLs and carbapenem-resistant organisms were found in fruits and vegetables that were sold in India and AMR *Cronobacter* spp. were found in cereals and cereal products in China (Li et al. 2014).

Humans can also be exposed to AMR organisms through animals while handling. There is a risk of getting exposure to AMR organisms when humans pet companion animals such as cats and dogs (Gwenzi et al. 2021). Also, abattoir workers and farmers have a high chance of getting infected by AMR organisms in their working premises (Manyi-Loh et al. 2018). Inanimate objects such as mobile phones can act as a reservoir of AMR and transmission of it between human (Olsen et al. 2020).

Several routes have been found for AMR bacteria to be released into the environment as a result of human activities. Human excreta and wastewater have been identified and documented as important sources of AMR bacteria. Soil and water can be directly contaminated by AMR bacteria that are present in the human feces and urine where communities have insufficient sanitation facilities. For example, informal settlements (slums) that are mainly found in LMIC are identified as a hotspot of AMR mainly due to their poor sanitation (Nadimpalli et al. 2020).

Wastewater would be discharged untreated into the environment due to a lack of sufficient facilities to manage municipal and domestic wastes that may carry AMR bacteria and AMR genes (Fouz et al. 2020; Osińska et al. 2020). Furthermore, aging infrastructure such as leaking sewers are typically found alongside municipal water distribution pipelines. As a result, AMR organisms are freely emitted into the water. Not only does the wastewater originate from the household, but wastewater that is released from hospital premises is also identified as a hotspot for AMR (Kaur et al. 2020). Further, a significant prevalence of *Klebsiella pneumoniae* carbapenemase gene was found in hospital wastewater, whereas it was not found in non-hospital wastewater AMR (Loudermilk et al. 2022).

On the other hand, farm animals can be exposed to AMR bacteria through contaminated drinking water and feeds. A variety of AMR organisms can emerge in farms animals. Because farmland is contaminated by animal excreta, farms associated environments can act as a reservoir for resistant organisms ultimately. Several studies were reported that soil and water from dairy farmland were highly contaminated by clinically important resistant organisms (He et al. 2020). Very recently, Amoafo et al. (2022) reported that the prevalence of AMR *E. coli* isolated from soil was lower in organic dairy farming compared to conventional dairy farming systems. Not only cattle manure but also poultry litter was identified as a key source of AMR organisms (Ngogang et al. 2020). The effluent of slaughterhouses and animal-originated food processing plants carried resistant organisms and can cause environmental contamination of AMR bacteria and genes (Neyra et al. 2012).

Aquaculture farms were identified as a hotspot of resistant organisms. Shrimp farms can spread AMR organisms to wild water bodies through effluent water. Further, both surface water and groundwater can be contaminated by AMR organisms from ornamental aquaculture settings (Dhanapala et al. 2021).

Animal and human excreta and wastewater are widely used in fruit and vegetable farms as sources of water and plant nutrients. Therefore, it leads to contamination of farmlands by AMR organisms that originated from humans (Manyi-Loh et al. 2018). Further, AMR bacteria were found in soil from both conventional and organic farming operations (Armalytė et al. 2019). Food crops and associated environments can be contaminated by AMR organisms due to manure and slurry application. Further, according to Guo et al. 2021 slurry application showed the high potential of contamination of AMR genes compared to manure application to the agricultural land (Guo et al. 2021).

Unlike farm animals and humans, wild animals are rarely treated with antimicrobials but, due to their extensive home range and feeding habits, wild animals act as a reservoir and transmission route of AMR within an ecosystem (Bamunusinghage et al. 2022). Moreover, wild animals who live in or around the farmlands have access to and consume animal waste such as dead carcasses. Also, their drinking water sources might be contaminated with resistant organisms through wastewater that arises from farmlands. Rats and shrews are common animal species that are found around the farms, and a study reported that the AMR pattern of rats and shrews was closely associated with the AMR pattern of livestock animals in respective farms (Nhung et al. 2015). Similarly, wild animals can be exposed to human-originated resistant organisms (Lagerstrom and Hadly 2021). An interesting study was carried out by Jaelle C. Brealey et al. 2021 to determine the abundance and repertoire of AMR genes in the oral microflora of Swedish brown bears collected, and the results revealed that gene diversity of bears' oral microbiome was related to national antibiotic consumption patterns in humans of respective periods (Brealey et al. 2021). Compared to the herbivorous wild animals, omnivorous and carnivorous wild animals have a high potential to get infected by the resistant organism through human and animal waste and wastewater (Vittecoq et al. 2016; Bamunusinghage et al. 2022).

Invertebrate animals can act as a vector for the spread of AMR bacteria between animals and between animals and humans or within humans. For example, multidrug-resistant *E.coli* were isolated in the exoskeleton of flies who were found in farm environments (dos Santos Alves et al. 2018). Migratory animals, especially migratory birds, are identified as a key route of transmission of AMR throughout the world (Yuan et al. 2021). Animal-originated foods can carry AMR bacteria from one corner of the world to another corner (Cahill et al. 2017) (Figure 22.4).

As health of humans, animals, and environment are all strongly interconnected, drug-induced AMR in animals can have a negative influence on human health and vice versa. Furthermore, antimicrobials used in humans and animals ultimately end up in the environment posing a threat to ecosystem health while also possibly serving as a reservoir for resistant microbes. Therefore, in order to have a better grasp of the current situation, the AMR crisis should be explored through the "One Health" lens.

22.7 One Health Approach for Tackling AMR

"One Health is an approach that recognizes that the health of people is closely connected to the health of animals and our shared environment" (CDC 2022). A significant One Health issue that is causing concern is AMR. The vast majority of antimicrobials used to treat humans and animals are the same. In addition, environment can act as a reservoir and mediator for transmission of AMR microbes. To tackle this global health issue systematically, a multisectoral collaborative strategy is required, which must include medical, veterinary, and environmental health specialists, as well as economic, social, political, and legal professionals. The WHO, Food and Agricultural Organization of the United Nations (FAO), and OIE have united to fight against AMR and have identified the necessity of One Health in combating the issue, hence several action plans have been developed (OIE).

22.7.1 Action Plan by WHO

In May 2015, WHO announced a global action plan based on the One Health concept, in response to the urgent need for a plan to address the AMR crisis (WHO 2015b). Many governments have established their unique implementation plan based on the WHO action plan while keeping in view their particular country's requirements, which is a constructive trend in addressing this global crisis.

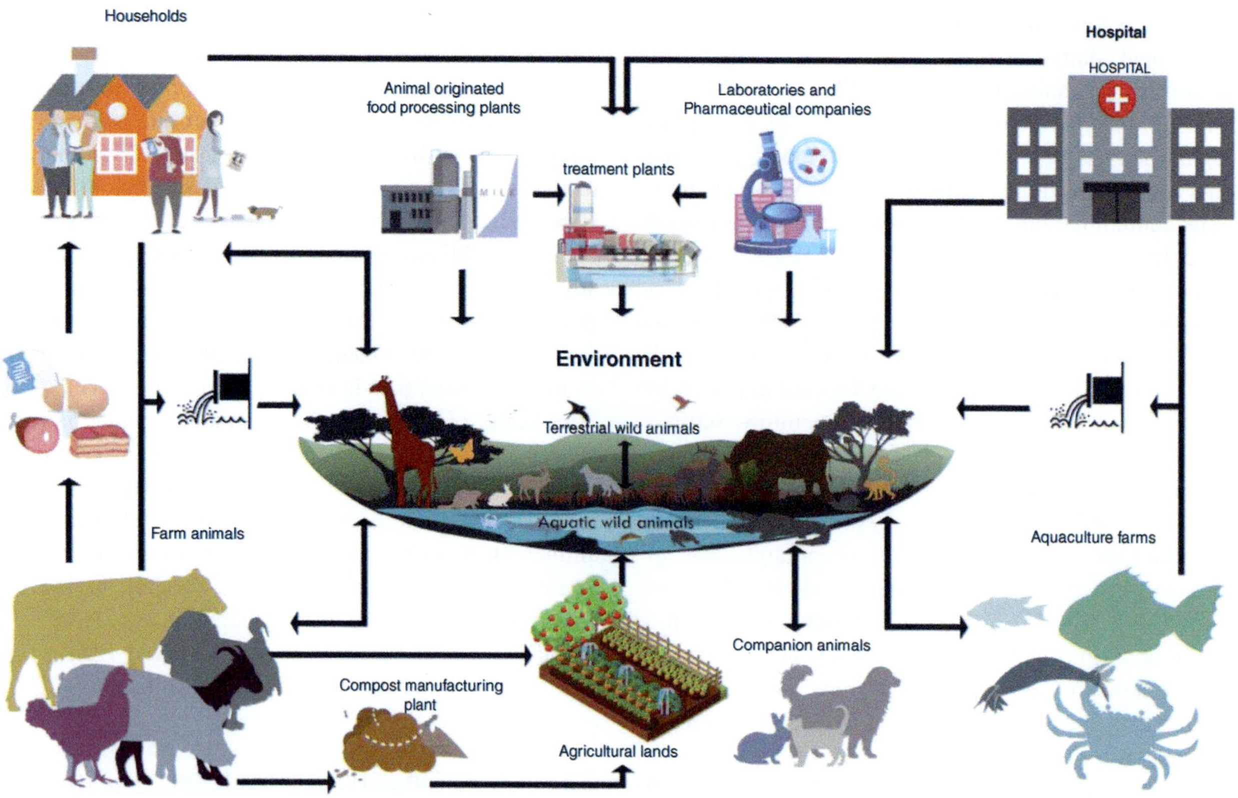

Figure 22.4 Spread of AMR among different components of an ecosystem. AMR microbes are found in humans, animals, food, and the environment (in water, soil, and air). They can spread between humans and animals and the environment through various pathways. Humans and animals are exposed to AMR organisms mainly through foods and water, while environmental contamination occurs by their excreta. Wild animals can act as sentinels of environmental contaminations of AMR bacteria due to the exposure to AMR organisms through the environment.

The WHO action plan has five strategic objectives. The first objective is to maximize AMR awareness and comprehension via effective communication, education, and training. Under this objective, both health professionals and community members will be educated on AMR, and behavioral adjustments toward antibiotic consumption will be encouraged. Furthermore, in order to achieve their primary goal, WHO conducted a multicounty public awareness questionnaire survey, the findings of which revealed a lack of understanding of antimicrobials and AMR among participants (WHO 2015a). Not only the community members but health professionals have also shown poor awareness regarding AMR. Furthermore, the introduction of antimicrobial agents and resistance in the school curriculum is mentioned under the first aim, which will facilitate greater knowledge and awareness from a young age. However, there has yet to be a meaningful proof of concept implementation. Hence, the authors are keen to emphasize it because the advancement of this goal is so crucial.

As a second objective; effective surveillance and research will be used to improve the knowledge and evidence regarding AMR to fill the knowledge gap. Moreover, AMR incidence, prevalence, range among pathogens, and spatial variations must all be investigated. Research and surveillance priority must be given to LMIC because it is identified as a hotspot of AMR. The identification of novel emerging AMR pathogens in this region may be underreported due to financial and research facility constraints. As a result, significant policy implications should be made to address the problem.

When it concerns AMR, prevention is preferable to cure the infection. They have established their third objective in tandem with this approach; reduce the spread of AMR infection by implementing appropriate sanitation, hygiene, and infection-prevention strategies such as immunization.

Antimicrobial drug utilization in human and animal health should be optimized since it has been established as one of the primary factors of the emergence of AMR. This factor was considered in the fourth objective. The WHO has established recommendations for the use of antibiotics in hospitals in order to ensure that they are used appropriately. Furthermore, they have divided human medically relevant antimicrobials into three categories: critically important antimicrobials, highly important antimicrobials, and important antimicrobials. The critically important antimicrobials are further split into two subcategories: highest priority critically important and high priority critically important (WHO 2016) (Table 22.2).

On the other hand, they have published protocols to use antibiotics in food-producing animals. The necessity to reduce the negative human health implications of using medically important antimicrobials in food-producing animals prompted the creation of these guidelines (WHO 2017). The first recommendation they propose is that all classes of medically important antimicrobials be used less often in food-producing animals. Their second recommendation is to ban the use of all classes of medically important antimicrobials in food-producing animals

Table 22.2 Categorization of human medically relevant antimicrobials.

Group	Antimicrobial class	Examples of antimicrobial
Critically important antimicrobials	**Highest priority critically important**	
	Cephalosporins (third,fourth, and fifth generation)	Ceftriaxone, cefepime, cefazoline, ceftobiprole
	Glycopeptides	Vancomycin
	Macrolides and ketolides	Azithromycin, erythromycin, telithromycin
	Polymyxins	Colistin
	Quinolones	Ciprofloxacin
	High priority critically important	
	Aminoglycosides	Gentamicin
	Ansamycins	Rifampicin
	Carbapenems and other penems	Meropenem
	Glycyclines	Tigecycline
	Lipopeptides	Daptomycin
	Monobactams	Aztreonam
	Penicillins (antipseudomonal, aminopenicillin, aminopenicillin with β-lactamase inhibitors)	Ampicillin, amoxicillin, amoxicillin-clavulanic acid
Highly important antimicrobials	Amphenicols	Chloramphenicol, thiamphenicol
	Cephalosporins (first and second generation)	Cefazolin
	Lincosamides	Clindamycin
	Penicillin (aminopenicillins, anti-staphylococcal, narrow spectrum)	Mecillinam, flucloxacillin, benzathine-benzylpenicillin
	Pseudomonic acids	Mupirocin
	Riminofenazines	Clofazimine
	Steroid antibacterials	Fusidic acid
	Streptogramins	Guinupristin
	Sulfonamides	Sulfamethoxazole
	Sulfones	Dapsone
	Tetracyclines	Chlortetracycline
Important antimicrobials	Aminocyclitols	Spectinomycin
	Cyclic polypeptides	Bacitracin
	Nitrofuran derivatives	Nitrofurantoin
	Nitroimidazoles	Metronidazole
	Pleuromutilins	Retapamulin

Source: Adapted from WHO (2016).

for the purpose of growth promotion. In addition to that, all classes of medically important antimicrobials should not be used in food-producing animals as a prophylactic treatment to prevent infectious diseases that have not yet been clinically confirmed is mentioned as their third recommendation. Fourth recommendation is regarding uses of antimicrobials that are categorized as critically important and high priority antimicrobials for human medicine. Furthermore, critically important antimicrobials should not be used to prevent infections in livestock animals, and high priority antimicrobials should not be used to treat livestock animals that have been diagnosed with an infectious disease. Many governments have established laws and regulations that make it more difficult to use animal growth promoters as well as prophylactic treatments as a result of these recommendations. However, due to insufficient surveillance, unauthorized usage may still occur.

Last but not least, increasing investment in novel medicines, diagnostic tools, vaccinations, and other treatments by developing an economic rationale for a long-term investment that considers the needs of all countries is a timely needed goal. This will also take into account the WHO while implementing the action plan.

22.7.2 Tripartite (WHO, FAO, and OIE Working Together)

To combat the threat posed by AMR, international multisectoral partnerships are an urgently needed step. Furthermore, such cooperation will avoid individual efforts from overlapping, and collaborative efforts will aid in having a large impact on tackling the problem that has arisen globally. For example, the AMR Multi-Partner Trust Fund supports the long-standing tripartite partnership between FAO, OIE, and WHO to tackle the expanding global challenge of AMR. Moreover, the WHO/UN Interagency Coordination Group on AMR (IACG) has provided their recommendation to tackle AMR through One Health lens (IACG 2019).

Knowledge and understanding of socioeconomic and legal aspect of AMR is still poorly understood. Hence, to close this knowledge gap, more research is urgently required.

22.8 Constraints in Implementing One Health Approach

In the human and animal health sectors, poor data quality and a lack of AMR data are major obstacles to reliable comparisons between human and livestock populations, as well as between countries and regions. Therefore, proper surveillance methods are timely. Multisectoral collaboration is very important. However, to establish successful multisectoral collaboration, all relevant sectors must develop trust, transparency, equal representation, and consensus. Otherwise, it will lead to a misunderstanding among partners. Evidence suggests that antibiotic usage and misuse are linked to larger sociocultural and sociodemographic determinants. Therefore, strategic plan should concern all sociodemographic level in the society.

22.9 Conclusion

Besides the huge demand for new antibiotics in both human and animal clinical settings, introducing them into the market is negligible mainly due to two reasons: (i) discovering and releasing antibiotics into the market is often not economical for private drug manufacturers and (ii) developing new antibiotics has become harder since bacteria have evolved additional methods to escape antibiotics within a short period when they began to be used in therapeutic contexts. The last fully novel antibiotic class was discovered in the late 1980s.

With preceding limitations there is an urgent need to safeguard the usage of existing antimicrobials and the collective actions of the members of the One Health sectors. Ultimately it is imperative to ensure that action plans, policies, and regulations are implemented without delay.

References

Abraham, E.P. and Chain, E. (1940). An enzyme from bacteria able to destroy penicillin. *Nature* 146: 837–837.

Alawi, M., Torrijos, T.V., and Walsh, F. (2022). Plasmid-mediated antimicrobial resistance in drinking water. *Environmental Advances* 8: 100191.

Al-Harbi, H., Ranjbar, S., Moore, R.J., and Alawneh, J.I. (2021). Bacteria isolated from milk of dairy cows with and without clinical mastitis in different regions of Australia and their AMR profiles. *Frontiers in Veterinary Science* 8: 743725.

Allcock, S., Young, E., Holmes, M. et al. (2017). Antimicrobial resistance in human populations: challenges and opportunities. *Global Health, Epidemiology and Genomics* 2: e4.

Amoafo, O.Y., Malekar, V., Jones, E., and On, S.L. (2022). Antibiotic resistance and phylogenetic profiling of *Escherichia coli* from dairy farm soils; organic versus conventional systems. *Current Research in Microbial Sciences* 3: 100088.

Antonoplis, A., Zang, X., Wegner, T. et al. (2019). Vancomycin–arginine conjugate inhibits growth of carbapenem-resistant *E. coli* and targets cell-wall synthesis. *ACS Chemical Biology* 14: 2065–2070.

Armalytė, J., Skerniškytė, J., Bakienė, E. et al. (2019). Microbial diversity and antimicrobial resistance profile in microbiota from soils of conventional and organic farming systems. *Frontiers in Microbiology* 10: 892.

Authority, E. F. S., Prevention, E. C. F. D. & Control (2021). The European Union summary report on antimicrobial resistance in zoonotic and indicator bacteria from humans, animals and food in 2018/2019. *EFSA Journal* 19: e06490.

Ayukekbong, J.A., Ntemgwa, M., and Atabe, A.N. (2017). The threat of antimicrobial resistance in developing countries: causes and control strategies. *Antimicrobial Resistance and Infection Control* 6: 1–8.

Bamunusinghage, N., Neelawala, R., Magedara, H. et al. (2022). Antimicrobial resistance patterns of fecal *Escherichia coli* in wildlife, urban wildlife and livestock in Eastern region of Sri Lanka and their differences between carnivores, omnivores and herbivores. *Journal of Wildlife Diseases* 58 (2): 380–383.

Brealey, J.C., Leitão, H.G., Hofstede, T. et al. (2021). The oral microbiota of wild bears in Sweden reflects the history of antibiotic use by humans. *Current Biology* 31: 4650–4658. e6.

Bush, K. and Bradford, P.A. (2016). β-Lactams and β-lactamase inhibitors: an overview. *Cold Spring Harbor Perspectives in Medicine* 6: a025247.

Cahill, S.M., Desmarchelier, P., Fattori, V. et al. (2017). Global perspectives on antimicrobial resistance in the food chain. *Food Protection Trends* 37: 353–360.

Capita, R., Vicente-Velasco, M., Rodríguez-Melcón, C. et al. (2019). Effect of low doses of biocides on the antimicrobial resistance and the biofilms of cronobacter sakazakii and yersinia enterocolitica. *Scientific Reports* 9: 1–12.

CDC (2019). 2019 AR Threats Report.

CDC (2022). https://www.cdc.gov/onehealth/basics/index.html (accessed 14 March 2020)

Chattopadhyay, M.K. (2014). Use of antibiotics as feed additives: a burning question. *Frontiers in Microbiology* 5: 334.

Chibabhai, V., Duse, A., Perovic, O., and Richards, G. (2020). Collateral damage of the COVID-19 pandemic: exacerbation of antimicrobial resistance and disruptions to antimicrobial stewardship programmes? *South African Medical Journal* 110: 572–573.

Davies, R. and Wales, A. (2019). Antimicrobial resistance on farms: a review including biosecurity and the potential role of disinfectants in resistance selection. *Comprehensive Reviews in Food Science and Food Safety* 18: 753–774.

Dhanapala, P.M., Kalupahana, R.S., Kalupahana, A.W. et al. (2021). Characterization and antimicrobial resistance of environmental and clinical aeromonas species isolated from fresh water ornamental fish and associated farming environment in Sri Lanka. *Microorganisms* 9: 2106.

Dos Santos Alves, T., Lara, G.H.B., Maluta, R.P. et al. (2018). Carrier flies of multidrug-resistant *Escherichia coli* as potential dissemination agent in dairy farm environment. *Science of the Total Environment* 633: 1345–1351.

Fillol-Salom, A., Alsaadi, A., Sousa, J.A.M.D. et al. (2019). Bacteriophages benefit from generalized transduction. *PLoS Pathogens* 15: e1007888.

Fletcher, S. (2015). Understanding the contribution of environmental factors in the spread of antimicrobial resistance. *Environmental Health and Preventive Medicine* 20: 243–252.

Founou, L.L., Founou, R.C., and Essack, S.Y. (2016). Antibiotic resistance in the food chain: a developing country-perspective. *Frontiers in Microbiology* 7: 1881.

Fouz, N., Pangesti, K.N., Yasir, M. et al. (2020). The contribution of wastewater to the transmission of antimicrobial resistance in the environment: implications of mass gathering settings. *Tropical Medicine and Infectious Disease* 5: 33.

Galarce, N., Arriagada, G., Sánchez, F. et al. (2021). Antimicrobial use in companion animals: assessing veterinarians' prescription patterns through the first national survey in Chile. *Animals* 11: 348.

Guo, X., Akram, S., Stedtfeld, R. et al. (2021). Distribution of antimicrobial resistance across the overall environment of dairy farms–A case study. *Science of the Total Environment* 788: 147489.

Gwenzi, W., Chaukura, N., Muisa-Zikali, N. et al. (2021). Insects, rodents, and pets as reservoirs, vectors, and sentinels of antimicrobial resistance. *Antibiotics* 10: 68.

He, Y., Yuan, Q., Mathieu, J. et al. (2020). Antibiotic resistance genes from livestock waste: occurrence, dissemination, and treatment. *NPJ Clean Water* 3: 1–11.

Holmes, A.H., Moore, L.S., Sundsfjord, A. et al. (2016). Understanding the mechanisms and drivers of antimicrobial resistance. *The Lancet* 387: 176–187.

Hooper, D.C. and Jacoby, G.A. (2015). Mechanisms of drug resistance: quinolone resistance. *Annals of the New York Academy of Sciences* 1354: 12–31.

Huemer, M., Mairpady Shambat, S., Brugger, S.D., and Zinkernagel, A.S. (2020). Antibiotic resistance and persistence – implications for human health and treatment perspectives. *EMBO Reports* 21: e51034.

Hutchings, M.I., Truman, A.W., and Wilkinson, B. (2019). Antibiotics: past, present and future. *Current Opinion in Microbiology* 51: 72–80.

IACG (2019). No Time to Wait-Securing the Future from Drug-Resistant Infections. Report to the Secretary General of the Nations.

Ibrahim, M., Ahmad, F., Yaqub, B. et al. (2020). Current trends of antimicrobials used in food animals and aquaculture. In: *Antibiotics and Antimicrobial Resistance Genes in the Environment* (ed. M.Z. Hashmi), 39–69. Elsevier.

James, C., Dixon, R., Talbot, L. et al. (2021). Assessing the impact of heat treatment of food on antimicrobial resistance genes and their potential uptake by other bacteria – a critical review. *Antibiotics* 10: 1440.

Jans, C., Sarno, E., Collineau, L. et al. (2018). Consumer exposure to antimicrobial resistant bacteria from food at Swiss retail level. *Frontiers in Microbiology* 9: 362.

Karp, B.E., Tate, H., Plumblee, J.R. et al. (2017). National antimicrobial resistance monitoring system: two decades of advancing public health through integrated surveillance of antimicrobial resistance. *Foodborne Pathogens and Disease* 14: 545–557.

Kaur, R., Yadav, B., and Tyagi, R. (2020). Microbiology of hospital wastewater. In: *Current Developments in Biotechnology and Bioengineering* (ed. R.D. Tyagi, B. Sellamuthu, B. Tiwari, et al.), 103–148. Elsevier.

Lagerstrom, K.M. and Hadly, E.A. (2021). The under-investigated wild side of *Escherichia coli*: genetic diversity, pathogenicity and antimicrobial resistance in wild animals. *Proceedings of the Royal Society B* 288: 20210399.

Lerminiaux, N.A. and Cameron, A.D. (2019). Horizontal transfer of antibiotic resistance genes in clinical environments. *Canadian Journal of Microbiology* 65: 34–44.

Li, Y., Chen, Q., Zhao, J. et al. (2014). Isolation, identification and antimicrobial resistance of Cronobacter spp. isolated from various foods in China. *Food Control* 37: 109–114.

Loudermilk, E.M., Kotay, S.M., Barry, K.E. et al. (2022). Tracking klebsiella pneumoniae carbapenemase gene as an indicator of antimicrobial resistance dissemination from a hospital to surface water via a municipal wastewater treatment plant. *Water Research* 213: 118151.

Manyi-Loh, C., Mamphweli, S., Meyer, E., and Okoh, A. (2018). Antibiotic use in agriculture and its consequential resistance in environmental sources: potential public health implications. *Molecules* 23: 795.

Mateus, A., Takahashi, E., Elkholly, D. et al. (2016). *A Systematic Review of AMR Bacteria in Pork, Poultry, Dairy Products, Seafood and Fresh Produce at UK Retail Level.* Food Standards Agency.

Michael, C.A., Dominey-Howes, D., and Labbate, M. (2014). The antimicrobial resistance crisis: causes, consequences, and management. *Frontiers in Public Health* 2: 145.

Monger, X.C., Gilbert, A.-A., Saucier, L., and Vincent, A.T. (2021). Antibiotic resistance: from pig to meat. *Antibiotics* 10: 1209.

Nadimpalli, M.L., Marks, S.J., Montealegre, M.C. et al. (2020). Urban informal settlements as hotspots of antimicrobial resistance and the need to curb environmental transmission. *Nature Microbiology* 5: 787–795.

Neyra, R.C., Vegosen, L., Davis, M.F. et al. (2012). Antimicrobial-resistant bacteria: an unrecognized work-related risk in food animal production. *Safety and Health at Work* 3: 85–91.

Ngogang, M.P., Ernest, T., Kariuki, J. et al. (2020). Microbial contamination of chicken litter manure and antimicrobial resistance threat in an urban area setting in Cameroon. *Antibiotics* 10: 20.

Nhung, N., Cuong, N., Campbell, J. et al. (2015). High levels of antimicrobial resistance among *Escherichia coli* isolates from livestock farms and synanthropic rats and shrews in the Mekong Delta of Vietnam. *Applied and Environmental Microbiology* 81: 812–820.

OIE (2022) Antimicrobial resistance. https://www.oie.int/en/what-we-do/global-initiatives/antimicrobial-resistance (accessed 13 March 2022).

Olsen, M., Campos, M., Lohning, A. et al. (2020). Mobile phones represent a pathway for microbial transmission: a scoping review. *Travel Medicine and Infectious Disease* 35: 101704.

Osińska, A., Korzeniewska, E., Harnisz, M. et al. (2020). Small-scale wastewater treatment plants as a source of the dissemination of antibiotic resistance genes in the aquatic environment. *Journal of Hazardous Materials* 381: 121221.

Pandra, S.B., Otilia, D., Banji, J. et al. (2010). Antibiotic resistance: overview and mechanisms. *International Journal of Pharmaceutical Sciences and Research* 1: 17–27.

Peterson, E. and Kaur, P. (2018). Antibiotic resistance mechanisms in bacteria: relationships between resistance determinants of antibiotic producers, environmental bacteria, and clinical pathogens. *Frontiers in Microbiology* 9: 2928.

Prestinaci, F., Pezzotti, P., and Pantosti, A. (2015). Antimicrobial resistance: a global multifaceted phenomenon. *Pathogens and Global Health* 109: 309–318.

Purssell, E. (2020). Antimicrobials. In: *Understanding Pharmacology in Nursing Practice* (ed. P. Hood and E. Khan), 147–165. Springer.

Sah, S.K. and Hemalatha, S. (2015). Extended spectrum beta lactamase (ESBL) mechanism of antibiotic resistance and epidemiology. *International Journal of Pharmtech Reserach* 7: 303–309.

Scott, H.M., Acuff, G., Bergeron, G. et al. (2019). Critically important antibiotics: criteria and approaches for measuring and reducing their use in food animal agriculture. *Annals of the New York Academy of Sciences* 1441: 8–16.

Seitz, P. and Blokesch, M. (2013). Cues and regulatory pathways involved in natural competence and transformation in pathogenic and environmental Gram-negative bacteria. *FEMS Microbiology Reviews* 37: 336–363.

Stanaway, J.D., Reiner, R.C., Blacker, B.F. et al. (2019). The global burden of typhoid and paratyphoid fevers: a systematic analysis for the Global Burden of Disease Study 2017. *The Lancet Infectious Diseases* 19: 369–381.

Thanner, S., Drissner, D., and Walsh, F. (2016). Antimicrobial resistance in agriculture. *MBio* 7: e02227–e02215.

Ventola, C.L. (2015). The antibiotic resistance crisis: part 1: causes and threats. *Pharmacy and Therapeutics* 40: 277.

Vestergaard, M., Frees, D., and Ingmer, H. (2019). Antibiotic resistance and the MRSA problem. *Microbiology Spectrum* 7: 7–2.

Vikesland, P., Garner, E., Gupta, S. et al. (2019). Differential drivers of antimicrobial resistance across the world. *Accounts of Chemical Research* 52: 916–924.

Virolle, C., Goldlust, K., Djermoun, S. et al. (2020). Plasmid transfer by conjugation in Gram-negative bacteria: from the cellular to the community level. *Genes* 11: 1239.

Vittecoq, M., Godreuil, S., Prugnolle, F. et al. (2016). Antimicrobial resistance in wildlife. *Journal of Applied Ecology* 53: 519–529.

WHO (2015a). Antibiotic Resistance: Multi-Country Public Awareness Survey.

WHO (2015b). Global Action Plan on Antimicrobial Resistance. WHO Report.

WHO (2016). Critically important antimicrobials for human medicine. https://apps.who.int/iris/bitstream/handle/10665/312266/9789241515528-eng.pdf (accessed 13 March 2022).

WHO (2017). *WHO Guidelines on Use of Medically Important Antimicrobials in Food-Producing Animals: Web Annex A: Evidence Base*. World Health Organization.

von Wintersdorff, C.J., Penders, J., van Niekerk, J.M. et al. (2016). Dissemination of antimicrobial resistance in microbial ecosystems through horizontal gene transfer. *Frontiers in Microbiology* 7: 173.

Yuan, Y., Liang, B., Jiang, B. et al. (2021). Migratory wild birds carrying multidrug-resistant Escherichia coli as potential transmitters of antimicrobial resistance in China. *PLoS One*. 10.1371/journal.pone.0261444.

23

Eco-epidemiology of Tick-Borne Pathogens

Role of Tick Vectors and Host Animal Community Composition in Their Circulation and Source of Infections

Rupika S. Rajakaruna[1] *and Marina E. Eremeeva*[2]

[1] *Department of Zoology, University of Peradeniya, Peradeniya, Sri Lanka*
[2] *Jiann-Ping Hsu College of Public Health, Georgia Southern University, Statesboro, GA, USA*

23.1 General Features of Tick Biology

23.1.1 Ticks as Ectoparasites

Ticks are hematophagous ectoparasites of terrestrial vertebrates. They may impact their animal host in two ways: directly by sucking an excessive volume of blood and indirectly by transmitting and maintaining a variety of disease-causing pathogens. In 2010, Guglielmone et al. listed 896 valid species of ticks, some of which are distributed globally in warm and moist climates (Guglielmone et al. 2010). There are many genera and species of ticks in the family Ixodidae (hard ticks) and Argasidae (soft ticks) that are of public health and veterinary importance. Both soft and hard ticks feed on their hosts for only a short period of time compared to the duration of their life cycle. They both can have long off-host periods during which their survival depends greatly on their ability to cope with environmental conditions. Soft ticks have remarkable longevity and an ability to withstand starvation for many years (some up to 18 years) without a blood meal (Sonenshine 1993; Sonenshine and Roe 2013).

Ticks infest a wide range of vertebrate species, while humans are typically only an accidental host (except for some soft tick pathogens), which can be attacked by some questing ticks when entering in tick-infested habitats. Views on host specialization by ticks have evolved. Early research based on tick morphology (Hoogstraal and Aeschlimann 1982) proposed that most tick species and stages were specialists, but later work suggested that ticks can often be generalists who will feed on a variety of locally available hosts (Cumming 1999). Moreover, McCoy et al. (2013) re-evaluated the spatial and temporal scales of host use and found evidence supporting both views. Most tick species have the potential to feed on a wide range of phylogenetically diverse host species that share the same ecological habitats but may have preferences dictated by host availability and habitat seasonality (Krasnov et al. 2010; McCoy et al. 2013).

23.1.2 Tick Life Cycle

The life cycle of all ticks has four phases: eggs and three active parasitic stages (larva, nymph, and the adult stages, male and female). Except for the eggs, ticks need a blood meal during each stage of their life, when they may acquire microbes from infected hosts and/or transmit them to naïve hosts. Ixodid (hard) ticks have a single nymph stage, while the number of nymphal instars in argasid (soft) ticks is always more than one and varies from two to eight depending on species and temperature and degree of engorgement during previous stages or instars.

Four different life cycle patterns have been described for ticks: one, two, three, and multi-host cycles. Ixodid ticks undergo either one-, two-, or three-host life cycles (Figure 23.1).

During the one-host life cycle, ticks remain on the same host for the larval, nymphal, and adult stages, only leaving the host prior to laying eggs. A few ixodid ticks of public health importance have this life cycle; one example is the cattle tick, *Rhipicephalus annulatus*, which may be infected with *Babesia bigemina*, *Babesia bovis*, and/or *Anaplasma marginale*. During the two-host life cycle, larval feeding, molting, and nymphal feeding occur on one host and then engorged nymphs drop off and molt in the natural environment into adults, which will feed and mate on a second host. *Hyalomma marginatum*, a vector of Crimean–Congo viral hemorrhagic fever, is an example of an ixodid tick with a two-host cycle. Its immatures prefer to feed on small mammals (lagomorphs and insectivores) or ground-foraging

One Health: Human, Animal, and Environment Triad, First Edition. Edited by Meththika Vithanage and Majeti Narasimha Vara Prasad.

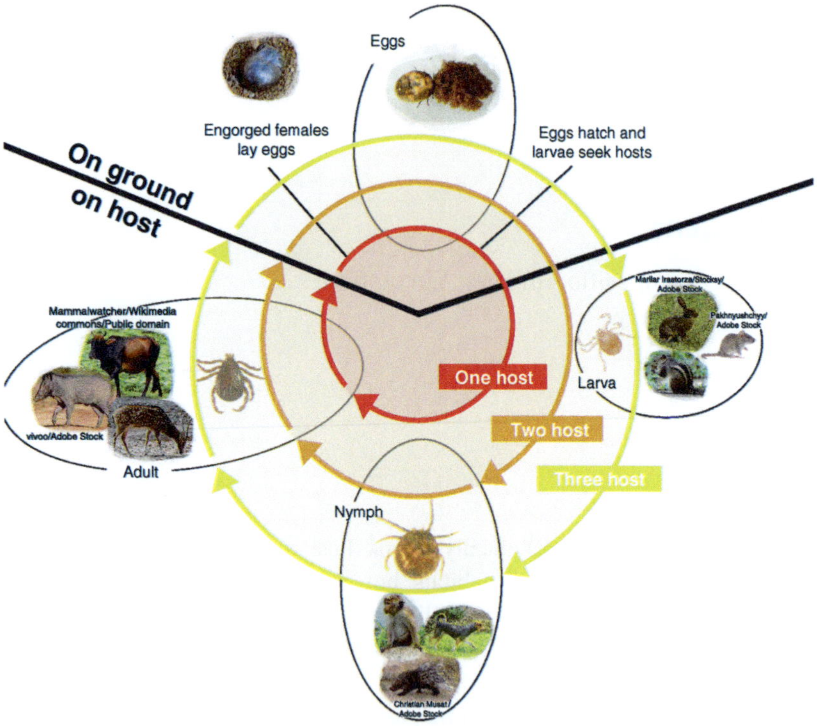

Figure 23.1 A generalized life cycle of ixodid ticks. Ticks with a one-host life cycle remain on the same host for the larval, nymphal, and adult stages, with only gravid females leaving the host prior to laying eggs. Ticks with a two-host life cycle: the larva molts to nymph on the first host but engorged nymphs will drop off the host to molt into adults. The second host may be the same animal as the first host, the same species, or a different animal species. Ticks with three-host life cycle: the engorged larvae, nymphs, and gravid females drop of the host after their blood meals; hosts may be the same species, or even the same individual, or three different animal species depending on host availability. Humans may serve as incidental first, second, or third stage hosts.

birds, while adults feed on large animals. Most ticks of public health importance have a three-host life cycle, which can span three years; however, it may be completed more quickly depending on environmental conditions. Questing larvae attach to the first host, feed to repletion, and drop off to molt into nymphs. The nymphs quest for a second host, the same or a different species, and then feed and drop off to molt to adults. The adults find the third host, mate and feed, and drop off to lay eggs and die.

Humans may serve as incidental first, second, or third stage hosts and, respectively, become infected depending on the nature of the tick-borne pathogen (TBP) vectored by a particular species of the tick and agent susceptibility of animal hosts. These multi-host ticks belong to the genera *Amblyomma*, *Dermacentor*, *Ixodes*, *Haemaphysalis*, *Hyalomma*, and *Rhipicephalus*, and they transmit diversity of bacterial, parasitic, and viral agents.

Members of the family Argasidae undergo a multi-host life cycle with two or more nymphal stages, each requiring a blood meal from a host. Unlike ixodid ticks, which stay attached to their hosts for up to several days while feeding, argasid ticks are adapted to feeding rapidly (about an hour) and then drop off. Adults of the majority argasid ticks can feed up to six times and females oviposit after each blood meal; however, the number of eggs in each cluster is no more than several hundred compared to the thousands of eggs laid by ixodid females. As an example, argasid ticks from the genera *Ornithodoros* are vectors of tick-borne relapsing fever spirochetes (Herms and Wheeler 1936).

The tick life cycles are dictated by seasonal events, especially in the temperate regions. Sonenshine and Roe (2013) explain how the length of life cycles may vary as a result of the complex interplay among photoperiod, temperature, moisture, and availability of suitable hosts and mates, acting on the genetic variability of each species. Photoperiodicity influences the seasonal adaptations of ticks, as it entrains their circadian rhythms for host seeking, feeding, drop-off, and oviposition. Moreover, seasonal rhythms ensure that critical activities of ticks are synchronized with appropriate climatic conditions, and this adaptation is mediated via diapause that may occur in any or all stages of the tick life cycle. Ticks take large blood meals of about 200–600 times their unfed bodyweight (Sonenshine 1991). This flow permits pathogens to migrate from the host feeding site to the tick's midgut, and subsequently to invade the reproductive organs (ovary) and salivary glands so the tick can become a competent vector for particular microbe (Dantas-Torres and Otranto 2016).

23.1.3 Tick-Borne Infections (TBIs) and Tick-Borne Pathogens

Among the arthropod vectors of diseases, ticks are second only to the mosquitoes in carrying the etiological agents of human diseases (Sonenshine and Roe 2013); however, overall ticks transmit the most diverse array of infectious agents when all human and domestic animal diseases are considered (Jongejan and Uilenberg 2004; Colwell et al. 2011; Pfäffle et al. 2013). As many as 808 tick–pathogen associations that are of medical and/or veterinary significance have been identified (Jongejan and Uilenberg 2004; Nijhof et al. 2005), and this inventory is continuously growing. On the global scale, these are mainly caused by pathogenic bacteria, viruses, and protozoans. Among them, diverse tick-borne bacterial infections are caused by *Anaplasma* (anaplasmoses), *Borrelia* (Lyme disease), *Rickettsia* (rickettsioses), and *Ehrlichia* (ehrlichioses); viral infections include tick-borne encephalitis and Crimean–Congo hemorrhagic fever, and protozoan infections are due to different species of *Babesia* (babesiosis) and *Theileria* (theileriosis).

Transmission of these pathogens between or in ticks may occur in various ways, including cofeeding, trans-stadial (horizontal transmission, from one developing stage to another stage; e.g. larva to nymph or nymph to adult), sexual, and transovarial transmission (vertical transmission, female ovaries to eggs). Although the relative importance of these modes to the evolutionary success of each agent is not well understood, their efficiency may be defined by host genetics, physiology, or environmental conditions as well as agent-specific factors (Rochlin and Toledo 2020). Examples of trans-stadially transmitted microorganisms are *Theileria, Borrelia*, and *Ehrlichia*; transovarially transmitted pathogens include Nairobi sheep virus; and various species of *Rickettsia* and *Babesia* can be transmitted by both trans-stadial and transovarial mechanisms (Hauck et al. 2020). Furthermore, Sambado et al. (2020) reported that all three feeding stages of *Ixodes pacificus* can carry *Borellia miyamotoi* and the prevalence of infection increases with each life stage. Their data indicate that in western United States, *B. miyamotoi* is maintained in natural populations by both transovarial transmission and transmission from blood meal hosts and that synchronous phenology of juvenile stages of *I. pacificus* may facilitate the transmission dynamics of *B. miyamotoi* and other vertically transmitted, vector-borne pathogens.

Globally, the frequency and severity of infectious disease outbreaks in humans, wildlife, and domesticated animals are increasing (Jones et al. 2008). Since 1990's much attention has been paid to laboratory and field studies of TBIs, but their incidence continues to rise. Some of this increase is due to the recognition of new agents in new sites (Parola et al. 2005, 2013; Szabo et al. 2013); their varied pathogenicity and epidemiological attributes present new surveillance challenges to the medical and public health communities (Parola et al. 2013). Among the contributing factors that may have affected this increase are ecological factors particularly those driven by climate change, human population increases, and behavioral aspects of recreational activities and nature tourism (Obsomer et al. 2013; Ogden et al. 2013). Increases in human outdoor activities underlie the increased contacts with tick vectors necessary for emergence of TBIs (Jongejan and Uilenberg 2004). A better understanding of the interactions between animal reservoirs and agents of TBIs with tick vectors in different ecological settings (eco-epidemiology) will be necessary to improve surveillance, and to evaluate disease risk and prevent future outbreaks.

23.2 Ecological Factors Affecting Tick-Borne Agents

23.2.1 Reservoirs of TBIs: Domestic and Sylvatic Cycles

Ticks and their pathogens coevolved with various wild reservoirs and often exist in a state of equilibrium consisting of a natural cycle involving wild or peridomestic vertebrates and their ticks (Ostfeld et al. 2014). The enzootic cyclic stability of transmission in the wild can easily change to the unstable epizootic transmission through human alterations of habitat by urbanization and agricultural interactions enhanced by increased stocks of domestic animals (Ogden et al. 2013). Ticks inhabit many natural landscapes, but landscape changes can cause them to spread to new areas. When domestic and livestock animals share feeding grounds or grazing pastures with peridomestic or wild animals, ticks and TBPs can be introduced to those domestic animals and through those sources to humans. Although wild animals typically do not exhibit marked clinical disease unless they are immune compromised or in stressed conditions, humans and domestic animals can exhibit clinical disease when bitten by infected ticks or by coming into contact with infected animal tissues or blood. Tick infestations and TBIs of pets and livestock are a major health concern, globally (Millan et al. 2016; Tabor et al. 2018; Cicculli et al. 2019; Weaver et al. 2022). Moreover, companion animals like dogs and cats infested with ticks can play a significant role in human exposure to TBPs (Maia et al. 2014, 2015).

There are many factors affecting the emergence of zoonotic TBIs and their continuing circulation in sylvatic cycles so most are not understood completely. Identifying potential sylvatic reservoirs and their ecological characteristics are important to identify regions that could be vulnerable to outbreaks (Ostfeld et al. 2014). Among the vertebrate hosts, the non-volant small mammals are the most important hosts for the subadult stages (larva and nymph) of many tick species. Small mammals have high metabolic and reproductive rates with relatively large body surfaces compared to their body weights; they can be present in high densities in the natural as well as domestic and peri-domestic habitats and are therefore suitable hosts for ticks and essential reservoirs for many TBPs (Ostfeld et al. 2014). Birds play an important role in the ecology of TBI globally. In a quantitative review of the role of birds in carrying ticks and TBPs, Loss et al. (2016) gave a very comprehensive account of interactions between avian foraging and migratory strategies; these, in turn, can influence the prevalence and intensity of TBIs. Birds are involved in not only local transmission of TBIs but also long-distance dispersal of pathogens (Loss et al. 2016).

Infection risk to humans is determined by the population of reservoir-competent animal species and the local density of the tick population. As this can be seasonal, varying from month to month or year to year, it is not easy to accurately predict the level of infection risk in a specific geographic location (Lewis et al. 2021).

23.2.2 Biodiversity and the Dilution Effect Model

Higher biodiversity resulting in lower human disease risk has been termed "the Dilution Effect." Ostfeld and Keesing (2000) were among the first to describe the dilution effect model using a TBI as an example. They hypothesized that Lyme disease risk for humans in North America was reduced where there is higher host species richness and evenness (Ostfeld and Keesing 2000; Schmidt and Ostfeld 2001). Lyme disease agent *Borrelia burgdoferri* is mainly transmitted by the ixodid tick, *Ixodes scapularis*, and the main reservoir for this spirochete is the white-footed mouse, *Peromyscus leucopus*. According to Ostfeld and Keesing (2000) when the biodiversity of the reservoir host community of a pathogen like *Borrelia* is high, there is expected to be a reduction in tick infection of the preferred host reservoir; pathogen transmission is frequency dependent as there are more "wasted" bites on non-competent hosts such as humans and particularly non-productive animal hosts. Hawlena et al. (2012) reported that the pathogen community composition of ticks varies with the tick life stage but less so for vertically transmitted pathogens. Many studies have investigated the interactions between pathogen transmission, disease risk, and biodiversity due to increased deforestation and environmental degradation (Levy 2013; Salkeld et al. 2013; Pfaeffle et al. 2015; Hartemink and Takken 2016); these are probably the primary ecological factors that drive pathogen eco-epidemiological dynamics and disease emergence or re-emergence (Rogalski et al. 2017). On the contrary to the "Dilution Effect Model," some argue that pristine natural areas with high biodiversity have been considered as likely sources of new zoonotic pathogens, suggesting that such high biodiversity could negatively impact human health as a source of emerging disease agents (Jones et al. 2008; Wood et al. 2017). These are obviously conflicting ideas but even a few new agents could have drastic effects, as seen with coronaviruses. Consequently, Keesing and Ostfeld (2021) in a new analysis showed that some taxa are more likely to be zoonotic hosts, and if these animals are common in human-dominated habitats, then these scenarios may result in increased likelihood of host spillovers. They also showed that in less-disturbed areas these zoonotic reservoir hosts are less abundant and non-reservoirs predominate; therefore, loss of biodiversity appears to increase the risk of human disease due to both new and established pathogens.

Wild animals that are adapted to urban and peri-urban areas can serve as tick-maintenance hosts as well as reservoirs of TBPs (Niemelä 2011; Pfäffle et al. 2013). Spillovers from wildlife into humans is more likely to occur in fragmented forests and in public parks, gardens, peri-urban leisure areas, and cemeteries where humans and domestic animals can encounter potentially infected questing ticks (Ginsberg and Faulde 2008). In peri-urban areas in Europe, there are rodents (mice, voles, dormice, squirrels, and rats), hedgehogs, shrews, birds, lizards, and companion animals (dogs and cats), but also medium-sized and larger mammals like foxes, roe deer, and wild boars. The larger animals play the major role as tick-maintenance hosts and reservoirs of TBPs because they can harbor very large numbers of ticks (Dautel et al. 1991; Dauntel and Khal 1999; Pfäffle et al. 2013). Urbanization leads to increased contacts of humans and companion animals with nature and contributes to changing epidemiological and epizootiological conditions in those urban and peri-urban areas (Neiderud 2015).

23.3 Ticks and Tick-Transmitted Pathogens in the United States

23.3.1 Ticks are the Most Prevalent Sources of Vector-Borne Infections in the United States

Tick-borne infectious agents currently recognized in the United States are summarized in Table 23.1; this table also contains information pertinent to their specific vectors and animal reservoirs as well as the known impact of these pathogens on pets and companion animals, livestock, and wild animals. At least 90 tick species are known in the United States; however, just two tick species, *I. scapularis* and *Amblyomma americanum*, carry the largest number of pathogens responsible for human and veterinary diseases (Eisen et al. 2017; Eisen and Paddock 2021). It is important

Table 23.1 Tick-borne diseases of public health and veterinary significance in the United States.

			Vertebrate Impact					
Disease	**Agent**	**Tick**	**Humans**	**Dogs**	**Cats**	**Horses**	**Livestock**	**Wild animals**
Lyme disease	*B. burgdorferi* *B. mayonii*	*I. scapularis* *I. pacificus*	• Acute febrile illness • Arthritis, carditis, meningitis, and neuritis in late untreated cases • Post-treatment Lyme disease syndrome	• Susceptible to *Borrelia burgdorferi* • 5–10% exposed dogs develop clinical borreliosis • Manifests as self-limiting polyarthritis	• Seroconvert to *Borrelia burgdorferi* • No documented cases of clinical disease	• Rare • Broad spectrum of clinical symptoms	• Uncommon • Occurs as a herd problem	• White-tailed deer host for adult ticks • Competent larval hosts for *B. burgdorferi*: – white-footed mice, shrews, chipmunks, tree squirrels, and woodrats
Rocky Mountain spotted fever	*R. rickettsii*	*D. andersoni* *D. variabilis* *R. sanguineus* *A. canjennese* *H. leporispalustris*	• Acute febrile illness • 12.5–73.3% fatality	• Acute febrile illness • Asymptomatic persisting rickettsiemia	Unknown	• Seroconversion without acute infection	Unknown	Asymptomatic rickettsiemia in lagomorphs, opossum, voles, and cotton rats
Rickettsia parkeri rickettsiosis	*R. parkeri*	*A. maculatum*	• Acute febrile illness with an eschar • Non-fatal	• Asymptomatic persisting rickettsiemia	Unknown	• Seroconversion without acute infection	Unknown	Short-term transient bacteremia in small rodents and marsupials (experimental)
Human granulocytic anaplasmosis	*A. phagocytophilum*	*I. scapularis* *I. pacificus*	• Acute febrile illness • <1% fatality	• No clinical symptoms in most dogs • Asymptomatic persistence	• Nonspecific clinical signs of lethargy, anorexia, fever, and dehydration • Under-recognized condition • Seroconversion • Bacteriemia	• Equine anaplasmosis	Bovine anaplasmosis Ovine anaplasmosis Carpine anaplasmosis	Transient bacteremia white-footed mice, raccoons, and squirrels
Canine cyclic thrombocytopenia	*A. platys*	*R. sanguineus*	• Persistent bacteriemia with variable clinical symptoms • Very rare condition	• Commonly asymptomatic cyclic parasitemia and concomitant thrombocytopenia at one- to two-week intervals	Bacteriemia	Unknown	Unknown	Unknown

(*Continued*)

Table 23.1 (Continued)

Disease	Agent	Tick	Vertebrate Impact					
			Humans	Dogs	Cats	Horses	Livestock	Wild animals
Human monocytic ehrlichiosis	*E. chaffeensis*	*A. americanum*	• Acute febrile illness • 2–5% fatality	• Acute, subclinical, and chronic infection • May be fatal	• Nonspecific febrile illness • Seroconversion • Bacteremia	Seroconversion	Seroconversion	White-tailed deer is source of infection for *A. americanum*
E. ewingii ehrlichiosis	*E. ewingii*	*A. americanum*	Acute febrile illness	• Acute, subclinical, and chronic infection • May be fatal	• Nonspecific febrile illness • Seroconversion • Bacteremia	Seroconversion	Seroconversion	White-tailed deer is source of infection for *A. americanum*
Ehrlichiosis	*E. muris eauclairensis*	*I. scapularis*	Acute febrile illness	Acute febrile illness	Unknown	Unknown	Unknown	Systemic infection and transient bacteremia in *Peromyscus leucopus*
Canine monocytic ehrlichiosis	*E. canis*	*R. sanguineus*	Acute febrile illness	• Acute, subclinical, and chronic infection • May be fatal	Bacteremia, seroconversion	Unknown	Unknown	Red foxes bacteremic, jackals
Tularemia	*Francisella turalensis*	*D. andersoni* *D. variabilis* *A. americanum*	• Acute febrile illness • Clinical manifestations depend on the route of infection and other factors	• Nonspecific clinical signs including lethargy, pyrexia, and anorexia • Moderate to severe illness, often self-limiting	• Highly susceptible • Acute highly fatal illness • Most common through oropharyngeal route	Unknown	Seroconversion	• Diverse terrestrial and aquatic animals [re-phrase] are susceptible and develop bacteremia • Enzootic rabbit tularemia is most recognized reservoir of infection
Babesiosis	*Babesia microti*	*I. scapularis*	• Asymptomatic to life threatening	• Azotemia, anemia, and high mortality due to *B. microti*-like infection • More susceptible to other species of *Babesia*	More susceptible to other species of *Babesia*	More susceptible to other species of *Babesia*	More susceptible to other species of *Babesia*	• Diverse animals are susceptible to different species of zoonotic *Babesia* and develop parasitemia
Borrelia miyamotoi disease (hard tick relapsing fever)	*Borrelia miyamotoi*	*I. scapularis*	• Nonspecific febrile illness • Chronic meningitis in immunocompromised individuals	Unknown	Unknown	Unknown	Unknown	Small wild rodents may serve as a reservoir

Tick-borne relapsing fever	• *Borrelia hermsii* • *B. turicatae*	*O. hermsii* *O. turicatae*	Febrile illness with recurring episodes	• Canine relapsing fever • Also susceptible to other species of relapsing fever spirochetes	Feline relapsing fever caused by other species of relapsing fever spirochetes	Unknown	Unknown	Pine squirrels and other small animals serve as a reservoir
Colorado tick fever	Colorado tick fever virus (Coltivirus)	*D. andersoni*	• Acute febrile illness • Recurrent symptoms in 50% of cases	Unknown	Unknown	Unknown	Unknown	Black-tailed jackrabbit (*Lepus californicus*) develops bacteremia and serves as a reservoir and many other small wild animal species
Heartland and Bourbon viral diseases	*Heartland virus* (Plebovirus)	*A. americanum*	• Acute febrile illness with nonspecific symptoms • May be fatal	Seroconversion	Unknown	Seroconversion	Unknown	Seroconversion most observed in raccoons and white-tail deer
Powassan virus disease	*Powassan virus (Flavivirus)*	*I. scapularis* *D. andersoni*	• Acute illness progressing to meningoencephalitis • Fatal encephalitis	Unknown	Unknown	Widespread encephalitis (animal model)	Unknown	*Marmota momax, Tamiasciurus hudsonicus*, and *Peromyscus leucopus* are the most likely reservoirs
Cytauxzoonosis (bobcat fever)	*Cytauxzoon felis*	*A. americanum* *D. variabilis*	• Unknown	None	• Acute severe to potentially lethal infection • Manifests with depression, lethargy, fever, hemolytic crisis, and icterus	Unknown	Unknown	Infected bobcats (*Lynx rufus*) serve as wild animal reservoirs

to underscore that humans are most often accidental victims and a dead-end host in the natural cycle of their TBPs (even for transfusion-mediated transmission of etiological agents persisting in blood cells). Most of the ticks are active during the warm months of the year – spring, summer, and fall, although ticks may remain active year round in warmer parts of the country. Nymphs and adult females are the most aggressive human biting stages, and when infected are responsible for transmitting TBPs. Risk of human encounters with infected ticks varies based on the prevalence of infection in ticks and the densities of the host-seeking infected ticks (Eisen and Eisen 2018; Eisen and Paddock 2021). Dogs and cats are bitten by at least 14 and 12 different species of ticks, respectively, although *A. americanum*, *I. scapularis*, and *Dermacentor variabilis*, which also commonly bite people, are most often reported along with *Rhipicephalus sanguineus* that most frequently parasitizes dogs (Little et al. 2018; Saleh et al. 2021).

In the United States, the recognition of a tick association with human and animal diseases dates back to the nineteenth century. Cattle fever (also called Texas cattle fever) has been a long-term concern for livestock producers; however, it was not until work performed by Theobald Smith and Frederic L. Kilborne demonstrated the protozoan *B. (Piroplasma) bigemina* was present in the erythrocytes of infected cattle (Smith and Kilborne 1893). They then showed that the tick, *Rhipicephalus (Boophilus) bovis (R. annulatus)*, is necessary for transmission of the cattle fever agent (Smith and Kilborne 1893). Their colleague, Cooper Curtice, determined that *R. annulatus* is a single host tick. The important outcome of those investigations is that they provided the first evidence that an infectious disease agent may not be contagious by itself, rather it may be transmitted to a susceptible animal or human through an intermediate host such as a tick. The interaction between Smith, a physician, and Kilborne, a veterinarian, is a fine example of an aspect of what we now term One Health (Bulloch 1935).

Clinically first described in 1899, Rocky Mountain spotted fever (RMSF) was the earliest recognized human tick-borne disease in the United States. It was first reported in the northwestern Rocky Mountains and especially known in the Bitterroot Valley of Montana. The specific symptoms of RMSF – the blue-black rash, high fever, and delirium – and a high mortality rate among healthy young adults produced anxiety in prospective residents of western frontiers (Harden 1990). Work pioneered by the American physician Howard Taylor Ricketts provided evidence that this deadly disease is caused by a bacterium, *Rickettsia rickettsii*, and that it is transmitted by the wood tick, *Dermacentor andersoni* (Ricketts 1906, 1909). Originally it was thought that the disease was limited to the Rocky Mountain region; however, as the disease became nationally reportable due to its morbidity and mortality, clinical cases were also recognized in eastern and southeastern parts of the country as well as other parts of the western territories. Since the early 1970s, a majority of cases have occurred in the mid-central parts of the United States, from Oklahoma to North Carolina and adjacent states (Burgdorfer 1975; Adjemian et al. 2009; Alkishe et al. 2021). During the early days of recognition of RMSF, particularly in the pre-antibiotic era, a much greater case-fatality rate was reported relative to disease incidence compared to the present time (Figure 23.2a). Beside *D. andersoni* other tick species either tested positive for or were a source of *R. rickettsii* isolates; however, the natural prevalence of *R. rickettsii* in US ticks is typically less than 1% (Ribeiro et al. 2021). Endemic peridomestic associations of *R. rickettsii* with the brown dog tick, *R. sanguineus*, is an exception as tick infection rates varying as high as 4–10% have been determined (Demma et al. 2005; Ribeiro et al. 2021).

The current upward trend in the incidence of rickettsial infections in the United States has been counteracted by a steady decline in the case-fatality rate (Figure 23.2a, b). Some of this decline may be due to confusion of RMSF cases with other spotted fever group (SFG) rickettioses when cross-reactive serology is used as the basis for the diagnosis of the infection (Raoult and Parola 2008; Openshaw et al. 2010). Several other objective and subjective causes include true or perceived changes in the geographic distribution of traditionally diagnosed rickettsioses. Description of new etiologic agents co-circulating in these areas may also be important factors contributing to the current epidemiological situation in the United States, and similar situations are observed worldwide (Parola et al. 2013). The recent findings of highly prevalent carriage of *Rickettsia amblyommatis* by the lone star tick, *A. americanum* and *Rickettsia montanensis* by *D. variabilis*, may actually contribute to an incorrect number of cases previously counted as RMSF in Central and Atlantic states (Ammerman et al. 2004; Moncayo et al. 2010; Stromdahl et al. 2011; Trout Fryxell et al. 2015, 2017; Duncan et al. 2021). Because these other tick-borne agents may cause mild rickettsiosis, they could contribute to the apparent numerical decline of fatal cases of RMSF in the United States (Apperson et al. 2008; McQuiston et al. 2012; Yen et al. 2021).

First discovered in the 1980s in New England, Lyme disease is caused by a spirochete, *Borrelia burgdorferi sensu stricto*, and nowadays is the most prevalent TBD in the United States (Eisen et al. 2017; Barbour and Benach 2019). The disease has received a high clinical recognition level due to its unusual manifestations of a bull-eye rash (erythema chronicum migrans) in the acute stage, numerous symptoms affecting various organ systems during the disseminated stage of illness, and lingering and debilitating neurologic and musculoskeletal conditions in up to 10–35% individuals including children in the post-treatment period (Rebman and Aucott 2020). It is still primarily reported from a relatively small region in the Upper Midwest and

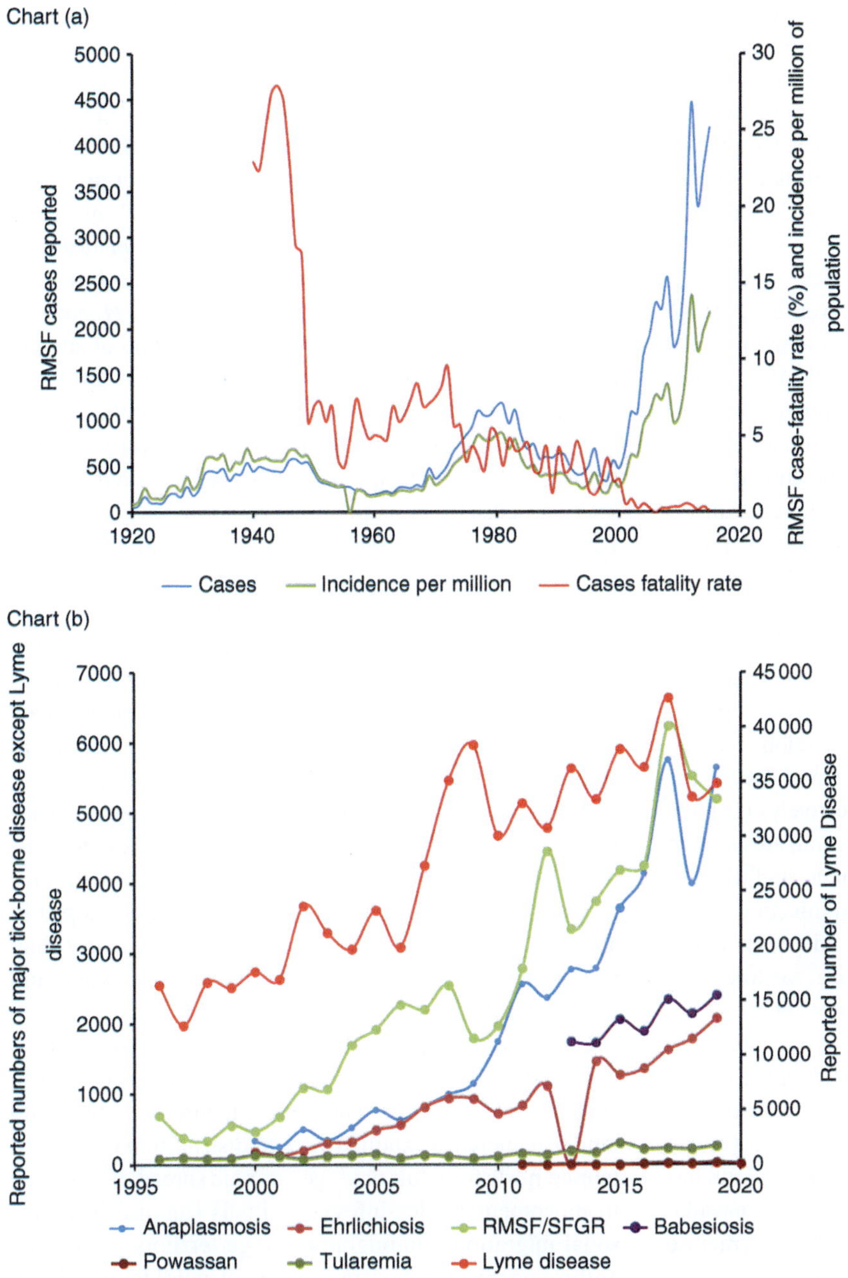

Figure 23.2 Historic and recent trends in incidence of tick-borne diseases reported in the United States. (a) National incidence and case-fatality rate of Rocky Mountain spotted fever in the United States. (b) Incidence of reportable tick-borne diseases in the United States, 1995–2020. *Source:* Centers for Disease Control and Prevention. Graphs were made using publicly available data downloaded from www.cdc.gov.

New England states of the United States, where it is transmitted by the black-legged deer tick *I. scapularis* and along the Pacific coast, where it is vectored by *I. pacificus* (Eisen et al. 2016a). It is estimated to cause over 300,000 cases annually. *Borrelia mayonii* is another *Borrelia* species discovered and recognized as a new etiological agent of Lyme disease in the United States, where it circulates in *I. scapularis* in Minnesota and Wisconsin (Pritt et al. 2016). Patients infected with *B. mayonii* present with primary clinical symptoms differing from patients infected with *B. burgdorferi* s.s. including the development of a diffuse macular rash instead of erythema migrans and nausea or vomiting and symptoms consistent with neurological involvement. Laboratory testing detected high levels of spirochetemia (up to 10^5/ml of blood), which is more typical for relapsing fever borreliosis in which spirochete loads range from 10^5 to $>10^6$/ml of blood (Dworkin et al. 2008).

Although ixodid ticks are widespread across the United States, the reported distribution of *B. burgdorferi* and *B. mayonii* in ixodid ticks is more limited compared to the distribution of reported Lyme disease cases (Fleshman et al. 2021). *I. scapularis* or *I. pacificus* is present in 35 eastern and 6 western states (Eisen et al. 2016b); however, Lyme disease spirochetes were only reported from 26 (74%) and 2 (33%) states, respectively. Detection of *B. burgdorferi* s.s. in questing *I. scapularis* nymphs or adults is rare in southern states (Diuk-Wasser et al. 2006, 2012; Lane et al. 2013; Arsnoe et al. 2015).

Human anaplasmosis and ehrlichioses were first described during the early 1990s; however, knowledge about related veterinary diseases existed for many years prior to these discoveries (Anderson et al. 1991, 1992; Bakken et al. 1994). *Anaplasma phagocytophilum* is transmitted by *Ixodes* ticks; this agent causes human, equine, and canine granulocytic anaplasmosis in the United States and tick-borne fever in cattle and sheep in Europe (Woldehiwet 2010). It exists as diverse genetic variants, some of which circulate exclusively among ticks and wildlife and are not known to cause human illness (Poitout et al. 2005; Michalski et al. 2006; Morissette et al. 2009; Trost et al. 2018). *A. phagocytophilum* has been detected in ticks from every region of the United States except the Southeast, with the highest prevalence of infection recorded in the northeast (5.76% [CI 4.62–7.17%] and 8.07% [CI 6.99–9.30%] in nymphs and adults, respectively) (Lehane et al. 2021). Other related species of *Anaplasma* are adapted to a wide range of livestock, wildlife animals, and dogs, in which they cause either acute or persistent infection with a broad range of different outcomes (Woldehiwet 2010). Many of these *Anaplasma* species are vectored by *Amblyomma* and *Dermacentor* ticks (Lane et al. 2010; Clark 2012; Francis et al. 2020) and are not known to cause human illness. *Anaplasma platys* is vectored by the brown dog tick, *R. sanguineus*; it may infect people and cause a persistent infection, similar to the canine disease (Maggi et al. 2013; Breitschwerdt et al. 2014). Because *A. platys* has not been cultured, accurate serological tests are unavailable; therefore, it is typically detected using polymerase chain reaction (PCR) or other molecular approaches.

Three *Ehrlichia* species pathogenic to humans, *Ehrlichia chaffeensis*, *Ehrlichia ewingii*, and *Ehrlichia muris eauclarensis*, are known in the United States (Pritt et al. 2011; Ismail and McBride 2017). *E. chaffeensis* and *E. ewingii* are both transmitted by *A. americanum* and their natural cycle involves white-tailed deer (Paddock and Yabsley 2007). The true prevalence for each infection is not well known because *E. ewingii* has not been cultured, yet its definitive etiological diagnosis can be established only by using molecular methods, while serological diagnosis relies on *E. chaffeensis* as a surrogate antigen. Both are known etiological agents of canine illnesses, whose infections may be also misdiagnosed as a disease due to *Ehrlichia canis*, vectored by broadly distributed *R. sanguineus*, and with *Anaplasma* infections (Nair et al. 2016). On rare occasions, *E. canis* or *Ehrlichia* with a similar genotype may infect humans (Perez et al. 2006). In contrast, *E. muris eauclarensis* is transmitted by *I. scapularis* and circulates in the Midwest and Northeast geographic locations (Murphy et al. 2017). The natural prevalence of *E. chaffeensis* and *E. ewingii* is typically higher in adults than in nymphs of *A. americanum*; however, a wide range of infection prevalence has been reported (0–53.6% for *E. chaffeensis* and 0–46.4% for *E. ewingii*) depending on the geographic locations, duration of surveillance, and tick sample size and stage (Wright et al. 2014).

Human infections by *Babesia* are rare in the United States and only limited to the northeast and North-Central counties where *Babesia microti* has been detected in host-seeking ticks (Fleshman et al. 2022; Johnston et al. 2022). Powassan virus infection (POWVI) is the only tick-borne encephalitis known in North America (Hermance and Thangamani 2017). Over 100 human infections due to POWVI have been reported since the description of the index case in 1958; however, an apparent increase in disease incidence has been observed in the last 20 years (Hermance and Thangamani 2017). The causes of recent changes in POWVI epidemiology are not fully understood, and POWVI is found only in 1–4% of host-seeking ticks; however, this is an agent of concern since a tick can transmit POW virus within 15 minutes of attachment to a person, and long-term neurological sequelae developed in about half the reported cases, and it causes greater than a 10% fatality rate in infected individuals (Ebel and Kramer 2004; Hermance and Thangamani 2017).

The ongoing expansion of ticks and increases in tick-transmitted diseases are congruent with many changes in climate and landscape. These include altered habitat and land use, increased abundance and distribution of key vertebrate hosts for adult ticks, geographic spread of ticks due to movement of tick-infested animals (natural host seasonal migration, nonmigratory range/territory expansion, anthropogenic planned movement of wildlife, and inadvertent importation of tick-infested animals) (Diuk-Wasser et al. 2010; Eisen et al. 2016a, b; Diuk-Wasser et al. 2021; Alkishe et al. 2021; Mathisson et al. 2021) Animals also contribute in various ways to enzootic maintenance of different TBPs and thus increased risk of human infection. Wildlife animals contribute to increases in tick-borne diseases of companion animals (Nicholson et al. 2010; Saleh et al. 2021). Wildlife animals are also responsible for increasing incidences of tick-borne diseases of livestock, a significant problem in the northwestern portion of the United States where wildlife ungulates and domestic stock may share habitat and various ticks, including *Dermacentor occidentalis*, *D. variabilis*, and *Dermacentor albipictus*, each competent vector for *A. marginale* and *Anaplasma ovis* (Tsao et al. 2021).

23.3.2 A New Concern in the Study of Tick-Borne Agents in the United States

In 2017, the US Department of Agriculture (USDA) confirmed the presence of the Asian longhorned tick (*Haemaphysalis longicornis*) in the eastern United States. This species is native to eastern Asia and is capable of reproduction without mating (parthenogenesis). Since it readily bites humans, there are significant concerns about its vectorial capacity for various pathogens. Recent field studies reported findings of *H. longicornis* in the highest proportions compared with other native tick species on raccoons (55.4%), Virginia opossums (28.9%), and white-tailed deer (11.5%). Tissue, blood, and engorged larvae were tested for 17 different pathogens using a nanoscale PCR platform. Five pathogens (*B. burgdorferi*, *A. phagocytophilum*, *Rickettsia* spp., *Mycoplasma haemocanis*, and *Bartonella* spp.) were detected in nymph and adult samples, but no pathogens were found in any larval samples. These results suggest that although large and medium-sized mammals can serve as hosts for *H. longicornis* in the environment, there is presently a low potential for *H. longicornis* to acquire pathogens from these wildlife hosts (Tufts et al. 2021). At the same time, these acquisition events may occur in various geographic locales, as indicated by the recent detection of human variant of *A. phagocytophilum* in *H. longicornis* collected in Pennsylvania (Price et al. 2022). One experimental study found that this tick is not likely to contribute to the spread of Lyme disease bacteria in the United States (Rainey et al. 2018). Another laboratory study found that this tick has the ability to carry and spread *R. rickettsii*; however, *R. rickettsii* have not yet been found in these ticks in nature (Stanley et al. 2020).

23.4 Ticks and Tick-Transmitted Pathogens in Sri Lanka

23.4.1 Current Knowledge About Ticks and their Hosts in Sri Lanka

Sri Lanka has a very diverse tick fauna consisting of at least 31 formally described species of ticks belonging to 11 genera. Over 20 different tick species are known to infest diverse wild animals including tortoises and reptiles (Liyanaarachchi et al. 2015a), 8 species on goats (Diyes and Rajakaruna 2015), 19 species on livestock and peridomestic animals, and 12 tick species commonly attach to people (Liyanaarachchi et al. 2013, 2015b, c). While records of human tick infestations are very scarce, diagnosis of intra-aural tick infestation, called otoacariasis (Ariyaratne et al. 2016; Bandaranayaka et al. 2021), and associated facial palsy have become commonplace in the hilly regions of Sri Lanka in the past two decades (Kularatne et al. 2018). Among the widely distributed tick species, *R. sanguineus*, *Rhipicephalus haemaphysaloides*, *Haemaphysalis intermedia*, and *Haemaphysalis bispinosa* are common ticks infesting cattle, goats, and dogs in both the dry and wet zones (Diyes and Rajakaruna 2015; Bandaranayaka et al. 2022) while *Rhipicephalus microplus* is common in both wet and dry zones infesting cattle and goat island-wide. Common widely distributed reptile ticks are *Amblyomma clypeolatum*, *Amblyomma varanense*, and *Amblyomma trimaculatum* found in both dry and wet zones (Liyanaarachchi et al. 2015a). *Hyalomma turturis* is a rare tick species infesting reptiles but has also been recorded in dogs (Liyanaarachchi et al. 2015a; Bandaranayaka et al. 2022).

23.4.2 Tick-Borne Disease Agents and Human Diseases in Sri Lanka

TB infectious agents and corresponding clinical diseases are reported in humans, domesticated animals, and wildlife in Sri Lanka (Table 23.2). The first record of clinical and laboratory diagnosis of spotted fever group rickettsioses (SFGR) in Sri Lanka described 10 acute patients and 11 cases of seroconversion in individuals from the central hills, many of whom reported regular contact with arthropods, most likely ticks (Kularatne et al. 2003). A 2002–2003 hospital-based study in Colombo North Teaching Hospital identified eight acute cases with possible SFGR etiology in the lowland Western Province (Premaratna et al. 2008). More recently, the occurrence of SFGR has been demonstrated serologically and with genus-specific PCR in different regions of Sri Lanka (Table 23.2). Occurrence of SFGR among Sri Lankan patients with acute febrile illness is accounted for 17.7% of cases with IFA antibodies to SFG rickettsiae and 38.7% of cases with antibodies to both SFG and typhus group rickettsiae (Reller et al. 2012). These human cases were initially attributed to *Rickettsia conorii* based on results of cross-reactive serological tests; however, western blotting data suggested circulation of and patient exposure to different species of SFG rickettsiae in Sri Lanka (Angelakis et al. 2012). These laboratory observations are consistent with reports of SFGR with variable clinical manifestations including forms such as fern leaf skin necrosis, arthritis, and acute vasculitis (Luke et al. 2017). Since these cases have occurred in both local residents and travelers to Sri Lanka, the ubiquitous occurrence of ticks carrying SFG rickettsiae and various scenarios of their transmission to humans are probable. Because

Table 23.2 Tick-borne organisms and tick-borne infections reported in humans, wild and domestic animals, and ticks in Sri Lanka.

Disease	Agent (method)	Tick species	Host	References
Spotted fever group rickettsiosis	*Rickettsia conorii* (serology)	Not collected/tested	Human (resident)	Kularatne et al. (2003, 2013, 2018), Premaratne et al. (2008, 2009, 2012, 2014), Nagalingam et al. (2009), Dissanayake and Madegedara (2011), Weerakoon et al. (2014), Dahanayaka et al. (2017), Herath et al. (2018), Ehelepola et al. (2019), Kariyawasam et al. (2019), Warnasooriya et al. (2021)
	Rickettsia sp. (serology)	Not collected/tested	Human (resident)	Luke et al. (2017), Reller et al. (2012)
	R. conorii (serology)	Not collected/tested	Human (traveler)	Stokes and Walters (2009)
	R. sibirica mongolitimonae (PCR)	Not collected/tested	Human (traveler)	Cordier et al. (2017)
	R. conorii (serology)	Not collected/tested	Domestic dog	Nanayakkara et al. (2013)
	SFG *Rickettsia* (serology)	Not collected/tested	Human (resident)	Liyanapathirana and Thevanesam (2011)
	SFG *Rickettsia* (serology)	Not collected/tested	Human (resident)	Angelakis et al. (2012)
	SFG *Rickettsia* (serology)	Not collected/tested	Human (resident)	Kovácová et al. (1996)
	Rickettsia sp. (PCR)	*Dermacentor auratus*	Human (resident)	Bandaranayaka et al. (2021)
	Rickettsia sp. (PCR)	*Rhipicephalus* sp.	Human (resident)	Kularatne et al. (2018)
	Rickettsia sp. (PCR)	*Rhipicephalus sanguineus*	Domestic dog	Liyanaarachchi et al. (2015a)
	Rickettsia sp. (PCR)	*Amblyomma testudinarium*	Wild boar	Liyanaarachchi et al. (2015a)
	Rickettsia sp. (PCR)	*Amblyomma clypeolatum*	Star tortoise	Liyanaarachchi et al. (2015a)
	Rickettsia sp. (PCR)	*Amblyomma javanense*	Pangolin	Liyanaarachchi et al. (2015a)
	Rickettsia sp. SriLankaAT31-R (PCR)	*Amblyomma trimaculatum*	Snake (*Boiga fortesi*)	Andoh et al. (2015)
	Rickettsia sp. (PCR)	*R. haemaphysaloides*	Rat (*Rattus rattus*)	Yathramullage et al. (2018)
	Rickettsia sp. (PCR)	*Ixodes ceylonensis*	Mouse (*Mus fernandoni*)	Yathramullage et al. (2018)
	Rickettsia sp. (PCR)	*Haemaphysalis spinigera*	Rat (*R. rattus*)	Yathramullage et al. (2018)
	Rickettsia sp. (PCR)	*Haemaphysalis* sp.	Rat (*R. rattus*); bandicoot (*Bandicota indica*)	Yathramullage et al. (2018)
	R. africae (PCR)	*Amblyomma* sp.	Unknown	Dasch et al. (2022)
	R. kellyi (PCR)	R. haemaphysaloides	Goat	Dasch et al. (2022)
	R. massiliae (PCR)	*Rhipicephalus* sp.	Domestic dog	Dasch et al. (2022)
	R. massiliae-like (PCR)	*Rhipicephalus* sp.	Domestic dog, cattle	Dasch et al. (2022)
	Rickettsia sp. SL94 (PCR)	*Rhipicephalus* sp.	Domestic dog	Dasch et al. (2022)

Babesiosis	*Babesia gibsoni* (microscopy)	Not collected/tested	Domestic dog	Seneviratna (1953, 1965a, b)
	B. gibsoni (PCR)	Not collected/tested	Domestic dog	Zahler et al. (2000)
	B. gibsoni (microscopy)	Not collected/tested	Domestic dog	Weeratunga et al. (2019)
	B. gibsoni (microscopy, PCR)	Not collected/tested	Domestic and military dogs	Jayathilake et al. (2020)
	B. gibsoni (microscopy, PCR)	Not collected/tested	Domestic dog	Neelawala et al. (2021)
	B. gibsoni (microscopy, PCR)	Not collected/tested	Domestic dog	Ranatunga et al. (2022)
	Babesia canis (PCR)	Not collected/tested	Domestic dog	Kumara et al. (2013)
	B. canis (microscopy)	Not collected/tested	Domestic dog	Weeratunga et al. (2019)
	B. canis (microscopy, PCR)	Not collected/tested	Domestic and military dogs	Jayathilake et al. (2020)
	Babesia sp. (PCR)	*Otobius megnini*	Racehorse	Diyes et al. (2018)
	Babesia perroncitoi (PCR)	Not collected/tested	Pig (*Sus domesticus*)	Ranatunga et al. (2021)
	Babesia sp. Mymensingh (PCR)	Not collected/tested	Cattle, buffalo	Sivakumar et al. (2020)
	Babesia bigemina (PCR)	Not collected/tested	Cattle	Sivakumar et al. (2016)
	Babesia bovis (culture)	*Rhipicephalus annulatus*	Unknown	Weilgama et al. (1989)
	Babesia bovis (PCR)	Not collected/tested	Cattle	Sivakumar et al. (2012, 2018)
	Babesia divergens (PCR)	Not collected/tested	Cattle	Sivakumar et al. (2018)
	Babesia bigemina (PCR)	Not collected/tested	Cattle	Gunasekara et al. (2019)
	Babesia ovata (PCR)	Not collected/tested	Cattle	Sivakumar et al. (2018)
Anaplasmosis	*Anaplasma platys* (PCR)	Not collected/tested	Domestic and military dogs	Bennett et al. (2005), Jayathilake et al. (2020)
	Anaplasma marginale (PCR)	Not collected/tested	Cattle, buffalo	Zhyldyz et al. (2019), Sivakumar et al. (2012, 2014), Jorgensen et al. (1992), Dasch et al. (2022)
	Anaplasma sp. (serology)	Not collected/tested	Cattle, buffalo	
	Anaplasma sp. (PCR)	*Amblyomma* sp.	Tortoise	
Ehrlichiosis	*Ehrlichia canis* (microscopy)	Not collected/tested	Domestic dog	MacGaughey et al. (1962)
	E. canis (PCR)	Not collected/tested	Domestic dog	Bennett et al. (2005)
	E. canis (microscopy)	Not collected/tested	Domestic dog	Kumara et al. (2013)
	E. canis (microscopy)	Not collected/tested	Domestic dog and military dogs	Weeratunga et al. (2019)
	Ehrlichia sp. (PCR)	*Rhipicephalus annulatus*	Cattle	Jayathilake et al. (2020)
				Dasch et al. (2022)
Hepatozoonosis	*Hepatozoon canis* (PCR, microscopy)	Not collected/tested	Domestic dog	Atapattu et al. (2017), Weeratunga et al. (2019), Jayathilake et al. (2020)
	H. canis (microscopy)	Not collected/tested	Domestic dog	
	H. canis (microscopy)	Not collected/tested	Domestic and military dogs	
Borreliosis	*Borrelia* sp. (serology)	Not tested/collected	Human	Jeker et al. (2005)
Theileriosis	*Theileria annulata* (PCR)	Not collected/tested	Cattle, water buffalo	Sivakumar et al. (2012, 2014, 2019), Gunasekara et al. (2019)
	Theileria orientalis (PCR)	Not collected/tested	Cattle, water buffalo	Sivakumar et al. (2012, 2014), Gunasekara et al. (2019), Ahedor et al. (2022)
	Theileria equi (PCR)	Not collected/tested	Donkey (*Equus africanus asinus*)	

Indirect Fluorescent Antibody test (IFA) and PCR testing is only available through a few research-focused laboratories, while routine clinical laboratory diagnosis is limited to the archaic Weil–Felix test, the exact etiology and prevalence of human cases due to SFG rickettsiae and other related organisms is unknown and should be a priority for proper patient management.

Some rickettsioses with low pathogenicity may be accounted for only a few cases but specific tests are not available to define their relative incidence. Otoacariasis patients exhibit seroconversion too (Kularatne et al. 2018) and tested PCR-positive for DNA (Bandaranayaka et al. 2021) of SFG rickettsiae and defervesce quickly after doxycycline treatment.

23.4.3 Animal Reservoirs of Tick-Borne Disease Agents in Sri Lanka

The host reservoirs of TB disease agents in Sri Lanka are poorly known, but their zoonotic potential cannot be ruled out. DNA of SFG rickettsiae was detected in *Amblyomma testudinarium* collected from a wild boar, *R. sanguineus* from a domestic dog, *A. clypeolatum* from a star tortoise, and *Amblyomma javanense* from a pangolin (Liyanaarachchi et al. 2015c; Table 23.2). Except for *A. javanense*, the other three tick species are generalists infesting humans as well as domestic and wild animals, so there is a high potential that various pathogens can be transmitted easily to humans via ticks from infested domesticated animals. A recent study by Dasch et al. (2022) reported five genotypes of SFG rickettsiae: a *Rickettsia africae*-like agent in *Amblyomma larvae*, *Rickettsia massiliae* and a related genotype identified in *R. sanguineus* and *R. haemaphysaloides* from dogs and cattle, and *Candidatus* Rickettsia kellyi and another novel genotype (SL94) in *R. haemaphysaloides*. Moreover, the study also presented the first records for yet unidentified one *Anaplasma* agent and two *Ehrlichia* genotypes in Sri Lankan ticks.

Sri Lanka has a large canine population with an estimated 1 : 6.7 dog to human ratio that includes an estimated three million street dogs, 120,000 owned dogs, and 500 military and working dogs (Pimburage et al. 2017; The Kennel Association of Sri Lanka n.d.). Therefore, TB infectious agents are a significant health concern for dogs in Sri Lanka with canine babesiosis due to *Babesia gibsoni* and *B. canis* being the most reported clinical condition (summarized in Table 23.2). As early as 1953, Seneviratna studied piroplasmosis in dogs in Sri Lanka, describing *B. gibsoni*, the small canine *Babesia* agent (Seneviratna 1965a), its treatment (Seneviratna and Jayawickrama 1961), and pathology (Seneviratna 1965b). Prevalence of canine babesiosis and its etiological agents appears to vary in different climatic regions of the country. A microscopy study carried out in the North Central Province recorded a low prevalence of *B. canis* (1.25%) and a higher percentage of 15.04% of *B. gibsoni* (Weeratunga et al. 2019). A more recent, island-wide study carried out microscopically and with DNA analysis reported 0.3 and 13.8% of *B. canis* and *B. gibsoni* (Jayathilake et al. 2020). Clinical manifestations and morbidity of babesiosis differ between pedigreed and stray dogs. Mostly young adults of pedigreed dog breeds like German shepherds, Dobermann, and Pomeranians have the highest susceptibility, while Rottweilers, Labradors, Boxers, and crossbred dogs of any age are more susceptible to both babesiosis and ehrlichiosis compared to other breeds (Silva 2016). Non-pedigree, mixed breeds, and stray dogs show more resistance and tolerance to these infections, most probably due to their diverse ancestry and resultant genetic diversity (Silva 2016). A very high prevalence of canine babesiosis (78.6%) due to *B. gibsoni* was diagnosed among dogs treated at one veterinary teaching hospital, and 66.7% of these dogs were asymptomatic (Ranatunga et al. 2022). Moreover, only 19 out of 42 blood samples were microscopically positive for babesiosis while 33 (78.6%) tested PCR positive, a significant difference in the two methods of diagnosis. Impact of TBI on the health of military working dogs is another emerging issue much as it was previously recognized in other tropical and subtropical countries (Personal communication with the military kennel veterinarian, Katunayake; Huxsoll et al. 1970; Keefe et al. 1982; Suksawat et al. 2001). There are over 500 working dogs in the Sri Lanka Army, Navy, Air Force, and Police. Most of these dogs are imported from various countries, mainly from the United Kingdom, Germany, and the Netherlands, but some are locally bred (Personal communication with the veterinarians in the military and Police). In general, the majority of dogs in the developing world are short-lived (Pimburage et al. 2017). Even the Sri Lanka Police working dogs, with more adequate maintenance and health care, die at an average age of 6.1 years (Jayathilake et al. 2020). Moreover, 75% of the dogs belonging to the Sri Lanka Air Force (SLAF) and Army have died as young animals, presumably due to TBIs; although suspected, these have not been confirmed or properly diagnosed (personal communication with the Squadron leader and the Manager of the Animal Husbandry Project at the SLAF, Katunayake). Since there is a quarantine and screening process for all hemoparasites of all dogs before introducing them to the military unit, they probably acquire the diseases from arthropod vectors once they are brought to the country.

Babesia infections have been recorded in livestock like cattle, buffalo, and pigs (Table 23.2). Bovine babesiosis is common among cattle in Sri Lanka. In 1970, the morphology of *Babesia argentina* (*B. bovis*) and the clinical manifestations of the experimental disease were described in cattle slaughtered in various parts of Sri Lanka, 10 of 44 brains were infected, indicating that it is a much more common parasite than was thought at the time (Abeysena and Seneviratna 1970). More recently, PCR-based testing has determined that bovine babesiosis in Sri Lanka is mainly caused by *B. bovis* and *B. bigemina* island-wide (Sivakumar et al. 2012), although *B. divergens* has been known to cause clinical babesiosis (Zintl et al. 2003). A novel *Babesia* species, designated *Babesia* sp. Mymensingh, causing clinical bovine babesiosis was also reported in cattle (1.5%; $n = 672$) and buffalo (1.2%; $n = 327$) tested across different provinces of Sri Lanka (Sivakumar et al. 2020). Bovine babesiosis was originally concentrated mainly in the wet zone of Sri Lanka and was not common in the dry zone (Jorgensen et al. 1992). Serological studies showed that antibodies to *B. bovis* are high (100%) in cattle from localities below 1200 m and more variable in herds from the hill country (5–100%); these differences were attributed in part to differing cattle breed and management practices (Jorgensen et al. 1992). Since the beginning of the past decade, bovine babesiosis has become common in both wet and dry zones (Department of Animal Production and Health, Sri Lanka 2012). *Babesia* DNA has been detected in 18% of spinose ear ticks, *Otobius megnini* removed from the ear canal of racehorses in Nuwara Eliya (Diyes et al. 2018) and DNA of *Babesia perroncitoi* was detected in blood samples collected from pigs in a piggery (Ranatunga et al. 2021). These observations indicate that diverse populations of *Babesia* species circulate and may negatively impact other livestock and peridomestic animals in Sri Lanka.

Other TB agents causing anaplasmosis, ehrlichiosis, hepatozoonosis, and theileriosis are also reported in studies to a lesser extent, mostly in dogs and livestock (Table 23.2). In contrast to countries with temperate climates, Lyme disease is not known in Sri Lanka. However, a 44-year-old man who traveled to Sri Lanka and returned to Germany was diagnosed with multilocular erythema migrans based on clinical observations and detection of serum IgM against *B. burgdorferi* (Jeker et al. 2005). Although cases of borreliosis have not been diagnosed yet, there is a possibility that it may be overlooked because Lyme neuroborreliosis and erythema multiforme occur in India (Vasudevan and Chatterjee 2013).

23.4.4 Ecological Considerations Affecting Tick-Borne Disease Agents and Their Transmission in Sri Lanka

The transmission dynamics of TB agents in Sri Lanka is influenced by the active management of forests. Timber harvesting near new human settlements has resulted in a recent significant reduction in the natural forest cover. The main causes of this reduction have been the clearing of forests for agricultural development, shifting cultivation practices, and new settlements. These changes led to increased wildlife introduction near neighborhoods. Some vertebrate taxa are more likely to be zoonotic hosts than others, and in human-altered habitats these reservoir animals often proliferate increasing the likelihood of tick and disease agent spillover (Ellwanger and Chies 2021). The intensity and frequency of human interactions with livestock, pets, and wildlife create opportunities for the occurrence of spillover events.

In Sri Lanka, the livestock management systems in the dry and wet zone vary substantially; in the dry zone, the cattle are fed in communal grazing lands during the daytime (Abeygunawardena et al. 1997; Figure 23.3a) and brought back home in the evening and kept in a paddock near the farmers' dwellings. The usual grazing lands are catchments of the village tank or tank beds (Figure 23.3a), shrub jungle, and paddy fields after the harvest. Sometimes, the animals also walk to distant places in search of grazing lands that are close to forested areas. In the wet zone, however, the animals are kept and maintained in stall-fed conditions (Figure 23.3b). Farmers feed them with cut grass from nearby forests, roadsides, riverbanks, state reservations, and uncultivable terrains. The difference in cattle management appears to be a determining factor for the extent of tick infestations of pets and humans. As an example, the main risk factors of otoacariasis were identified as engagement in outdoor activities within the presence of domestic animals in the dry zone and the presence of wildlife in and around the household in the wet zone (Bandaranayaka et al. 2021). This can be related to the livestock management system as the cattle coming back home from grazing pastures can bring ticks in the dry zone, whereas wildlife is present in the home gardens in the wet zone. The home garden system in the wet zone is known as the "Kandyan home garden system," which is an age-old traditional agroforestry system practiced in the central hilly areas and in some other districts in the wet zone. It is the globally recognized oldest agroforestry system in Asia and used as an alternative household income source. This system combines agriculture, forestry, and livestock; trees are grown in a multilayer arrangement and mixed cropping of trees yielding timber, small wood, fuelwood, fodder, food, fruits, and medicines together with crops yielding food and medicine is practiced (Figure 23.4). The forest garden is used by the household members for collecting firewood, rearing animals, cutting grass for livestock, etc. Women and children are mostly involved in these activities. There is a high chance that while engaged in outdoor activities, questing ticks on vegetation are encountered.

(a)

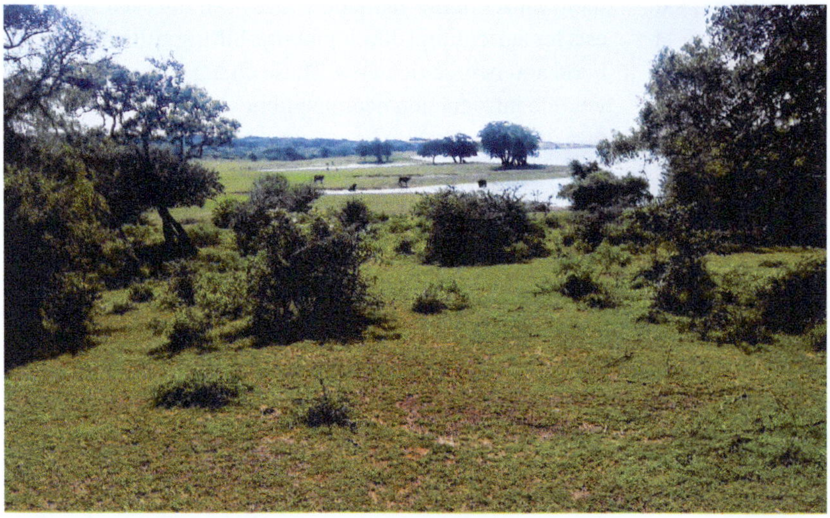

(b)

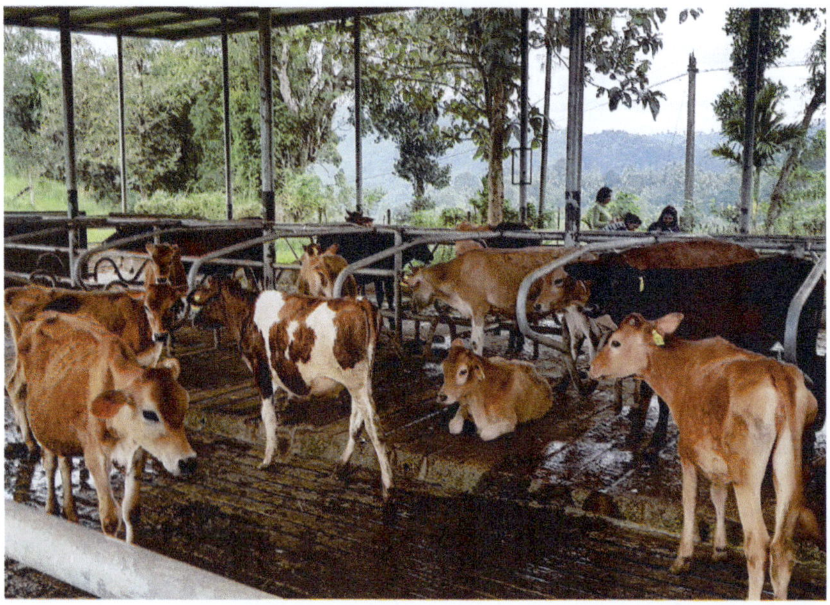

Figure 23.3 Cattle in the Dry Zone are fed in communal grazing lands near tanks and tank beds during the daytime, brought back home in the evening, and kept in a paddock near the farmers' house (a). Cattle in the Wet Zone are kept in stall-fed conditions and fed with cut grass (b).

These forested gardens attract many wildlife species such as rodents, wild boars, monkeys, peacocks, barking deer, and porcupines. Wild boar is a very frequent visitor to home gardens and is the primary host of *Dermacentor auratus,* the causative agent of human otoacariasis (Bandaranayaka et al. 2021). These communities have experienced an increase in the number of wild boars in recent years (personal communication with villages). Among the questing ticks collected from the houses are immature stages of *D. auratus*, which were acquired from farm paddocks (Liyanaarachchi et al. 2015b).

23.5 The One Health Approach to Understanding Tick-Borne Disease Agents

Many factors need to be considered to understand the emergence and transmission of TB disease agents because of their complexity and interconnectedness with deforestation, climate change, population growth, habitat alterations, increased transportation, tourism, and trade. Although considerable progress has been made in our understanding

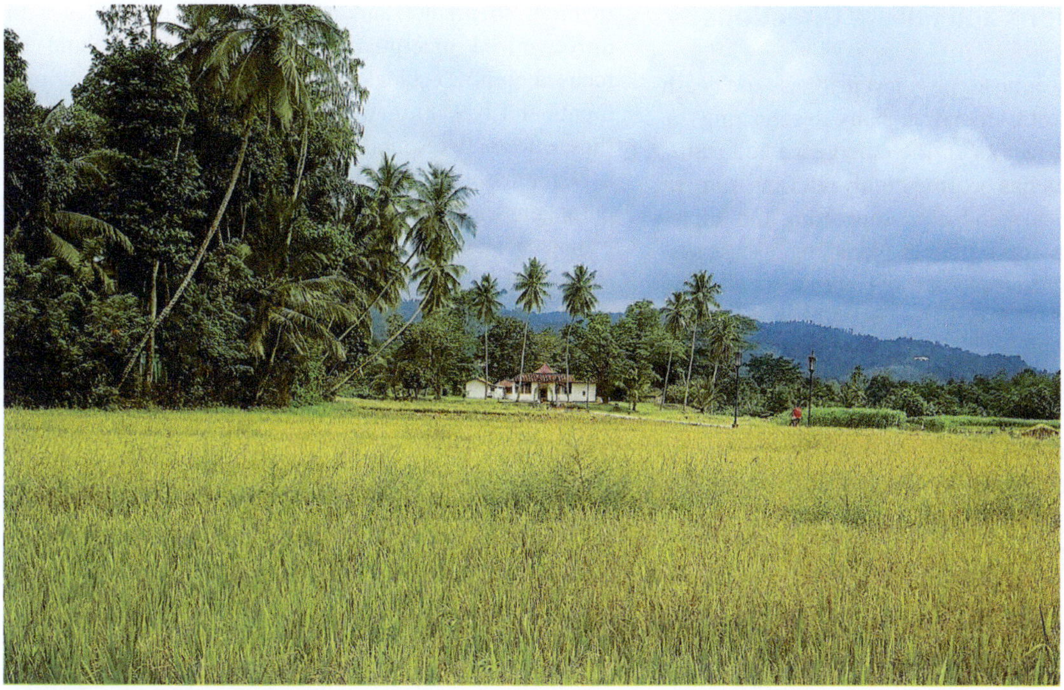

Figure 23.4 Kandyan Home garden system: an age-old traditional agroforestry system practiced in the central hilly areas and in some other districts in the Wet Zone of Sri Lanka. This system combines agriculture, forestry, and livestock; trees are grown in a multilayer arrangement and mixed cropping of trees yield timber, small wood, fuelwood, fodder, food, fruits, and medicines together with crops yielding food. Maximum utilization of space, both vertical and horizontal, is ensured in this system.

of the transmission of tick-borne infectious agents in recent years, controlling them is highly challenging.

One Health is a collaborative, multisectoral, and transdisciplinary approach – working at the local, regional, national, and global levels – with the goal of achieving optimal health outcomes by recognizing the interconnection between people, animals, plants, and their shared environment (CDC). Expansion in tick populations has led to the increased risk of infection for humans and animals by both established tick-borne agents and newly recognized ones, creating a serious One Health problem. There are many potential benefits to applying a One Health approach to control TBIs. One Health research on ticks and TBI not only addresses multidisciplinary medical and veterinary issues but also promotes research on the basic biology, ecology, monitoring, and management of ticks. Dantas Torres and Otranto (2016) point out that the natural divisions present between human and veterinary medicine are major obstacles that have resulted in a fragmented patchwork of disease surveillance, communication, and control systems. They highlight that veterinarians can play an important role in notifying public health authorities of TB disease outbreaks in pets and livestock that can act as sentinels for human TBIs. Likewise, clinicians and veterinarians dealing with infection should not only treat the owner or animal but record such data in a shared platform to inform epidemiologists of disease risk and current treatment. This bilateral approach to the exchange of information improves understanding of TBIs and their distribution. The integration of such data with ecological surveillance would then inform other disciplines and improve entomological, epidemiological, and public health efforts to refine control strategies. Such increased regional public awareness could reduce the burden of controlling and treating disease on physicians and veterinarians (Baneth 2014). Torina et al. (2018) proposed a geographical information system (GIS)-based approach for integrated strategies of tick surveillance and control, which is of benefit for public health actions. Indeed, Europe CDC (ECDC) established a network for medical and veterinary entomology (VectorNet 2014), which is expected to contribute to improving preparedness and response to vector-borne diseases. Information on geographic spread and prevalence of ticks of public, medical, and veterinary interests are published as a part of this joint effort. (see here: https://www.ecdc.europa.eu/en/about-us/partnerships-and-networks/disease-and-laboratory-networks/vector-net).

23.6 Conclusions and Future Directions

Today, TB agents continue to cause severe illness and death in humans and domestic animals globally. Recognizing the impact of ecological factors on the emergence and transmission of pathogens has become highly relevant from an economic and practical standpoint. Supporting and implementing One Health approaches to managing disease systems is perhaps the most important step needed for tackling the big questions of the next decade. Although a One Health approach works best for simple human/animal TB disease, the paradigm for those vectors carrying multiple pathogens and feeding on multiple hosts is more complex. Future studies should be carried out to obtain data on the abundance, diversity, and vector capacity of tick taxa that are shared with wild and domestic animals that carry zoonotic TB pathogens. As Ostfeld et al. (2014) point out, in order to predict and prevent future epidemics with unrecognized emerging pathogens, studies should be focused on how ecological changes affect human environments and how human behaviors mitigate or exacerbate these effects. To respond to these concerns, Sri Lanka needs a better baseline inventory of circulating ticks and the pathogens they transmit so subsequent environmental and ecological studies can be performed to mitigate tick transmission of various pathogens and outbreaks of associated diseases.

Acknowledgments

We thank Gregory A. Dasch for reading and providing practical suggestions and acknowledge Mevan Rajakaruna for illustration on tick life cycle.

References

Abeygunawardena, H.A., Rathnayaka, D., and Jayathilaka, W.M.A.P. (1997). Characteristics of cattle farming systems in Sri Lanka. *Journal of the National Science Foundation of Sri Lanka* 25 (1): 25–38. https://doi.org/10.4038/jnsfsr.v25i1.5016.

Abeysena, F.A. and Seneviratna, P. (1970). Studies of *Babesia argentina* in cattle in Ceylon. *Ceylon Veterinary Journal* 18: 76–85.

Adjemian, J.Z., Krebs, J., Mandel, E., and McQuiston, J. (2009). Spatial clustering by disease severity among reported Rocky Mountain spotted fever cases in the United States, 2001–2005. *The American Journal of Tropical Medicine and Hygiene* 80 (1): 72–77. https://doi.org/10.4269/ajtmh.2009.80.72.

Ahedor, B., Kothalawala, H., Kanagaratnam, R. et al. (2022). First detection of *Theileria equi* in free-roaming donkeys (*Equus africanus asinus*) in Sri Lanka. *Infection, Genetics and Evolution* 99: 105244. https://doi.org/10.1016/j.meegid.2022.105244.

Alkishe, A., Raghavan, R.K., and Peterson, A.T. (2021). Likely geographic distributional shifts among medically important tick species and tick-associated diseases under climate change in North America: A review. *Insects* 12 (3): 225. https://doi.org/10.3390/insects12030225.

Ammerman, N.C., Swanson, K.I., Anderson, J.M. et al. (2004). Spotted-fever group *Rickettsia* in *Dermacentor variabilis*, Maryland. *Emerging Infectious Diseases* 10 (8): 1478–1481. https://doi.org/10.3201/eid1008.030882.

Anderson, B.E., Dawson, J.E., Jones, D.C., and Wilson, K.H. (1991). *Ehrlichia chaffeensis*, a new species associated with human ehrlichiosis. *Journal of Clinical Microbiology* 29 (12): 2838–2842. https://doi.org/10.1128/jcm.29.12.2838-2842.1991.

Anderson, B.E., Greene, C.E., Jones, D.C., and Dawson, J.E. (1992). *Ehrlichia ewingii* sp. nov., the etiologic agent of canine granulocytic ehrlichiosis. *International Journal of Systematic Bacteriology* 42 (2): 299–302. https://doi.org/10.1099/00207713-42-2-299.

Andoh, M., Sakata, A., Takano, A. et al. (2015). Detection of *Rickettsia* and *Ehrlichia* spp. in ticks associated with exotic reptiles and amphibians imported into Japan. *PLoS One* 10 (7): e0133700. https://doi.org/10.1371/journal.pone.0133700.

Angelakis, E., Munasinghe, A., Yaddehige, I. et al. (2012). Detection of rickettsioses and Q fever in Sri Lanka. *The American Journal of Tropical Medicine and Hygiene* 86 (4): 711–712. https://doi.org/10.4269/ajtmh.2012.11-0424.

Apperson, C.S., Engber, B., Nicholson, W.L. et al. (2008). Tick-borne diseases in North Carolina: Is '*Rickettsia amblyommii*' a possible cause of rickettsiosis reported as Rocky Mountain spotted fever? *Vector Borne and Zoonotic Diseases* 8 (5): 597–606. https://doi.org/10.1089/vbz.2007.0271.

Ariyarathne, S., Apanaskevich, D.A., Amarasinghe, P.H., and Rajakaruna, R.S. (2016). Diversity and distribution of tick species (Acari: Ixodidae) associated with human otoacariasis and socio-ecological risk factors of tick infestations in Sri Lanka. *Experimental and Applied Acarology* 70 (1): 99–123. https://doi.org/10.1007/s10493-016-0056-z.

Arsnoe, I.M., Hickling, G.J., Ginsberg, H.S. et al. (2015). Different populations of blacklegged tick nymphs exhibit differences in questing behavior that have implications for human Lyme disease risk. *PLoS One* 10 (5): e0127450. https://doi.org/10.1371/journal.pone.0127450.

Atapattu, U., Dissanayake, D.R.A., Silva, I.D. et al. (2017). Acute heaptozoonosis caused by *Hepatozoon canis* in dogs in Sri Lanka. *Sri Lanka Veterinary Journal* 64 (1A): 8. https://doi.org/10.4038/slvj.v64i1a.19.

Bakken, J.S., Dumler, S.M., Chen, M.R. et al. (1994). Human granulocytic ehrlichiosis in the upper Midwest United States. A new species emerging? *The Journal of the American Medical Association* 272 (3): 212–218. https://doi.org/10.1001/jama.272.3.212.

Bandaranayaka, K.O., Kularatne, S.A.M., Rajapakse, R.P.V.J. et al. (2021). Human otoacariasis in two climatically diverse districts in Sri Lanka: seasonality, risk factors, and case notes. *Acta Parasitologica* 66 (4): 1326–1340. https://doi.org/10.1007/s11686-021-00372-w.

Bandaranayaka, K.O., Dissanyakae, U.I., and Rajakaruna, R.S. (2022). Diversity and geographic distribution of dog tick species in Sri Lanka and the life cycle of brown dog tick, *Rhipicephalus sanguineus* under laboratory conditions. *Acta Parasitologica* 67: 1708–1718. https://doi.org/10.1007/s11686-022-00622-5.

Baneth, G. (2014). Tick-borne infections of animals and humans: a common ground. *International Journal for Parasitology* 44 (9): 591–596. https://doi.org/10.1016/j.ijpara.2014.03.011.

Barbour, A.G. and Benach, J.L. (2019). Discovery of the Lyme disease agent. *MBio* 10 (5): e02166–e02119. https://doi.org/10.1128/mbio.02166-19.

Bennett, S.R., Quinn, R.L., Telford, S. et al. (2005). The prevalence and significance of canine ehrlichiosis in Colombo, Sri Lanka. *Sri Lanka Veterinary Journal* 52: 1–8.

Breitschwerdt, E.B., Hegarty, B.C., Qurollo, B.A. et al. (2014). Intravascular persistence of *Anaplasma platys, Ehrlichia chaffeensis,* and *Ehrlichia ewingii* DNA in the blood of a dog and two family members. *Parasites & Vectors* 7 (1): 298. https://doi.org/10.1186/1756-3305-7-298.

Bulloch, W. (1935). Theobald Smith. *The Journal of Pathology and Bacteriology* 40 (3): 621–635. https://doi.org/10.1002/path.1700400318.

Burgdorfer, W. (1975). A review of Rocky Mountain spotted fever (tick-borne typhus), its agent, and its tick vectors in the United States. *Journal of Medical Entomology* 12 (3): 269–278. https://doi.org/10.1093/jmedent/12.3.269.

Centers for Disease Control and Prevention. One Health Office Fact Sheet. https://www.cdc.gov/onehealth/who-we-are/one-health-office-fact-sheet.html (accessed 22 January 2022).

Cicculli, V., Capai, L., Quilichini, Y. et al. (2019). Molecular investigation of tick-borne pathogens in ixodid ticks infesting domestic animals (cattle and sheep) and small rodents (black rats) of Corsica, France. *Ticks and Tick-borne Diseases* 10 (3): 606–613. https://doi.org/10.1016/j.ttbdis.2019.02.007.

Clark, K.L. (2012). *Anaplasma phagocytophilum* in small mammals and ticks in northeast Florida. *Journal of Vector Ecology* 37 (1): 262–268. https://doi.org/10.1111/j.1948-7134.2012.00226.x.

Colwell, D.D., Dantas-Torres, F., and Otranto, D. (2011). Vector-borne parasitic zoonoses: emerging scenarios and new perspectives. *Veterinary Parasitology* 182 (1): 14–21. https://doi.org/10.1016/j.vetpar.2011.07.012.

Cordier, C., Tattevin, P., Leyer, C. et al. (2017). *Rickettsia sibirica mongolitimonae* infection, Sri Lanka. *The Journal of Infection in Developing Countries* 11 (8): 668–671. https://doi.org/10.3855/jidc.8743.

Cumming, G.S. (1999). Host distributions do not limit the species ranges of most African ticks (Acari: Ixodida). *Bulletin of Entomological Research* 89 (4): 303–327. https://doi.org/10.1017/s0007485399000450.

Dahanayaka, N.J., Semage, S.N., Weerakoon, K.G. et al. (2017). An unusual outbreak of Rickettsial infection among army soldiers engaged in reconnaissance mission in Northern Sri Lanka. *Ceylon Medical Journal* 62 (2): 108. https://doi.org/10.4038/cmj.v62i2.8477.

Dantas-Torres, F. and Otranto, D. (2016). Best practices for preventing vector-borne diseases in dogs and humans. *Trends in Parasitology* 32 (1): 43–55. https://doi.org/10.1016/j.pt.2015.09.004.

Dasch, G.A., Eremeeva, M.E., Zambrano, M.L. et al. (2022). Molecular characterization of rickettsial agents in ticks (Acari: Ixodidae) from Sri Lanka. *The American Journal of Tropical Medicine and Hygiene* 106 (6): 1613–1623. https://doi.org/10.4269/ajtmh.21-0995.

Dautel, H., Kahl, O. (1999). Ticks *(Acari: Ixodoidea)* and their medical importance in the urban environment. In *Proceedings of the 3rd International Conference on Urban Pests* (ed. W.H. Robinson, F. Rettich, G.W. Rambo). 73–82.

Dautel, H., Kahl, O., and Knülle, W. (1991). The soft tick *Argas reflexus* (F.) (Acari, Argasidae) in urban environments and its medical significance in Berlin (West). *Journal of Applied Entomology* 111 (1–5): 380–390. https://doi.org/10.1111/j.1439-0418.1991.tb00338.x.

Demma, L.J., Traeger, M.S., Nicholson, W.L. et al. (2005). Rocky Mountain spotted fever from an unexpected tick vector in Arizona. *New England Journal of Medicine* 353 (6): 587–594. https://doi.org/10.1056/nejmoa050043.

Department of Animal Production and Health and Lanka, S. (2012). Bovine babesiosis. *Veterinary Epidemiological Bulletin of Sri Lanka* 5: 1–3.

Dissanayake, N.L.A. and Madegedara, D. (2011). An unusual case of fatal pulmonary hemorrhage in pregnancy. *Lung India* 28 (3): 205–208. https://doi.org/10.4103/0970-2113.83979.

Diuk-Wasser, M.A., Gatewood, A.G., Cortinas, M.R. et al. (2006). Spatiotemporal patterns of host-seeking *Ixodes scapularis* nymphs (Acari: Ixodidae) in the United States. *Journal of Medical Entomology* 43 (2): 166–176. https://doi.org/10.1093/jmedent/43.2.166.

Diuk-Wasser, M.A., Vourc'h, G., Cislo, P. et al. (2010). Field and climate-based model for predicting the density of host-seeking nymphal *Ixodes scapularis*, an important vector of tick-borne disease agents in the eastern United States. *Global Ecology and Biogeography* 19: 504–514. https://doi.org/10.1111/j.1466-8238.2010.00526.x.

Diuk-Wasser, M.A., Hoen, A.G., Cislo, P. et al. (2012). Human risk of infection with *Borrelia burgdorferi*, the Lyme disease agent, in Eastern United States. *The American Journal of Tropical Medicine and Hygiene* 86 (2): 320–327. https://doi.org/10.4269/ajtmh.2012.11-0395.

Diuk-Wasser, M.A., VanAcker, M.C., and Fernandez, M.P. (2021). Impact of land use changes and habitat fragmentation on the eco-epidemiology of tick-borne diseases. *Journal of Medical Entomology* 58 (4): 1546–1564. https://doi.org/10.1093/jme/tjaa209.

Diyes, G. and Rajakaruna, R. (2015). Diversity and distribution of tick species infesting goats with two new host records from Sri Lanka. *Journal of the National Science Foundation of Sri Lanka* 43 (3): 225. https://doi.org/10.4038/jnsfsr.v43i3.7951.

Diyes, G.C.P., Rajapakse, R.P.V.J., and Rajakaruna, R.S. (2018). Molecular evidence of *Babesia* infections in Spinose ear tick, *Otobius megnini* infesting stabled horses in Nuwara Eliya racecourse: a case study. *Ceylon Journal of Science* 47 (4): 405. https://doi.org/10.4038/cjs.v47i4.7559.

Duncan, K.T., Grant, A., Johnson, B. et al. (2021). Identification of *Rickettsia* spp. and *Babesia conradae* in *Dermacentor* spp. collected from dogs and cats across the United States. *Vector Borne and Zoonotic Diseases* 21 (12): 911–920. https://doi.org/10.1089/vbz.2021.0047.

Dworkin, M.S., Schwan, T.G., Anderson, D.E., and Borchardt, S.M. (2008). Tick-borne relapsing fever. *Infectious Disease Clinics of North America* 22 (3): 449–468. https://doi.org/10.1016/j.idc.2008.03.006.

Ebel, G.D. and Kramer, L.D. (2004). Short report: duration of tick attachment required for transmission of Powassan virus by deer ticks. *The American Journal of Tropical Medicine and Hygiene* 71 (3): 268–271. https://doi.org/10.4269/ajtmh.2004.71.3.0700268.

Ehelepola, N.D.B., Kumara, G.D.N.R., Sapurugala, S.A.C.S. et al. (2019). An atypical case of rickettsial spotted fever myocarditis mimicking weil's disease. *Case Reports in Infectious Diseases* 9620245, pp. 1–6. https://doi.org/10.1155/2019/9620245.

Eisen, R.J. and Eisen, L. (2018). The blacklegged tick, *Ixodes scapularis*: an increasing public health concern. *Trends in Parasitology* 34 (4): 295–309. https://doi.org/10.1016/j.pt.2017.12.006.

Eisen, R.J. and Paddock, C.D. (2021). Tick and tickborne pathogen surveillance as a public health tool in the United States. *Journal of Medical Entomology* 58 (4): 1490–1502. https://doi.org/10.1093/jme/tjaa087.

Eisen, R.J., Eisen, L., and Beard, C.B. (2016a). County-scale distribution of *Ixodes scapularis* and *Ixodes pacificus* (Acari: Ixodidae) in the continental United States. *Journal of Medical Entomology* 53 (2): 349–386. https://doi.org/10.1093/jme/tjv237.

Eisen, R.J., Eisen, L., Ogden, N.H., and Beard, C.B. (2016b). Linkages of weather and climate with *Ixodes scapularis* and *Ixodes pacificus* (Acari: Ixodidae), enzootic transmission of *Borrelia burgdorferi*, and Lyme Disease in North America. *Journal of Medical Entomology* 53 (2): 250–261. https://doi.org/10.1093/jme/tjv199.

Eisen, R.J., Kugeler, K.J., Eisen, L. et al. (2017). Tick-borne zoonoses in the United States: persistent and emerging threats to human health. *ILAR Journal* 58 (3): 319–335. https://doi.org/10.1093/ilar/ilx005.

Ellwanger, J.H. and Chies, J.A.B. (2021). Zoonotic spillover: Understanding basic aspects for better prevention. *Genetics and Molecular Biology* 44 (1 Suppl. 1): e20200355. https://doi.org/10.1590/1678-4685-GMB-2020-0355.

Fleshman, A.C., Graham, C.B., Maes, S.E. et al. (2021). Reported county-level distribution of Lyme disease spirochetes, *Borrelia burgdorferi sensu stricto* and *Borrelia mayonii* (Spirochaetales: Spirochaetaceae), in host-seeking *Ixodes scapularis* and *Ixodes pacificus* ticks (Acari: Ixodidae) in the contiguous United States. *Journal of Medical Entomology* 58 (3): 1219–1233. https://doi.org/10.1093/jme/tjaa283.

Fleshman, A.C., Foster, E., Maes, S.E., and Eisen, R.J. (2022). Reported county-level distribution of seven human pathogens detected in host-seeking *Ixodes scapularis* and *Ixodes pacificus* (Acari: Ixodidae) in the contiguous United States. *Journal of Medical Entomology* 59 (4): 1328–1335. https://doi.org/10.1093/jme/tjac049.

Francis, L., Paddock, C.D., Dykstra, E.A., and Karpathy, S.E. (2020). *Rickettsia* and *Anaplasma* species in *Dermacentor andersoni* ticks from Washington. *Ticks and Tick-borne Diseases* 11 (4): 101422. https://doi.org/10.1016/j.ttbdis.2020.101422.

Ginsberg, H.S. and Faulde, M.K. (2008). Ticks. In: *Public Health Significance of Urban Pests* (ed. X. Bonnefoy, H. Kampen and K. Sweeney), 303–345. Copenhagen: World Health Organization.

Guglielmone, A.A., Robbins, R.G., Apanaskevich, D.A. et al. (2010). The Argasidae, Ixodidae and Nuttalliellidae (Acari: Ixodida) of the world: a list of valid species names. *Zootaxa* 2528 (1): 1–28. https://doi.org/10.11646/zootaxa.2528.1.1.

Gunasekara, E., Sivakumar, T., Kothalawala, H. et al. (2019). Epidemiological survey of hemoprotozoan parasites in cattle from low-country wet zone in Sri Lanka. *Parasitology*

International 71: 5–10. https://doi.org/10.1016/j.parint.2019.03.004.

Harden, V.A. (1990). A blight on the Bitterroot, chapter 2. In: *Rocky Mountain spotted fever. History of a twentieth-century disease,* 9–22. Baltimore, MD: Johns Hopkins University Press.

Hartemink, N. and Takken, W. (2016). Trends in tick population dynamics and pathogen transmission in emerging tick-borne pathogens in Europe: an introduction. *Experimental and Applied Acarology* 68 (3): 269–278. https://doi.org/10.1007/s10493-015-0003-4.

Hauck, D., Jordan, D., Springer, A. et al. (2020). Transovarial transmission of *Borrelia* spp., *Rickettsia* spp. and *Anaplasma phagocytophilum* in *Ixodes ricinus* under field conditions extrapolated from DNA detection in questing larvae. *Parasites & Vectors* 13 (1): 176. https://doi.org/10.1186/s13071-020-04049-7.

Hawlena, H., Rynkiewicz, E., Toh, E. et al. (2012). The arthropod, but not the vertebrate host or its environment, dictates bacterial community composition of fleas and ticks. *The ISME Journal* 7 (1): 221–223. https://doi.org/10.1038/ismej.2012.71.

Herath, H.M.L.Y., Jayasundara, J.M.H.D., Senadhira, S.D.N. et al. (2018). Spotted fever rickettsioses causing myocarditis and ARDS: a case from Sri Lanka. *BMC Infectious Diseases* 18 (1): 705. https://doi.org/10.1186/s12879-018-3631-6.

Hermance, M.E. and Thangamani, S. (2017). Powassan virus: an emerging arbovirus of public health concern in North America. *Vector Borne and Zoonotic Diseases* 17 (7): 453–462. https://doi.org/10.1089/vbz.2017.2110.

Herms, W.B. and Wheeler, C.M. (1936). *Ornithodoros hermsi* Wheeler as a vector of relapsing fever in California. *The Journal of Parasitology* 22 (3): 276. https://doi.org/10.2307/3271536.

Hoogstraal, H. and Aeschlimann, A. (1982). Tick-host specificity. *Bulletin de la Société Entomologique Suisse* 55: 5–32.

Huxsoll, D.L., Hildebrandt, P.K., Nims, R.M. et al. (1970). Epizootiology of tropical canine pancytopenia. *Journal of Wildlife Diseases* 6 (4): 220–225. https://doi.org/10.7589/0090-3558-6.4.220.

Ismail, N. and McBride, J.W. (2017). Tick-borne emerging infections. *Clinics in Laboratory Medicine* 37 (2): 317–340. https://doi.org/10.1016/j.cll.2017.01.006.

Jayathilake, P.S., Rajakaruna, R.S., Fernando, A.D.S. et al. (2020). *Canine Vector-Borne Diseases of Working Military Dogs of Sri Lanka Air Force, Free-Roaming and Owned Dogs*, 140. *PGIS (Postgraduate Institute of Science) Research Congress, RESCON. University of Peradeniya.*

Jeker, K., Weber, R., Schulthess, G., and Furrer, J. (2005). Multilokuläre grosse Erytheme und Fieber. *Praxis* 94 (46): 1815–1819. https://doi.org/10.1024/0369-8394.94.46.1815.German.

Johnston, D., Kelly, J.R., Ledizet, M. et al. (2022). Frequency and geographic distribution of *Borrelia miyamotoi, Borrelia burgdorferi*, and *Babesia microti* infections in New England residents. *Clinical Infectious Diseases* 1–6. https://doi.org/10.1093/cid/ciac107.

Jones, K.E., Patel, N.G., Levy, M.A. et al. (2008). Global trends in emerging infectious diseases. *Nature* 451 (7181): 990–993. https://doi.org/10.1038/nature06536.

Jongejan, F. and Uilenberg, G. (2004). The global importance of ticks. *Parasitology* 129 (Suppl): S3–S14. https://doi.org/10.1017/s0031182004005967.

Jorgensen, W.K., Weilgama, D.J., Navaratne, M., and Dalgliesh, R.J. (1992). Prevalence of *Babesia bovis* and *Anaplasma marginale* at selected localities in Sri Lanka. *Tropical Animal Health and Production* 24 (1): 9–14. https://doi.org/10.1007/bf02357227.

Kariyawasam, A.G.T.A., Palangasinghe, D.R., Fonseka, C.L. et al. (2019). Bilateral sensorineural deafness in a young pregnant female presenting with a fever: a rare complication of a reemerging disease – spotted fever group rickettsioses. *Case Reports in Infectious Diseases* 2019: 5923146, pp. 1–5. https://doi.org/10.1155/2019/5923146.

Keefe, T.J., Holland, C.J., Salyer, P.E., and Ristic, M. (1982). Distribution of *Ehrlichia canis* among military working dogs in the world and selected civilian dogs in the United States. *Journal of the American Veterinary Medical Association* 181 (3): 236–238.

Keesing, F. and Ostfeld, R.S. (2021). Impacts of biodiversity and biodiversity loss on zoonotic diseases. *Proceedings of the National Academy of Sciences* 118 (17): e2023540118. https://doi.org/10.1073/pnas.2023540118.

Kováčová, E., Sixl, W., Stünzner, D. et al. (1996). Serological examination of human and animal sera from six countries of three continents for the presence of rickettsial antibodies. *European Journal of Epidemiology* 12 (1): 85–89. https://doi.org/10.1007/bf00144434.

Krasnov, B.R., Mouillot, D., Shenbrot, G.I. et al. (2010). Similarity in ectoparasite faunas of Palaearctic rodents as a function of host phylogenetic, geographic or environmental distances: which matters the most? *International Journal for Parasitology* 40 (7): 807–817. https://doi.org/10.1016/j.ijpara.2009.12.002.

Kularatne, S.A.M., Edirisingha, J.S., Gawarammana, I.B. et al. (2003). Emerging rickettsial infections in Sri Lanka: the pattern in the hilly Central Province. *Tropical Medicine and International Health* 8 (9): 803–811. https://doi.org/10.1046/j.1365-3156.2003.01108.x.

Kularatne, S.A.M., Rajapakse, R.P.V.J., Wickramasinghe, W.M.R.S. et al. (2013). Rickettsioses in the central hills of Sri Lanka: serological evidence of increasing burden of spotted fever group. *International Journal of Infectious Diseases* s17: e988–e992.

Kularatne, S.A.M., Fernando, R., Selvaratnam, S. et al. (2018). Intra-aural tick bite causing unilateral facial nerve palsy in 29 cases over 16 years in Kandy, Sri Lanka: is rickettsial aetiology possible? *BMC Infectious Diseases* 18 (1): 418. https://doi.org/10.1186/s12879-018-3338-8.

Kumara, K.A.A.S., Wickramasinghe, S., Kulanayake, S.M.P., and Rajapakse, R.P.V.J. (2013). Molecular identification and prevalence of vector-borne infections in dogs from Western Province in Sri Lanka. *Symp. 2nd Annual Conference and Scientific sessions of Sri Lankan Society for Microbiology (SSM)* (25 October 2013). PGIS, University of Peradeniya, 25.

Lane, R.S., Mun, J., Peribáñez, M.A., and Fedorova, N. (2010). Differences in prevalence of *Borrelia burgdorferi* and *Anaplasma* spp. infection among host-seeking *Dermacentor occidentalis, Ixodes pacificus*, and *Ornithodoros coriaceus* ticks in northwestern California. *Ticks and Tick-borne Diseases* 1 (4): 159–167. https://doi.org/10.1016/j.ttbdis.2010.09.004.

Lane, R.S., Fedorova, N., Kleinjan, J.E., and Maxwell, M. (2013). Eco-epidemiological factors contributing to the low risk of human exposure to ixodid tick-borne borreliae in southern California, USA. *Ticks and Tick-borne Diseases* 4 (5): 377–385. https://doi.org/10.1016/j.ttbdis.2013.02.005.

Lehane, A., Maes, S.E., Graham, C.B. et al. (2021). Prevalence of single and coinfections of human pathogens in Ixodes ticks from five geographical regions in the United States, 2013–2019. *Ticks and Tick-borne Diseases* 12 (2): 101637. https://doi.org/10.1016/j.ttbdis.2020.101637.

Levy, S. (2013). The Lyme disease debate host biodiversity and human disease risk. *Environmental Health Perspectives* 121 (4): A120–A125. https://doi.org/10.1289/ehp.121-a120.

Lewis, J., Kirby, A.M., Harris, K.D. et al. (2021). Monitoring risk: tick and *Borrelia burgdorferi* public participatory surveillance in the Canadian Maritimes, 2012–2020. *Pathogens* 10 (10): 1284. https://doi.org/10.3390/pathogens10101284.

Little, S.E., Barrett, A.W., Nagamori, Y. et al. (2018). Ticks from cats in the United States: patterns of infestation and infection with pathogens. *Veterinary Parasitology* 257: 15–20. https://doi.org/10.1016/j.vetpar.2018.05.002.

Liyanaarachchi, D.R., Jinadasa, H.R.N., Dilrukshi, P.R.M.P., and Rajapakse, R.P.V.J. (2013). Epidemiological study on ticks in farm animals in selected areas of Sri Lanka. *Tropical Agricultural Research* 24: 336–346.

Liyanaarachchi, D.R., Rajakaruna, R.S., Dikkumbura, A.W. et al. (2015a). Ticks (Acarina: Ixodida) infesting five reptile species in Sri Lanka with sixteen new host records. *Zootaxa* 3964 (1): 146. https://doi.org/10.11646/zootaxa.3964.1.11.

Liyanaarachchi, D.R., Rajakaruna, R.S., Dikkumbura, A.W., and Rajapakse, R.P.V.J. (2015b). Ticks infesting wild and domestic animals and humans of Sri Lanka with new host records. *Acta Tropica* 142: 64–70. https://doi.org/10.1016/j.actatropica.2014.11.001.

Liyanaarachchi, D.R., Rajakaruna, R.S., and Rajapakse, R.P.V.J. (2015c). Spotted fever group rickettsia in ticks infesting humans, wild and domesticated animals of Sri Lanka: one health approach. *Ceylon Journal of Science (Biological Sciences)* 44 (2): 67. https://doi.org/10.4038/cjsbs.v44i2.7351.

Liyanapathirana, V.C. and Thevanesam, V. (2011). Seroepidemiololgy of rickettsioses in Sri Lanka: a patient-based study. *BMC Infectious Diseases* 11 (1): 328. https://doi.org/10.1186/1471-2334-11-328.

Loss, S.R., Noden, B.H., Hamer, G.L., and Hamer, S.A. (2016). A quantitative synthesis of the role of birds in carrying ticks and tick-borne pathogens in North America. *Oecologia* 182 (4): 947–959. https://doi.org/10.1007/s00442-016-3731-1.

Luke, N., Munasinghe, H., Balasooriya, L., and Premaratna, R. (2017). Widespread subcutaneous necrosis in spotted fever group Rickettsioses from the coastal belt of Sri Lanka – a case report. *BMC Infectious Diseases* 17 (1): 278. https://doi.org/10.1186/s12879-017-2375-z.

MacGaughey, C.A., Seneviratna, P., and Mahalingam, S. (1962). Rickettsiosis of dogs in Ceylon. *Ceylon Veterinary Journal* 10: 82–87.

Maggi, R.G., Mascarelli, P.E., Havenga, L.N. et al. (2013). Co-infection with *Anaplasma platys, Bartonella henselae* and *Candidatus* Mycoplasma haematoparvum in a veterinarian. *Parasites & Vectors* 6 (1): 103. https://doi.org/10.1186/1756-3305-6-103.

Maia, C., Ramos, C., Coimbra, M. et al. (2014). Bacterial and protozoal agents of feline vector-borne diseases in domestic and stray cats from southern Portugal. *Parasites & Vectors* 7 (1): 115. https://doi.org/10.1186/1756-3305-7-115.

Maia, C., Almeida, B., Coimbra, M. et al. (2015). Bacterial and protozoal agents of canine vector-borne diseases in the blood of domestic and stray dogs from southern Portugal. *Parasites & Vectors* 8 (1): 138. https://doi.org/10.1186/s13071-015-0759-8.

Mathisson, D.C., Kross, S.M., Palmer, M.I., and Diuk-Wasser, M.A. (2021). Effect of vegetation on the abundance of tick vectors in the Northeastern United States: a review of the literature. *Journal of Medical Entomology* 58 (6): 2030–2037. https://doi.org/10.1093/jme/tjab098.

McCoy, K.D., Léger, E., and Dietrich, M. (2013). Host specialization in ticks and transmission of tick-borne diseases: a review. *Frontiers in Cellular and Infection Microbiology* 3 (Article 57): 1–12. https://doi.org/10.3389/fcimb.2013.00057.

McQuiston, J.H., Zemtsova, G., Perniciaro, J. et al. (2012). Afebrile spotted fever group *Rickettsia* infection after a bite from a *Dermacentor variabilis* tick infected with *Rickettsia montanensis*. *Vector Borne and Zoonotic Diseases* 12 (12): 1059–1061. https://doi.org/10.1089/vbz.2012.1078.

Michalski, M., Rosenfield, C., Erickson, M. et al. (2006). *Anaplasma phagocytophilum* in central and western Wisconsin: a molecular survey. *Parasitology Research* 99 (6): 694–699. https://doi.org/10.1007/s00436-006-0217-9.

Millán, J., Proboste, T., Fernández de Mera, I.G. et al. (2016). Molecular detection of vector-borne pathogens in wild and domestic carnivores and their ticks at the human–wildlife interface. *Ticks and Tick-borne Diseases* 7 (2): 284–290. https://doi.org/10.1016/j.ttbdis.2015.11.003.

Moncayo, A.C., Cohen, S.B., Fritzen, C.M. et al. (2010). Absence of *Rickettsia rickettsii* and occurrence of other spotted fever group rickettsiae in ticks from Tennessee. *The American Journal of Tropical Medicine and Hygiene* 83 (3): 653–657. https://doi.org/10.4269/ajtmh.2010.09-0197.

Morissette, E., Massung, R.F., Foley, J.E. et al. (2009). Diversity of *Anaplasma phagocytophilum* strains, USA. *Emerging Infectious Diseases* 15 (6): 928–931. https://doi.org/10.3201/eid1506.081610.

Murphy, D.S., Lee, X., Larson, S.R. et al. (2017). Prevalence and distribution of human and tick infections with the *Ehrlichia muris*-like agent and *Anaplasma phagocytophilum* in Wisconsin, 2009–2015. *Vector Borne and Zoonotic Diseases* 17 (4): 229–236. https://doi.org/10.1089/vbz.2016.2055.

Nagalingam, K., Rolain, J.M., Thevanesam, V. et al. (2009). Spotted fever rickettsioses in children in Sri Lanka. *Clinical Microbiology and Infection* 15 (Suppl. 2): 330–331. https://doi.org/10.1111/j.1469-0691.2008.02262.x.

Nair, A.D.S., Cheng, C., Ganta, C.K. et al. (2016). Comparative experimental infection study in dogs with *Ehrlichia canis, E. chaffeensis, Anaplasma platys* and *A. phagocytophilum*. *PLoS One* 11 (2): e0148239. https://doi.org/10.1371/journal.pone.0148239.

Nanayakkara, D.M., Rajapakse, R.P.V.J., Wickramasinghe, S., and Kularatne, S.A.M. (2013). Serological evidence for exposure of dogs to *Rickettsia conorii*, *Rickettsia typhi*, and *Orientia tsutsugamushi in* Sri Lanka. *Vector Borne and Zoonotic Diseases* 13 (8): 545–549. https://doi.org/10.1089/vbz.2012.1049.

Neelawala, D., Dissanayake, D.R.A., Prasada, D.V.P., and Silva, I.D. (2021). Analysis of risk factors associated with recurrence of canine babesiosis caused by *Babesia gibsoni*. *Comparative Immunology, Microbiology and Infectious Diseases* 74: 101572. https://doi.org/10.1016/j.cimid.2020.101572.

Neiderud, C.J. (2015). How urbanization affects the epidemiology of emerging infectious diseases. *Infection Ecology & Epidemiology* 5 (1): 27060. https://doi.org/10.3402/iee.v5.27060.

Nicholson, W.L., Allen, K.E., McQuiston, J.H. et al. (2010). The increasing recognition of rickettsial pathogens in dogs and people. *Trends in Parasitology* 26 (4): 205–212. 10.1016/j.pt.2010.01.007.

Niemelä, J. (2011). *Urban Ecology, Patterns, Processes, and Applications*, 392. New York, NY: Oxford University Press.

Nijhof, A., Guglielmone, A.A., Horak I. et al. (2005). A global tick host-pathogen database (THPbase) *Newsletter on ticks and tick-borne diseases of livestock in the tropics (ICTTD-3)* 28: 3.

Obsomer, V., Wirtgen, M., Linden, A. et al. (2013). Spatial disaggregation of tick occurrence and ecology at a local scale as a preliminary step for spatial surveillance of tick-borne diseases: general framework and health implications in Belgium. *Parasites & Vectors* 6 (1): 190. https://doi.org/10.1186/1756-3305-6-190.

Ogden, N.H., Mechai, S., and Margos, G. (2013). Changing geographic ranges of ticks and tick-borne pathogens: drivers, mechanisms and consequences for pathogen diversity. *Frontiers in Cellular and Infection Microbiology* 3 (Article 46): 1–11. https://doi.org/10.3389/fcimb.2013.00046.

Openshaw, J.J., Swerdlow, D.L., Krebs, J.W. et al. (2010). Rocky Mountain spotted fever in the United States, 2000–2007: interpreting contemporary increases in incidence. *The American Journal of Tropical Medicine and Hygiene* 83 (1): 174–182. https://doi.org/10.4269/ajtmh.2010.09-0752.

Ostfeld, R.S. and Keesing, F. (2000). Biodiversity series: the function of biodiversity in the ecology of vector-borne zoonotic diseases. *Canadian Journal of Zoology* 78: 2061–2078.

Ostfeld, R.S., Levi, T., Jolles, A.E. et al. (2014). Life history and demographic drivers of reservoir competence for three tick-borne zoonotic pathogens. *PLoS One* 9 (9): e107387. https://doi.org/10.1371/journal.pone.0107387.

Paddock, C.D. and Yabsley, M.J. (2007). Ecological havoc, the rise of white-tailed deer, and the emergence of *Amblyomma americanum*-associated zoonoses in the United States. *Current Topics in Microbiology and Immunology* 315: 289–324. https://doi.org/10.1007/978-3-540-70962-6_12.

Parola, P., Paddock, C.D., and Raoult, D. (2005). Tick-borne rickettsioses around the world: emerging diseases challenging old concepts. *Clinical Microbiology Reviews* 18 (4): 719–756. https://doi.org/10.1128/CMR.18.4.719-756.2005.

Parola, P., Paddock, C.D., Socolovschi, C. et al. (2013). Update on tick-borne rickettsioses around the world: a geographic approach. *Clinical Microbiology Reviews* 26 (4): 657–702. https://doi.org/10.1128/CMR.00032-13.

Perez, M., Bodor, M., Zhang, C. et al. (2006). Human infection with *Ehrlichia canis* accompanied by clinical signs in Venezuela. *Annals of the New York Academy of Sciences* 1078 (1): 110–117. https://doi.org/10.1196/annals.1374.016.

Pfaeffle, M., Littwin, N., and Petney, T.N. (2015). The relationship between biodiversity and disease transmission risk. *Research and Reports in Biodiversity Studies* 4: 9–20. https://doi.org/10.2147/rrbs.s52433.

Pfäffle, M., Littwin, N., Muders, S.V., and Petney, T.N. (2013). The ecology of tick-borne diseases. *International Journal for Parasitology* 43 (12–13): 1059–1077. https://doi.org/10.1016/j.ijpara.2013.06.009.

Pimburage, R.M.S., Harischandra, P.A.L., Gunatilake, M. et al. (2017). A cross-sectional survey on dog ecology and dog anti-rabies vaccination coverage in selected areas in Sri Lanka. *Sri Lanka Veterinary Journal* 64 (1A): 1. https://doi.org/10.4038/slvj.v64i1a.18.

Poitout, F.M., Shinozaki, J.K., Stockwell, P.J. et al. (2005). Genetic variants of *Anaplasma phagocytophilum* infecting dogs in Western Washington State. *Journal of Clinical Microbiology* 43 (2): 796–801. https://doi.org/10.1128/jcm.43.2.796-801.2005.

Premaratna, R., Loftis, A.D., Chandrasena, T.G.A.N. et al. (2008). Rickettsial infections and their clinical presentations in the Western Province of Sri Lanka: a hospital-based study. *International Journal of Infectious Diseases* 12 (2): 198–202. https://doi.org/10.1016/j.ijid.2007.06.009.

Premaratna, R., Chandrasena, T.G.A.N., Rajapakse, R.P.V.J. et al. (2009). Rickettsioses presenting as major joint arthritis and erythema nodosum: description of four patients. *Clinical Rheumatology* 28 (7): 867–868. https://doi.org/10.1007/s10067-009-1166-3.

Premaratna, R., Liyanaarachchi, E., Rajapakse, R. et al. (2012). A patient with spotted fever group rickettsiosis mimicking connective tissue disease. *Ceylon Medical Journal* 57 (3): 127. https://doi.org/10.4038/cmj.v57i3.4707.

Premaratna, R., Ariyaratna, N., Attanayake, C. et al. (2014). Rickettsial infection among military personnel deployed in Northern Sri Lanka. *BMC Infectious Diseases* 14 (1): 3864. https://doi.org/10.1186/s12879-014-0688-8.

Price, K.J., Ayres, B.N., Maes, S.E. et al. (2022). First detection of human pathogenic variant of *Anaplasma phagocytophilum* in field-collected *Haemaphysalis longicornis*, Pennsylvania, USA. *Zoonoses and Public Health* 69 (2): 143–148. https://doi.org/10.1111/zph.12901.

Pritt, B.S., Sloan, L.M., Johnson, D.K.H. et al. (2011). Emergence of a new pathogenic *Ehrlichia* species, Wisconsin and Minnesota, 2009. *New England Journal of Medicine* 365 (5): 422–429. https://doi.org/10.1056/nejmoa1010493.

Pritt, B.S., Respicio-Kingry, L.B., Sloan, L.M. et al. (2016). *Borrelia mayonii* sp. nov., a member of the *Borrelia burgdorferi sensu lato* complex, detected in patients and ticks in the upper midwestern United States. *International Journal of Systematic and Evolutionary Microbiology* 66 (11): 4878–4880. https://doi.org/10.1099/ijsem.0.001445.

Rainey, T., Occi, J.L., Robbins, R.G., and Egizi, A. (2018). Discovery of *Haemaphysalis longicornis* (Ixodida: Ixodidae) parasitizing a sheep in New Jersey, United States. *Journal of Medical Entomology* 55 (3): 757–759. https://doi.org/10.1093/jme/tjy006.

Ranatunga, R.A.S., Bodahewa, A.P., Peiris, K.H.A.T.D et al. (2021). First detection and molecular identification of *Babesia peroncitoi* in pigs in Sri Lanka Peradeniya University International Research Sessions (iPURSE), Peradeniya, Sri Lanka.

Ranatunga, R.A.S., Dangolla, A., Sooriyapathirana, S.D.S.S., and Rajakaruna, R.S. (2022). High Asymptomatic cases of babesiosis in dogs and comparison of diagnostic performance of conventional PCR vs blood smears. *Acta Parasitologica* https://doi.org/10.1007/s11686-022-00549-x.

Raoult, D. and Parola, P. (2008). Rocky Mountain spotted fever in the USA: a benign disease or a common diagnostic error? *The Lancet Infectious Diseases* 8 (10): 587–589. https://doi.org/10.1016/s1473-3099(08)70210-x.

Rebman, A.W. and Aucott, J.N. (2020). Post-treatment Lyme disease as a model for persistent symptoms in Lyme disease. *Frontiers in Medicine* 7 (Article 57): 1–16. https://doi.org/10.3389/fmed.2020.00057.

Reller, M.E., Bodinayake, C., Nagahawatte, A. et al. (2012). Unsuspected rickettsioses among patients with acute febrile illness, Sri Lanka, 2007. *Emerging Infectious Diseases* 18 (5): 825–829. https://doi.org/10.3201/eid1805.111563.

Ribeiro, C.M., de Carvalho, J.L.B., de Santis Bastos, P.A. et al. (2021). Prevalence of *Rickettsia rickettsii* in ticks: systematic review and meta-analysis. *Vector Borne and Zoonotic Diseases* 21 (8): 557–565. https://doi.org/10.1089/vbz.2021.0004.).

Ricketts, H.T. (1906). The transmission of rocky mountain spotted fever by the bite of the wood-tick (*Dermacentor occidentalis*). *JAMA: The Journal of the American Medical Association* XLVII (5): 358. https://doi.org/10.1001/jama.1906.25210050042002j.

Ricketts, H.T. (1909). A micro-organism which apparently has a specific relationship to Rocky Mountain spotted fever: A preliminary report. *JAMA: The Journal of the American Medical Association* LII (5): 379–380. https://doi.org/10.1001/jama.1909.02540320063015.

Rochlin, I. and Toledo, A. (2020). Emerging tick-borne pathogens of public health importance: a mini-review. *Journal of Medical Microbiology* 69 (6): 781–791. https://doi.org/10.1099/jmm.0.001206.

Rogalski, M.A., Gowler, C.D., Shaw, C.L. et al. (2017). Human drivers of ecological and evolutionary dynamics in emerging and disappearing infectious disease systems. *Philosophical Transactions of the Royal Society, B: Biological Sciences* 372 (1712): 20160043. https://doi.org/10.1098/rstb.2016.0043.

Saleh, M.N., Allen, K.E., Lineberry, M.W. et al. (2021). Ticks infesting dogs and cats in North America: biology, geographic distribution, and pathogen transmission. *Veterinary Parasitology* 294: 109392. https://doi.org/10.1016/j.vetpar.2021.109392.

Salkeld, D.J., Padgett, K.A., and Jones, J.H. (2013). A meta-analysis suggesting that the relationship between biodiversity and risk of zoonotic pathogen transmission is idiosyncratic. *Ecology Letters* 16 (5): 679–686. https://doi.org/10.1111/ele.12101.

Sambado, S., Salomon, J., Crews, A., and Swei, A. (2020). Mixed transmission modes promote persistence of an emerging tick-borne pathogen. *Ecosphere* 11 (6): e03171. https://doi.org/10.1002/ecs2.3171.

Schmidt, K.A. and Ostfeld, R.S. (2001). Biodiversity and the dilution effect in disease ecology. *Ecology* 82 (3): 609–619. https://doi.org/10.1890/0012-9658(2001)082[0609:BATDEI]2.0.CO;2.

Seneviratna, P. (1953). Piroplasmosis of dogs in Ceylon. *Ceylon Veterinary Journal* 1: 95–98.

Seneviratna, P. (1965a). Studies of *Babesia gibsoni* (Patton, 1910) Infections in the dog. *British Veterinary Journal* 121 (6): 263–271. https://doi.org/10.1016/s0007-1935(17)41153-5.

Seneviratna, P. (1965b). The pathology of *Babesia gibsoni* (Patton, 1910) infection in the dog. *Ceylon Veterinary Journal* 13: 107–110. https://doi.org/10.1016/0014-4894(72)90057-4.

Seneviratna, P. and Jayawickrama, S.D. (1961). Treatment of *Babesia gibsoni* infections in dogs with Spirotrypan hoeschst. *The Indian Veterinary Journal* 38: 465–474.

VectorNet (2014). European network for medical and veterinary entomology. https://www.ecdc.europa.eu/en/about-us/partnerships-and-networks/disease-and-laboratory-networks/vector-net (accessed 9 January 2022).

Silva, I. (2016). Complex clinical presentations of tick-borne diseases in dogs in Sri Lanka. *Sri Lanka Veterinary Journal* 63 (2): 1. https://doi.org/10.4038/slvj.v63i2.9.

Sivakumar, T., Fujita, S., Tuvshintulga, B. et al. (2019). Discovery of a new *Theileria* sp. closely related to *Theileria annulata* in cattle from Sri Lanka. *Scientific Reports* 9 (1): 16132. https://doi.org/10.1038/s41598-019-52512-y.

Sivakumar, T., Kothalawala, H., Abeyratne, S.A.E. et al. (2012). A PCR-based survey of selected *Babesia* and *Theileria* parasites in cattle in Sri Lanka. *Veterinary Parasitology* 190 (1–2): 263–267. https://doi.org/10.1016/j.vetpar.2012.05.014.

Sivakumar, T., Kothalawala, H., Weerasooriya, G. et al. (2016). A longitudinal study of *Babesia* and *Theileria* infections in cattle in Sri Lanka. *Veterinary Parasitology: Regional Studies and Reports* 6: 20–27. https://doi.org/10.1016/j.vprsr.2016.11.009.

Sivakumar, T., Tattiyapong, M., Fukushi, S. et al. (2014). Genetic characterization of *Babesia* and *Theileria* parasites in water buffaloes in Sri Lanka. *Veterinary Parasitology* 200 (1–2): 24–30. https://doi.org/10.1016/j.vetpar.2013.11.029.

Sivakumar, T., Tuvshintulga, B., Kothalawala, H. et al. (2020). Host range and geographical distribution of *Babesia* sp. Mymensingh. *Transboundary and Emerging Diseases* 67: 2233–2239. https://doi.org/10.1111/tbed.13546.

Sivakumar, T., Tuvshintulga, B., Zhyldyz, A. et al. (2018). Genetic analysis of *Babesia* isolates from cattle with clinical babesiosis in Sri Lanka. *Journal of Clinical Microbiology* 56 (11): e00895–e00818. https://doi.org/10.1128/JCM.00895-18.

Smith, T. and Kilborne, F.L. (1893). Investigations into nature, causation, and preventions of Texas or Southern cattle fever. *Washington Government Printing Office* 1893: http://resource.nlm.nih.gov/62350480R.

Sonenshine, D.E. (1991). *Biology of Ticks*. New York Oxford University Press.

Sonenshine, D.E. (1993). *Biology of Ticks*, vol. 2. New York Oxford: Oxford University Press.

Sonenshine, D.E. and Roe, R.M. (2013). *Biology of Ticks*, 2e. Oxford University Press: New York Oxford.

Stanley, H.M., Ford, S.L., Snellgrove, A.N. et al. (2020). The ability of the invasive Asian Longhorned tick *Haemaphysalis longicornis* (Acari: Ixodidae) to acquire and transmit *Rickettsia rickettsii* (Rickettsiales: Rickettsiaceae), the agent of Rocky Mountain spotted fever, under laboratory conditions. *Journal of Medical Entomology* 57 (5): 1635–1639. https://doi.org/10.1093/jme/tjaa076.

Stokes, P.H. and Walters, B.J. (2009). Spotted fever rickettsiosis infection in a traveler from Sri Lanka. *Journal of Travel Medicine* 16 (6): 436–438. https://doi.org/10.1111/j.1708-8305.2009.00360.x.

Stromdahl, E.Y., Jiang, J., Vince, M., and Richards, A.L. (2011). Infrequency of *Rickettsia rickettsii* in *Dermacentor variabilis* removed from humans, with comments on the role of other human-biting ticks associated with spotted fever group rickettsiae in the United States. *Vector Borne and Zoonotic Diseases* 11 (7): 969–977. https://doi.org/10.1089/vbz.2010.0099.

Suksawat, J., Pitulle, C., Arraga-Alvarado, C. et al. (2001). Coinfection with three *Ehrlichia* species in dogs from Thailand and Venezuela with emphasis on consideration of 16S ribosomal DNA secondary structure. *Journal of Clinical Microbiology* 39 (1): 90–93. https://doi.org/10.1128/jcm.39.1.90-93.2001.

Szabó, M.P.J., Pinter, A., and Labruna, M.B. (2013). Ecology, biology and distribution of spotted-fever tick vectors in Brazil. *Frontiers in Cellular and Infection Microbiology* 3: 27, pp. 1–9. https://doi.org/10.3389/fcimb.2013.00027.

Tabor, A.E., Graves, S.R., Rodriguez Valle, M., and Stenos, J. (2018). 'One Health' solutions for ticks and tick-borne diseases, and rickettsial pathogens of humans, domestic animals and wildlife. *Ticks and Tick-borne Diseases* 9 (6): 1604–1605. https://doi.org/10.1016/j.ttbdis.2018.08.006.

The Kennel Association of Sri Lanka (n.d.). http://www.kasl.lk/ (accessed 3 November 2021).

Torina, A., Blanda, V., Blanda, M. et al. (2018). A geographical information system based approach for integrated strategies of tick surveillance and control in the Peri-Urban Natural Reserve of Monte Pellegrino (Palermo, Southern Italy). *International Journal of Environmental Research and Public Health* 15: 404.

Trost, C.N., Lindsay, L.R., Dibernardo, A., and Chilton, N.B. (2018). Three genetically distinct clades of *Anaplasma phagocytophilum* in *Ixodes scapularis*. *Ticks and Tick-borne Diseases* 9 (6): 1518–1527. https://doi.org/10.1016/j.ttbdis.2018.07.002.

Trout Fryxell, R.T., Hendricks, B.M., Pompo, K. et al. (2017). Investigating the adult ixodid tick populations and their associated *Anaplasma*, *Ehrlichia*, and *Rickettsia* bacteria at a Rocky Mountain spotted fever hotspot in Western Tennessee. *Vector Borne and Zoonotic Diseases* 17 (8): 527–538. https://doi.org/10.1089/vbz.2016.2091.

Trout Fryxell, R.T., Steelman, C.D., Szalanski, A.L. et al. (2015). Molecular detection of *Rickettsia* species within ticks (Acari: Ixodidae) collected from Arkansas United States. *Journal of Medical Entomology* 52 (3): 500–508. https://doi.org/10.1093/jme/tjv027.

Tsao, J.I., Hamer, S.A., Han, S. et al. (2021). The contribution of wildlife hosts to the rise of ticks and tick-borne diseases in North America. *Journal of Medical Entomology* 58 (4): 1565–1587. https://doi.org/10.1093/jme/tjab047.

Tufts, D.M., Goodman, L.B., Benedict, M.C. et al. (2021). Association of the invasive *Haemaphysalis longicornis* tick with vertebrate hosts, other native tick vectors, and tick-borne pathogens in New York City, USA. *International Journal for Parasitology* 51 (2–3): 149–157. https://doi.org/10.1016/j.ijpara.2020.08.008.

Vasudevan, B. and Chatterjee, M. (2013). Lyme borreliosis and skin. *Indian Journal of Dermatology* 58 (3): 167–174. https://doi.org/10.4103/0019-5154.110822.

Warnasooriya, S., Kularatne, D., Kularatne, S., and Weerakoon, K. (2021). Massive tick bites causing spotted fever rickettsial infection: a hazard in a tea plantation, Sri Lanka. *Wilderness & Environmental Medicine* 32 (4): 499–502. https://doi.org/10.1016/j.wem.2021.05.003.

Weaver, G.V., Anderson, N., Garrett, K. et al. (2022). Ticks and tick-borne pathogens in domestic animals, wild pigs, and off-host environmental sampling in Guam, USA. *Frontiers in Veterinary Science* 8: 803424, pp. 1–12. https://doi.org/10.3389/fvets.2021.803424.

Weerakoon, K., Kularatne, S.A.M., Rajapakse, J. et al. (2014). Cutaneous manifestations of spotted fever rickettsial infections in the Central Province of Sri Lanka: a descriptive study. *PLoS Neglected Tropical Diseases* 8 (9): e3179. https://doi.org/10.1371/journal.pntd.0003179.

Weerathunga, D., Amarasinghe, A., Iddawela, D., and Wickramasinghe, S. (2019). Prevalence of canine tick-borne haemoparasites in three Divisional Secretariat Divisions (Rambewa, Tirappane, and Galenbidunuwewa) in the Anuradhapura district, Sri Lanka. *Sri Lankan Journal of Infectious Diseases* 9 (2): 111–119. https://doi.org/10.4038/sljid.v9i2.8254.

Weilgama, D.J., Jorgensen, W.K., Dalgliesh, R.J. et al. (1989). Comparison between Sri Lankan and Australian strains of *Babesia bovis* in the vaccination of imported cattle in Sri Lanka. *Tropical Animal Health and Production* 21 (2): 141–145. https://doi.org/10.1007/bf02236195.

Woldehiwet, Z. (2010). The natural history of *Anaplasma phagocytophilum*. *Veterinary Parasitology* 167 (2–4): 108–122. https://doi.org/10.1016/j.vetpar.2009.09.013.

Wood, C.L., McInturff, A., Young, H.S. et al. (2017). Human infectious disease burdens decrease with urbanization but not with biodiversity. *Philosophical Transactions of the Royal Society, B: Biological Sciences* 372 (1722): 20160122. https://doi.org/10.1098/rstb.2016.0122.

Wright, C.L., Gaff, H.D., and Hynes, W.L. (2014). Prevalence of *Ehrlichia chaffeensis* and *Ehrlichia ewingii* in *Amblyomma americanum* and *Dermacentor variabilis* collected from southeastern Virginia, 2010–2011. *Ticks and Tick-borne Diseases* 5 (6): 978–982. https://doi.org/10.1016/j.ttbdis.2014.07.023.

Yathramullage, S., Rajapakse, J., and Boyagoda, S. (2018). Rickettsiae reservoirs among small mammals (rats, mice and shrews) and their arthropod vectors in Sri Lanka. *Ceylon Journal of Science* 47 (2): 175–183. 10.4038/cjs.v47i2.7514.

Yen, W.-Y., Stern, K., Mishra, S. et al. (2021). Virulence potential of *Rickettsia amblyommatis* for spotted fever pathogenesis in mice. *Pathogens and Disease* 79 (5): ftab024. https://doi.org/10.1093/femspd/ftab024.

Zahler, M., Rinder, H., Zweygarth, E. et al. (2000). '*Babesia gibsoni*' of dogs from North America and Asia belong to different species. *Parasitology* 120 (4): 365–369. https://doi.org/10.1017/s0031182099005557.

Zhyldyz, A., Sivakumar, T., Igarashi, I. et al. (2019). Epidemiological survey of *Anaplasma marginale* in cattle and buffalo in Sri Lanka. *Journal of Veterinary Medical Science* 81 (11): 1601–1605. https://doi.org/10.1292/jvms.19-0242.

Zintl, A., Mulcahy, G., Skerrett, H.E. et al. (2003). *Babesia divergens*, a bovine blood parasite of veterinary and zoonotic importance. *Clinical Microbiology Reviews 16*: 622–636. https://doi.org/10.1128/CMR.16.4.622-636.2003.

24

Natural Enemies Against Dengue

Opportunities and Constraints on Biological Control of Dengue Vectors in Sri Lanka

Lahiru Udayanga[1], Sandun J. Perera[2], and Tharaka Ranathunge[3]

[1] *Department of Bio-Systems Engineering, Faculty of Agriculture & Plantation Management, Wayamba University of Sri Lanka, Kuliyapitiya, Sri Lanka*
[2] *Department of Natural Resources, Faculty of Applied Sciences, Sabaragamuwa University of Sri Lanka, Belihuloya, Sri Lanka*
[3] *Department of Zoology, Faculty of Science, Eastern University of Srilanka, Chenkaladi, Sri Lanka*

24.1 Dengue: The Fastest Spreading Vector-Borne Disease

Dengue is a major life-threatening infectious disease, which is reported as the most common and rapidly spreading mosquito-borne viral disease in the world. At present epidemics of dengue are being reported from more than 100 countries in the world, emerging as a challenge to both health and economic sectors in the world. According to the estimates, around 50–100 million cases of dengue are being reported annually (Gubler 1998). Dengue comprises of three main stages as dengue fever (DF), dengue hemorrhagic fever (DHF), and its consecutive dengue shock syndrome (DSS). The situation has become extremely serious especially due to unplanned urbanization, global warming, spatial and temporal co-circulation of different dengue virus serotypes, and international trade and transportation (Lourenço and Recker 2014).

Dengue is caused by a single-stranded RNA virus (DENV), which includes four antigenically distinct and closely related serotypes, namely, DENV-1, DENV-2, DENV-3, and DENV-4. Dengue virus belongs to the family Flaviviridae and genus Flavivirus (Lourenço and Recker 2014). *Aedes aegypti* and *Aedes albopictus* mosquitoes act as the major vectors of dengue, while *A. aegypti,* which initiates the disease outbreak, acts as the primary vector, especially in urban areas (Gubler 2002). Multiple factors such as, characteristics of the vulnerable populations, vector dynamics and ecology, local environmental conditions, circulating strain of the dengue virus, urbanization, poor waste management practices, degree of population mobilization, water storage, and inadequate water supply influence the occurrence of dengue outbreaks (Ali 2013; Udayanga et al. 2020). Since the late 1960s, the World Health Organization (WHO) has encouraged endemic countries to engage in routine entomological surveillance and seroprevalence studies to estimate the dengue prevalence in order to recognize risk populations (WHO 2009).

Sri Lanka, as a tropical island located in the South Asian region, has reported its first dengue incidence in 1962, while the first island-wide epidemic was reported in 1965 (Messer et al. 2002). Since then, dengue has imposed a growing risk on the Sri Lankan population, causing 30,000–55,000 average annual cases during the past decade. The most severe outbreak of dengue in Sri Lanka was experienced in 2017, reporting around 186,101 suspected dengue cases, along with over 390 deaths. This number of dengue cases was three times higher than that in previous years (Epidemiology Unit 2022). In 2018, 51,586 dengue cases were reported, of which the majority were accounted from Colombo, Gampaha, Kalutara, and Kandy districts.

24.2 Management Strategies of Dengue

At the global level dengue epidemics are managed through several major approaches, such as vector management, patient care, environmental management, and controlling human–mosquito contact (Udayanga et al. 2020). In Sri Lanka, vector controlling entities mainly focus on the elimination of breeding sites (mechanical/physical and chemical) and controlling of human–mosquito contact (through adulticides and chemical fogging) to prevent and manage dengue epidemics (Udayanga et al. 2018a). Annually, considerable amounts of financial, human, medical, and

One Health: Human, Animal, and Environment Triad, First Edition. Edited by Meththika Vithanage and Majeti Narasimha Vara Prasad.

infrastructural allocations are made for dengue epidemic management, causing dengue to be recognized as a priority health issue in Sri Lanka (Udayanga et al. 2018a).

The simplest form of DF control is through proper practice of personal protective measures to avoid the bites of infected *Aedes* mosquitoes. A variety of methods such as use of physical barriers against mosquito bites (mosquito nets and screens), wearing suitable clothing and applying effective insect repellents, use of vaporizers or mosquito coils, and creation of smoke (with coconut husks and dry plant leaves) are practiced within Sri Lanka as personal protection measures (Udayanga et al. 2018b). With the recent advancement in technology, novel physical protection tools such as insecticide-treated materials (insecticide-treated window curtains and long-lasting insecticidal fabric covers) and nanoparticle-based repellants have been introduced to facilitate this aspect (WHO 2009).

Early detection of dengue patients, supportive treatment of severe dengue cases, and prevention of further transmission of dengue from patients are continued to manage dengue epidemics under patient care (Sirisena and Noordeen 2014; Udayanga et al. 2020). Among numerous methods used for controlling of vector breeding, physical measures are quite simple to be implemented and inexpensive. Routine search for vector breeding sites in the homesteads, removal of such potential breeding sites, and maintenance of a breeding site free environment are some of the simple strategies that could be implemented to control vector breeding, mechanically (Udayanga et al. 2018b). Chemical vector control methods are often used to control vector breeding and to suppress vector populations of dengue, especially when rapid elimination of vectors is necessary. Conventionally, fumigation, residual spraying, and the elimination of breeding sites are used to control *Aedes* mosquitoes (WHO 2009). Houses provide a favorable environment for human–vector contact and dengue transmission, while providing apposite resting sites for adult mosquitoes. Therefore, indoor residual spraying has become a widely practiced method to control the adult vector populations, while eliminating the chances of vector–human contact (Bath et al. 2021).

Larvicides are also widely applied to control the breeding of dengue vectors. Insecticides such as chlorinated hydrocarbons like dichloro-diphenyl-trichloroethane (DDT) or dieldrin, organophosphates like diazinon or bensolid, and carbamates like carbofuran and carboxyl are often used to treat potential breeding containers via perifocal treatment approach, which provides both larviciding and residual adulticiding characteristics. In this case, the used larvicides should possess low toxicity to other sensitive species and should not considerably change the color, taste, or odor of the water, which could reduce the oviposition preference of gravid *Aedes* females (WHO 2009). Proper environmental management is also a key strategy to minimize vector propagation and human–vector contact. Modification, alteration, or manipulation of the environment is often practiced to restrict vector populations. Destroying, altering, or removing nonessential containers and other potential larval habitats, modification of water supply and water storage systems, proper solid waste management, and cautiously conducted construction activities would immensely contribute for the source reduction of *Aedes* vector breeding sites (WHO 2009).

Apart from the above approaches, several novel vector control strategies, namely sterile insect technique (SIT), incompatible insect technique (IIT), application of chitosan-synthesized silver nanoparticles (Ch–AgNP), green-fabricated nanoparticles, have provided highly promising results for controlling different *Aedes* species (Kalimuthu et al. 2017; Murugan et al. 2017; Benelli et al. 2018). In Sri Lanka, all the aforementioned approaches are being utilized to manage dengue epidemics, with special emphasis on vector control, environmental management, and personal protection (Sirisena et al. 2017). However, irresistible drawbacks of chemical-based vector control methods such as short-term efficacy, practical difficulties faced in implementation, insecticide resistance development (Walker and Lynch 2007), retention of insecticide residues in the natural environment (Paaijmans et al. 2008; Nájera et al. 2011), ill effects on humans and other biota (Hemingway and Ranson 2000), and unbalancing the delicate balance in ecosystems act as limitations of chemical-based vector control methods (Yasuoka et al. 2006; Araújo et al. 2015).

24.3 Biological Control of Dengue

Due to the unavailability of effective drugs or a vaccine for all dengue serotypes, many countries rely upon patient management and vector control strategies to manage dengue epidemics (Harrington et al. 2005). However, development of insecticide-resistant strains and unintended side effects on human and ecosystem health have led to concerns about the long-term use of chemical-based vector control approaches (Seixas et al. 2017). Hence, application of chemical insecticides is no longer considered as an effective solution to suppress dengue vector populations. Hence, effective, environmentally friendly, and sustainable strategies of dengue epidemic management are in need to be practiced in Sri Lanka. Under such conditions, biological control remains a highly viable option to control dengue vectors (Bock et al. 2005; Sintupachee et al. 2006). Biocontrol strategies utilize locally available natural predators to eliminate immature or adult stages of vector mosquitoes or exploit mosquito behavior to induce the mosquito mortality.

Use of a natural predator for biological controlling of *Aedes* would provide an economic yet efficient mechanism for *Aedes* vector control with minimal impacts on the environment (Kalimuthu et al. 2017). However, selection of a natural predator should be done with care, while respecting the prey-predator interactions, evolutionary, environmental, and behavioral characteristics to predict possible scenarios (Lima and Dill 1990; Romano et al. 2019). At the global level, a wide range of natural predators, ranging from microscopic to macroscopic (dytiscid beetles, crustaceans, notonectids, belostomatids, Odonata, larvivorous fish, and amphibians), have been used as biological control agents against different mosquito vectors (WHO 1992). Many studies have recommended larvivorous fish (Subramaniam et al. 2016), parasitic nematodes (Georgis et al. 2006), beetle larvae (WHO 1992), certain fly larvae (WHO 1992), aquatic bugs (WHO 1992), dragonflies and damselflies (odonates) (Benelli et al. 2016), dragonfly/damselfly nymphs (WHO 1992), cyclopoid copepods (Benelli et al. 2016), bacteria (Benelli et al. 2016), protozoans (Benelli et al. 2016), and fungus (Benelli et al. 2016) as effective biological agents to control *Aedes* mosquito populations. These biocontrol agents target different stages of the mosquito life cycle, with minimum impacts on the natural ecosystems.

24.4 Biological Control of Dengue in Sri Lanka

Many organisms have been evaluated as potential biological control agents for *Aedes* mosquito larvae in the world as well as in Sri Lanka. Within the recent years, actions have been taken to promote the use of few of these agents for *Aedes* vector control (Ranathunge et al. 2021). Currently, careful introduction of natural predators and proper environmental management have become a prioritized approach for vector control in Sri Lanka. Based on recent studies following species could be identified as effective biological control agents of *Aedes* vectors.

24.4.1 Larvivorous Fish

Biological control approaches of mosquitoes have mostly focused on the role of larvivorous fish that consume the aquatic larval stage of mosquitoes. Predation of mosquito larvae by fish has been recorded in many habitats, from small ponds to complex natural ecosystems, including coastal wetland environments (Ranathunge et al. 2021). Up to now, biocontrol efficacy of a variety of larvivorous fish species have been evaluated against *Aedes* larvae in Sri Lanka. Ranathunge et al. (2021) provide an insight into six locally abundant fish species as predators against *Aedes* mosquito larvae. In fact, all tested fish in the laboratory have preyed on *A. aegypti* mosquito larvae, with different consumption rates. Among the considered varieties, juvenile stage of *Oreochromis mossambicus* has shown the highest predatory efficiency over of *A. aegypti* larvae, while *Rasbora daniconius* has recorded the least under laboratory settings. Despite being smaller in body size, *Aplocheilus dayi* and *Poecilia reticulata* have been recommended as the ideal candidates for biological control of *Aedes* larvae under both laboratory and field settings. In addition, the survival and reproductive ability of *Aplocheilus* sp. and *P. reticulata* remain at a relatively higher level, due to their wider ecological elasticity, which allows them to tolerate different habitat and environmental conditions (Wijesinghe et al. 2009). Another recent study conducted using both native and introduced larvivorous fish has recommended both *Puntius bimaculatus* and *Aplocheilus dayi* as potential candidates for biological control of *A. aegypti* larvae (Sandupama et al. 2019). Since both the aforementioned fish species are native, the possible ecological impacts of using them are expected to be minimum. Meanwhile, another study conducted by Surendran et al. (2008) has recommended the use of *O. mossambicus* for *Aedes* larval control, especially in cement tanks and ponds. National Dengue Control Unit in Sri Lanka has also recommended the use of aforementioned larvivorous fish to control a variety of medically important mosquito larvae, including *Aedes* (National Dengue Control Unit 2019).

24.4.2 Cyclopoid Copepods

Majority of omnivorous copepods (small aquatic cyclopoid crustaceans) can prey on young mosquito larval stages (Marten et al. 1989). Often copepods could be considered as more effective agents for biological control, due to their higher abundance and reproductive rates, which enable easy and cost-effective mass rearing. However, the larval predation rates of copepods strongly depend on the size of the *Aedes* larvae and the nature of the breeding site, which act as limiting factors. After considering five copepod species, *Mesocyclops leuckarti* and *Mesocyclops scrassus* have been reported as excellent predators of *A. aegypti* and *A. albopictus* larvae under laboratory settings (Udayanga et al. 2019) in Sri Lanka. However, further studies on the predatory efficacy of above copepods under field settings have not been conducted up to now. Due to the high diversity of copepods in Sri Lanka, further studies could be recommended to identify more suitable copepod species to be used as biological control agents.

24.4.3 Dragonfly Nymphs

Nymphal and the adult stages of dragonflies (Infraorder Anisoptera) and damselflies (Suborders Zygoptera) that belong to the order Odonata are also considered as potential predators of a variety of mosquito larvae (Shad and Andrew 2013). Despite the remarkable diversity of the order Odonata in Sri Lanka, the potential of locally available dragonfly nymphs for *Aedes* mosquito control has been barely investigated (Samanmali et al. 2018). A recent study has evaluated the biocontrol efficacy of five locally available dragonfly nymphs over *A. aegypti* larvae, where *Anax indicus* and *Pantala flavescens* have been recommended as excellent candidates in Belihuloya area. Among them *P. flavescens* indicates a relatively wider distribution along with high feasibility for adaptation, while *A. indicus* is also not an uncommon species. Therefore, focusing on these species would be immensely important to support the *Aedes* vector control requirements. However, dragonflies go through 10–15 instars of nymphal stages, which requires around one year or more in a waterbody for a dragonfly to emerge as an adult (Chatterjee et al. 2007). Therefore, maintenance of mass cultures of dragonflies under laboratory conditions could be challenging. As a solution, natural environmental conditions should be maintained to promote the diversity and abundance of dragonflies naturally. However, further studies should be conducted on the ability of *P. flavescens* and *A. indicus* as well as other potential species of Odonata to suppress dengue mosquito populations under field conditions (Figure 24.1).

24.4.4 Bacillus Strains

Initially isolated in 1976, *Bacillus thuringiensis* var. *israelensis* (Bti) is currently one of the most widely used mosquito larvicides. Bti is a Gram-positive, spore-forming bacterium that releases insecticidal toxins and virulence factors that selectively target larval stages of insects. Application of Bti has been used to suppress *A. aegypti* and *A. albopictus* larval populations through mechanisms that result in minimum adverse effects on non-target invertebrates and vertebrates (Lacey 2007). However, long-term use of Bti could lead to the development of resistance, while the use of Bti in an urban environment could be logistically demanding (Tissera et al. 2018). As a result of a collaborative project between the Medical Research Institute and the Industrial Technology Institute, a commercial formulation of Bti (Bacto Bti) has been developed in Sri Lanka from a local *B. thuringiensis* strain (Baragamaarachchi et al. 2019; MRI 2021).

In addition, Induwara et al. (2018) have demonstrated that *Bacillus cereus* could also be used as an effective biocontrol agent of *Aedes* larvae, residual effect of which may last for around 12 days. However, the toxicity of microbial insecticides are often specific, and external factors such as heat, desiccation, and exposure to ultraviolet radiation could influence their larvicidal efficiency. Therefore, further studies should be conducted to assess the efficacy of *B. cereus* for *Aedes* larval control in different geographical areas in Sri Lanka.

24.5 Carnivorous Mosquito Larvae

Certain mosquitoes that fulfill their nutrient requirements from plant nectar without depending on blood meals while acting as predators of *Aedes* larvae could also be used as biological control agents. Larvae of genus *Toxorhynchites* have been recognized as a potential biocontrol agent of many mosquito larvae, including those of *Aedes* due to their aggressive feeding behavior (Donald et al. 2020). However, the cannibalistic tendency of *Toxorhynchites* and difficulties in maintaining large colonies have been identified as limitations. Two species of *Toxorhynchites* have been reported from Sri Lanka, i.e. *T. splendens* and *T. minimus* (Gunathilaka 2018). A previous study conducted by Wijesinghe et al. (2009) has reported a satisfactory predation level of *A. albopictus* larvae (10 larvae within 5 hours and 30 minutes) by *T. splendens*, followed by *T. minimus* under laboratory settings. Further, some field-based investigations have indicated that *T. splendens* and *T. minimus* breed in water-filled barrels (Wijesinghe et al. 2009). Based on the above evidence, *T. splendens* has been recommended as a potential biocontrol agent of *Aedes* mosquitoes in peridomestic breeding sites.

Culex (Lutzia) *fuscanus* (Diptera: Culicidae) is another predatory mosquito, whose larva feed mainly on the larvae of other mosquito species. *C. fuscanus* has shown a promising predatory efficacy over *Aedes* larvae (Surendran et al. 2013). Adult females of *C. fuscanus* prefer birds as their main blood source, and therefore they are not considered to be medically important for human health. Despite cannibalism being demonstrated in the absence of alternative prey, *C. fuscanus* larvae could also be used as a potential biological agent in integrated vector control approaches of dengue. However, a limited number of studies have been conducted in Sri Lanka focusing on this aspect, which have mainly been restricted to laboratory-based evaluations.

24.6 Carnivorous Aquatic Plants

Being a carnivorous angiosperm, genus *Utricularia,* belongs to the family Lentibulariaceae, which includes approximately 235 species. They usually grow in nutrient-poor shallow habitats with standing water, such as small lakes,

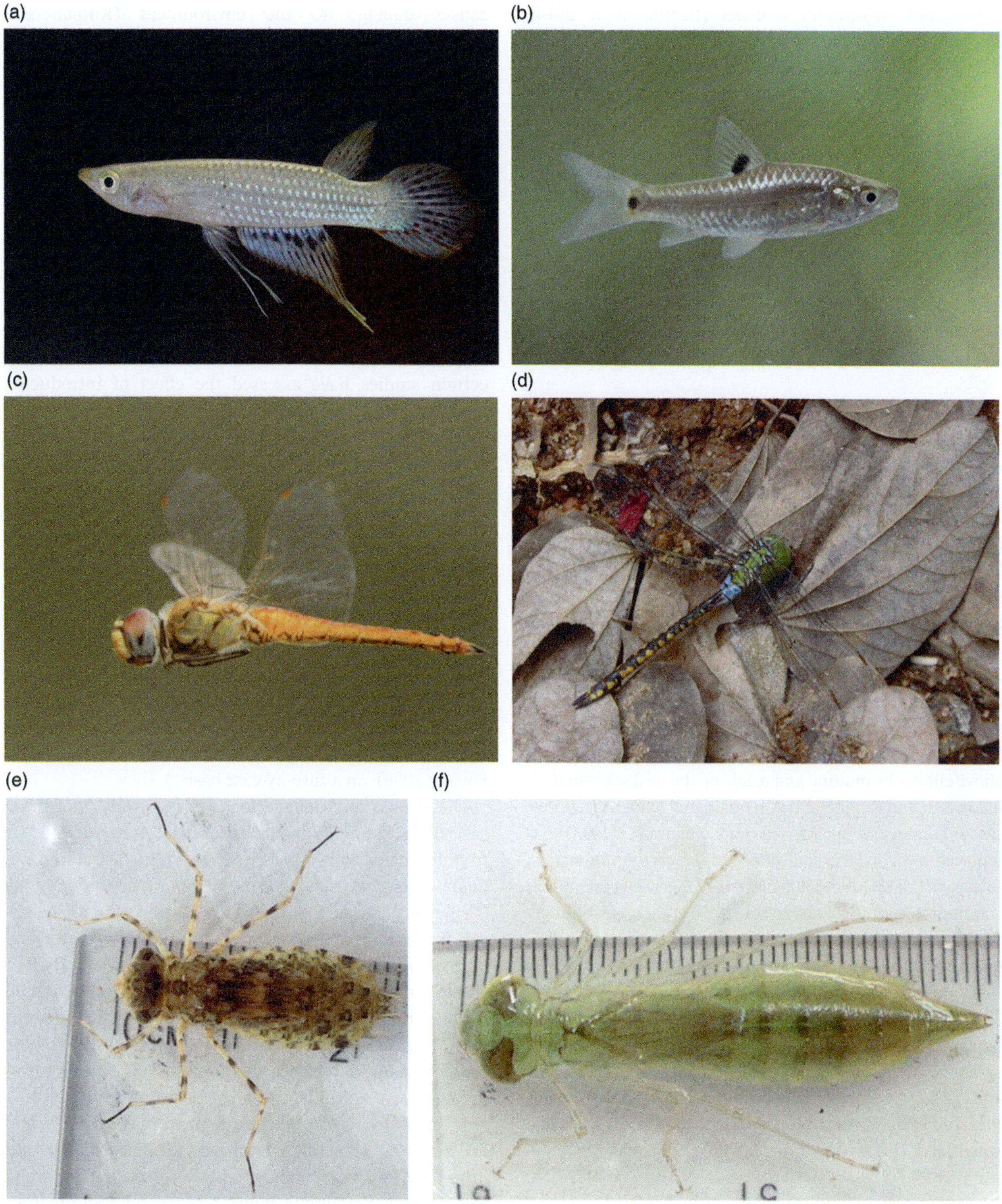

Figure 24.1 A few selected potential biological control agents of dengue among the native fauna in Sri Lanka: (a) *Aplocheilus dayi* (Ceylon killifish) endemic to Sri Lanka, (b) *Puntius bimaculatus* (two-spot barb), (c) adult and (e) nymph of *Pantala flavescens* (Wandering Glider), and (d) adult and (f) nymph of *Anax indicus* (Elephant Emperor). *Source:* Photo credits: Samantha Gunasekara (a), W. P. Naalin Perera (b, c), Sandun J. Perera (d), and W. R. Chathurika Samanmali (e, f).

ponds, and oligotrophic marshes (Beretta et al. 2014). *Utricularia species* have evolved to directly take up required nutrients either from water using shoots or from aquatic animal preys through bladder traps. Due to this trapping behavior of *Utricularia,* it can be considered as potential biological control agents for a variety of mosquito larvae. Until now, only one study has been conducted in Sri Lanka on this aspect, where *Utricularia vulgaris* and *Utricularia reticulata* have denoted a satisfactory predation rate against *A. aegypti* larvae (Perera et al. 2021). *U. reticulata* is an endemic species and bears an attractive bright blue colored flower, further increasing its dual potential of ornamental use while contributing to its conservation, catering at the same time for biological control of dengue in Sri Lanka.

24.7 Endoparasitic Ciliates with Antagonistic Effect

Endoparasitic ciliates (Protista: Ciliophora) such as *Lambornella stegomyiae*, *Lambornella clarki*, and *Tetrahymena pyriformis* have reported to demonstrate parasitic effects over a variety of mosquito larvae including *Aedes* and *Anopheles* (Corliss and Coats 1976; Washburn 1995; Arshad and Sulaiman 1995). These ciliates can also infect adult mosquitoes and thereby disperse easily. In addition, the ability of them to form desiccation-resistant cysts makes them an effective biological control agent (Washburn 1995). However, some larvae may survive from the infection of above ciliates by molting and reaching the next stage in their life cycle (Ranasinghe and Amarasinghe 2020). A previous study conducted by Arshad and Sulaiman (1995) has reported a high larvicidal effect of *L. stegomyiae* against *A. aegypti* (90.8%) and *A. albopictus* (99.5%) under laboratory conditions. In the Sri Lankan context, the antagonistic effect of ciliates (*Zoothamnium* sp., *Chilodinella* sp., and *Vorticella microstoma*) has been evaluated under laboratory settings by Ranasinghe (2020) against larvae of few medically important mosquitoes. According to the findings, *V. microstoma* has been recommended as a potential biological control agent for the larvae of *Culex tritaeniorhynchus, Culex gelidus*, and *Anopheles subpictus* (Ranasinghe 2020). Therefore, further studies have to be conducted to investigate the larvicidal potential of ciliates over *Aedes* larvae in Sri Lanka.

24.8 Ecological Perspective of Biological Control

Biological control of mosquito larvae using biocontrol agents has been proven to be an ecofriendly approach as it significantly reduces the use of synthetic chemicals, which causes damage to the environment (Kumar and Hwang 2006). In general understanding, biological control involves the use of natural enemies including parasites, pathogens, and predators in declining target vector populations in natural environments (Venkatesh and Tyagi 2013), which could lead to unforeseen ecological imbalances of aquatic ecosystems. Such phenomena may affect the aquatic as well as the adjoining terrestrial food webs, population dynamics of native and more importantly range-restricted endemic species, and all-in-all the functionality of essential ecosystem services (Ellis and Wilcox 2009; Kiruba-Sankar et al. 2018; Weterings et al. 2018). Although biological control typically focuses on the introduction of a natural enemy of the adult or larval stages of mosquitoes, certain studies have assessed the effect of introducing selected phytoplankton species that are unable to be digested by mosquito larvae. Such approaches may utilize around 200 species of planktonic green algae that can induce mortality of *Aedes*, *Anopheles*, and *Culex* larvae (Marten 1987), which could cause further ecological imbalances as the intervention affects the base of the aquatic food web. Hence, although the biological control can be considered a feasible alternative to battle against the medically important mosquitoes, characters of biocontrol agents such as their mode and the rate of reproduction, adaptability to the introduced environment, preference for the target population, existence of alternative natural prey, and overall interaction with native organisms need a careful consideration, when selecting a biocontrol agent (Kumar and Hwang 2006), on a case-by-case basis.

The structure of aquatic food webs as well as of those cascades into adjoining terrestrial habitats are defined by trophic interactions among species within the communities and determined by the amount of primary productivity (Begon and Parker 1986). This directly determines the larval mosquito population in a given lentic waterbody (Washburn 1995). Unfortunately, a limited number of studies on biological control of *Aedes* vectors have focused on how mosquito abundance is regulated by food webs (Weterings et al. 2018). Poor understanding of the trophic status and the role played by mosquitoes in food webs of the wider ecological landscape is a reason for limited success in many *Aedes* biocontrol programmes (Ellis and Wilcox 2009). Hence, it is important to consider inter- and intra-specific interactions of *Aedes* (predation on them and competition among them) and the optimal environmental factors for those interactions when planning biological control strategies (Moore et al. 2010). For instance, after studying food web trophic cascades in both aquatic and terrestrial environments, Weterings et al. (2018) have concluded that mosquito predators in the terrestrial environment play a major role in regulating mosquito populations. This clearly indicates that the current practice of introducing an aquatic predator to control mosquito larval populations in breeding sites alone may not provide best results. Hence, integrated vector management strategies in biological control (Rodríguez-pérez et al. 2012) are necessary without ignoring the pivotal role played by naturally occurring aquatic and terrestrial predators (Weterings et al. 2018).

The prey-predator interactions play a vital role in regulating the population dynamics and keeping the ecosystem in balance. As predatory and anti-predatory traits, respectively, of the predator and prey evolve in response to environmental changes, the introduction of an alien predator may lead to an artificial selection distracting the stabilized food webs of the aquatic ecosystem. Further, the alien predator may find easier to prey among native biota in the introduced ecosystem than the target prey, causing extirpations of local populations of native species. At the same time the alien predator could have advantageous predatory traits to over compete existing native predators in the system. Both the above phenomena can make the introduced biocontrol agent to suppress non-target native populations (Abrams 2000). Such impacts on population dynamics of native species and more importantly the range-restricted endemic spices could even lead to species extinctions of narrow endemics. Hence, it is apparent that biocontrol agents can become a threat to non-target native species, especially when predators with board diets are used (Strong and Pemberton 2001). However, existing knowledge in this regard is still patchy and restricted only to a few species of vertebrates.

Both the guppy (*P. reticulata*) and western mosquito fish (*Gambusia affinis*) initially introduced to Sri Lanka as predators of mosquito larva to prevent mosquito-borne diseases has eventually become alien-invasive species in the island (Bambaradeniya 2002; Silva and Kurukulasuriya 2010; Marambe et al. 2011). *P. reticulata*, which is native to northern south America, has well naturalized in Sri Lanka even reaching upper catchment areas above 1000 m elevations above mean sea level in some river basins, while *G. affinis*, native to south-eastern United States and northern Mexico, has become established in the lowland wet zone of the island (Pethiyagoda 1991; Silva and Kurukulasuriya 2010). Although *P. reticulata* has been reported to successfully control mosquito populations in Sri Lanka (Rodrigo and De Silva 2004, Kusumawathie et al. 2008) and elsewhere, its behavioral ecology (Deacon 2011) has made it invasive in its introduced range. It is a prolific breeder and has become increasingly carnivorous in Sri Lanka, even been reported to feed on eggs of native amphibians, which shows a remarkably high percentage endemism of above 90% in the island (De Silva 1996; Bambaradeniya 2002; Shirantha et al. 2008).

Therefore, understanding the relationship between specific prey such as the adults, larvae, and eggs of mosquitoes and their predators is becoming essential in selecting potential biocontrol agents to combat mosquito-borne diseases (Shad and Andrew 2013). Those predators should effectively influence target mosquito populations by consuming their immature stages or adults, while disturbing their rates of development, hence affecting mosquito densities (Ellis and Ladeau 2013). Such assessments should also note the apparent predominance of evolutionary responses of the prey to predators over those of predators to prey (Abrams 2000), which could cause biological control using a predator to fail in case of a rapidly evolving prey.

In looking for alternatives for fish as *Aedes* biocontrol agents, recent studies highlight odonates, especially dragonflies, as mosquito predators, the ecology of which has not yet been fully understood (Ellis and Ladeau 2013). Odonates are harmless to humans, while being ecologically beneficial as voracious predators of mosquitoes, where adult odonates as well as their nymphal stages effectively prey upon respective mosquito life stages. Further, the life cycle of dragonflies can last up to one to six years, while their nymphal stage usually goes through more than 10 instars (Ellis and Ladeau 2013), hence acting as efficient predators for several generations of mosquito larvae. The knowledge of the ecology of odonate larvae including their inter- and intra-specific competition and reproductive strategies has proven them to be excellent *Aedes* mosquito control agents with supreme potential (Córdoba-Aguilar and Lee 1994). Therefore, acquiring a complete understanding of the native prey ecology and the dynamics of prey-predator interactions among native species can be identified as a matter of utmost importance in selecting biocontrol agents for the suppression of *Aedes* vectors.

Further, biological control of mosquito larvae is always best to be considered as a part of an integrated vector management programme (Manna et al. 2011), together with other, as much as non-chemical, means of controlling mosquito populations. Recent studies in Sri Lanka have looked at various natural enemies of mosquitoes including freshwater fish (Sandupama et al. 2019; Ranathunge et al. 2021), tadpoles (Bowatte et al. 2013), dragonfly larvae (Samanmali et al. 2018), and copepods (Anukulan et al. 2015; Udayanga et al. 2019) for the control of eggs and larvae of *A. aegypti*, while many of the other potential biocontrol agents may be of non-native origins. The integration of biological measures in an integrated mosquito control programme involves a cautious selection of the predators in a way to ensure human protection without affecting the ecology, biodiversity, and the balance of ecosystem (Venkatesh and Tyagi 2013).

A major drawback in usage of fish as *Aedes* vector control agents is that some fishes such as *P. reticulata* and *G. affinis* affect the native aquatic community as invasive species, which leads to the failure of the satisfactory mosquito control. This urges the need to assess the predatory potency of the native larvivorous fish such as the killifish of the genus *Aplocheilus* (Manna et al. 2011). In this regard, the findings of Fernando et al. (2018) indicate a prominent active selection of prey insects and insect larvae by *Aplocheilus parvus* native in Sri Lanka, in contrast to the alien *P. reticulata* consuming the most readily available food items regardless of the target prey for which it has been used as a biocontrol agent.

The concept of integrated vector management has recently given much attention to native predatory aquatic insects (Shaalan and Canyon 2009). However, narrow ecological elasticity of many potential biocontrol agents in their aquatic habitat requirements such as pH, temperature, and the degree of organic pollution (biological oxygen demand) stands as a limitation in their versatile use for biological control of *Aedes* larvae. Further, none of the aforementioned potential predators have been evaluated through a detailed ecological assessment before selecting them as biocontrol agents. Therefore, it is imperative to conduct a careful ecological assessment, which especially is a must when considering the introduction of an alien predator to the island. Recent efforts in Sri Lanka to conduct national pre-entry risk assessments of potential invasive alien species, not yet recorded in Sri Lanka, that have invaded ecosystems in the region and thereby preparing black lists of potential invasive alien species (Silva and Kurukulasuriya 2010) can therefore be identified as an important proactive intervention in this regard.

24.9 Opportunities, Constraints, and Way Forward

Despite the availability of a variety of dengue epidemic management strategies, controlling the dengue transmission remains a challenge for many countries, including Sri Lanka. At present, vector control is the mostly focused strategy to manage dengue epidemics, and under this main attention has been placed on the use of chemical-based vector control strategies. However, the higher costs, potential of insecticide resistance development, unintended impacts on the environment and non-target species, higher persistence of insecticides, health hazards on humans, and necessity of labor for routine applications have led to rethink about the usefulness and effectiveness of chemical-based vector control methods. Therefore, much attention is being placed on the use of effective, environmentally friendly, cost-effective, and sustainable solutions to control *Aedes* vectors.

Biological control approaches provide an ideal solution for above requirements, whereby a variety of non-modified natural organisms such as larvivorous fish, copepods, dragonfly/damselfly nymphs, carnivorous mosquito larvae and aquatic plants, endoparasitic ciliates, and certain *Bacillus* strains could be used as effective candidates for control of *Aedes* larvae and adults. At present, several studies have been conducted to evaluate the biological control potential of aforementioned organisms to control *Aedes* vectors. However, most of them have been restricted to laboratory-based evaluations, while field or semi-field applications are hardly documented in Sri Lanka. Being a country with a unique biodiversity and a remarkable degree of endemism, Sri Lanka has a high potential to excel in biological control of dengue vectors. Therefore, further studies should be encouraged within the country. In addition, selection of an ideal biological control agent is not a simple task. Characteristics such as growth and development, survival, reproduction, predatory potential, and alternate food preferences of the selected candidate should be carefully considered under field conditions, along with ecosystem level impacts. Lack of attention on the above aspects have caused several biological control programmes to end as failures, while introducing invasive species that threaten the native biota in Sri Lanka. Therefore, in-depth ecological assessments have to be accompanied along with predation trials in selection of a potential biological control agent for *Aedes* vector control. Further, the knowledge synthesized through these assessments and field trials should be adequately disseminated among the public, scientific community, and most importantly with the government vector controlling entities and policy makers, enabling them to incorporate biological control strategies into National Vector Control Programmes.

However, regardless of the sustainable nature and higher efficacy, biological control approaches require more time for complete ecological assessment and face challenges in maintaining large cultures or colonies of selected biocontrol agents, as well as practical difficulties associated with the release and monitoring of the candidates in the field. In addition, biological control agents might require a certain period of time to establish themselves in the natural environment. Therefore, biological control approaches cannot solely manage dengue epidemics. For this an integrated vector control strategy should be adopted, where adequate environmental management, physical control (breeding site elimination and alteration), and chemical-based vector control strategies (with least impacts on the environment) are accompanied with biological control. Especially, sudden outbreaks of dengue should be managed through chemical-based control measures.

Based on the current status in biological control strategies of *Aedes* vectors in Sri Lanka, more studies should be conducted to further evaluate the biocontrol efficacy of already selected candidates under field conditions, while paying attention to develop standard protocols and guidelines to practically use them in dengue vector control at the national level. In addition, the health policy makers should be encouraged to further incorporate such strategies in National Vector Control Programmes of dengue as a pillar of integrated vector management. With the current challenges faced during dengue epidemic management such as poor coordination among the government institutes; high cost; limited availability of technical, financial, and human resources; poor knowledge on the socioeconomic determinants of dengue risk and knowledge gaps in risk communities; and adoption of biological control-based integrated vector management strategy could ensure successful dengue management in Sri Lanka.

Acknowledgments

All authors who have contributed to the field of biological control of dengue in Sri Lanka are acknowledged for disseminating their valuable findings. Ms. Chathurika Samanmali and Ms. Aroshani Sandupama are acknowledged for their field and laboratory trials, especially Chathurika for bringing up the novel aspect of the use of odonate nymphs as larval predators of mosquitoes into our research agenda. The photographers mentioned for each photograph are thanked for their generosity.

References

Abrams, P.A. (2000). The evolution of predator – prey interactions: theory and evidence. *Annual Review of Ecology and Systematics* 31: 79–105.

Ali, M. (2013). Dengue: factors driving the emerging epidemic. *Clinical Epidemiology* 5: 461.

Anukulan, J.W., Ratnayake, R.M.A.S., Perera, R.S.M., Hapukotuwa, R.B. and Iqbal, M.C.M. (2015). Biology and diversity of copepods in Sri Lanka and their potential use as predator of *Aedes* larvae. *Proceedings of the Current Research Activities on Dengue Conducted by the Faculty of Medicine*. University of Kelaniya, Sri Lanka. p. 37.

Araújo, H.R., Carvalho, D.O., Ioshino, R.S. et al. (2015). *Aedes aegypti* control strategies in Brazil: incorporation of new technologies to overcome the persistence of dengue epidemics. *Insects* 6 (2): 576–594.

Arshad, H.H. and Sulaiman, I. (1995). Infection of *Aedes albopictus* (Diptera: Culicidae) and *Ae. aegypti* with *Lambornella stegomyiae* (Ciliophora: Tetrahymenidae). *Journal of Invertebrate Pathology* 66 (3): 303–306.

Bambaradeniya, C.N.B. (2002). The status and implications of invasive alien species in Sri Lanka. *Zoos Print Journal* 17 (11): 930–935.

Baragamaarachchi, R.Y., Samarasekera, J.K.R.R., Weerasena, O.V.D.S.J. et al. (2019). Identification of a native *Bacillus thuringiensis* strain from Sri Lanka active against Dipel-resistant *Plutella xylostella*. *PeerJ* 7: e7535.

Bath, D., Cook, J., Govere, J. et al. (2021). Effectiveness and cost-effectiveness of reactive, targeted indoor residual spraying for malaria control in low-transmission settings: a cluster-randomised, non-inferiority trial in South Africa. *The Lancet 397* (10276): 816–827.

Begon, M. and Parker, G.A. (1986). Should egg size and clutch size decrease with age? *Oikos* 293–302.

Benelli, G., Jeffries, C.L., and Walker, T. (2016). Biological control of mosquito vectors: past, present, and future. *Insects* 7 (4): 52.

Benelli, G., Maggi, F., Pavela, R. et al. (2018). Mosquito control with green nanopesticides: towards the One Health approach? A review of non-target effects. *Environmental Science and Pollution Research* 25 (11): 10184–10206.

Beretta, M., Rodondi, G., Adamec, L., and Andreis, C. (2014). Pollen morphology of European bladderworts (*Utricularia* L., Lentibulariaceae). *Review of Palaeobotany and Palynology* 205: 22–30.

Bock, G.W., Zmud, R.W., Kim, Y.G., and Lee, J.N. (2005). Behavioral intention formation in knowledge sharing: examining the roles of extrinsic motivators, social-psychological forces, and organizational climate. *MIS Quarterly* 29: 87–111.

Bowatte, G., Perera, P., Senevirathne, G. et al. (2013). Tadpoles as dengue mosquito (*Aedes aegypti*) egg predators. *Biological Control* 67: 469–474.

Chatterjee, S.N., Ghosh, A., and Chandra, G. (2007). Eco-friendly control of mosquito larvae by *Brachytron pratense* nymph. *Journal of Environmental Health* 69 (8): 44–49.

Córdoba-Aguilar, A. and Lee, M. (1994). Prey size selection by *Orthemis ferruginea* (Fabricius) larvae (Odonata: Libellulidae) over mosquito instars. *Folia Entomologica Mexicana* 30: 91323.

Corliss, J.O. and Coats, D.W. (1976). A new cuticular cyst-producing tetrahymenid ciliate, *Lambornella clarki* n. sp., and the current status of ciliatosis in culicine mosquitoes. *Transactions of the American Microscopical Society* 725–739.

De Silva, A. (1996). *The Herpetofauna of Sri Lanka: A Brief Review*, 99. Gampola: Published by the author.

Deacon, A.E. (2011). The behavioural ecology of the *Trinidadian guppy, Poecilia reticulata,* as an invasive species. PhD thesis. University of St Andrews.

Donald, C.L., Siriyasatien, P., and Kohl, A. (2020). *Toxorhynchites* species: a review of current knowledge. *Insects* 11 (11): 747.

Ellis, M.R. and Ladeau, S. (2013). Influence of dragonfly larvae on mosquito development and survival. *Cary Institute of Ecosystem Studies* 12545: 8.

Ellis, B.R. and Wilcox, B.A. (2009). The ecological dimensions of vector-borne disease research and control. *Cadernos de Saúde Pública* 25: S155–S167.

Epidemiology Unit, Ministry of Health (2022). Dengue update. www.epid.gov.lk/web/index.php?Itemid=448# (accessed 9 March 2022).

Fernando, G.K., Jayakody, S., Wijenayake, W.M. et al. (2018). A comparison of the larvivorous habits of exotic *Poecilia reticulata* and native *Aplocheilus parvus*. *BMC Ecology* 18 (1): 1–12.

Georgis, R., Koppenhöfer, A.M., Lacey, L.A. et al. (2006). Successes and failures in the use of parasitic nematodes for pest control. *Biological Control 38* (1): 103–123.

Gubler, D.J. (1998). Dengue and dengue hemorrhagic fever. *Clinical Microbiology Reviews* 11 (3): 480–496.

Gubler, D.J. (2002). Epidemic dengue/dengue hemorrhagic fever as a public health, social and economic problem in the 21st century. *Trends in Microbiology* 10 (2): 100–103.

Gunathilaka, N. (2018). The potential strength of eco-friendly non-modified biological control approaches as additional tools in integrated management of dengue vectors in Sri Lanka. In: *Marching Towards a Bioeconomy*, 27–41. Colombo: Institute of Biology.

Harrington, L.C., Scott, T.W., Lerdthusnee, K. et al. (2005). Dispersal of the dengue vector *Aedes aegypti* within and between rural communities. *The American Journal of Tropical Medicine and Hygiene* 72 (2): 209–220.

Hemingway, J. and Ranson, H. (2000). Insecticide resistance in insect vectors of human disease. *Annual Review of Entomology* 45 (1): 371–391.

Induwara, R., Fernando, M., Ranathunge, R. et al. (2018). Isolation of potential microbial agent for controlling dengue mosquitoes in Sri Lanka. *International Postgraduate Research Conference* 19: 47.

Kalimuthu, K., Panneerselvam, C., Chou, C. et al. (2017). Predatory efficiency of the copepod *Megacyclops formosanus* and toxic effect of the red alga *Gracilaria firma*-synthesized silver nanoparticles against the dengue vector *Aedes aegypti*. *Hydrobiologia* 785 (1): 359–372.

Kiruba-Sankar, R., Praveen Raj, J., Saravanan, K. et al. (2018). Invasive species in freshwater ecosystems – threats to ecosystem services. In: *Biodiversity and Climate Change Adaptation in Tropical Islands* (ed. S. Chandrakasan, A. Velmurugan, A. Singh and I. Jaisankar), 257–296. USA: Elsevier Inc. Academic Press.

Kumar, R. and Hwang, J.-S. (2006). Larvicidal efficiency of aquatic predators: a perspective for mosquito biocontrol. *Zoological Studies* 45: 447–466.

Kusumawathie, P.H.D., Wickremasinghe, A.R., Karunaweera, N.D., and Wijeyaratne, M.J.S. (2008). Larvivorous potential of the guppy, *Poecilia reticulata*, in anopheline mosquito control in riverbed pools below the Kotmale dam, Sri Lanka. *Asia-Pacific Journal of Public Health* 20 (1): 56–63.

Lacey, L.A. (2007). *Bacillus thuringiensis serovariety israelensis* and *Bacillus sphaericus* for mosquito control. *Journal of the American Mosquito Control Association* 23 (sp2): 133–163.

Lima, S.L. and Dill, L.M. (1990). Behavioral decisions made under the risk of predation: a review and prospectus. *Canadian Journal of Zoology* 68 (4): 619–640.

Lourenço, J. and Recker, M. (2014). The 2012 Madeira dengue outbreak: epidemiological determinants and future epidemic potential. *PLoS Neglected Tropical Diseases* 8 (8): e3083.

Manna, B., Aditya, G., and Banerjee, S. (2011). Habitat heterogeneity and prey selection of *Aplocheilus panchax*: an indigenous larvivorous fish. *Journal of Vector Borne Diseases* 48: 144.

Marambe, B., Silva, P., Ranwala, S. et al. (2011). Invasive alien fauna in Sri Lanka: national list, impacts and regulatory framework. In: *Island Invasives: Eradication and Management* (ed. C.R. Veitch, M.N. Clout and D.R. Towns), 445–450. Gland: IUCN.

Marten, G.G. (1987). The potential of mosquito-indigestible phytoplankton for mosquito control. *Journal of the American Mosquito Control Association* 3: 105–106.

Marten, G.G., Astaiza, R., SuÁRez, M.F. et al. (1989). Natural control of larval *Anopheles albimanus* (Diptera: Culicidae) by the predator *Mesocyclops* (Copepoda: Cyclopoida). *Journal of Medical Entomology* 26 (6): 624–627.

Messer, W.B., Vitarana, U.T., Sivananthan, K. et al. (2002). Epidemiology of dengue in Sri Lanka before and after the emergence of epidemic dengue hemorrhagic fever. *The American Journal of Tropical Medicine and Hygiene* 66 (6): 765–773.

Moore, S.M., Borer, E.T., and Hosseini, P.R. (2010). Predators indirectly control vector-borne disease: linking predator–prey and host–pathogen models. *Journal of the Royal Society Interface* 7 (42): 161–176.

Murugan, K., Anitha, J., Suresh, U. et al. (2017). Chitosan-fabricated Ag nanoparticles and larvivorous fishes: a novel route to control the coastal malaria vector *Anopheles* sundaicus? *Hydrobiologia* 797 (1): 335–350.

Nájera, J.A., González-Silva, M., and Alonso, P.L. (2011). Some lessons for the future from the Global Malaria Eradication Programme (1955–1969). *PLoS Medicine* 8 (1): e1000412.

National Dengue Control Unit, Sri Lanka (2019). Vector surveillance and integrated vector management. http://www.dengue.health.gov.lk/web/index.php/en/activities-andservices/vector-surveillance-and-integrated-vector-management (accessed 8 May 2022).

Paaijmans, K.P., Takken, W., Githeko, A.K., and Jacobs, A.F.G. (2008). The effect of water turbidity on the near-surface water temperature of larval habitats of the malaria mosquito *Anopheles gambiae*. *International Journal of Biometeorology* 52 (8): 747–753.

Perera, K.R.N., Gunathilaka, P.A.D.H.N., Amerasinghe, L.D. and Udayanga, N.W.B.A.L., (2021). Potential of aquatic carnivorous plants; *Utricularia vulgaris* and *Utricularia reticulata* as biological control agents for the larval stages of dengue vector, *Aedes aegypti*. In: *Proceedings of the 41st Annual Sessions of Institute of Biology*, Sri Lanka. p. 24.

Pethiyagoda, R. (1991). *Freshwater Fishes of Sri Lanka*. Colombo, Sri Lanka: Wildlife Heritage Trust.

Ranasinghe, H.A.K. (2020). Diversity of microbiota in mosquito breeding habitats in selected districts in Sri Lanka and screening of bacteria in the midgut of dengue transmitting vectors. PhD thesis, University of Kelaniya, Sri Lanka.

Ranasinghe, H.A.K. and Amarasinghe, L.D. (2020). Naturally occurring microbiota associated with mosquito breeding habitats and their effects on mosquito larvae. *BioMed Research International* 4065315: 11 pp.

Ranathunge, T., Kusumawathie, P.H.D., Abeyewickreme, W. et al. (2021). Biocontrol potential of six locally available fish species as predators of *Aedes aegypti* in Sri Lanka. *Biological Control* 160: 104638.

Rodrigo, W.W.P. and De Silva, S.D. (2004). Feeding behavior Guppy fish (*Poecilia reticulata,*) on mosquito larvae. *Proceedings of the 2nd Annual Academic Sessions*. Open University of Sri Lanka, Colombo, Sri Lanka. p. 26.

Rodríguez-pérez, M.A., Howard, A.F., and Reyes-Villanueva, F. (2012). Biological control of dengue vectors. In: *Integrated Pest Management and Pest Control-Current and Future Tactics* (ed. M.L. Larramendy and S. Soloneski), 241–270. Rijeka: InTech-Open Access Publisher.

Romano, D., Benelli, G. and Stefanini, C., 2019. Encoding lateralization of jump kinematics and eye use in a locust via bio-robotic artifacts. Journal of Experimental Biology, 222(2), jeb187427.

Samanmali, C., Udayanga, L., Ranathunge, T. et al. (2018). Larvicidal potential of five selected dragonfly nymphs in Sri Lanka over *Aedes aegypti* (Linnaeus) larvae under laboratory settings. *BioMed Research International* 2018: 8759459. 10 pp.

Sandupama, T.V.A., Udayanga, N.W.B.A.L., Perera, S.J., Walpita, C.N., Ranathunge, R.M.T.B., Priyadarshana, M.K.C., and Hapugoda, M. (2019). A preliminary investigation on the predatory potency of selected native and introduced fish species over *Aedes aegypti* mosquito larvae. *Abstracts of 7th International Conference of Sabaragamuwa University of Sri Lanka*, Belihuloya, Sri Lanka (14 and 15 November 2019). Belihuloya, Sri Lanka: Sabaragamuwa University of Sri Lanka. p. 156.

Seixas, G., Grigoraki, L., Weetman, D. et al. (2017). Insecticide resistance is mediated by multiple mechanisms in recently introduced *Aedes aegypti* from Madeira Island (Portugal). *PLoS Neglected Tropical Diseases* 11 (7): e0005799.

Shaalan, E.A.-S. and Canyon, D.V. (2009). Aquatic insect predators and mosquito control. *Tropical Biomedicine* 26: 223–261.

Shad, A. and Andrew, J. (2013). Original research article a study on the predatory potency of dragonfly, *Bradinopyga geminata* nymphs over the immature stages of the filarial vector, *Culex quinquefasciatus* say. *International Journal of Current Microbiology and Applied Sciences* 2: 172–182.

Shirantha, R.R.A.R., Amarathunga, A.A.D., and Weerasekara, K.A.W.S. (2008). Do feral populations of *Poecilia reticulata* ready to bring its overall efficacy as a mosquito bio-*control* agent or pose threats to aquatic biodiversity in Sri Lanka. *National Symposium on Invasive Alien Species*, Colombo, Sri Lanka (11 November 2008).

Silva, P. and Kurukulasuriya, M. (2010). Invasive alien fauna in Sri Lanka – introduction, spread, impacts and management. In: *Invasive Alien Species in Sri Lanka – Strengthening Capacity to Control Their Introduction and Spread* (ed. B. Marambe, P. Silva, S. Wijesundara and N. Atapattu), 39–61. Colombo: Biodiversity Secretariat of the Ministry of Environment.

Sintupachee, S., Milne, J.R., Poonchaisri, S. et al. (2006). Closely related Wolbachia strains within the pumpkin arthropod community and the potential for horizontal transmission via the plant. *Microbial Ecology* 51 (3): 294–301.

Sirisena, P.D.N.N. and Noordeen, F. (2014). Evolution of dengue in Sri Lanka – changes in the virus, vector, and climate. *International Journal of Infectious Diseases* 19: 6–12.

Sirisena, P.D.N.N., Noordeen, F., Kurukulasuriya, H. et al. (2017). Effect of climatic factors and population density on the distribution of dengue in Sri Lanka: a GIS based evaluation for prediction of outbreaks. *PLoS One* 12 (1): e0166806.

Strong, D.R. and Pemberton, R.W. (2001). Food webs, risks of alien enemies and reform of biological control.

In: *Evaluating Indirect Ecological Effects of Biological Control* (ed. E. Wajnberg, J.K. Scott and P.C. Quimby), 57–79. Wallingford: CAB International Publishing.

Subramaniam, J., Murugan, K., Panneerselvam, C. et al. (2016). Multipurpose effectiveness of Couroupita guianensis-synthesized gold nanoparticles: high antiplasmodial potential, field efficacy against malaria vectors and synergy with *Aplocheilus lineatus* predators. *Environmental Science and Pollution Research* 23 (8): 7543–7558.

Surendran, S.N., Kajatheepan, A., Jude, P.J., and Ramasamy, R. (2008). Use of tilapia, *Oreochromis mossambicus*, for the control of mosquito breeding in water storage tanks in the Jaffna district of Sri Lanka. *Tropical Medicine and Health* 36 (2): 107–110.

Surendran, S.N., Jude, P.J., Thavaranjit, A.C. et al. (2013). Predatory efficacy of *Culex* (Lutzia) *fuscanus* on mosquito vectors of human diseases in Sri Lanka. *Journal of the American Mosquito Control Association* 29 (2): 168–170.

Tissera, H.A., Samaraweera, P.C., Jayamanne, B.D.W. et al. (2018). Use of *Bacillus thuringiensis israelensis* in integrated vector control of *Aedes* sp. in Sri Lanka: a prospective controlled effectiveness study. *Tropical Medicine & International Health* 23 (2): 229–235.

Udayanga, L., Gunathilaka, N., Iqbal, M.C.M. et al. (2018a). Empirical optimization of risk thresholds for dengue: an approach towards entomological management of *Aedes* mosquitoes based on larval indices in the Kandy district of Sri Lanka. *Parasites & Vectors* 11 (1): 1–12.

Udayanga, L., Gunathilaka, N., Iqbal, M.C.M. et al. (2018b). Comprehensive evaluation of demographic, socio-economic and other associated risk factors affecting the occurrence of dengue incidence among Colombo and Kandy districts of Sri Lanka: a cross-sectional study. *Parasites & Vectors* 11 (1): 1–18.

Udayanga, L., Ranathunge, T., Iqbal, M.C.M. et al. (2019). Predatory efficacy of five locally available copepods on *Aedes* larvae under laboratory settings: an approach towards bio-control of dengue in Sri Lanka. *PLoS One* 14 (5): e0216140.

Udayanga, L., Gunathilaka, N., Iqbal, M.C.M., and Abeyewickreme, W. (2020). Climate change induced vulnerability and adaption for dengue incidence in Colombo and Kandy districts: the detailed investigation in Sri Lanka. *Infectious Diseases of Poverty* 9 (1): 1–17.

Venkatesh, A. and Tyagi, B.K. (2013). Predatory potential of *Bradinopyga geminata* and *Ceriagrion coromandelianum* larvae on dengue vector *Aedes aegypti* under controlled conditions (anisoptera: libellulidae; zygoptera: coenagrionidae; diptera: culicidae). *Odonatologica* 42: 139–149.

Walker, K. and Lynch, M. (2007). Contributions of *Anopheles* larval control to malaria suppression in tropical Africa: review of achievements and potential. *Medical and Veterinary Entomology* 21 (1): 2–21.

Washburn, J.O. (1995). Regulatory factors affecting larval mosquito populations in container and pool habitats: implications for biological control. *Journal of the American Mosquito Control Association-Mosquito News* 11 (2): 279–283.

Weterings, R., Umponstira, C., and Buckley, H.L. (2018). Landscape variation influences trophic cascades in dengue vector food webs. *Science Advances* 4 (2): eaap9534.

WHO (2009). *Dengue: Guidelines for Diagnosis, Treatment, Prevention and Control*, http://whqlibdoc.who.int/publications/2009/9789241547871_eng.pdf. World Health Organization (accessed 12 May 2022).

WHO Expert Committee on Vector Biology and Control and World Health Organization (1992). *Vector Resistance to Pesticides: Fifteenth Report of the WHO Expert Committee on Vector Biology and Control* (meeting held in Geneva from 5 to 12 March 1991). World Health Organization.

Wijesinghe, W.M.G.S., Wickramasinghe, M.B., Kusumawathie, P.H.D. et al. (2009). Studies on the efficacy of *Toxorhynchites* larvae and three larvivorous fish species for the control of *Aedes* larval populations in water-storage tanks in the Matale district of Sri Lanka. *Dengue Bulletin* 33 (1): 40–147.

Yasuoka, J., Levins, R., Mangione, T.W., and Spielman, A. (2006). Community-based rice ecosystem management for suppressing vector anophelines in Sri Lanka. *Transactions of the Royal Society of Tropical Medicine and Hygiene* 100 (11): 995–1006.

Section III

Futuristic Approach for One Health

25

Planetary Health

Rethinking Health

Novil Wijeskara

Humphrey Fellowship Program, Department of Global Health, Rollins School of Public Health, Emory University, Atlanta, GA, USA
Disaster Preparedness and Response Division, Ministry of Health, Colombo, Sri Lanka

25.1 Impact of Humans on the Planet

In the history of the Earth, the geological epoch that started 11,700 years ago is named the Holocene. A need to coin a new epoch marking the end of the Holocene led to the term "Anthropocene" (Crutzen 2002, p. 415:23) being proposed, which demarcates when human activities started making a substantial impact on the Earth's natural systems. Though the start of the Anthropocene is yet to be recognized as a formal geological epoch, the scientific consensus notes that it may have started around the 1950s.

During the Anthropocene, socioeconomic trends show rapid changes corresponding with an increased use of natural resources almost tangentially over this period, which is sometimes called the Great Acceleration (McNeill and Engelke 2014). Figure 25.1 illustrates the aforementioned pattern of excessive consumption of natural resources.

According to the 2015 global assessment report on biodiversity and ecosystem services, nature's potential to sustain contributions to an acceptable quality of life has declined for 14 of the 18 categories of nature's contributions to people from 1970 to the present as shown in Figure 25.2.

The planetary boundaries framework (Steffen et al. 2015, p. 347) with nine domains has been used to explain the biological and physical systems that are vital for the survival and sustenance of human beings on the Earth. It is clear that we are already encroaching on four out of nine planetary boundaries as shown in Figure 25.3 and Table 25.1 (Rockström et al. 2009, p. 461).

Humans have overrun the boundaries of climate change, rate of biodiversity loss, and the nitrogen cycle (biochemical flows). Furthermore, the boundary associated with ocean acidification is reaching its threshold value, while global freshwater use has already breached regional thresholds in areas of low water availability and high consumption (Steffen et al. 2015, p. 347).

25.1.1 Climate Change

Climate change is an alarming environmental trend that has been observed in the contemporary decades (IPCC 2013). An increase in atmospheric concentrations of greenhouse gases such as carbon dioxide, methane, and nitrous oxide, as well as black carbon, is noted to cause a substantial increase in atmospheric global temperatures, due to the greenhouse effect. It is becoming increasingly clear that human activity, such as the burning of fossil fuels and the altering of natural ecosystems for human benefit, is the primary source of these emissions. As such the resulting global emissions trajectory exceeds the IPCC's Representative Concentration Pathway (RCP 8) for gauging climate change by a significant margin (Sanford et al. 2014, pp. 164–166).

Effects of climate change have been studied profusely. Ice sheets in Greenland and Antarctica are melting due to rising global temperatures. As such, since 1900, there has been a 0.19-m rise in mean sea level, which is expected to climb between 0.52 and 0.98 m by 2100. While the global mean surface temperature has risen by 0.85° C since 1800, it is anticipated to climb by 2.6–4.8° C by the end of the twenty-first century, using the 1986–2005 period as a baseline. The frequency and length of heatwaves, as well as excessive rains, are projected to increase, as land areas warm faster than marine areas (IPCC 2013). Nonetheless, in many mid-latitude and subtropical dry regions, mean rainfall may decline, posing major health risks to humans and animals (Intergovernmental Panel on Climate Change 2015, p. 1134).

One Health: Human, Animal, and Environment Triad, First Edition. Edited by Meththika Vithanage and Majeti Narasimha Vara Prasad.

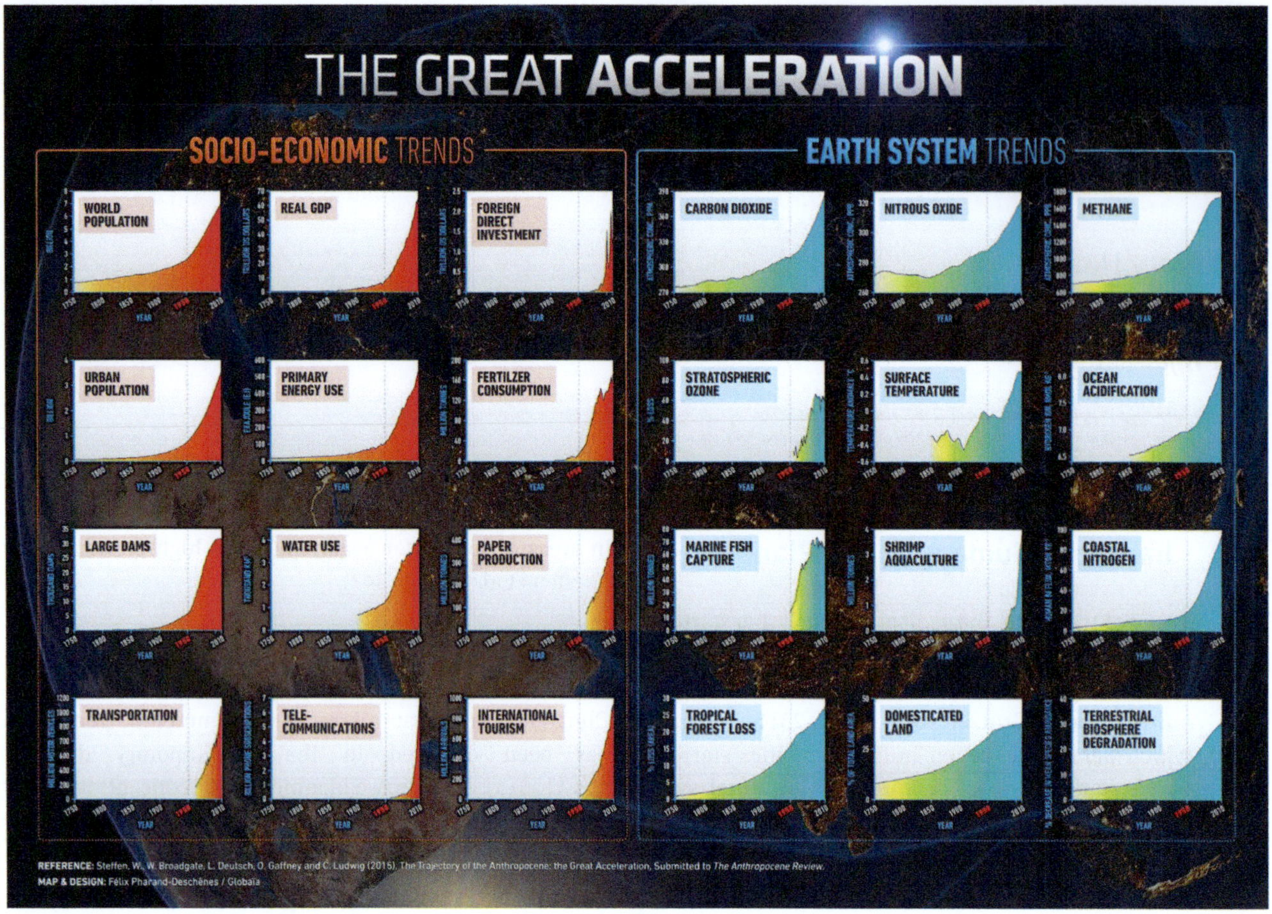

Figure 25.1 The Great Acceleration. *Source:* Steffen et al. 2015/with permission of SAGE publications.

25.1.2 Ocean Acidification

Due to the rising carbon dioxide levels in the atmosphere, more carbon dioxide will be dissolved in the ocean. As a result, ocean acidity will increase. Since the beginning of the Industrial Revolution, the pH of the seas has dropped by 0.1 pH. However by 2100, ocean acidity is expected to rise by up to 170% (IGBP, IOC, SCOR 2013). The saturation of certain kinds of oceanic calcium carbonate utilized by marine animals such as mussels, clams, and corals to construct their shells or skeletons would be reduced as a result of ocean acidification. Reduced survival rates and decreased growth and development of marine organisms, rapid global loss of coral reefs, and loss of the ability to form and maintain shells are all projected outcomes of ocean acidification (IGBP, IOC, SCOR 2013).

Due to the impact of fluctuating acidity levels on hatching success of shelled animals, it has been estimated that the whole population of Antarctic krill (*Euphausia superba*) may perish within 300 years if carbon dioxide emissions continue to rise (Kawaguchi et al. 2013, pp. 843–847). However, it has been noted that some organisms, such as sea grasses and fleshy algae, can withstand ocean acidification, while others may even profit from increased carbon availability. While such animals may stand to benefit, the balance of the ecosystem and habitat may change significantly thereby causing negative consequences for complex natural systems.

25.1.3 Freshwater

Water is all around us as our planet is 70% water. However, all humans and land animals have access to only about 2.5% of the total water reserves as freshwater. The majority of available freshwater is in the form of ice or permanent snow cover. Renewable (rivers, surface water, and groundwater) and nonrenewable (groundwater) freshwater resources exist (e.g. deep aquifers, which have a negligible rate of replenishment on human timescales) (Food and Agriculture Organization of the United Nations 2003). Groundwater is used to satisfy 50% of household needs, 40% of non-piped industrial water, and 20% of irrigation needs. In many parts of the world, groundwater is being depleted faster than it can be replenished. The rate of extraction doubled between 1960 and 2000 (OECD 2012).

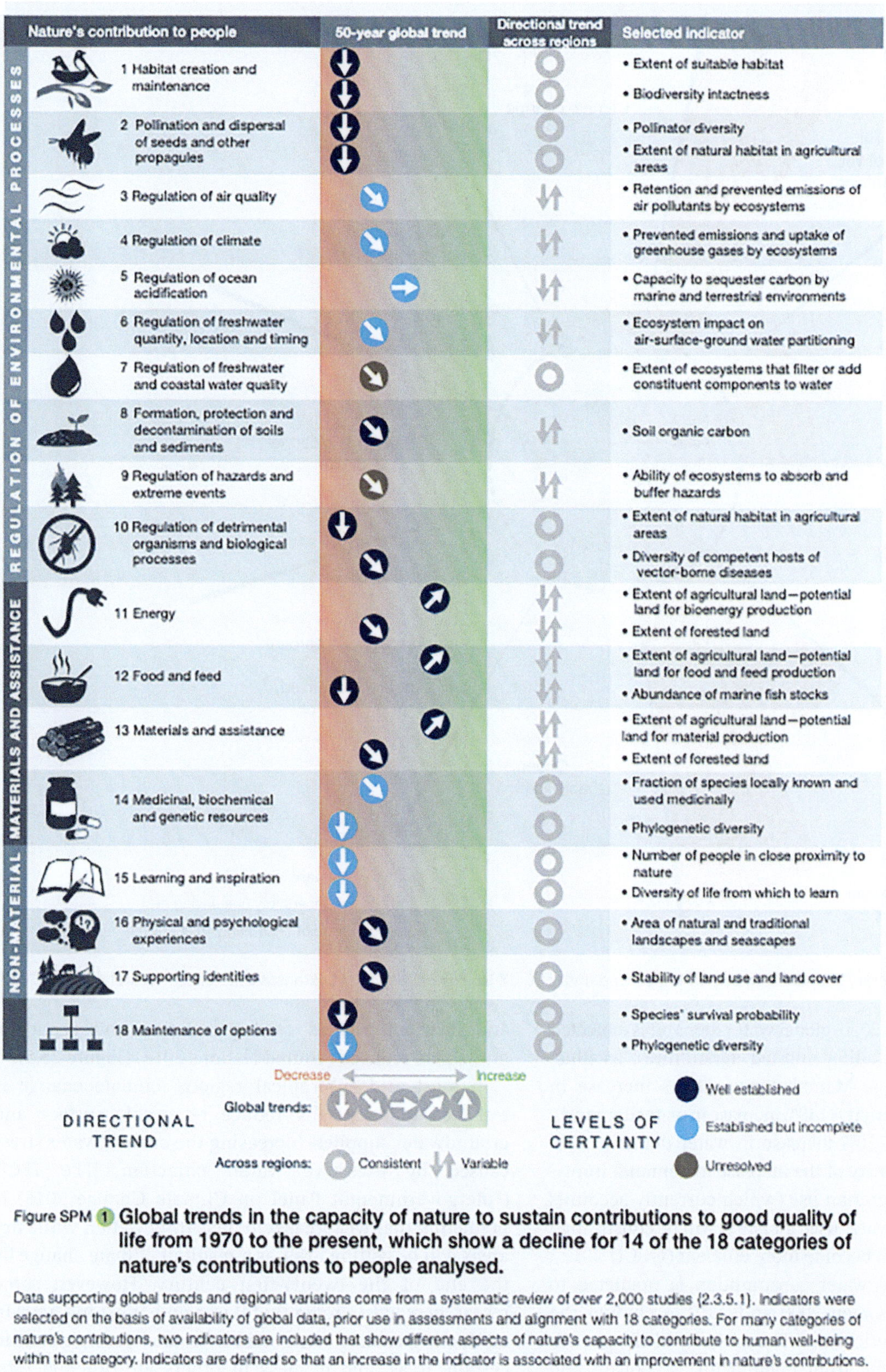

Figure 25.2 Global trends in capacity for nature to sustain good quality life. *Source:* IPBES (2019).

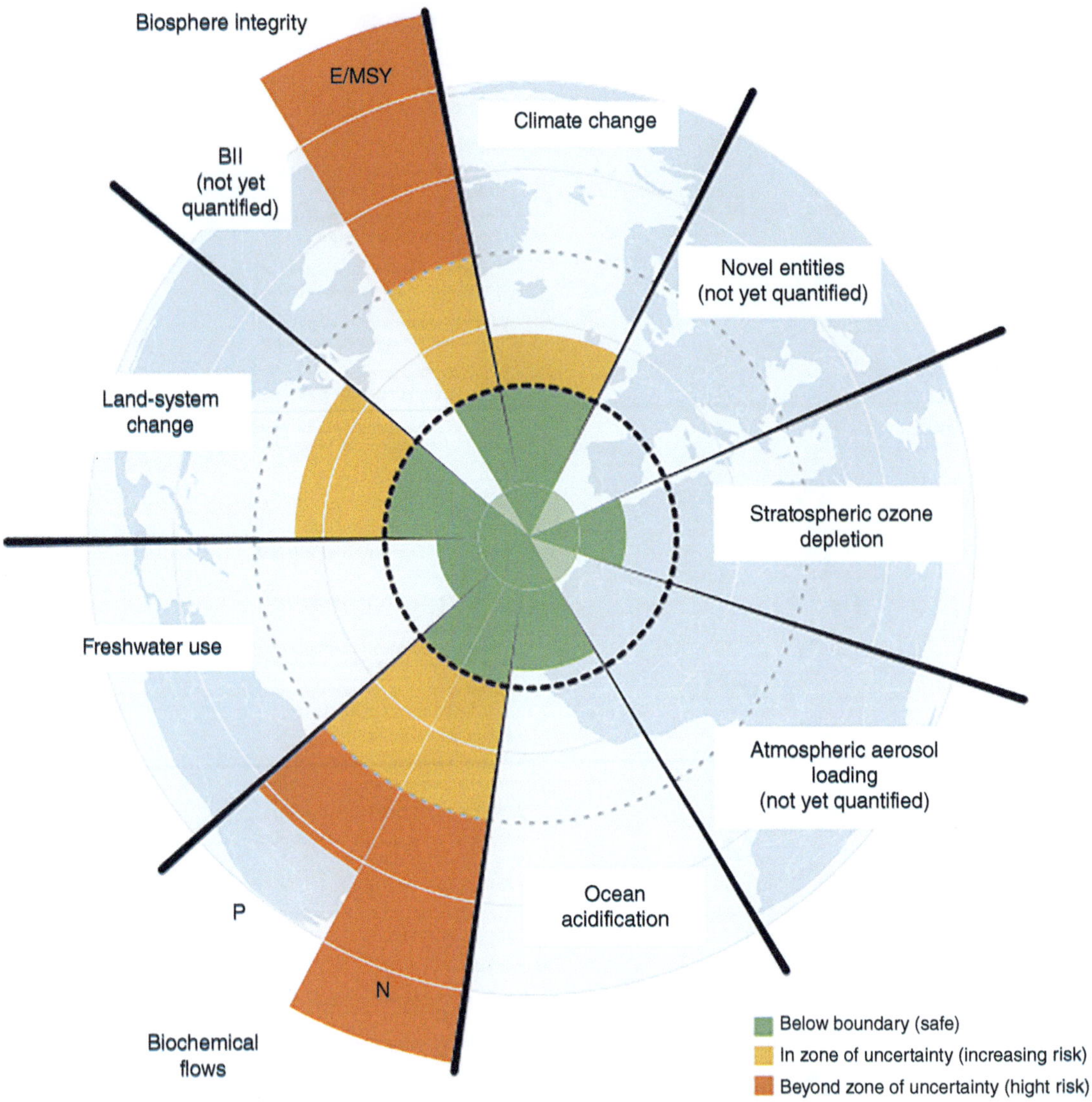

Figure 25.3 The planetary boundaries framework. Licenced under CC BY-NC-ND 3.0. *Source:* J. Lokrantz/Azote based on Steffen et al. 2015.

Between 2000 and 2050, global water demand is expected to rise by 55% (excluding rain-fed agriculture), as illustrated in Figure 25.4. Manufacturing (400% increase in water demand), electricity (140% increase in water demand), and domestic use (130% increase in water demand) will account for the majority of the increase in demand, implying that water for agrarian use (which currently accounts for about 70% of all water used globally) will be constrained and thus will need to become more efficient (OECD 2012). Furthermore, global water consumption is predicted to increase by 55% between 2000 and 2050, excluding the needs for rain-fed agriculture. The majority of the growth in demand will come from manufacturing, power, and home consumption.

As such, water scarcity will have significant and long-lasting indirect health consequences, both procedurally and distributively, as food production and economic growth are reduced (United Nations 2014) (Figure 25.5).

In most arid subtropical regions, climate change is expected to drastically reduce renewable surface and groundwater supplies, increasing the current water stress caused by excessive water extraction. The IPCC (Intergovernmental Panel on Climate Change 2015) is predicting that wet areas will be getting wetter, while dry areas will be getting drier as a result of climate change by the end of the twenty-first century. However, some researchers have shown that it is even happening now. In addition, greater glacier melt, increased precipitation in certain areas, and dryness in others are other factors. Many water sources are also impacted by habitat loss and pollution around the world. By the end of the century, over 70% of the world's wetlands that existed in 1900

Table 25.1 Planetary boundaries framework.

Planetary boundaries				
Earth-system process	**Parameters**	**Proposed boundary**	**Current status**	**Preindustrial value**
Climate change	i) Atmospheric carbon dioxide concentration (parts per million by volume)	350	387	280
	ii) Change in radiative forcing (watts per meter squared)	1	1.5	0
Rate of biodiversity loss	Extinction rate (number of species per million species per year)	10	>100	0.1–1
Nitrogen cycle (part of a boundary with the phosphorus cycle)	Amount of N_2 removed from the atmosphere for human use (millions of tons per year)	35	121	0
Phosphorus cycle (part of a boundary with the nitrogen cycle)	Quantity of P flowing into the oceans (millions of tons per year)	11	8.5–9.5	−1
Stratospheric ozone depletion	Concentration of ozone (Dobson unit)	276	283	290
Ocean acidification	Global mean saturation state of aragonite in surface sea water	275	2.90	3.44
Global freshwater use	Consumption of freshwater by humans (km^3 per year)	4000	2600	415
Change in land use	Percentage of global land cover converted to cropland	15	11.7	Low
Atmospheric aerosol loading	Overall particulate concentration in the atmosphere, on a regional basis	To be determined		
Chemical pollution	For example, amount emitted to or concentration of persistent organic pollutants, plastics, endocrine disrupters, heavy metals, and nuclear waste in the global environment or the effects on ecosystem and functioning of earth system thereof	To be determined		

Boundaries for processes in red have been crossed.
Data sources: Ref. 10 and supplementary information. Steffen et al. 2015/Springer Nature.

had vanished, with considerably greater losses in Asia (Davidson 2014, p. 65: 934)

25.1.4 Changes in Land Use and Soil Erosion

Most of the world's territory was wilderness for much of human history, with woods, meadows, and shrubbery dominating its landscapes. This has altered considerably over the past few centuries, as wild habitats have been driven out by conversion to agricultural land (Masundire et al. 2005) (Figure 25.6).

Figure 25.6 depicts the current state of global land area. Glaciers cover 10% of the Earth, whereas barren area – deserts, arid salt flats, beaches, sand dunes, and exposed rocks – cover the remaining 19%. This leaves us with what we refer to as "habitable land." Agriculture occupies half of all habitable land. This leaves only 37% for forests, 11% for shrubs and grasslands, 1% for freshwater coverage, and 1% for built-up urban areas, which includes cities, towns, villages, highways, and other human infrastructure. Natural environments have been converted to agricultural or other uses in many regions of the world over the decades, as a response to human population increase and development. With the exception of Oceania and Antarctica, around 25% of natural habitats have been converted to other land. This conversion rate can be as high as 50% in some parts of the world, such as in Southeast Asia. Many temperate areas in North America and Europe have been cultivated and developed already. Despite this, due to the scarcity of natural habitats, only a minor increase in the extension of agricultural areas has been noticed over the past four decades.

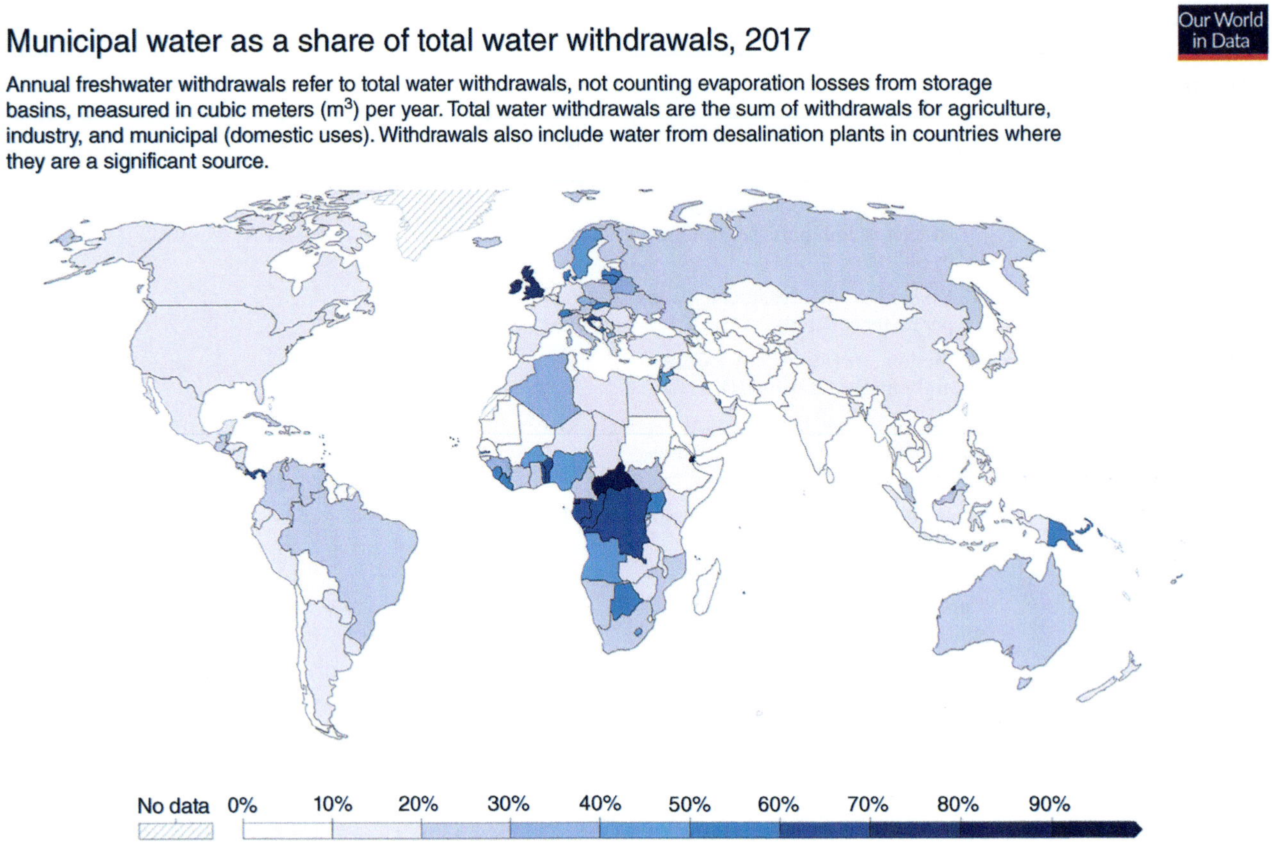

Figure 25.4 Annual global water withdrawals in 2017. *Source:* Ritchie and Roser (2017).

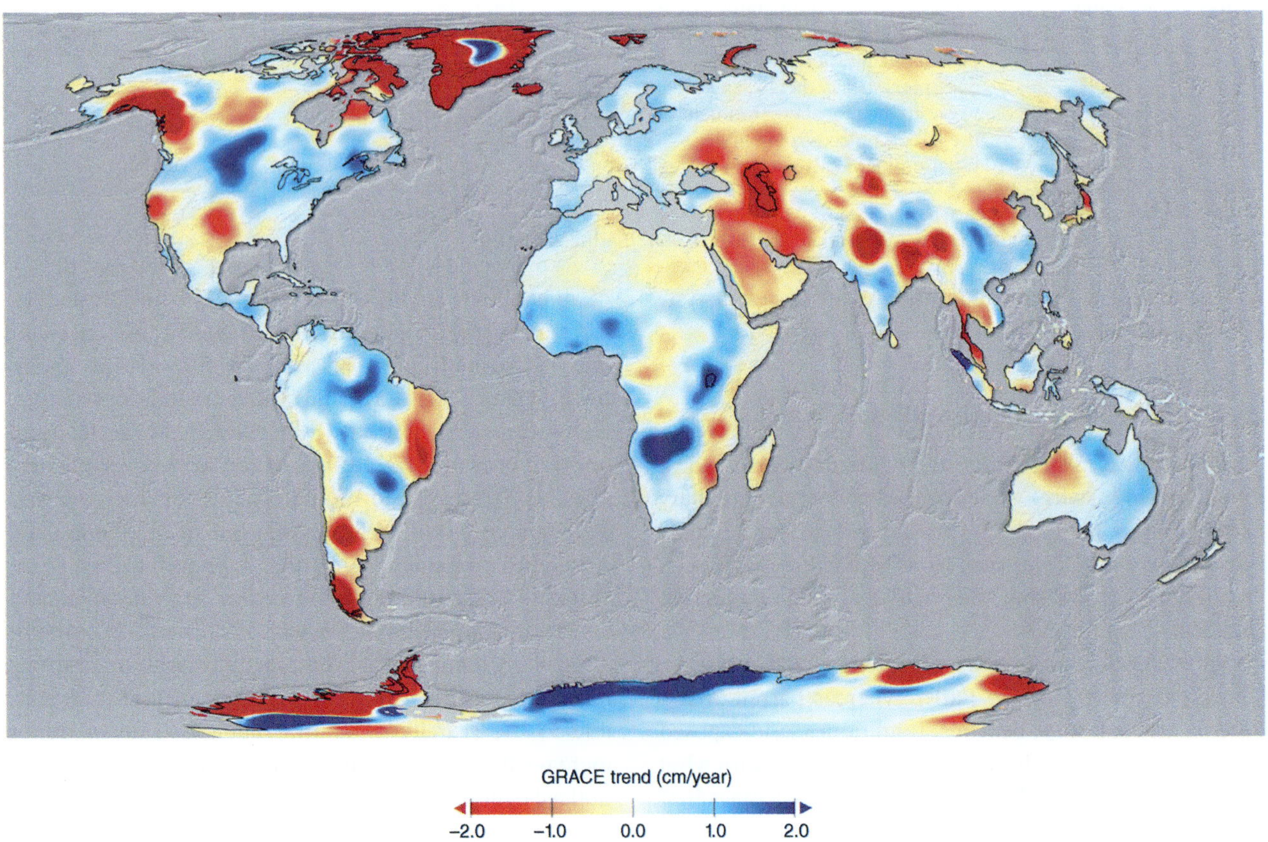

Figure 25.5 Total groundwater storage map, NASA GRACE 2018.

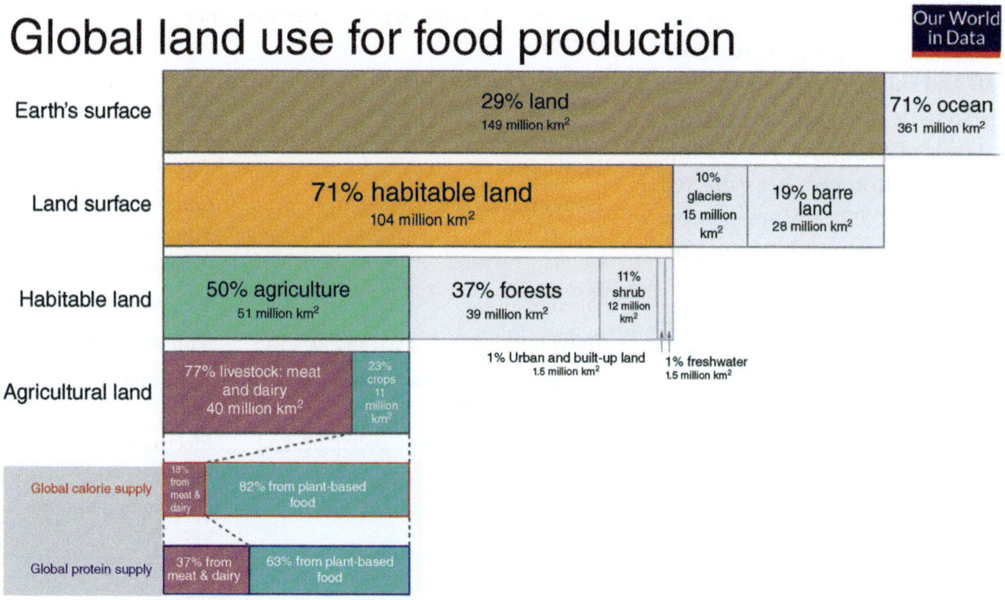

Figure 25.6 Global land use for food production. *Source:* UN Food and Agriculture Organization (FAO).

Growing food is not the only motive of humans to consume land. The conversion of natural habitats to grow non-food crops (e.g. maize, sugarcane, and oil palm) for biofuel and cosmetics continues at a rapid pace in many places, particularly in tropical and subtropical regions. The depreciation of environmental sustainability maybe driven by rising global wealth and globalization, as the demand for animal products grow as populations grow wealthier, thus the need for non-food crops for biofuel and cosmetics increase (Tilman and Clark 2014, pp. 518–522).

At the global level, the land use for oil crops has grown from 113.62 million hectares to 301.95 million hectares in 2014. Demand for biofuels in Europe and food in India, Indonesia, and China is driving an increase in oil palm (*Elaeis guineensis*) growth of 9% per year (World Health Organization and Convention on Biological Diversity 2015). Monoculture plantations such as oil palm have many derogatory effects on biodiversity, as they contain around half the number of vertebrate species as primary forests and have a lower species richness than secondary forests (Savilaakso et al. 2014). Furthermore, the deforestation of primary and secondary forests in creating monoculture plantations, especially in the tropics, is threatening native species to extinction (Foley et al. 2005, pp. 570–574)

In addition to threatening native species, the conversion of natural habitat to agricultural land is increasing the deposition of nitrogen and phosphorus due to agricultural run-off, thereby contributing to soil degradation. Forest fires caused by land clearance activities with the intention of agriculture will add to the air pollution at the local level, while contributing to greenhouse gas emissions, aggravating the climate change (Kemf and United Nations Environment Programme 2013).

There has been a fine balance between the processes of soil formation and degradation over the millennia. Nevertheless, due to human activity, natural soil degradation processes are being disproportionately accelerated by land clearance and intensive agricultural techniques (Van and Oldeman 1998). Such degradation maybe aggravated by urban growth that consumes clearance of topsoil and unsustainable land usage by industry. It has been shown that tillage agriculture causes erosion rates that are one to two orders of magnitude higher than soil formation, which itself is a lengthy process (Montgomery 2007, p. 104).

Soil degradation is fast making once used agricultural land into deserts (Lambin and Meyfroidt 2011). Fifty-five percent of global land degradation is attributed to human action (Lal 2010), which contributes to increased flood risks and loss of soil microbiological density (Koch et al. 2013). Soil functions as a carbon sink, and soil of natural habitats have twice the carbon capacity as their agricultural counterparts (Lal 2010). Thus, soil degradation means loss of carbon sink too, aggravating the problem of rising greenhouse gases. As a result of changes in rainfall and temperature-driven changes in plant biomass, future climate change is projected to affect the amount, frequency, and amplitude of soil erosion (Mullan 2013).

Nitrogen and phosphorous are two of the large number of elements that go through a cyclical process and are in fine balance in natural habitats, in their own as well as in combination. In the past 60 years, as a result of upscaling food production to feed the expanding human population, increased levels of nitrogen and phosphorus entering the environment synthetically. Such an inorganic increase via agricultural fertilizer run-off and soil erosion have become significant drivers of ecosystem change (Rockström et al. 2009). In the future, levels of biologically accessible nitrogen and phosphorus in the environment are expected to rise dramatically (Masundire et al. 2005). Humans now produce accessible nitrogen than all natural nitrogen production mechanisms put together (Masundire et al. 2005).

Due to the same reason of increased use of agricultural fertilizer extracted from mined reserves, in addition to livestock slurry and dung, the prevalence of phosphorous in water runoffs and agrarian land is three times that of preindustrial age (Bennett et al. 2001). Excess nitrogen in terrestrial ecosystems such as temperate grasslands, shrublands, and forests can reduce plant diversity while conversely, excessive nitrogen and phosphorus in water bodies, such as rivers and other wetlands, can cause algal blooms and eutrophication in inland waters and coastal areas (Masundire et al. 2005).

25.1.5 Toxic Chemical Pollution and Exposure

Humans are using many chemicals either directly or indirectly in many domains of their life such as production of food, consumer goods, and health. In parallel with other trends observed since 1950, the global production and consumption of most types of chemicals has increased dramatically (UNEP 2013). It is estimated that more than 140,000 chemicals are in existence in the EU market alone, and chemical sales are expected to grow at a rate of roughly 3% per year through 2050 (UNEP 2013). In addition, there will be a shift in the majority of the production of chemicals from high-income nations to low- and middle-income ones (Daughton and Ternes 1999) (Table 25.2).

In many parts of the world, the total amount of chemicals released into the environment as waste is unknown (Kemf and United Nations Environment Programme 2013), largely due to the lack of systems for environmental accountability, as a result of information and governance challenges (Whitmee et al. 2015). However, for a sense of scale, the United States, Canada, and Mexico alone released 4.9 million tons of chemicals into the environment in 2009. Such chemicals included persistent, bioaccumulative, and toxic chemicals and known or suspected carcinogens.

The effects of chemical pollution on humans could be direct and indirect. For example, human carcinogenesis could be taken as a direct effect on humans due to chemical pollution, such as from substances like asbestos. On the other hand, the reactions on humans could be indirect, as a product of chemical effects on the ecosystem. In such, chemical pollution can contribute to loss of biodiversity, which could have impacts on food chains, and may contribute to bioaccumulation of chemicals throughout the food chain (Kemf and United Nations Environment Programme 2013). Aforementioned phenomena in marine ecosystems could in turn affect humans due to consumption of seafood. Furthermore, changes to the native environment, such as through the feminization of fish, development delays, and malformations in amphibians have been reported due to ecosystem toxicity (Kemf and United Nations Environment Programme 2013). While it is good news that pollution in relation to polychlorinated biphenyl and dioxins in wildlife is decreasing, brominated fire retardants and per fluorinated compounds have increased in the same (Kemf and United Nations Environment Programme 2013). Furthermore, climate change has added to the complexity of the problem of chemical pollution since the dispersion of these substances is inconsistent due to the effects of climate change. In the meantime, the effects of mixtures of different chemicals on individuals is another challenge that needs to be addressed. There is a possibility that there exists a mixture of chemicals, where even if each of the individual chemicals are in concentrations below the non-toxic standards, there could be an adverse effect in their cumulative number (Diamond et al. 2015).

Table 25.2 Major sources of chemical contaminants and their sources.

Chemical	Source
Pesticides	Agriculture
Heavy metals such as mercury	Cement production Mining Coal combustion
Dioxins	Electronics recycling
Butyl tins, heavy metals, and asbestos	Ship breakage
Mutagenic dyes, heavy metals, and other pollutants	Textile industry
Toxic metals, solvents, polymers, and flame retardants	Electronic manufacturing
Pharmaceuticals	Human and animal use

25.1.6 Biodiversity Loss

As per the 2015 Global Assessment Report on Biodiversity and Ecosystem Services, human actions are putting more species on the verge of extinction than ever before (World Health Organization and Convention on Biological Diversity 2015). As such, around 25% of species in the examined animal and plant groupings are threatened, implying that around one million species are currently on the verge of extinction with many within decades, unless action is taken to lessen the intensity of causes of biodiversity loss. Without such action, the global rate of species extinction, which is now tens to hundreds of times faster than it has averaged over the past 10 million years, would accelerate even further (World Health Organization and Convention on Biological Diversity 2015)

Five direct and five indirect drivers of change of biodiversity has been identified in the aforementioned report:

- Direct drivers: changes in ecosystems on land and in sea, direct exploitation of organisms, climate change, pollution and increase in foreign chemicals, and invasion of alien species.
- Indirect drivers: changes in human production and consumption patterns, human population dynamics and trends, trade and global interdependence, technological innovations, and distributive capacities of local and global governance institutions.

It should be noted that the indirect drivers are determining the direct drivers. Both types of drivers differ among regions and countries widely.

The effects of alterations in biodiversity could have negative consequences on the structure and function of the ecosystem and may have differing impacts around the world. While in the local level, the ecosystem services could be compromised, but at the global level, the beneficial effects of biodiversity in buffering climate change and the removal of pollutants will be affected (World Health Organization and Convention on Biological Diversity 2015)

So far, we have discussed the effects of linear changes of individual environmental threats. However, multiple such threats could interact at the same time to produce detrimental consequences. It must be noted that some environmental systems' response to rising environmental services by humans may be sudden, instead of being gradual. Such sudden shifts in social-ecological systems could create regime changes. Regime shifts are defined as large, persistent changes in the structure and function of social-ecological systems, with substantive impacts on the suite of ecosystem services provided by these systems (see Table 25.3) (Barnosky et al. 2014).

It is important to be cognizant of the complexity of the operations of the environmental systems in the wake of rising demands by humans for their ecosystem services. Some complicated issues that are seen today, with no identifiable causes, could be traced to such complexities of interaction rather than a lack of etiology (Rocha et al. 2015).

Key factors that drive human-induced environmental changes are closely linked to population growth, unsustainable consumption patterns, and the indiscriminate use of technology. Increasing population means the rising

Table 25.3 Examples of well-known regime shifts and their impacts.

Regime shift	Regime A	Regime B	Impacts of shift from A to B	Evidence	Source of evidence
Freshwater eutrophication	Non-eutrophic	Eutrophic	Reduced access to recreation, reduced drinking water quality, risk of fish loss	Strong	Observations, experiments, models
Bush encroachment	Open grassland	Closed woodland	Reduced grazing for cattle, reduced mobility, increased fuelwood	Medium	Observations, experiments, models
Soil salinization	High productivity	Low productivity	Yield declines, salt damage to infrastructure and ecosystems, contamination of drinking water	Strong	Observations, experiments, models
Coral reef degradation	Diverse coral reef	Reef dominated by macro-algae	Reduced tourism, fisheries, biodiversity	Strong	Observations, experiments, models
Coastal hypoxia	Non-hypoxic	Hypoxic	Fishery decline, loss of marine biodiversity, toxic algae	Strong	Observations, models
River channel position	Old channel	New channel	Damage to trade and infrastructure	Strong	Observations, models
Wet savanna-dry savanna	Wet savanna	Dry savanna or desert	Loss of productivity, yield declines, droughts/dry spells	Medium	Models

Information from the Regime Shifts Database www.regimeshifts.org.

demand for goods and services (Affairs 2013). This rise of demand for goods and services is often coupled with unsustainable consumption of limited planetary resources over short periods of time (Bradshaw et al. 2010). This means the exploitation of resources that are meant to be used by future generations as well (Gerland et al. 2014). While it may be noted that technology may allow for more efficient and less invasive exercise of natural systems, it is not ubiquitous, is a privileged commodity, and its use in developing countries is less prevalent over the developed due to structural disadvantages (Al-Kalbani et al. 2014). It is thus understood that the use of technology has been instrumental in extracting natural resources faster, especially in areas where it was once not possible, and this has occurred at the expense of harmful effects on the environment (Alcott 2005). Thus, it is clear that the human-induced environmental changes are closely driven by the above three key facts. Another important factor that could either positively or negatively affect environment effects is urbanization. Urbanization refers to the concentration of human populations into discrete areas. Unplanned urbanization could increase the effects of environmental effects by humans (Campbell-Lendrum and Corvalán 2007), whereas planned urbanization that use sustainable technology could minimize such negative effects while catering to the consumption needs of a large number of people in the meantime (McMichael 2014).

It is evident that planetary health is a complex issue that needs a systemic approach to addressing it. This is based on the fact that human health outcomes arise from the complex interaction between natural and social systems, which demands the engagement of diverse stakeholders for addressing it. It is important to note that the linkages between human-driven environmental change and effects on human health could not necessarily be linear and may have delayed feedback loops cutting across social, economic, and environmental dimensions (Intergovernmental Panel on Climate Change 2015).

25.2 Paradigm Shift: Human to Planetary Health

From the point of human health, several improvements also have occurred over the same period of time in human history. Few selected indicators of human health are presented in Figure 25.7.

As per Figure 25.7, life expectancy increased from an average of 29 in 1950 to 73 years in 2019. Maternal mortality has declined from 385 per 100,000 live births to 216 per 100,000 live births in 2019. Showing the same pattern, the child mortality rate has also declined from 12.5 million in 1990 to 5.2 million in 2019. In 1950, diarrheal diseases killed 1.7 million children while by 2019, this number has reduced to 1.5 million children.

As humans, we are extracting natural resources to an exceptional level and exerting extensive pressure on natural systems. Yet, human health is increasing, while the health of the global ecosystem is decreasing. Therein lies a paradox, as there would be definite, complex and serious effects on human health due to the environmental impacts. Planetary health is a novel idea that emphasizes the connection between human health, animal health, and environmental health. One of the focuses of planetary health is enhancing the understanding of the effects of environmental degradation on human health (Intergovernmental Panel on Climate Change 2015; World Health Organization and Convention on Biological Diversity 2015).

Large number of negative consequences of a disturbed planetary system have been identified at least partially, while still there is a large deficit in understanding in this area. The following Table 25.4 summarizes some of the known adverse health effects that result from the aforementioned disturbed system that have been already identified (Elbehri and Food and Agriculture Organization of the United Nations 2015).

Some milestones in the evolution of the concept of planetary health is summarized in Fact Box 25.1.

The concept of planetary health refers to an inclusive holistic approach to health, wherein the term "health" is considered in its broadest definition. It involves not only humans but also animals, plants, and the natural systems. Further, planetary health attempts to explain the determinants of both health and ill-health. First bought into the mainstream in *The Lancet* report of March 2014 (Whitmee et al. 2015), planetary health encompasses multiple streams of medical health, socioeconomic parameters, political incentives, and structural deficits to provide the said holistic approach. A wide approach allows the concept to appreciate the nuances that the normative streams do not and marry such streams to examine their intersections. Furthermore, such a wide range allows the concept to be fitted into existing and established schools of thought. The overreaching message remains, however, which is that there exists a causal relationship between the well-being of humans and the well-being of our planet, with all its life-forms and systems.

Planetary health considers the health of the people as well as the health of the planet and its systems because they are closely interdependent. Any changes in the health of natural systems of the planet could create serious human health repercussions (Watts et al. 2015). The concept further focuses on reversing these trends of environmental degradation by combining human demands with environmental preservation in order to ensure future generations' health and well-being (Whitmee et al. 2015). To do this, a multidisciplinary, cross-sector, and transnational strategy to change attitudes and behaviors at all levels, from global to local, is required. As such, the concept of planetary health is unique; it is built on and integrates several comparable concepts that address the intersections of several disciplines and approaches as shown in Figure 25.8

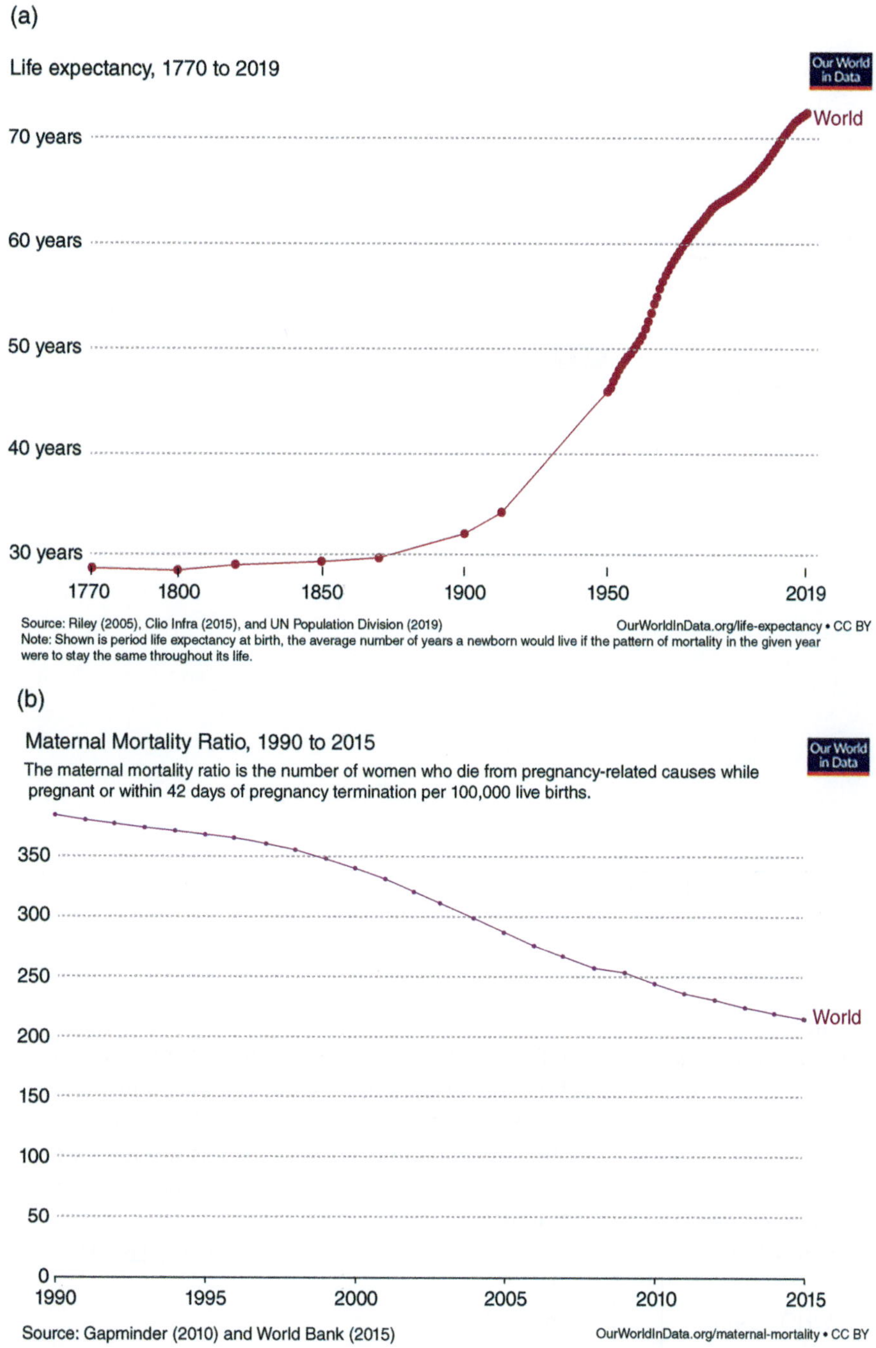

Figure 25.7 Selected trends in human health 1950–2019. (a) Life expectancy, 1770 to 2019. *Source:* Roser et al. (2013a). (b) Maternal mortality, 1990 to 2015. *Source:* Roser and Ritchie (2013). (c) Number of child deaths, 1900–2019. *Source:* Roser et al. (2013b). (d) Number of child deaths by diarrheal diseases, by age, world, 1990–2019. *Source:* Roser et al. (2013b).

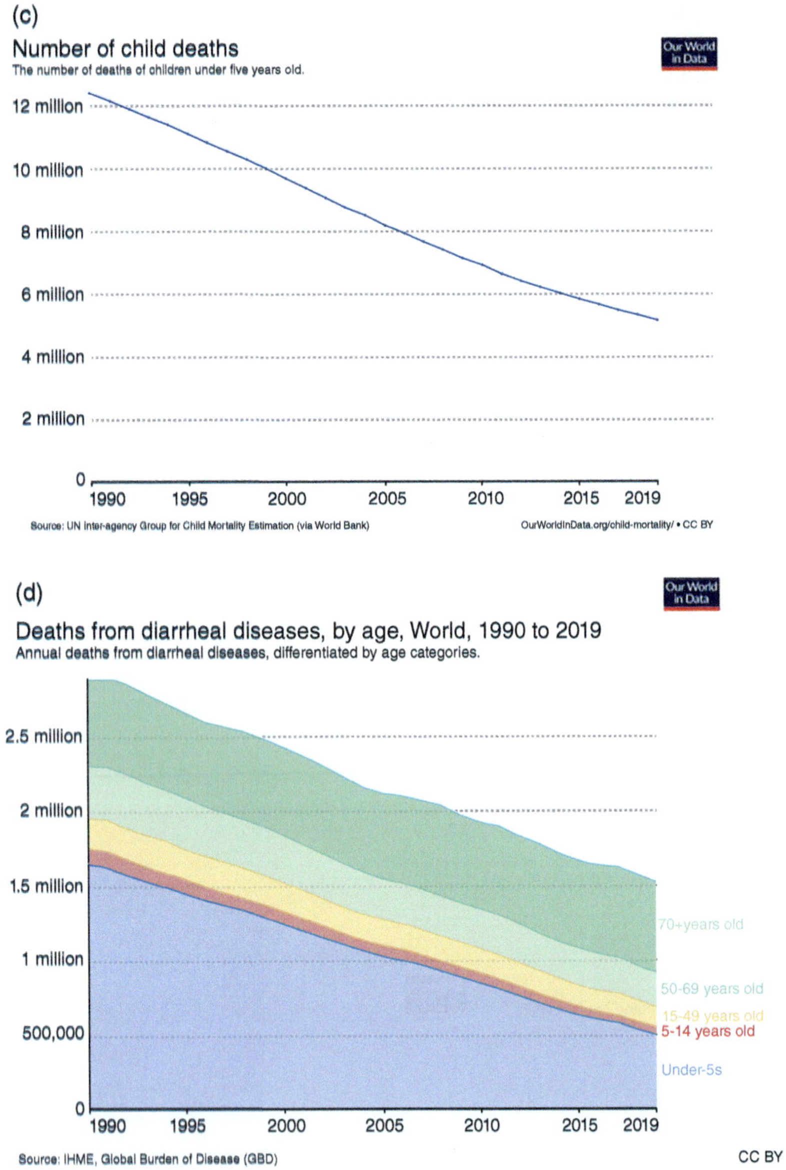

Figure 25.7 (Continued)

Health has been a concept that has been used to denote a positive state of well-being, not merely the absence of disease or infirmity.

> WHO Definition of Health
>
> "A state of complete physical, mental and social well-being and not merely the absence of disease or infirmity."
>
> –(WHO 1948).
>
> Planetary Health Definition
>
> Planetary health is the achievement of the highest attainable standard of health, wellbeing, and equity worldwide through judicious attention to the human systems – political, economic, and social – that shape the future of humanity and the Earth's natural systems that define the safe environmental limits within which humanity can flourish
>
> –(Horton and Lo 2015).
>
> Simple definition:
>
> Planetary health is the health of human civilization and the state of the natural systems on which it depends

Table 25.4 Adverse health effects as a result of disturbed planetary system.

Effect	Mechanism
Loss of food security and undernutrition	Compromised agricultural yield due to land degradation and soil erosion. The global environmental changes can affect the quality and quantity of agricultural yield, often adversely. Land degradation due to erosion, desertification, salination, and urban land development further contributes to the loss of agricultural yield (Bai et al. 2008).The poor yield can reduce food availability, food accessibility, food utilization, and food system stability. Furthermore, there is growing evidence correlating the reduction the nutritional value of food with environmental changes, such as rising carbon levels and temperatures in the atmosphere (Bai et al. 2008). In addition, negative impacts of land use and ownership, soil erosion, fertilizer leakage, food wastage, and spoilage all contribute to undernutrition, particularly in the global south (Sanchez 2002) (United Nations 2014). Loss of pollinators Pollinators, both wild and domesticated, play a critical role in ensuring successful agricultural harvests. There is evidence to suggest that the population of pollinators such as bees is declining due to increased exposure to pests, parasites, and agrochemicals (Godfray et al. 2014). In addition to the quantity of food produced, different food varieties would be affected diversely as a result of the loss of pollinators. It has been estimated that the resulting food shortage due to a 50% loss of pollinators could lead to an increase of 0.7 million deaths annually (Klein et al. 2007). Unsustainable fisheries Fish is an important source of proteins, with 2.9 billion people getting 20% of their annual protein from fish (FAO 2020). In addition, fish is an important source of vitamins, iron, zinc, and omega-three fatty acids (Sheeshka and Murkin 2002). The factors that contribute to unsustainable fishing include overfishing, warming, and acidification of water bodies due to climate change and marine habitat degradation (McCauley et al. 2015). In addition, due to climate change, changes in the ecosystem distribution of some fish as well as invertebrates that are crucial in the marine food chains could also contribute to fish catch. Effects of the environmental stressors such as ocean acidification, overfishing, and pollution can have negative impacts on coral reefs, which will deprive commercially fished fish species of food (Intergovernmental Panel on Climate Change 2015). Aquaculture, which has contributed to increased demand for fish, has its own set of negative environmental effects. For example, aquaculture could result in marine pollution due to organic and toxic waste, while irrational use of antibiotics in aquaculture could contribute toward antimicrobial resistance (Roberts 2013) Climate change It has been predicted that climate change will have larger negative impacts on global food production, despite a smaller positive yield on crop and food production in some areas (Intergovernmental Panel on Climate Change 2015). Different crops will be responding differently to climate change, while the effects would vary widely across different geographic regions of the world. Increased variability of temperature is identified as a worse threat than the rising temperature for agriculture (Huybers et al. 2014). The rising carbon dioxide concentrations do not show promising results on the number of crops produced, as it may affect the content of protein in and iron by different crop types (Ainsworth and Long 2005). Furthermore, both rising methane levels and ground-level ozone levels have been shown to be non-conducive for plant growth (Avnery et al. 2011). Another mechanism by which climate change would impact food security is through the increase of plant diseases due to infectious agents such as aflatoxin. Aflatoxin production is found to rise with increasing water stress, atmospheric carbon dioxide, and temperature (Chakraborty and Newton 2011). Loss of freshwater availability World's agriculture is largely dependent on irrigated water or groundwater (United Nations 2014). As the availability of freshwater would reduce due to climate change, this could impact agricultural food production as well. In addition, with the economic development of communities, protein consumption increases. This means more freshwater is needed for the production of meat and dairy products (Rosegrant et al. 2009). Climate change will aggravate water scarcity among water-rich regions, which in turn would in turn stress water import-dependent regions (Suweis et al. 2013).
Poor sanitation and rise of water-borne diseases	Loss of freshwater availability It is estimated that in 2015 alone, upwards of 500,000 children died from diarrheal illnesses across the world, most of which are caused by unsafe water, poor sanitation, and inadequate hygiene (Prüss-Ustün et al. 2014). Reducing the availability of freshwater can have serious negative consequences on sanitation. Water is used by all civilizations, especially those in the global south, to clean themselves as well as their facilities including toilets. Furthermore, due to the lack of technology and structural disadvantages, the developing world is at a higher risk of the adverse effects of the lack of freshwater availability than the developed world (Guynup 2010). Hence, loss of freshwater availability could compromise human sanitation and health (Myers and Patz 2009).

(*Continued*)

Table 25.4 (Continued)

Effect	Mechanism
Occurrence and spread of zoonotic and vector-borne diseases	Increased human exposure to animals and vectors The rapid urbanization causing land-use change resulting from intensified agriculture and livestock production, the trade in wildlife, and wild meat consumption have contributed in the increase in human exposure to animals (Keesing et al. 2010). In addition, climate change have brought disease transmitting vectors into close contact with human beings. As a result, vector-borne diseases such as malaria, dengue, and zika virus disease are increasing in their frequency (Brown et al. 2014).
Air pollution-related health effects	Household air pollution Globally, air pollution is responsible for more than one out of every nine deaths. In 2019, it is expected to have caused 6.67 million fatalities worldwide (95% UI: 5.90–7.49 million) (Lim et al. 2012). In 2019, air pollution was the world's fourth-biggest cause of mortality. Children and the elderly have been recognized as the most vulnerable groups of air-quality-related illnesses (Lim et al. 2012). In 2018, indoor air pollution was blamed for 2.31 million deaths. Indoor air pollution was responsible for 4.1% of all fatalities worldwide. Nevertheless, since 1990, the number of annual deaths due to indoor air pollution has decreased dramatically around the world. However, the number of illnesses and deaths due to indoor air pollution is found to be highest in low-income countries (Campbell-Lendrum and Corvalán 2007). In addition, forest fires in many parts of the world contribute to air pollution. For example, fire scientists in California believe that forest fires in October 2017 generated more CO_2 in one week than all of California's vehicles do in a year (Johnston et al. 2012). Forest fires are further known to increase lung diseases in vulnerable groups. Asthma, bronchitis, and emphysema sufferers may experience a worsening of their symptoms as a result of ground-level ozone. Ozone also has been linked to inflammation of the respiratory tract and shortness of breath, particularly during outdoor activities. Tropospheric ozone, also known as ground-level ozone, is produced by chemical interactions between nitrogen oxides (NO_x) and volatile organic molecules (VOC). When pollutants from automobiles, power plants, industrial boilers, refineries, chemical plants, and other sources react chemically in the presence of sunshine, generation of ground-level ozone occurs (Sitch et al. 2007).
Exposure to toxic chemicals	Water and soil pollution Water contamination has a significant impact on aquatic life. Animals and plants in contaminated water sources could die, and if they survive, they may have negative impacts on their reproduction (Kemf and United Nations Environment Programme 2013). For example, mercury could concentrate in tuna and other larger fish toward the end of food chains. Further, high concentrations of nitrates and phosphates could create algal blooms. Plastic pollution is harmful to marine life and takes up to 500 years to degrade, while it could be carcinogenic (Kemf and United Nations Environment Programme 2013). Chemicals in drinking water in harmful quantities could create health problems such as blue baby syndrome (nitrate), neurological problems (lead poisoning), and cancer (nitrate) (Prüss-Ustün et al. 2011). Soil pollution is a definite path by which contaminants can come into contact with human beings; however, data on soil-related health exposures are lacking globally (Landrigan and Etzel 2014).
Health effects due to extreme weather events	In 2020, extreme weather displaced over 30 million people around the world. Due to climate change, the frequency and the magnitude of extreme weather events will rise, increasing the displacement, deaths, and injuries. In addition, other health effects such as those due to food and water insecurity are going to be aggravated due to extreme weather events.
Health consequences of conflict and displacement	Persecution, conflict, and violence displaced approximately 61 million people by the end of 2013, according to the United Nations (United Nations 2014). Furthermore, the environmental crisis could create new conflicts or aggravate existing ones, especially in the global south (Hsiang et al. 2013).
Mental health effects	Rising NO_x (nitrous oxides) have proven to compromise the nervous system (Agyeman et al. 2009). Fine particulate matter ($PM_{2.5}$) levels also have been identified to affect mental health. Nitrogen derivatives in a combination of carbon monoxide have been linked with suicides and psychotic behaviors (Albrecht et al. 2007). The children could have permanent effects on their brain and nervous system development. However, in addition to such direct toxic effects of pollutants, all environmental problems discussed as well as their contributory factors could have serious impacts on mental health.

Fact Box 25.1 Key Milestones in the Evolution of the Concept of Planetary Health

- The term "planetary health" was first coined by Per Fugelli in 1993, where he described the Earth as a "patient" as "Global environmental disruptions can have serious consequences for human health. It's time for doctors to give a world diagnosis and advise on treatment." (Casassus 2017)
- The March 2014 issue (Whitmee et al. 2015) of *The Lancet* was a watershed event in the history of planetary health, which called for a departure from the traditional and procedural focus on human health to a more inclusive approach that considered secondary factors and distributions of effects.
- The planetary health was understood as the "achievement of the highest attainable standard of health, well-being, and equity worldwide through judicious attention to the human systems – political, economic, and social – that shape the future of humanity and the Earth's natural systems that define the safe environmental limits within which humanity can flourish." (Horton and Lo 2015)
- *The Lancet* report (Whitmee et al. 2015) provides a qualitative prescription of the three challenges humanity is facing in addressing the lack of planetary health: conceptual challenges, information challenges, and governance challenges.
- The term "planetary health" is used to denote the understanding that the procedural meaning of the word "Global Health does not fully take into account the natural foundation on which humans live – the planet itself. Nor does it factor in the force and fragility of human civilizations" (Horton in 2014).
- It should be noted that the effects of a subpar planetary health system are not distributed equally among the global population. One must remain cognizant that developing states of the global south are affected disproportionately due to lack of technology, funding, governance, and other structural causes (Campbell-Lendrum and Corvalán 2007).
- It may be interpreted that the concept of planetary health advocates, in essence, for an enhanced quality of life for all through the deliverance of improved health for all constituents of our planet, animal, plant, or system.
- It may be noted that the concept of planetary health has distributive challenges, wherein tracking accountability and noncooperation in the study of health, climate, and sociopolitical governance remains gray (Horton and Lo 2015).
- In 2015, the Planetary Health Alliance, led by the University of Harvard, the Wildlife Conservation Society, and other allied organizations, was founded to support the "rigorous, policy-focused, transdisciplinary field of applied research aimed at understanding and addressing the human health implications of accelerating change in the structure and function of Earth's natural systems" (Planetary Health Alliance 2016).

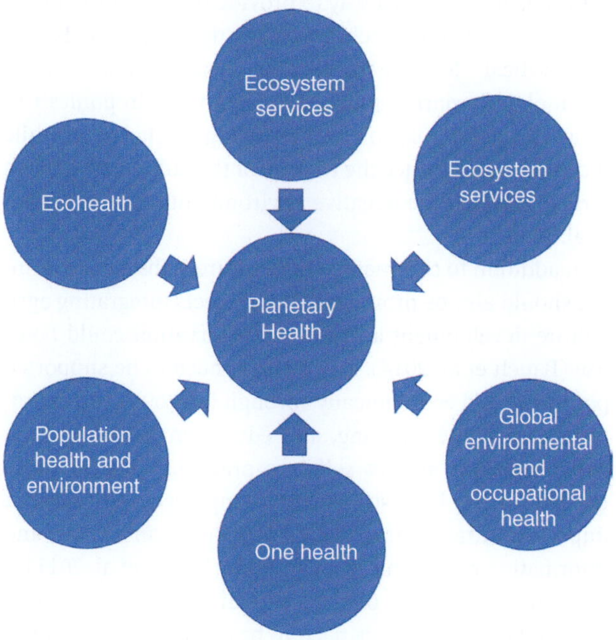

Figure 25.8 Intersectionality of planetary health with other disciplines and approaches.

Though the definition of health involves multiple dimensions from which it could be looked at, it is focusing primarily on the procedural health of human beings. As such, it does not take into consideration the complex distributive interactions between human beings and the other components of nature upon which the normative health of a human is quite dependent on.

As planetary health is defined as "the health of human civilization and the state of the natural systems on which it depends," by the Rockefeller Foundation–Lancet Commission, it calls for a paradigm shift in the human health focused approach to a holistic approach that includes all natural systems on which humankind is dependent for survival.

A key concept that is central to the development and application of planetary health is systems thinking, which demands the holistic examination of the inherent interconnectedness of different components of closed-loop systems.

Systems thinking is defined as a holistic approach for understanding the dynamic interactions among complex economic, environmental, and social systems for evaluating the potential consequences of interventions.

The systems approach has been used by intergovernmental and national organizations in addressing environmental issues. Green Economy Initiative of the UN Environment, US Environmental Protection Agency, and Future Earth and Urban Health and Wellbeing Program of the International Council of Science are some examples of organizations that use systems thinking to explore the complex relationship between the human, health, and environment.

The systems thinking approach has been useful in bringing the values into the equation of planetary health. Values are an integral part of the complex-rule-based interaction of humans and their environment. Due to the complexity of the systems, there is a need for unlearning some values and redefining others, if planetary health is to be advanced in practice.

Further, systems thinking can help to engage diverse stakeholders across the ecosystem of planetary health at all stages of the use of the planetary health approach. The stakeholders of planetary health are as complex as the systems that are involved. Thus, system thinking helps to identify as well as prioritize the stakeholders that need to be engaged. The community members, both as the contributors of pollution and the victims of the negative health effects of environmental damage, need to be actively engaged as key stakeholders as the systems thinking can help visualize their complex role in the phenomenon of planetary health.

The systems approach could be used in addressing complex planetary health problems. The planetary health calls for the adaption of systems approach in three ways:

1) To generate evidence demonstrating the complex links between global environmental changes and human health.
2) To carry out transboundary system-based research involving diverse stakeholders including end users.
3) To collectively create solutions that would lead to a transformative change.

25.3 Approaches to Promote Planetary Health

The summary of planetary health science is that humans can no longer safeguard their own health unless the current course of human action is changed (Whitmee et al. 2015). As such planetary health is an urgent call for action for urgent and deep structural changes in all dimensions of human activity.

25.3.1 Food

The rising demand for food production has to be addressed cautiously within the subtle limits of environmental balance. Sustainable intensification of global food production needs to be exercised since the available land is reaching its limits (Bai et al. 2008). Some options available include molecular breeding, the use of companion plants, and genetic modification.

Efficient water and fertilizer use in the contemporary has become an important area (Gibson 2020). Technologies such as drip and trickle irrigation, though more expensive at the beginning than traditional irrigation systems, have been proven that they could be around 33% more efficient in water use and effective in delivering the fertilizer directly to the roots of the crops.

Reduction of food wastage and spoilage is an urgent concern that needs to be addressed. It is estimated that around 30–50% of all food produced around the world is wasted, the loss is almost equally divided between the preharvest and postharvest periods (*Food wastage footprint: impacts on natural resources: summary report* 2013). Thus, there is a need to implement technologies and practices at all levels of the food supply chain, by not only engaging the food producers and suppliers but also the consumers.

Sustainable aquaculture and fisheries need to be taken into consideration as a way to provide not only protein but also micronutrients such as omega-three fatty acids that are critical for cardiovascular health (FAO 2020). Technologies marrying aquaculture and hydroponics can be a sustainable solution for increasing fish farming, while it could help to reduce the toxicity of the effluents from fish farms, reducing the negative environmental effects (Troell et al. 2014).

In addition to commercial agriculture, subsistence farming should also be promoted. The projects integrating agriculture development and forest conservation could be of use (Bauch et al. 2014). The farmers need to be supported politically and economically through improved social protection, awareness raising, and education not only about agriculture but also of self-care practices such as those needed during heat stress, improving access to markets, improved infrastructure such as irrigation and roads, and information communication systems (Weber et al. 2011).

Innovative sources of food and diversification of both food and diets and crops need to be considered. For example, it has been proposed to use insects as an alternative source of human food as well as a food item with lower greenhouse gas emissions during their production (Huis 2013). With regard to agriculture, it is necessary to increase the diversity of types of crops consumed by the human population, which can contribute to increasing the nutritious content of food (Penafiel et al. 2011). In the meantime, the introduction of food crops that could provide the highest nutrient content for the benefit of poor communities as well as using the same to raise the income of communities with a focus on women is needed. Biofortification could be practiced as a solution to address micronutrient deficiencies such as iron, vitamin A, and zinc especially among the poor communities (Nakanishi et al. 1976).

In addition, it is also necessary to promote healthy diets with low environmental impact (De Steur et al. 2015). While there are unresolved problems of malnutrition, the world is also facing problems due to overnutrition. Thus, while some communities of the world will benefit from more nutrients, others may need to restrict nutrient consumption to enhance their health. For example, a country with limited protein sources may benefit from the addition of proteins to the diet, and on the other hand, reduction of red meat consumption could lead to cardiovascular and anti-cancer health benefits (Milner et al. 2015).

It is a known fact that using crops to feed animals for human consumption could contribute to large greenhouse gas emissions (Cassidy et al. 2013). This shift to consuming legumes high in proteins could be a greener solution than eating meat produced after feeding animals with legumes.

25.3.2 Integrated Land Use Planning

Integrated land use planning could be used to optimize the effective use of resources, minimize environmental impacts, and enhance resilience to challenges such as flooding, drought, water scarcity, and heat stress (Angelsen et al. 2009). Some integrated land use planning techniques include zoning, green and disaster resilient building codes, and land use permits. The integrated land use planning demands interventions at all levels, starting off at policy and legislation level to consumer awareness and empowerment in relation to land use. On the other hand, a broad spectrum of stakeholders needs to be engaged in operationalizing such an approach as is common for many areas of action in relation to planetary health.

25.3.3 Female Empowerment

It is essential that women and girls are empowered in relation to all aspects of life including education, economy, and sexual and reproductive health rights (Royal Society (Great Britain) 2012). Empowerment of women and girls in sexual and reproductive health rights in specific and making contraceptives available can help in controlling population growth. This in turn could contribute toward reduction of maternal and child mortality, while improving the quality of life of the families in general (Connell 1987).

25.3.4 Energy

To avoid a hazardous rise in global temperatures, the IPCC (Intergovernmental Panel on Climate Change 2015) has concluded that global emissions must be reduced to zero within the next few decades. Affordable and dependable technologies can help us pass the peak in global emissions and begin the journey to net zero emissions (Jacobson 2002). Rapid emergence of renewable technology such as solar panels, wind turbines, and wave electricity that are at humanity's current disposal, and if deployed swiftly and on a large scale, can bring about the kind of reduction in energy-related emissions that will put the world on track to meet our long-term climate targets. Furthermore, it is essential to be cognizant of alternative energy sources such as biofuel in the context of total environmental effects (O'Neill et al. 2010). The environmental cost benefit of hydropower and nuclear energy needs to be clearly assessed. While trying to address the increase of energy supply, it is equally important to reduce the demand on nonrenewable fuels, as well as increase energy efficiency at all levels, in both industrial and residential levels. The efficient use of technology demands a driver, and thus there is a need for attitudinal change at global, country, community, and individual level toward energy accountability.

25.3.5 Manufacturing of Goods and Services

The planetary health discipline illustrates the deficiencies of the human centric and human-health centric approach humanity has adopted since 1950s, which have contributed toward the planetary health crisis that we are facing today (Kemf and United Nations Environment Programme 2013). It is important that the existing tools used in manufacturing goods and services such as environmental impact assessments, occupational health and safety assessment, disaster risk assessments, and health impact assessments all need to be integrated to broaden the scope of planetary health. Cleaner production technologies could be introduced not only to reduce the carbon footprint but also to address the broader environmental effects that could contribute toward planetary heath crisis (UNEP 2006). Planetary health impacts on goods and services, including greenhouse gas emissions, could be used to assess, audit, and improve manufacturing and service processes.

25.3.6 Sustainable and Resilient Cities

It is important that cities are provided with the guidance and tools to become both sustainable and resilient (De Silva et al. 2005). Introduction of sustainability and resilience to overcrowded and unplanned large cities could be challenging but not impossible. Several best practices in this regard could be learned from the 100 resilient cities initiative by the Rockefeller Foundation (Rockerfeller Foundation 2013). The challenge is to expand such initiatives beyond disaster or climate resilience, which on their behalf are not complete to planetary health resilience. The transdisciplinary research and innovation incorporating the systems thinking approach recommended by the planetary health approach could be used to make the cities more sustainable and resilient.

25.4 Measure Growth, Progress, and Development and Govern Ourselves

For all the aforementioned areas to be successful with regard to planetary health, the key is a paradigm shift in measuring growth, progress, and development and how we govern ourselves as human beings. This is the beauty and challenge of the planetary health approach. The hard science approach has to be backed with social science, philosophy, indigenous knowledge, and spirituality for such a paradigm shift to occur. We need to redefine our goals beyond per capita financial loss or gain to human happiness and planetary loss and gains. This is easier said than done, leading to the heavy demands that planetary health is making on us as a human nation.

1) It demands us to rethink our values and relationship within *nature* and to each other from human exceptionalism, domination, and scarcity to interdependence, equity, and regeneration.
2) It offers the possibility of a greater richness of experience, greater well-being, and an enhanced opportunity for all beings to thrive.
3) It takes the practitioners, scholars, and policy makers from all dimensions of human activity to work together.
4) It requires listening to, integrating, and amplifying the voices of all voices of the community.

The discipline of planetary health is making policy propositions and prescriptions in relation to three areas of concern of health of humans, environment, and the planet as a whole (Table 25.5).

In conclusion, the planetary health approach calls for an urgent relook at the relationship between the human actions, environmental effects, and human health. Human development and global economic capital since 1950 have been able to improve human health to the best possible levels in the history in the contemporary. However, it is important to realize that the action of the humans has shifted the natural balance of the ecosystems such that the negative health, social, and economic consequences of such alterations are imminent or present. The planetary health approach redefines human health as an entity that is not separable from the health of the environment and the health of the planet as a whole. The approach provides policy and operational propositions that the planners, policy makers, researchers, and implementers at global, national, and local level need to adopt in an urgent manner to hold escalating the impacts on the environment and return human health to precatastrophic levels.

Acknowledgement

The support extended by Banura Nadathilake in preparation of the manuscript is acknowledged with thanks.

Table 25.5 Propositions to address conceptual, research, and governance challenges.

Policy focus	Key policy propositions
1) Propositions to address imagination (conceptual) challenges	
Relationship between nature and economy	• Economy and nature are not separate. Keep account of the depreciation of natural capacity and nature's subsidy. • Balance social progress, environmental sustainability, and economy.
Need to support planetary health	• Address poverty that drives environmental health challenges. • Increase the resilience to emerging threats. • Tackle the drivers of environmental change, namely resource use, pollution, and technology.
Urgency of action prior to impending catastrophes	• Facilitate urgent action before irreversible changes to natural systems occur.

Table 25.5 (Continued)

Policy focus	Key policy propositions
Food and agricultural systems	• Strengthen resilient food and agricultural systems. • Reduce waste. • Diversify human diet. • Minimize environmental impacts.
Complementary nature of planetary health approach	• Complement the existing curative, biomedical, and molecular approaches to health. • Address environmental and root causes of ill health.
Health systems	• Develop more resilient health systems. • Integrate health care and environmental care to frontline primary level in addition to universal health coverage. • Integrate environmental health needs to budgeting and purchasing.
2) Propositions to address research and information challenges	
Urgency of need for transdisciplinary research	• Enhance transdisciplinary research activities and capacity substantially in an urgent manner. • Do not delay action in anticipation of research. • Assess technology and knowledge by implementing potential solutions with the aim of rapid scaling up.
Need to fill key evidence gaps	• Define links between health and environmental change. • Improve understanding of potential nonlinear state shifts in the natural systems underpinning human health. • Develop potential adaptation strategies for susceptible populations to environmental change.
Need for integrated surveillance systems	• Build integrated long-term surveillance systems in selected populations to collect rigorous health, socioeconomic, and environmental data to pick signals of emerging infectious diseases, burden of nutrition and non-communicable diseases, and integrated health, environmental, and socioeconomic effects of policies and technologies.
Relationship to Sustainable Development Goals (SGDs)	• Use the SGD monitoring indicators related to planetary health to report national and global progress.
Uncertainty	• Document and acknowledge uncertainty. • Embrace decision-making frameworks that operate under uncertainty to reduce planetary health risks.
Risk communication	• Improve risk communication to policy makers and to the public. • Increase capacity to do systematic reviews and policy briefs in relation to planetary health.
3) Propositions to address governance challenges	
Cross-sectionality	• Target for improved governance across global, national, and subnational levels • Push for a precautionary approach to reduce the risks to health and natural systems where vested interest contribute to disproportionate inequalities over marginalized groups.
Need for creative financing	• Implement creative financing options toward incentivizing a sustainable world economy. E.g. reduction of harmful subsidies, revenue recycling, payment of providers of ecosystem services, and taxation of polluters.
Need for transformative change	• Promote a transformative change using combination of approaches such as regulatory, fiscal, and tax policies; mass media campaigns; and individual behavior change interventions. • Use rigorous research to assess the effectiveness of implemented interventions.
Engagement of private sector	• Provide incentives and evidence-based methods to private sector to adopt higher levels of environmental stewardship and health protection in low- and middle-income countries.

References

Agyeman, J., Devine-Wright, P., and Prange, J. (2009). Close to the edge, down by the river? Joining up managed retreat and place attachment in a climate changed world. *Environment and Planning A: Economy and Space* 41 (3): 509–513. https://doi.org/10.1068/a41301.

Ainsworth, E.A. and Long, S.P. (2005). What have we learned from 15 years of free-air CO_2 enrichment (FACE)? A meta-analytic review of the responses of photosynthesis, canopy properties and plant production to rising CO_2. *New Phytologist* 165 (2): 351–372. https://doi.org/10.1111/j.1469-8137.2004.01224.x.

Albrecht, G., Sartore, G.-M., Connor, L. et al. (2007). Solastalgia: the distress caused by environmental change. *Australasian Psychiatry* 15 (1_suppl): S95–S98. https://doi.org/10.1080/10398560701701288.

Alcott, B. (2005). Jevons' paradox. *Ecological Economics* 54 (1): 9–21. https://doi.org/10.1016/j.ecolecon.2005.03.020.

Al-Kalbani, M.S., Price, M., Abahussain, A. et al. (2014). Vulnerability assessment of environmental and climate change impacts on water resources in Al Jabal Al Akhdar, Sultanate of Oman. *Water* 6 (10): 3118–3135. https://doi.org/10.3390/w6103118.

Angelsen, A., Brockhaus, M., and Center for International Forestry Research (ed.) (2009). *Realising REDD+: National Strategy and Policy Options*. Bogor: Center for International Forestry Research.

Avnery, S., Mauzerall, D.L., Liu, J. et al. (2011). Global crop yield reductions due to surface ozone exposure: 1. Year 2000 crop production losses and economic damage. *Atmospheric Environment* 45 (13): 2284–2296. https://doi.org/10.1016/j.atmosenv.2010.11.045.

Bai, Z.G., Dent, D.L., Olsson, L. et al. (2008). Proxy global assessment of land degradation. *Soil Use and Management* 24 (3): 223–234. https://doi.org/10.1111/j.1475-2743.2008.00169.x.

Barnosky, A.D., Brown, J.H., Daily, G.C. et al. (2014). Introducing the scientific consensus on maintaining humanity's life support systems in the 21st century: information for policy makers. *The Anthropocene Review* 1 (1): 78–109. https://doi.org/10.1177/2053019613516290.

Bauch, S.C., Sills, E.O., and Pattanayak, S.K. (2014). Have we managed to integrate conservation and development? ICDP impacts in the Brazilian Amazon. *World Development* 64: S135–S148. https://doi.org/10.1016/j.worlddev.2014.03.009.

Bennett, E.M., Carpenter, S.R., and Caraco, N.F. (2001). Human impact on erodable phosphorus and eutrophication: a global perspective: increasing accumulation of phosphorus in soil threatens rivers, lakes, and coastal oceans with eutrophication. *BioScience* 51 (3): 227–234. 10.1641/0006-3568(2001)051[0227:HIOEPA]2.0.CO;2.

Bradshaw, C.J.A., Giam, X., and Sodhi, N.S. (2010). Evaluating the relative environmental impact of countries. *PloS one*. Edited by S. Willis 5 (5): e10440. https://doi.org/10.1371/journal.pone.0010440.

Brown, L., Medlock, J., and Murray, V. (2014). Impact of drought on vector-borne diseases – how does one manage the risk? *Public Health* 128 (1): 29–37. https://doi.org/10.1016/j.puhe.2013.09.006.

Campbell-Lendrum, D. and Corvalán, C. (2007). Climate change and developing-country cities: implications for environmental health and equity. *Journal of Urban Health* 84 (1): 109–117. https://doi.org/10.1007/s11524-007-9170-x.

Casassus, B. (2017). Per Fugelli. *The Lancet* 390 (10107): 2032. https://doi.org/10.1016/S0140-6736(17)32737-X.

Cassidy, E.S., West, P.C., Gerber, J.S. et al. (2013). Redefining agricultural yields: from tonnes to people nourished per hectare. *Environmental Research Letters* 8 (3): 034015. https://doi.org/10.1088/1748-9326/8/3/034015.

Chakraborty, S. and Newton, A.C. (2011). Climate change, plant diseases and food security: an overview. *Plant Pathology* 60 (1): 2–14. https://doi.org/10.1111/j.1365-3059.2010.02411.x.

Connell, R. (1987). *Gender and Power: Society, the Person, and Sexual Politics*. Stanford, CA: Stanford University Press.

Crutzen, P.J. (2002). Geology of mankind. *Nature* 415 (6867): 23–23. https://doi.org/10.1038/415023a.

Daughton, C.G. and Ternes, T.A. (1999). Pharmaceuticals and personal care products in the environment: agents of subtle change? *Environmental Health Perspectives* 107 (suppl 6): 907–938. https://doi.org/10.1289/ehp.99107s6907.

Davidson, N.C. (2014). How much wetland has the world lost? Long-term and recent trends in global wetland area. *Marine and Freshwater Research* 65 (10): 934. https://doi.org/10.1071/MF14173.

De Silva, M.J., McKenzie, K., Harpham, T. et al. (2005). Social capital and mental illness: a systematic review. *Journal of Epidemiology and Community Health* 59 (8): 619. https://doi.org/10.1136/jech.2004.029678.

De Steur, H., Blancquaert, D., Strobbe, S. et al. (2015). Status and market potential of transgenic biofortified crops. *Nature Biotechnology* 33 (1): 25–29. https://doi.org/10.1038/nbt.3110.

Diamond, M.L. de Wit, C. A., Molander, S. *et al.* (2015) 'Exploring the planetary boundary for chemical pollution', Environment International, 78, pp. 8–15. doi:https://doi.org/10.1016/j.envint.2015.02.001.

Elbehri, A. and Food and Agriculture Organization of the United Nations (2015). Climate change and food systems: global assessments and implications for food securityandtrade.http://www.fao.org/3/714c5b59-9872-4b40-a971-b28b405349ea/i4332e.pdf (accessed 16 August 2022).

FAO (2013). *Food Wastage Footprint: Impacts on Natural Resources: Summary Report*. Rome: FAO.

FAO (2020). *The State of World Fisheries and Aquaculture 2020: Sustainability in Action*. Rome: FAO https://doi.org/10.4060/ca9229en.

Foley, J.A., DeFries, R., Asner, G.P. et al. (2005). Global consequences of land use. *Science* 309 (5734): 570–574. https://doi.org/10.1126/science.1111772.

Food and Agriculture Organization of the United Nations (ed.) (2003). *Review of World Water Resources by Country*, 23. Rome: Food and Agriculture Organization of the United Nations (Water reports.

Gerland, P., Raftery, A.E., Ševčíková, H. et al. (2014). World population stabilization unlikely this century. *Science* 346 (6206): 234–237. https://doi.org/10.1126/science.1257469.

Gibson, M. (ed.) (2020). Chapter 10 – global food waste. In: *Food and Society*, 223–240. Academic Press https://doi.org/10.1016/B978-0-12-811808-5.00010-6.

Godfray, H.C.J., Blacquière, T., Field, L.M. et al. (2014). A restatement of the natural science evidence base concerning neonicotinoid insecticides and insect pollinators. *Proceedings. Biological Sciences* 281 (1786): 20140558. https://doi.org/10.1098/rspb.2014.0558.

Guynup, S. (2010). *Dirty River*. Scientific American.

Horton in (2014). Planetary-Health-Special-Report the Economist. https://assets.rockefellerfoundation.org/app/uploads/20150625163005/Planetary-Health-Special-Report_06.25.14.pdf (accessed 25 June 2014).

Horton, R. and Lo, S. (2015). Planetary health: a new science for exceptional action. *The Lancet* 386 (10007): 1921–1922. https://doi.org/10.1016/S0140-6736(15)61038-8.

Hsiang, S.M., Burke, M., and Miguel, E. (2013). Quantifying the influence of climate on human conflict. *Science* 341 (6151): 1235367. https://doi.org/10.1126/science.1235367.

van Huis, A. (2013). *Edible Insects: Future Prospects for Food and Feed Security*, 171. Rome: Food and Agriculture Organization of the United Nations (FAO forestry paper.

Huybers, P., McKinnon, K.A., Rhines, A. et al. (2014). U.S. daily temperatures: the meaning of extremes in the context of nonnormality. *Journal of Climate* 27 (19): 7368–7384. https://doi.org/10.1175/JCLI-D-14-00216.1.

IGBP, IOC, SCOR (2013). *Ocean Acidification Summary for Policymakers*. IGBP, IOC, SCOR.

Intergovernmental Panel on Climate Change (2015). *Climate Change 2014: Impacts, Adaptation and Vulnerability, Global and Sectoral Aspects: Working Group II Contribution to the IPCC Fifth Assessment Report*, vol. 1. Cambridge: Cambridge University Press.

IPBES (2019). *Summary for Policymakers of the Global Assessment Report on Biodiversity and Ecosystem Services of the Intergovernmental Science-Policy Platform on Biodiversity and Ecosystem Services* (ed. S. Díaz, J. Settele, E.S. Brondízio, et al.), 56. Bonn, Germany: IPBES Secretariat.

IPCC (2013). *Climate Change 2013*. The Physical Science Basis Working Group.

Jacobson, M.Z. (2002). Control of fossil-fuel particulate black carbon and organic matter, possibly the most effective method of slowing global warming. *Journal of Geophysical Research: Atmospheres* 107 (D19): ACH 16-1–ACH 16-22. https://doi.org/10.1029/2001JD001376.

Johnston, F.H., Henderson, S.B., Chen, Y. et al. (2012). Estimated global mortality attributable to smoke from landscape fires. *Environmental Health Perspectives* 120 (5): 695–701. https://doi.org/10.1289/ehp.1104422.

Kawaguchi, S., Ishida, A., King, R. et al. (2013). 'Risk maps for Antarctic krill under projected Southern Ocean acidification. *Nature Climate Change* 3 (9): 843–847. https://doi.org/10.1038/nclimate1937.

Keesing, F., Belden, L.K., Daszak, P. et al. (2010). Impacts of biodiversity on the emergence and transmission of infectious diseases. *Nature* 468 (7324): 647–652. https://doi.org/10.1038/nature09575.

Kemf, E. and United Nations Environment Programme (2013). GCO – global chemicals outlook: towards sound management of chemicals. http://search.ebscohost.com/login.aspx?direct=true&scope=site&db=nlebk&db=nlabk&AN=993663 (accessed 15 August 2022).

Klein, A.-M., Vaissière, B.E., Cane, J.H. et al. (2007). Importance of pollinators in changing landscapes for world crops. *Proceedings of the Royal Society B: Biological Sciences* 274 (1608): 303–313. https://doi.org/10.1098/rspb.2006.3721.

Koch, A., McBratney, A., Adams, M. et al. (2013). Soil security: solving the global soil crisis. *Global Policy* 4 (4): 434–441. https://doi.org/10.1111/1758-5899.12096.

Lal, R. (2010). Managing soils and ecosystems for mitigating anthropogenic carbon emissions and advancing global food security. *BioScience* 60 (9): 708–721. https://doi.org/10.1525/bio.2010.60.9.8.

Lambin, E.F. and Meyfroidt, P. (2011). Global land use change, economic globalization, and the looming land scarcity. *Proceedings of the National Academy of Sciences* 108 (9): 3465–3472. https://doi.org/10.1073/pnas.1100480108.

Landrigan, P.J. and Etzel, R.A. (ed.) (2014). *Textbook of Children's Environmental Health*. Oxford; New York: Oxford University Press.

Lim, S.S., Vos, T., Flaxman, A.D. et al. (2012). A comparative risk assessment of burden of disease and injury attributable to 67 risk factors and risk factor clusters in 21 regions, 1990–2010: a systematic analysis for the global burden of disease study 2010. *The Lancet* 380 (9859): 2224–2260. https://doi.org/10.1016/S0140-6736(12)61766-8.

Masundire, M.G., Millennium, J., and Baillie, H. (2005). *Millennium Ecosystem Assessment*. Washington, DC: Island Press.

McCauley, D.J., Pinsky, M.L., Palumbi, S.R. et al. (2015). Marine defaunation: animal loss in the global ocean. *Science* 347 (6219): 1255641. https://doi.org/10.1126/science.1255641.

McMichael, A.J. (2014). Population health in the anthropocene: gains, losses and emerging trends. *The Anthropocene Review* 1 (1): 44–56. https://doi.org/10.1177/2053019613514035.

McNeill, J.R. and Engelke, P. (2014). *The Great Acceleration: an Environmental History of the Anthropocene Since 1945*. Cambridge, MA: The Belknap Press of Harvard University Press.

Milner, J., Green, R., Dangour, A.D. et al. (2015). Health effects of adopting low greenhouse gas emission diets in the UK. *BMJ Open* 5 (4): e007364. https://doi.org/10.1136/bmjopen-2014-007364.

Montgomery, D.R. (2007). Soil erosion and agricultural sustainability. *Proceedings of the National Academy of Sciences* 104 (33): 13268–13272. https://doi.org/10.1073/pnas.0611508104.

Mullan, D. (2013). Soil erosion under the impacts of future climate change: assessing the statistical significance of future changes and the potential on-site and off-site problems. *Catena* 109: 234–246. https://doi.org/10.1016/j.catena.2013.03.007.

Myers, S.S. and Patz, J.A. (2009). Emerging threats to human health from global environmental change. *Annual Review of Environment and Resources* 34 (1): 223–252. https://doi.org/10.1146/annurev.environ.033108.102650.

Nakanishi, S., Tanabe, T., Horikawa, S. et al. (1976). Dietary and hormonal regulation of the content of acetyl coenzyme a carboxylase-synthesizing polysomes in rat liver. *Proceedings of the National Academy of Sciences of the United States of America* 73 (7): 2304–2307. https://doi.org/10.1073/pnas.73.7.2304.

OECD (2012). *OECD Environmental Outlook to 2050: The Consequences of Inaction*. OECD (OECD Environmental Outlook) https://doi.org/10.1787/9789264122246-en.

O'Neill, B.C., Dalton, M., Fuchs, R. et al. (2010). Global demographic trends and future carbon emissions. *Proceedings of the National Academy of Sciences* 107 (41): 17521–17526. https://doi.org/10.1073/pnas.1004581107.

Penafiel, D., Lachat, C., Espinel, R. et al. (2011). A systematic review on the contributions of edible plant and animal biodiversity to human diets. *EcoHealth* 8 (3): 381–399. https://doi.org/10.1007/s10393-011-0700-3.

Planetary Health Alliance (2016). *Our Health Depends on Our Environment*. Planetary Health Alliance https://www.planetaryhealthalliance.org/pha-fellowship.

Prüss-Ustün, A., Vickers, C., Haefliger, P. et al. (2011). Knowns and unknowns on burden of disease due to chemicals: a systematic review. *Environmental Health* 10 (1): 9. https://doi.org/10.1186/1476-069X-10-9.

Prüss-Ustün, A. et al. (2014). Burden of disease from inadequate water, sanitation and hygiene in low- and middle-income settings: a retrospective analysis of data from 145 countries. *Tropical Medicine & International Health* 19 (8): 894–905. https://doi.org/10.1111/tmi.12329.

Hannah Ritchie and Max Roser (2017)."Water Use and Stress". OurWorldInData.org. 'https://ourworldindata.org/water-use-stress'.

Roberts, C. (2013). *Ocean of Life: How our Seas are Changing*. London: Penguin.

Rocha, J., Yletyinen, J., Biggs, R. et al. (2015). Marine regime shifts: drivers and impacts on ecosystems services. *Philosophical Transactions of the Royal Society B: Biological Sciences* 370 (1659): 20130273. https://doi.org/10.1098/rstb.2013.0273.

Rockerfeller Foundation (2013). 100-resilient-cities. https://www.rockefellerfoundation.org/100-resilient-cities (accessed 23 July 2022).

Rockström, J., Steffen, W., Noone, K. et al. (2009). A safe operating space for humanity. *Nature* 461 (7263): 472–475. https://doi.org/10.1038/461472a.

Rosegrant, M.W., Ringler, C., and Zhu, T. (2009). Water for agriculture: maintaining food security under growing scarcity. *Annual Review of Environment and Resources* 34 (1): 205–222. https://doi.org/10.1146/annurev.environ.030308.090351.

Max Roser and Hannah Ritchie (2013)."Maternal Mortality". OurWorldInData.org. 'https://ourworldindata.org/maternal-mortality'.

Max Roser, Esteban Ortiz-Ospina and Hannah Ritchie (2013a). "Life Expectancy". OurWorldInData.org. 'https://ourworldindata.org/life-expectancy'

Max Roser, Hannah Ritchie and Bernadeta Dadonaite (2013b). "Child and Infant Mortality". OurWorldInData.org. 'https://ourworldindata.org/child-mortality'

Royal Society (Great Britain) (2012). *People and the Planet*. London: The Royal Society.

Sanchez, P.A. (2002). Soil fertility and hunger in Africa. *Science* 295 (5562): 2019–2020. https://doi.org/10.1126/science.1065256.

Sanford, T., Frumhoff, P.C., Luers, A. et al. (2014). The climate policy narrative for a dangerously warming world.

Nature Climate Change 4 (3): 164–166. https://doi.org/10.1038/nclimate2148.

Savilaakso, S., Garcia, C., Garcia-Ulloa, J. et al. (2014). Systematic review of effects on biodiversity from oil palm production. *Environmental Evidence* 3 (1): 4. https://doi.org/10.1186/2047-2382-3-4.

Sheeshka, J. and Murkin, E. (2002). Nutritional aspects of fish compared with other protein sources. *Comments on Toxicology* 8 (4–6): 375–397. https://doi.org/10.1080/08865140215065.

Sitch, S., Cox, P.M., Collins, W.J. et al. (2007). Indirect radiative forcing of climate change through ozone effects on the land-carbon sink. *Nature* 448 (7155): 791–794. https://doi.org/10.1038/nature06059.

Steffen, W., Richardson, K., Rockström, J. et al. (2015). Planetary boundaries: guiding human development on a changing planet. *Science* 347 (6223): 1259855. https://doi.org/10.1126/science.1259855.

Suweis, S., Rinaldo, A., Maritan, A. et al. (2013). Water-controlled wealth of nations. *Proceedings of the National Academy of Sciences* 110 (11): 4230–4233. https://doi.org/10.1073/pnas.1222452110.

Tilman, D. and Clark, M. (2014). Global diets link environmental sustainability and human health. *Nature* 515 (7528): 518–522. https://doi.org/10.1038/nature13959.

Troell, M., Naylor, R.L., Metian, M. et al. (2014). Does aquaculture add resilience to the global food system? *Proceedings of the National Academy of Sciences* 111 (37): 13257–13263. https://doi.org/10.1073/pnas.1404067111.

UNEP (2006). *Strategic Approach to International Chemicals Management: Comprising the Dubai Declaration on International Chemicals Management, the Overarching Policy Strategy and the Global Plan Action: Resolution Of The International Conference on Chemicals Management.* Nairobi: United Nations Environment Programme.

United Nations (2014). *The Millennium Development Goals Report 2014.* United Nations https://doi.org/10.18356/bb4c0cc6-en.

United Nations Department of Economic and Social Affairs (2013). *World Population Prospects: The 2010 Revision, Volume II – Demographic Profiles.* United Nations https://doi.org/10.18356/02911eeb-en.

Van, B. and Oldeman, L.R. (1998). *Human-Induced Soil Degradation Activities.* International Agrophysics http://www.international-agrophysics.org/Human-induced-soil-degradation-activities,107006,0,2.html.

Watts, N., Adger, W.N., Agnolucci, P. et al. (2015). Health and climate change: policy responses to protect public health. *The Lancet* 386 (10006): 1861–1914. https://doi.org/10.1016/S0140-6736(15)60854-6.

Weber, J.G., Sills, E.O., Bauch, S. et al. (2011). Do ICDPs work? An empirical evaluation of Forest-based microenterprises in the Brazilian Amazon. *Land Economics* 87 (4): 661–681. https://doi.org/10.3368/le.87.4.661.

Whitmee, S., Haines, A., Beyrer, C. et al. (2015). Safeguarding human health in the Anthropocene epoch: report of the Rockefeller Foundation–Lancet Commission on planetary health. *The Lancet* 386 (10007): 1973–2028. https://doi.org/10.1016/S0140-6736(15)60901-1.

World Health Organization and Convention on Biological Diversity (2015). *Connecting Global Priorities: Biodiversity and Human Health: A State of Knowledge Review.* Geneva: World Health Organization https://apps.who.int/iris/handle/10665/174012 (accessed 15 August 2022).

26

SARS-CoV-2 and Other Pathogenic Organisms in Food and Water

Health Implications and Environmental Risk

Bhoirob Gogoi[1], Neehasri Kumar Chowdhury[2], Suprity Shyam[1], Reshma Choudhury[3], Mitali Chetia[4], Tanushree Basumatary[1], and Hemen Sarma[1]

[1] *Bioremediation Technology Research Group, Department of Botany, Bodoland University, Kokrajhar, Assam, India*
[2] *Department of Zoology, Gauhati University, Guwahati, Assam, India*
[3] *Department of Biotechnology, Royal Global University, Guwahati, Assam, India*
[4] *Department of Zoology, Nanda Nath Saikia College, Titabar, Assam, India*

26.1 Introduction

Food is an item that is processed and semiprocessed for human consumption (Akanele et al. 2015). Food is basically defined as a substance composed of carbohydrates, proteins, fats, vitamins, or minerals that boost our energy, health, and growth of the body (Jacobs et al. 2012). Despite its positive role in the body, it can also act as a channel for transmission of diseases leading to fatal consequences if it is infested with pathogenic microbes, harmful chemicals, or other forms of dirt (Akanele et al. 2015). As a part of food security measure and protection of human health, it is important to protect food sources from unwanted pathogens or toxins (Richard Gorham and Zurek 2005). In the meantime, it is also necessary to discriminate between harmful and useful microbes to register for the suitability of food consumption. However, there are multiple ways by means of which contamination can penetrate into the food chain. Apart from the serious health issues, contaminated food infested with hazardous components do have a damaging effect on the economy of a whole nation inflicting losses to food retailers and food companies (Willey et al. 2008). Although many types of microbes are responsible for food contamination leading to foodborne diseases, there are also microbes that work immensely well for the benefit of humankind. According to Council of Agricultural Science and Technology (CAST), there are more than 40 kinds of pathogens that are known to contaminate food and cause illness. Plant-based foods also pose a concern in terms of disease spread due to contamination (Foegeding et al. 1994). According to the World Health Organization (WHO), at least 1 out of 10 people fall sick each year from contaminated food resulting in around 420,000 deaths (Pascal 2012). Toxic chemicals, pathogens, and other forms of parasites may get into our food products at various stages of food preparation and processing (Allos et al. 2004). Irrigation water has been identified as a potential source of product contamination (Faour-Klingbeil et al. 2016) notwithstanding the fact that irrigation serves as one of the best supplements in areas of limited rainfall (Kirby et al. 2003). It has been pointed out during epidemiological studies of food poisoning and other experimental studies on pathogen contamination of fruits and vegetables that usage of wastewater for irrigation with little or no proper discharge system serves as an important source of germs found in food products. Inappropriate disposal of wastewater containing fecal matter or other pathogenic microbes into larger water bodies is also another source of germ transmission by means of getting into the system of drinking water (Cabral 2010).

In March 2020, the WHO announced that the outbreak of COVID-19 could be identified as an epidemic. Transmission from person to person is suspected as the primary cause of the spread of the SARS-CoV-2 virus. However, other possible modes of transmission through contaminated food or water is also being considered. SARS-CoV-2 belongs to the group Betacoronavirus, a type of virus already known medically as a common infective agent for both synanthropic and parasitic animals. Since the recent classification of the causal agent of COVID-19, several molecular studies have been conducted worldwide with the aim of determining the origin of the virus and the possible transmission pathways (Andersen et al. 2020). Phylogenetic analysis of the full-length genome sequence

One Health: Human, Animal, and Environment Triad, First Edition. Edited by Meththika Vithanage and Majeti Narasimha Vara Prasad.

from clinical classification has shown that SARS-CoV-2 is very similar to acute respiratory syndrome coronavirus (SARS-CoV) and may be using the same cell receptor, enzyme-2 converting angiotensin for the onset of the infection process (Leung et al. 2020). SARS-CoV-2 is identified to spread mainly through human to human contact or through respiratory droplets released when an infected person coughs or sneezes. Since droplets are usually airborne and fall below a few meters, the chances of transmission are reduced if a person stays at least 2 m apart (CDS 2021). In the meantime, ways of handling or use of contaminated food and water may contribute significantly to the spread of the virus (Coronavirus Disease [COVID-19]).

Our society has undergone major changes in terms of foodborne and waterborne diseases, especially over the past 20 years (Table 26.1). Certain diseases caused by food and water go unnoticed but the impact it can have on human health and the economy cannot be underestimated. In the past two decades, there has been an alarming increase in the appearance of a number of viruses called "germ infections" (Egli et al. 2002). In this case, one must keep in mind that the word "appearance" is used to denote that these viruses appear to be increasing in number in certain regions or in living organisms that have been neglected or difficult to identify. It also includes the species in which the role of food and water as transmission vehicles has recently been recognized. The extent of "emerging" virus appropriately through food and diet is different from that of water source. In case of diet, the members of the bacterium group seem to play a significant role in transmission (Egli et al. 2002). The primary objective of this review is to investigate the present state of research on SARS-CoV-2 and other pathogenic organisms, identify their routes of transmission while focusing on food and water as potential mediums, understanding the eradication strategies, and extracting the advantages and disadvantages of the various processes suggested.

26.2 SARS-CoV-2 and Other Pathogens in Food and Drinking Water

Foodborne and waterborne diseases caused by pathogens is a big threat to public health all over the world. Foodborne diseases can cause mild sickness, but they are also linked to acute gastrointestinal symptoms like diarrhea and vomiting (Blackburn and Mcclure 2002). Many foodborne pathogens are zoonoses, which means that they have non-human animal hosts that do not always make people sick. Most of the time, it is hard to figure out how many people have been sickened by foodborne pathogens because of the different reporting systems in different countries all over the world (Table 26.2). In the 1994 outbreak of foodborne diseases in Taiwan, 74% of it was caused by bacterial pathogens. *Vibrio parahaemolyticus, Staphylococcus aureus, Bacillus cereus*, and *Salmonellas* were the main pathogens found (Pan et al. 1996). There was a study done about diarrhea in South Eastern China between 1986 and 1987. The results showed that there were 730 cases of diarrhea per 1000 people in general (Kangchuan et al. 1991). Enterotoxigenic *Escherichia coli*, enteropathogenic *E. coli*, enteroinvasive *E. coli*, *Shigella* species, *Campylobacter jejuni*, and *Vibrio species* were most commonly isolated. These organisms along with *Entamoeba histolytica* are considered to be the main causes of diarrhea in developing countries (DuPont 1995). Other identified pathogens causing foodborne diseases especially in the United States are Norwalk-like viruses, *Campylobacters, Salmonellas, Clostridium perfringens, Giardia lamblia, Staphylococci, E. coli*, and *Toxoplasma gondii*. These pathogens are responsible for causing about 76 million illnesses, 325,000 hospitalizations, and approximately 5000 deaths each year (Mead et al. 1999).

The majority of waterborne infections, on the other hand, are constantly arising as a result of population increase, developmental activities, and expansion of commerce besides unchecked supply of contaminated food (Table 26.3). Again feces of humans and animals that are directly deposited into water bodies do contribute to the cause of various waterborne diseases (Arnone and Walling 2007). Although there exists ways of dealing with it, major evolution is noticed in the process of detection and tracking of pathogens, treatment of drinking water and in the direction of food supply procedures for the effective eradication of the disease causing pathogens transmitted through water (Nwachcuku and Gerba 2004).

The novel coronavirus infects humans throughout the world via different transmission routes. Among which the foodborne and waterborne routes are considered predominant modes of transmission causing morbidity and mortality (Bosch et al. 2016). According to recent report, viruses are not capable of toxin propagation in food that suggests that food acts as a mere route of virus transmission only (Petrović and D'Agostino 2016). Earlier, there was no evidence of the spread of COVID-19 through food sources (Han et al. 2020). This was a high held belief even by various organizations like the WHO (Mandal et al. 2020), the Centers for Disease Control and Prevention (CDC 2020), Food and Drug Administration (US Food and Drug Administration 2020) of the United States, and other regional regulatory bodies. But the detection of SARS-CoV-2 on frozen foods, packaging substances, and storage environments that were associated with the two

Table 26.1 Potential foods and waterborne organisms and their features.

Origin of foodborne/waterborne pathogen	Scientific name	Foodstuff contaminated	Mode of transmission	Carriers/host	Diseases caused	Incubation period	Clinical symptoms	Diagnosis	References
Foodborne pathogens of animal origin	*Salmonella* species	Red meat, eggs, fruits, vegetables, nuts, butter, chicken nuggets, and frozen pot pies	Contaminated food and contaminated water	Chicken, swine, turkeys, and cows	Septicemia, gastroenteritis and enteric fever	6–48 h	Fever, abdominal cramps, diarrhea, and typhoid fever	Widal test, ELISA (enzyme-linked immunosorbent assay), and RT-PCR (Reverse transcription polymerase chain reaction)	Gia (1996)
	Campylobacter species	Raw red meat, raw milk, food, and vegetables	Fecal and oral route	Poultry, cattle, swine, and sheep	Diarrhea	2–5 d	Fever, headache, diarrhea, and anorexia	RT-PCR, stool culture, EIA (enzyme immunoassay), and MALDI-TOF MS (matrix assisted laser desorption ionization-time of flight mass spectrometry)	Facciolà et al. (2017), Sibanda et al. (2018)
	Listeria monocytogenes	Cheese, raw milk, vegetables, fruits, meat, fish, and ice cream	Fecal and oral route	Animal	Self-limited febrile diarrhea	1–70 d	Fever, general malaise, and myalgia	PCR, immunological test, NASBA (nucleic acid sequence-based amplification), and LAMP (loop-mediated isothermal amplification)	Batt (2014)
	E. coli	Fruits, raw milk, raw flour, lettuce, beef, and cookie dough	Contaminated food and person to person	Cattle	Diarrhea	24–72 h	Malaise, vomiting, abdominal pain, and nausea	MUG (4-methylumbelliferyl-β-D glucuronide) testing, and toxin testing	Evans and Evans (1996)
	Clostridium perfringens	Raw meat and poultry, raw and processed food	Fecal and oral routes	Humans and domestic animals	Diarrhea	6–24 h	Abdominal pain, dehydration, and decrease in blood pressure	ELISA, RPLA (reversed passive latex agglutination), and SLAT (simultaneous laryngoscopy and abdominal thrusts)	Robertson et al. (2014)

(Continued)

Table 26.1 (Continued)

Origin of foodborne/ waterborne pathogen	Scientific name	Foodstuff contaminated	Mode of transmission	Carriers/host	Diseases caused	Incubation period	Clinical symptoms	Diagnosis	References
Foodborne illness related to seafood/ fish	*Vibrovalnificus*	Oyster, crab meat, and crawfish and fish	Consumption of contaminated seafood, and contaminated water, indirect contact with wound	Oyster and fish	Septicemia	12–72 h	Fever, diarrhea, headache, vomiting, and abdominal cramping	PCR, qPCR (quantitative polymerase chain reaction), RPA (recombinase polymerase amplification), labeled DNA probe, ELISA, and fatty acid profile	Oliver (2005)
	Vibrio parachaemolyticus	Shrimp, crab, shellfish, oyster, lobster, and fish	Ingestion, and direct contact of contaminated food	Fish and mussels	Gastrointestinal illness	4–96 h	Nausea, fever, vomiting, and abdominal cramping	Kanagawa test, PCR, and immunological detection	Rezny and Evans (2021)
	Shigella sp.	Potato salads, fish, oyster, ground beef, and raw vegetable	Fecal oral route, and direct contact with contaminated food		Shigellosis	1–7 d	Dysentery, mucus secretion, high fever, bloody stool, dehydration, and severe abdominal cramps	LA (Lupus anticoagulant testing), EIA, IMS (Infection Manager System), and PCR	Warren et al. (2006)
	Clostridium botulinum	Canned food and fish	Ingestion of contaminated food	Fish and mammals	Botulism intoxication	12–48 h	Double vision, slurred speech, difficulty in breathing, swallowing, and movement of the eye, vomiting, and diarrhea	Muse lethality assay, radioimmunoassays, ELISA, and PCR	Tiwari and Nagalli (2021)
	Staphylococcus aureus	Meat products, seafood, salads, milk, and milk products	Direct contact with contaminated food, and respiratory droplet	Human	Gastrointestinal illness	2–4 h	Pneumonia, meningitis, diarrhea phlebitis, nausea, vomiting, and hypotension	Catalase test, RT-PCR, and antimicrobial assay	Gillaspy et al. (2019)

Foodborne diseases: fruits and vegetables	*Aeromonas hydrophilia*	Fish, vegetable, meat, and their product, milk, and their products, and seafood	Fecal oral transmission	Human	Gastroenteritis and bacteremia	1–2 d	Fever, diarrhea, vomiting, and abdominal pain	Gene sequencing, fatty acid profiles, and PCR-positive oxidase test	Fernández-Bravo and Figueras (2020)
	Corynebacterium diptheriae	Fruits, vegetable, milk, meat, and seafood	Inhalation of aerosol and consumption of contaminated food	Human	Diptheria	2–5 d	Fever, weakness, sore throat, and malaise	Elek immunodiffusion test, and rabbit skin test	Murphy (1996)
Waterborne bacteria and virus	*Legionella*	Drinking water	Inhalation of contaminated aerosol		Legionellosis	2–14 d	Fever, muscle pain, cough, headache, and shortness of breath	Indirect immunofluorescence	Nazarian et al. (2014)
	Vibrio cholerae	Vegetable, meat, fruits, seafood, and crustaceans	Consumption of contaminated food and water	Copepods, chironomids	Gastroenteritis and cholera	6–48 h	Diarrhea, nausea, dehydration, muscle cramps, and vomiting	qPCR, RT-PCR, microarray, and ELISA	Albert et al. (1997), Finkelstein (1996)
	Adenovirus	Vegetable and fruits	Fecal oral route	Vertebrate	Gastroenteritis	2–14 d	Fever, common cold, sore throat, acute bronchitis, and pneumonia	qPCR and plaque assay	O'Shea et al. (2019)
	Rotaviruses	Drinking water and mussels	Fecal oral route	Human	Gastroenteritis	<48 h	Nausea, vomiting, fever, cramping, and diarrhea	qPCR, ELISA, complement fixation, and immunofluorescence	Kapikian and Shope (1996)
	Sapoviruses	Shellfish	Water, environment, direct contact, and food	Human and pigs	Gastroenteritis	Abdominal pain, headache, nausea, and malaise	1–4 days	ELISA, and PCR	Oka et al. (2015)

Table 26.2 Foodborne pathogens.

Pathogens		**Source**	**Disease**	**Symptoms/effects**
Bacteria	*Bacillus cereus*	Meat products, vegetables, and milk products	Diarrhea and emetic	Nausea, vomiting, and abdominal pain
	Campylobacter jejuni	Healthy domestic, and wild animals	Gastroenteritis and diarrhea	Nausea and vomiting
	Clostridium botulinum	Soils, freshwater, marine sediments, and intestinal tracts of animals	Botulism	Nausea, vomiting, visual impairment, and acute flaccid paralysis
	Escherichia coli	Feces of infected humans or animals	Diarrhea and hemolytic uremic syndrome (HUS)	Nausea, vomiting, abdominal pain, and profuse bleeding that can lead to kidney failure, and death
	Yersinia enterocolitica	Raw milk, sewage-contaminated water, soil, seafood, humans, and many warm-blooded animals	Intestinal yersiniosis	Watery, sometimes bloody stools or bloody diarrhea in conjunction with fever, vomiting, and abdominal pain
Virus	Hepatovirus	Shellfish	Hepatitis A	—
	Norovirus	Bivalve mollusks	Acute viral gastroenteritis	—
Parasite	*Cyclospora cayetanensis*	Small intestine of human	Prolonged illness (6 weeks or longer)	Non-bloody diarrhea, nausea, vomiting, anorexia, bloating, abdominal cramping, malaise, fever, and fatigue
	Toxoplasma gondii	Body tissues and tissue cysts	Toxoplasmosis	Fever, rash, headache, muscle aches, pain, and swelling of the lymph nodes
	Trichinella spiralis	Host of small intestine	Human trichinosis infections	Nonspecific gastroenteritis, nausea, vomiting, headaches, fever, visual deficiencies, difficulty in breathing, chills, night sweating, eosinophilia-myalgia, and circumorbital edema

Source: Adapted from Bintsis and Bintsis (2017).

re-emergent outbreaks of virus in China in early July 2020 pointed to the evidence of food as a possible carrier of the virus (Han et al. 2020). The detection of SARS-CoV-2 on the surface of frozen chicken from Shenzhen in Guangdong province and Brazil on 12 August 2020 confirmed the transmission of the coronavirus through food sources (Shenzhen Municipal Health Commission 2020). The process of bringing food from farm to table goes through a cycle of cold chain that involves conservation of food under refrigerated condition (Han et al. 2020). Contamination of cold chain acts as a vehicle for the transmission of coronavirus from one country to another as import of foodstuff is an important economic activity (Godoy et al. 2021). Incidents of COVID-19 spread have been found to occur during handling of food products by food workers infected with the SARS-CoV-2 virus. CDC identified 16,233 cases of COVID-19 in 23 states during April–May 2020 followed by 23 deaths among the food workers, working at 239 meat and poultry processing facilities (Waltenburg 2020). The same thing was also seen among field workers in the seafood industry with 117 crew members being positive for COVID-19 in the American seafood company (KUCB 2021). Temperature plays a crucial role in every step of cold chain (Figure 26.1). Frozen foods kept at low temperatures for cold transportation seem to provide a favorable condition for the survival of SARS-CoV-2 (Han et al. 2020). However, this virus is found to be very stable at 4 °C in comparison to its exposure at higher temperatures of 21 °C and above (Chin et al. 2020). Its viability has been shown to last up to 24–48 hours on disk surfaces.

Transmission may occur through various food sources like aquatic animals (Godoy et al. 2021), meat, vegetables,

Table 26.3 Waterborne pathogens.

Pathogens		Source	Disease	Symptoms/Effects
Bacteria	*Campylobacter*	Domestic and wild animal feces	Campylobacteriosis	Diarrhea
	Legionella pneumophilia	Aquatic environments	Legionellosis	Acute respiratory illness
	Leptospira interrogans	Urine of dogs, livestock, rodents, and wild animals	Leptospirosis (Weil's disease)	Jaundice and fever
	Salmonella typhi	Domestic and wild animal feces	Typhoid fever	High fever, diarrhea, and ulceration of small intestine
	Vibrio cholerae	Sediments, shellfish, and asymptomatic human carriers	Cholera	Extremely heavy diarrhea
Virus	Adenovirus	Humans	Respiratory disease and gastroenteritis	Acute respiratory disease, pneumonia, conjunctivitis, and gastroenteritis
	Astroviruses	Humans	Gastroenteritis	Vomiting and diarrhea
	Hepatitis E2	Humans and pigs	Infectious hepatitis	Jaundice and fever
	Rotavirus	Humans	Gastroenteritis	Vomiting and diarrhea
Protozoan	*Cryptosporidium*	Human, animal, and bird feces	Cryptosporidiosis	Diarrhea and death in susceptible populations
	Cyclospora	Human feces	Cyclosporiasis	Diarrhea
	Entamoeba histolytica	Human feces	Amoebiasis (amoebic dysentery)	Prolonged diarrhea with bleeding, abscesses of the liver, and small intestine
	Giardia lamblia	Human, animal, and bird feces	Giardiasis	Mild to severe diarrhea, nausea, and indigestion
	Naegleria fowleri	Bird, and aquatic mammal feces	Primary amoebic meningoencephalitis (PAM)	Inflammation of brain and meninges

Source: Adapted from Arnone and Walling (2007).

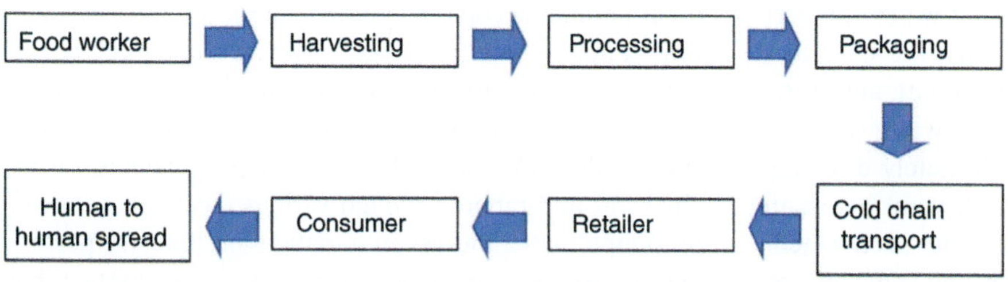

Figure 26.1 Survival of the SARS-CoV-2 during the entire sequence of events in the cold chain transportation and transmission of virus to its destination host.

fruits, dairy products, or bread (Yekta et al. 2021). The risk of exposure to SARS-CoV-2 through aquatic animals like fish, amphibians, mollusks, and crustaceans is quite low or negligible as they are cold-blooded animals and have a different ACE 2 cell receptor due to which the virus losses its ability to replicate in such animals. In a recent study, it has been revealed that vertebrate classes of animals excepting mammals cannot serve as host for SARS-CoV-2 (Damas et al. 2020). Therefore, it can be concluded that aquatic animals can only act as carriers of SARS-CoV-2 in case they are handled by infected workers (Bondad-Reantaso et al. 2020). Other meat and meat products are feasible for viral transmission. Therefore, it is necessary to subject them to heat treatment at >60 °C for at least 30 minutes before consumption (Yekta et al. 2021). Infection of rabbit and pig cells under in vitro condition has been detected (Chin et al. 2020). Dairy products like milk, yogurt, or ice cream can also act as a medium for virus transmission mainly from handlers. Thus, it becomes essential to take precautionary measures by the personnel at the processing level. Some industrial heat treatment precautions are already available for the viral unload, viz., high temperature short time (HTST), ultra-high temperature (UHT) at 71 °C for 15 seconds and at 130–150 °C for 3–5 seconds, respectively (Sarkar 2020). Commercial heat treatment plays a significant role for the fact that it does not decrease the nutritive value of foodstuff in comparison to the conventional domestic procedure of sterilization that is more likely to reduce its nutritive value (Yekta et al. 2021). Heat treatment of yogurt before fermentation stages at 90 °C for at least 15 minutes has shown to deactivate or kill SARS-CoV-2 (Yekta et al. 2021). Several vegetables and fruits are often seen to be contaminated by sewage during irrigation (Rusiñol et al. 2020). Mere disinfection under sunlight with ultraviolet A (UVA) spectrum (320–400 nm) is not enough to kill SARS-CoV-2 (Seyer and Sanlidag 2020). However, foodstuff with peel like bananas, oranges, or potatoes can restrict the spread by simply peeling or washing with water. But the commodities that cannot be peeled such as leafy vegetables and berries can go through enough household washing practices with appropriate disinfectants like chlorine solution, chlorine dioxide, and sodium hypochlorite (Quevedo-León et al. 2020). On the other hand, water sources may get contaminated by various ways. The main sources include saliva, sputum, vomit, urine samples, and feces (Giacobbo et al. 2021) that are discharged from several places like hospital sewage, waste from isolation plants, quarantine centers, contaminated surface, and other contaminated sewage (Sunkari et al. 2021). According to Water Framework Directive (WFD), the human use of water resources is connected with several water compartments that consist of all services right from the starting of abstraction, impoundment, storage, treatment, and distribution of surface water or groundwater to wastewater collection and treatment facilities that ultimately discharge into surface water (Langone et al. 2021). Several factors are responsible for the survival of virus in water such as temperature, sunlight, organic compounds, and some antagonistic microorganisms that enhance the virus survival. There exists only a little evidence of SARS-CoV-2 survival in freshwater. It becomes necessary to prevent these water resources from coming into contact with fecal matter that has high probability of SARS-CoV-2 infestation. Studies have confirmed the survivability and pathogenicity of the virus for 11 days in gastrointestinal tract of patients even after the samples from respiratory tract have tested negative. It has been confirmed that the virus remains active for up to 2–6 hr in adult feces and up to 48 hr in children's feces. This may act as a vehicle for outbreak of COVID-19 if it remains unobserved (Mahlknecht et al. 2021). 105–108, 106–1011 and 104–1014 copies/l were detected in urine, feces, and saliva or sputum, respectively, by various researchers, which are enough for an individual to shed billions of SARS-CoV-2 RNA fragments in wastewater at once. All this wastewater or sewage ultimately reaches a wastewater treatment plant (WWTP) for purification of water through sewage pipes (Haramoto et al. 2020). The untreated water may penetrate into the soil and act as a reservoir of SARS-CoV-2 for aerosol dispersion into the environment as a secondary element (Wiktorczyk-Kapischke et al. 2021). The 15 soil samples (20%) collected close to the WWTP and hospital areas were tested positive for COVID-19 with RNA copies ranging from 205 to 550 (Zhang et al. 2021). However, survival of the virus and its transmission has not been reported so far from soil samples (Table 26.4).

26.3 Food as a Non-Droplet Spreading Route of Pathogen

The novel coronavirus has zoonotic origin and spreads to healthy organisms through interspecies contact, sustained transmission, and cross-species viral transmission (Duda-Chodak et al. 2020). The virus supposedly enters the human body from fecal matter through oral route caused by inhalation of SARS-CoV-2 particles or ingestion of the virus along with infected food that includes milk, milk products, meat, bread, fruits, vegetables, and other junk food (Yekta et al. 2021). Bats are reported to be the primary natural reservoir of SARS-CoV-2. The aerosol from bats containing SARS-CoV-2 may directly get into humans and other animals. People may also acquire the viral particles from intermediate host like pigs, chickens, and horses through direct contact or by consuming their byproducts such as meat or milk (Fan et al. 2019). Some researchers suggest that SARS-CoV-2 can infect pigs, camels, civets, chickens, and rabbits through various means that involve presymptomatic and asymptomatic food industry personnel, shopkeepers, and consumers (Yekta et al. 2021). It has been observed in many Asian markets that selling of live animals takes place along with other foodstuffs like fresh vegetables, fruits, and other animal products. Live animals are kept in cramped cages and are killed to sell their flesh to customers. During such times, the virus if present has maximum chance to be transmitted to healthy individuals or plant sources. On the other hand, when infected bats and other potential intermediate hosts at the market place expel their excretory products, there are maximum chances for other consumable commodities getting contaminated through direct fall on them or through aerosol and thus become source of SARS-CoV-2 spread (Duda-Chodak et al. 2020).

Table 26.4 SARS-CoV-2 RNA concentrations in drinking water, wastewater, primary sludge, and secondary sludge across the world.

Continents	Sample locations	Sample type	Sample storage/ treatment before analysis	Genetic traces/ genes analyzed	Concentration (GC/ml)	Sample collection date	Main findings	References
Asia	Ahmedabad, Gujarat (India)	4 composite samples	4 °C; 19 d for first sampling campaign, <24 h	ORF1ab, N and S	<0.35	8–27 May 2020	2 out of 2 influent samples positive; 2 out of 2 effluent samples negative	Kumar et al. (2020)
	Lahore (Pakistan)	Untreated WW	Ice cooled/4 °C < 24 h	ORF1ab, N	0.267–36	13–25 July 2020	22 out of 28 positive	Yaqub et al. (2020)
	Israel	32 24-hours composite samples of raw WW	−80 °C or −20 °C	E	NA	10 March–21 April 2020	3 out of 6 WW samples in Tel Aviv positive; 2 out of 15 positive in different cities in March 2020; 8 out of 11 positive in different cities in April 2020	Bar-Or et al. (2020)
	Yamanashi prefecture (Japan)	Raw and treated WW	Ice; <6 h	N1 and N2	240 (1 treated WW sample)	17 March–7 May 2020	None of 5 raw samples positive; 1 out of 5 secondary treated samples positive; none out of 3 river water samples positive	Haramoto et al. (2020)
North America	Bozeman, Montana (USA)	Raw WW from 1 WWTP	NA	N1 and N2	ND to 5600	30 March–12 June 2020	13 out of 17 positive (1 out of 1 positive in March; 7 out of 7 positive in April; 0 out of 4 positive in May; 5 out of 5 positive in June)	Nemudryi et al. (2020)
	Monterrey (Mexico)	Groundwater from 3 aquifer units, 3 rivers, and 3 dams, raw WW from 1 WWTP	4 °C/<48 h (5 min at 5 °C)	N1 and N2	Groundwater <38.3; river water <7.0; dam water <3.8; raw WW < 3600	29 October–6 January 2021	22 out of 50 groundwater samples positive; 3 out of 24 river water samples positive, 2 out of 16 dam water samples positive, 3 out of 8 raw WW samples positive	Mahlknecht et al. (2021)

(Continued)

Table 26.4 (Continued)

Continents	Sample locations	Sample type	Sample storage/ treatment before analysis	Genetic traces/ genes analyzed	Concentration (GC/ml)	Sample collection date	Main findings	References
South America	Quito (Ecuador)	River water	4 °C; <6 h	N1 and N2	284–3190 (N1)	5 June 2020	3 out of 3 river water samples positive	Guerrero-Latorre et al. (2020)
Europe	Paris (France)	27 grab samples	4 °C; <24 h	RdRp	50 (5 March)–3000 (23 April)	5 March–23 April 2020	All samples found positive	Wurtzer et al. (2020)
	Netherlands	30 24-hours composite samples	Melting ice; <24 h	N1, N2, N3, and E	5–7 February: n.d.; 4/5 March: 2.6–30 GC/ml; 14–16 March: 8–2200 GC/ml; 25	5 February–25 March 2020	All negative on 5–7 February; 3 out of 7 WW samples positive on March 4/5; all samples positive in the middle of March	Medema et al. (2020)
	Murcia (Spain)	42 raw, 18 secondary, and 12 tertiary treated WW samples	4 °C; <24 h	N1, N2, and N3	ND to 5000 in raw WW	12 March–14 April 2020	35 out of 42 influent samples positive; 2 out of 18 secondary samples positive; none of 12 tertiary treated samples positive	Randazzo et al. (2020)
Australia	Southeastern Queensland	9 composite samples	−80 °C; <24 h	N and confirmation via Sanger and MiSeq Illumina sequencing	ND, 0.019 and 0.12	20 March–1 April 2020	2 out of 9 samples positive in raw WW	Ahmed et al. (2020)

Recent research has revealed that frozen food acts as a long-distance transmitting agent of SARS-CoV-2. It is established that consuming food served on contaminated surface, packing of food in contaminated room, or touching and sharing of food with an infected person may enhance the chance of spreading the virus. However, WHO and CDS (Clinical Decision Support) report shows lack of any evidence with regard to the spread of SARS-CoV-2 through food.

The COVID-19 illness of 2019 is a clinical condition brought about by extreme intense respiratory disorder caused by SARS-CoV-2. The spread of COVID-19 has been attributed to the adherence of the virus on contact surface, though endurance on foodstuff is yet to be completely deciphered. The likelihood of endurance and transmission of SARS-CoV-2 through food source and bundles is being examined based on information available for other respiratory infections like SARS-CoV and MERS-CoV (Yekta et al. 2021). The execution of food handling procedures of Hazard Analysis and Critical Control Points (HACCP) and Good Manufacturing Practices (GMP) is imperative to diminish the danger of COVID-19 disease.

The SARS-CoV-2 seems to be influenced by various parameters like water movement, pH, protein, fat, sugar, and minerals. Study shows that the COVID-19 virus is steady in a wide range of pH from 3 to 10, which is suggestive that the virus is steady in practically all food items. Avian flu virus was seen to be inactivated at low pH range from 3.80 to 4.70, which points toward the effectiveness of lower pH in combating virus elements. It was seen that the COVID-19 virus remains steady at 4 °C. With diminished pH, the unfavorable impacts of higher temperatures on the infection would be more articulated. Moreover, an immediate relationship between food protein content and viral solidness against warm treatment was additionally noticed. Rabenau et al. (2005a) observed that heat treatment of SARS-CoV-2 with and without protein showed decrease in viral titer.

The quick food varieties can prompt ongoing enactment of the inborn resistant framework and a restraint of the versatile safe framework. Momentarily, exorbitant SFA (seminal fluid analysis) utilization may incite a lipotoxic condition and evade the toll-like receptor 4 (TLR-4) expressed on macrophages, dendritic cells, and neutrophils. The actuation of these organic energizers produces proinflammatory effects on the natural safe framework. It was observed that use of high-fat diet (HFD) in rodents caused macrophage invasion to lung tissues, explicitly in the alveoli. HFD was also seen to build flu-like infection in mice causing cardiovascular damages (Goli 2020).

26.4 Water is a Carrier of SARS-CoV-2 With Other Pathogens

There are no evidences as yet to prove that the COVID-19 virus remains viable in drinking water and wastewater. Since there are close similarities in the morphology and chemical nature of the COVID-19 virus with the pre-existing corona viruses affecting human beings, presumably, their survival strategy and response to deactivation measures could be somewhat similar. Though persistence of the virus in drinking water is strongly suspected, experimental studies on surrogate human coronaviruses propose otherwise (Organization 2014). Therefore, the risk of the viral contraction from drinking water seems remote. However, studies reveal that water contaminated with fecal matter may serve as a haven for the virus wherein wastewater remedy workers have been found to catch the virus. Traces of SARS-CoV-2 coronavirus have been reported from WWTP-derived sludge, municipal wastewater, and wastewater from business passenger aircraft, river water, and non-portable water (Haramoto et al. 2020). Infection from such sources points toward the viability of the virus in such contaminated water sources. Apart from treating wastewater sewage systems with well-designed and properly managed centralized wastewater treatment procedures, it is also important to measure the viral load including the rate at which bacteria is infected in the wild. While the presence of infectious virus in wild samples has been demonstrated, there is still a lack of data at the cellular level (La Rosa et al. 2020). The virus is stated to be temperature dependent that prompts it to be viable longer in contaminated water during winter months as the sewage temperature would be lower. In such cases the history of sewage and the age of sewage need to be fully understood. Refugee camps or small towns located near water source with poor sanitation facilities could add to the woe of the spread of the virus through contaminated water buildup. Again, when it comes to UV ray efficacy on inactivation of SARS-CoV-2, it depends mostly on the nature of the surface to which the virus is attached (Derraik et al. 2020).

Whenever solid feces enter the sewage system, viral load is expected to be reduced through the purification process and environmental factors like temperature or pH in addition to the presence of degrading bacteria like *E. coli*, *Bacillus*, or *Clostridium*. Also, certain chemicals released into the sewage system from cleaners and disinfectants are found to contribute to the same (Carraturo et al. 2020). However, viruses and other microscopic pathogens may make their way into the source of drinking water through seepage from the sewage system inflicting waterborne diseases onto the consumers. Besides, it has been observed that natural streams are polluted by pathogenic bacteria present in fecal deposits that pose serious concern.

26.5 Eradication Methods of Pathogen for Safety and Sustainability

Eradication is the elimination of all members of a species from a geographical area that is sufficiently isolated in order to prevent reinvasion (Myers et al. 2003). This process involves various physical and chemical disinfection methods. In the present scenario, as there is no particular curative approach against the virus, prevention seems the key to avoid contraction of the disease that can be accomplished through available physical, chemical (Noorimotlagh et al. 2020), or mechanical approaches (Wiktorczyk-Kapischke et al. 2021). This operation will either help eliminate the virus or reduce the potential of pandemic infections. The key advantages of the eradication strategy are that if the disease is completely eradicated, additional control efforts may be abandoned, resulting in cost savings, unfavorable vaccine responses, and so on (Boslaugh 2012).

26.5.1 Chemical Disinfectant

Chemical disinfection is a multistep process that uses particular chemicals to eliminate hazardous germs from food products and their touch surfaces (Rai et al. 2020). Disinfectants are available in a variety of forms, each with its own set of activities, efficiency, and methods of action. Bacteriostatic disinfectants inhibit the growth of bacterial populations, whereas bactericidal disinfectants destroy bacterial cells by causing structural damage, autolysis, cell lysis, and cytoplasm leaking or coagulation (Sandle 2019). Some of the most commonly used chemical disinfectants are chlorine, iodophors, quaternary ammonium compounds, carboxylic acids, alcohol, and peroxy compounds among others (Kakurinov 2014). Alcohols (ethanol-70%), povidone-iodine (7.5%), chloroxylenol (0.05%), chlorhexidine (0.05%), and benzalkonium chloride (0.1%) are sprayed to surfaces (104 TCID50/ml) to deactivate SARS-COV-2. Chemical disinfectants such as iodine, per acetic acid, quaternary ammonia, and sodium hypochlorite are efficient against foodborne pathogens such as *S. aureus, Listeria monocytogenes*, and *E. coli* (Cabeça et al. 2012). Benzalkonium chloride (BZK), sodium hypochlorite (10% active chlorine; SYH), and per acetic acid (39% solution of per acetic acid in acetic acid; PAA) are excellent disinfectants against *Cronobacter sakazakii* and *Yersinia enterocolitica* (Capita et al. 2019).

26.5.2 Physical Disinfectant

Physical disinfection is a method of reducing microbial loads by disrupting normal microbial function or causing structural damage to them through the use of physical treatments such as UV light, high pressure, high-intensity ultrasound, ionizing radiation, pulsed light, high hydrostatic pressure, and cold plasma (Deng et al. 2019; Nguyen-Viet and Pham-Duc 2019). A 30-minute dry steam or heat treatment has shown to be sufficient to destroy viruses and other infectious organisms. Bacteria and protozoans such as *E. coli, S. aureus, L. monocytogenes, Salmonella* spp., *C. sakazakii, Cryptosporidium*, and *Giardia* are observed to be more susceptible to UV while most viruses and some bacterial spores are more resistant (Deng et al. 2019). Use of UV radiation is highly encouraged since spectrum UVC between 207 and 222 nm was successful in destroying H1N1 virus. Destruction of SARS-CoV-2 on clothing surfaces was also practiced with only a few minutes of UV irradiation (Cervino et al. 2020). Gamma radiation is seen to be effective in combating the SARS-CoV-2 infection. It acts by the dislocation of electrons, covalent bonds breakage, or release of free radicals causing harm to the viral particle (Ghernaout et al. 2020). Use of porous membranes having microfiltration capacity >50 nm and ultrafiltration capacity of 2–50 nm has proved to be effective against some pathogenic protozoan cysts and bacteria. However, these have shown low efficacy against viruses (Wiktorczyk-Kapischke et al. 2021).

26.6 Disadvantage of Chemical Remediation of Foodborne Pathogen

The primary function of a disinfectant is to diminish the surface population of pathogenic germs (Table 26.5). However, use of chemical disinfectants in foodstuffs especially the phenolics or metal-ion-based compounds is highly discouraged as these are associated with a number of disadvantages (Blackburn and Mcclure 2002). The following are some of the disadvantages of commonly used chemicals (Marriott and Williams 2018)

- Chlorine dioxide is very expensive, difficult to handle, has safety and toxicity issues, and is light as well as temperature sensitive.
- Chlorines become unstable when exposed to heat or organic materials. The effectiveness of the product is reduced with the rise in pH.
- Iodine vaporizes at around 50 °C (122 °F) and becomes less effective than chlorine against bacterial spores

Table 26.5 Various disinfection agents and their efficiencies against coronavirus.

Virus	Viral strain	Disinfectant	Concentration (%)	Exposure time	Reduction of viral infectivity (log10)	References
HCoV	Strain 229E (ATCC VR-740)	Sodium hypochlorite	0.5	10 min	≥4.50	Tyan et al. (2018)
	ATCC VR-759 (strain OC43)	Benzalkonium chloride	0.2	10 min	0.0	Wood and Payne (1998)
	Strain 229E	Ethanol	70	60 s	>3.0	Sattar et al. (1989)
		Benzalkonium chloride	0.04		<3.0	
		Sodium hypochlorite	0.1		>3.0	
		Sodium hypochlorite	0.01		<3.0	
		Glutaraldehyde	2		>3.0	
CCoV	Strain S378	Benzalkonium chloride	0.00175	3 d	3.0	Pratelli (2007)
		DDA	0.0025	3 d	>4.0	Pratelli (2007)
		Formaldehyde	0.009	24 h	>4.0	Pratelli (2008)
MHV	MHV1 and MHV-N	Ethanol	70	10 min	>3.9	Noorimotlagh et al. (2021)
		Benzalkonium chloride	0.05		>3.7	
		Formaldehyde	0.7		>3.5	
		2-Propanol	50		>3.7	
		Chlorhexidine digluconate	0.02		0.7–0.8	
		Sodium hypochlorite	0.01		2.3–2.8	
		Sodium hypochlorite	0.001		0.3–0.6	
	Strain MHV-1	Household bleach: sodium hypochlorite	0.21	30 s	≥4.40	Dellanno et al. (2009)
	Strain A59	The multiple-emitter, automated, continuous, whole-room UVC disinfection system		5 min	2.71	Bedell et al. (2016)
MERS-CoV	Strain EMC	Alcohol-based hand rubs (ethanol)	80	30 s	>4.0	Siddharta et al. (2017)
		Alcohol-based hand rubs (2-propanol)	75		≥4.0	
	MERS-CoV/Hu/Taif/SA/2015	Disinfection of virus in human plasma by amotosalen and ultraviolet A	—	—	>4.67	Hindawi et al. (2018)
	Hu/France–FRA2_130,569/2013 (FRA2)	Heat treatment at – Temperature 25 °C		2 h	0	Leclercq et al. (2014)
		Temperature 56 °C		25 min	4.0	
		Temperature 65 °C		1 min	4.0	
	Isolate HCoV-EMC/2012	PVP-I	75	15 s	4.6	Eggers et al. (2015)
			4.0		5.0	
			1.0		4.3	
			0.23		≥4.4	

(*Continued*)

Table 26.5 (Continued)

Virus	Viral strain	Disinfectant	Concentration (%)	Exposure time	Reduction of viral infectivity (log10)	References
SARS-CoV-1	Isolate FFM-1	Sterillium rub (ethanol)	80	30 s	≥4.25	Rabenau et al. (2005b)
		Sterillium gel (ethanol)	85		≥5.5	
		Sterillium virugard (ethanol)	95		≥5.5	
		Sterillium (iso-propanol, *n*-propanol)	45, 30		≥4.25	
		2-Propanol	100 and 70		≥3.31	
		Desderman *N* (ethanol, 2-biphenylol)	78, 0.2		≥5.01	
		Sterillium (2-propanol, 1-propanol)	45, 30		≥2.78	
		Formaldehyde	0.7 and 1.0	120 s	≥3.01	
		Glutaraldehyde	0.5		≥4.01	
		Incidin plus	2		≥1.68	
		Glucoprotamin	26		≥1.68	
		Temperature (4 °C)		30 min	0	
		Temperature (56 °C)			≥5.01	
		Temperature (60 °C)			≥5.01	
	Hanoi strain	Glutaraldehyde	2.5	5 min	>4.0	Kariwa et al. (2006)
		PVP-I	1	1 min	>4.0	
			0.47		3.8	
			0.25		>4.0	
			0.23		>4.0	
SARS-CoV-2		Plasma-activated water	—	10 min	69.7%	Xiling et al. (2021)
		Hydrogen peroxide	0.5	15 min	>99.9%	Mileto et al. (2021)
		Ethanol	75	0.30 min	>99.9%	Xiling et al. (2021)
		2-Propanol	75	0.30 min	50%	
		Di-*N*-decyl dimethyl ammonium bromide	0.02	0.5 min	>99.9%	Xiling et al. (2021)
		Di-*N*-decyl dimethyl ammonium chloride	0.02	0.5 min	>99.9%	

CCoV, canine coronavirus; DDA, didecyl-dimethyl-ammonium chloride; HCoV, human coronavirus; MERS-CoV, Middle East respiratory syndrome-coronavirus; MHV, mouse hepatitis virus; PVP-I, povidone-iodine; SARS-CoV, severe acute respiratory syndrome-coronavirus.

and bacteriophages. Iodine performs poorly at low temperature. It is sensitive. It discolors porous and plastic surfaces.

- Quaternary ammonium compounds are less effective against bacteriophage, and they develop a film on food handling and processing equipment.
- Dilute phosphoric acid is used as a disinfectant. But use in hand sanitizers can lead to skin irritations. It is also corrosive to some metals, such as mild and galvanized steel, which increases with rise in temperature.

26.6.1 Chlorine as Disinfectant to Remove SARS-CoV-2 and its Impact on Ecosystem (Chemical Remediation)

Chlorine solutions are oxidative in nature showing broad spectrum activity against a variety of microorganisms. It has also shown to be effective in eradicating human coronavirus that is almost similar to SARS-CoV-2 (Dev Kumar et al. 2020). Chlorine has the highest cost-effective advantage and can be used in multiple health units (de Andrade and de Bessa Pereira 2020). SARS-CoV-2 is an enveloped virus with a lipid membrane surrounding a capsule made up of protein and glycoprotein, and chlorine acts by interrupting and destroying the internal proteins while entering through the lipid membrane making the virus inactivate (Ye et al. 2016). According to WHO, chlorine compounds lead to denaturation of protein, inactivation of nucleic acids, and inhibition of enzyme activity. Therefore, it is highly recommended to use chlorine as a disinfectant for the control of viral infections such as COVID-19. WHO recommends cleaning of the environment following correct protocol for the eradication of the viral population. Such cleaning can be done commonly with disinfectants like water and detergent or NaClO. 5% hypochlorite in a 1 : 100 dilution (García-Ávila et al. 2020). In hospital wastewater, residual chlorine of 6 mg/l is used as a disinfectant while WHO suggests a concentration of 5 mg/l for tap water (Wang et al. 2020). A concentration of 0.5–1% of chlorine is found to be suitable for cleaning clothes contaminated with patient's secretions (blood, vomit, and others) by dipping it for at least 30 mins in the disinfectant solution. Patients' transporting vehicles can also be sanitized with the same concentration (de Andrade and de Bessa Pereira 2020). Cotton balls immersed in chlorine solution of 0.3–0.5% are used in plugging the mouth, ears, nostrils, and other open channels of cadavers infected by coronavirus (Fung and Liu 2019). 5000 mg/l or 0.5% solution of chlorine helps in disinfection of household objects and surfaces such as light switches, keys, tables, chairs, phones, and others (Fung and Liu 2019). Bathrooms and latrines can also be treated with chlorine disinfectant of strength 40 mg/l or 0.004% maintaining an exposure time of 1.5 hour making sure that residual chlorine reaches a level of concentration of 10 mg/l (Shereen et al. 2020). While chlorine is stated to be a potential disinfectant, it has been cited to have lots of disadvantages. Whenever chlorine reacts with the natural organic matters (coming from plant material and soil) of the water, generation of byproducts takes place (Li et al. 2019). In urban drinking water treatment plants, chlorine reacts with organic matters and produces small molecules as byproducts whose daily consumption may lead to cancer or reproductive issues (Bond et al. 2012). Respiratory problems may occur in workers who deal with chlorine-related works as chlorine causes an annoying and irritating effect on the mucous membrane (Zambrano-Monserrate et al. 2020). Disinfection byproducts (DBP) and halogenated organic compounds are also produced after reaction of chlorine with organic matter present in water that prove toxic to aquatic animals (García-Ávila et al. 2020). Chlorine released into the environment also causes depletion of ozone layer, further resulting in increase of global warming (Andersen et al. 2013; Brenna et al. 2019).

26.7 Biological Remediation and its Advantage

Biological methods are cost-effective, environmentally acceptable, and can be produced on a big scale for industrial applications, allowing them to make progress in the pathogen treatment process. The use of microbes or their enzymes in food preservation is a novel method in the field of science. For example, the fermentation process reduces food spoilage by keeping food free of dangerous microbes and metabolites (Singh 2018). The use of plant extracts for pathogen eradication (particularly fungus) is regarded as a favorable option since it contains more than one antifungal ingredients, resulting in lesser pathogen resistance development if the multiple compounds influence separate metabolic processes (Shuping and Eloff 2017).

26.7.1 The Application of Biosurfactant as Antiviral Agent Against COVID-19

The molecules with both hydrophobic and hydrophilic properties (amphipathic) that act between liquid and biphasic systems such as liquid/gas, liquid/liquid, and solid/liquid and help in the reduction of surface and interfacial tension occurring between them are called surfactants. There are two types of surfactants according to their origin: chemical surfactants and biosurfactants (BS) (Sarma and Prasad 2021). Biosurfactants are biomolecules that are mainly produced from several microorganisms (bacteria, yeasts, and fungi) and plants (Saikia et al. 2021). Figure 26.2 explains the mechanistic understanding of BS-assisted destruction of SARS-CoV-2 cell. The main advantage of using BS is that it is biodegradable and ecofriendly as compared with chemical surfactant. Also, it has unique characteristics like specificity, low toxicity, and smooth preparation for which it has now achieved great attention in commercial applications and in various other areas (Smith et al. 2020). The physiochemical reactions performed by BS are helpful in inactivating enveloped viruses. The acetyl group promotes the hydrophilic nature of the BS, which enhances its antiviral activity.

Antiviral activity is mainly based on the number of carbon atoms in the hydrophobic part. BS with 15 carbon atoms of fatty acid chain, a negative charge, and monomethyl esters show high inactivation of viruses in general and more specifically in Semliki forest virus. The same could be applicable in SARS-CoV-2, as it is an enveloped virus. When SARS-CoV-2 enters into the host cell, BS interacts with the cell membrane and enters the plasma membrane that results in the disintegration of viral envelope and capsid protein in the presence of high concentration of BS. Finally, the lipid envelope and spike protein are

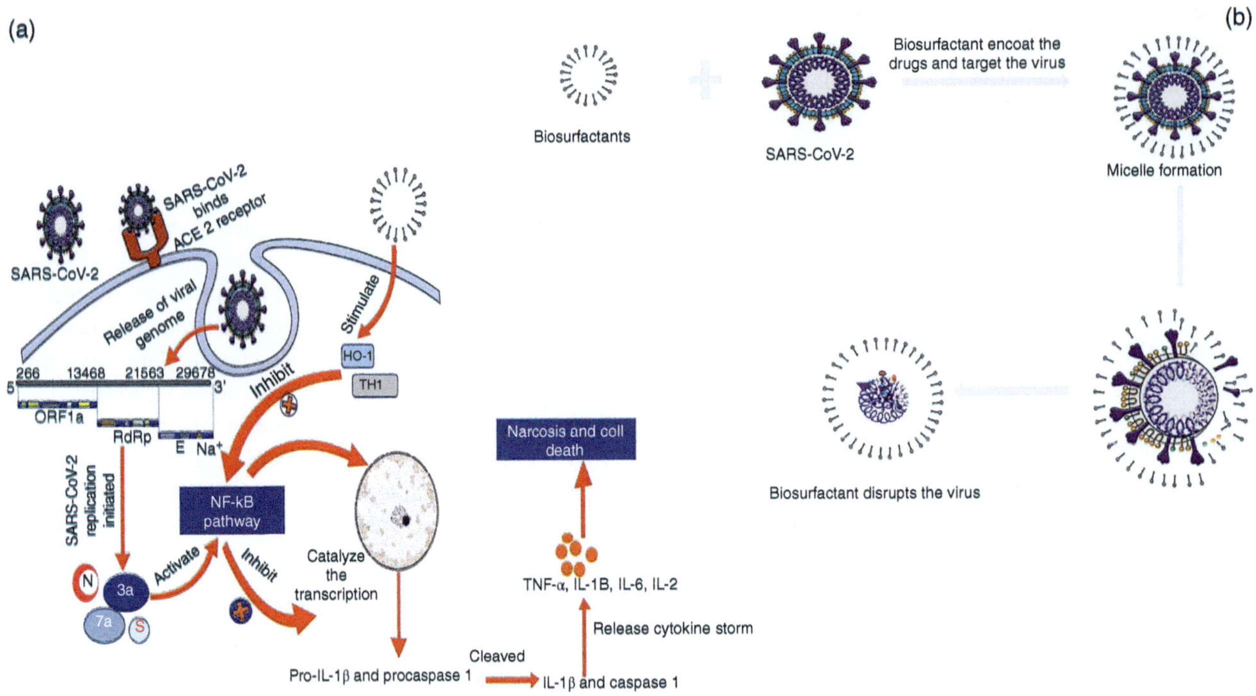

Figure 26.2 SARS-CoV-2 binds to the ACE 2 receptor of the human host cell, and the virus releases its genome into the cytoplasmic matrix, where it begins replication and eventually produces viral proteins (N, 3a, 7a, and S) that activate the NF-B pathway and catalyze the transcription of pro-IL-1 and procaspase 1. Cell necrosis occurs as a result of cytoplasmic storm. When infected cells were given biosurfactant in addition to medicines, it stimulated heme-oxidase 1 and TH1 macrophages, which blocked the NF-kB pathway and, as a result, turned off the release of cytoplasmic storm (a). The biosurfactant segregated around the virus and formed a micelle inside the host cell's cytoplasm, progressively disintegrating the viral lipid membrane and spike protein. Finally, the entire virus was destroyed (b).

enclosed into micelles and cause the virus to disintegrate (Subramaniam et al. 2020).

Drug delivery to the infection site can be treated with the micelle formation as it can act as liposome. Use of BS-based handwashes and hand sanitizers renders maximum protection shield against SARS-CoV-2. Moreover, its use is recommended in household cleaning products such as detergents or soaps as BS is ecofriendly and tends to be less harmful to the environment (Subramaniam et al. 2020). Rhamnolipids, sophorolipids, and surfactin are some of the most studied microbial BS of which surfactin is used as antiviral agents for the enveloped and nonenveloped viruses such as SARS-CoV-2, porcine epidemic diarrhea, herpes simplex virus, transmissible gastroenteritis virus, and Semliki forest virus (Vollenbroich et al. 1997; Yuan et al. 2018). Rhamnolipids and surfactins are mostly available in lip gloss formulations for being biodegradable and soothing BSs. Saikosaponin is a plant-based BS that prevents early phase of infection, viral attachment, and penetration in H-CoV-22E9 coronavirus (Lin et al. 2014). The gel obtained from *Aloe vera* plant contains aloin and aloe-emodin molecules that act against some enveloped viruses like SARS-CoV-1, influenza, and HIV viruses by disintegrating the lipid envelope or preventing replication (Mpiana et al. 2020), making it an attractive choice as a non-alcoholic sanitizer. Resveratrol (triterpenoid) obtained from grape seeds and skin is responsible for prevention of entry and inhibition of replication in SARS-CoV and MERS-CoV (Lin et al. 2017).

26.8 Conclusion

Navigating the COVID-19 circumstances needs considering diet aspects, strict follow-up of COVID-19 appropriate behavior, and effective handling of post-COVID-19 recuperation. The regularity of one's eating habits is crucial for sustaining good health. It needs to be composed of whole grain, unsaturated fats, and gut microbes' booster that actually helps in enhancing immunity buildup. Cleanliness regime needs to be followed at personal level and especially while handling food items at various stages, which we finally ingest. Cooking temperature and timing also play a very significant role. Cooking food items at or above 60 °C for not less than 30 minutes is suggestive. While these are precautionary measures to prevent from SARS-CoV infestation, still further investigation is needed to determine its authentic transmission route in order to combat this dreadful disease.

Acknowledgments

The authors would like to thank the Bodoland University, Kokrajhar (BTR), and all collaborating institutes for their logistical support.

Conflict of Interest

The authors declare that they have no known competing financial interests or personal relationships that could have appeared to influence the work reported in this paper.

Funding

This research did not receive any specific grant from funding agencies in the public, commercial, or not-for-profit sectors.

Credit Author Statement

BG: first draft, data compilation; NKC: assist in the preparation of the first draft, data compilation, SS and TB: assist in the preparation of the first draft, data compilation; RC: preparation of the first draft; MC: editing, proofreading; HS: prepare design, concept, final draft, all figures, and graphical abstract of the software as well as visualization.

References

Ahmed, W., Angel, N., Edson, J. et al. (2020). First confirmed detection of SARS-CoV-2 in untreated wastewater in Australia: a proof of concept for the wastewater surveillance of COVID-19 in the community. *Sci. Total Environ.* 728: 138764. https://doi.org/10.1016/J.SCITOTENV.2020.138764.

Akanele, E., Mgbo Otu Chukwu, S., and Mary Ahudie, C. (2015). Microbiological contamination of food the mechanisms impacts and prevention. *Int. J. Sci. Technol. Res.* 4: 65–78.

Albert, M.J., Neira, M., and Motarjemi, Y. (1997). The role of food in the epidemiology of cholera. *World Heal. Stat. Q.* 50 (1/2): 111–118.

Allos, B.M., Moore, M.R., Griffin, P.M., and Tauxe, R.V. (2004). Surveillance for sporadic foodborne disease in the 21st century: the FoodNet perspective. *Clin. Infect. Dis.* https://doi.org/10.1086/381577.

Andersen, S.O., Halberstadt, M.L., and Borgford-Parnell, N. (2013). Stratospheric ozone, global warming, and the principle of unintended consequences – an ongoing science and policy success story. *J. Air Waste Manage. Assoc.* 63: 607–647. https://doi.org/10.1080/10962247.2013.791349.

Andersen, K.G., Rambaut, A., Lipkin, W.I. et al. (2020). The proximal origin of SARS-CoV-2. *Nat. Med.* 264 (26): 450–452. https://doi.org/10.1038/s41591-020-0820-9.

de Andrade, F.P. and de Bessa Pereira, C. (2020). Use of chlorine solutions as disinfectant agents in health units to contain the spread of COVID-19. *J. Heal. Biol. Sci.* 8: 1–9. https://doi.org/10.12662/2317-3076jhbs.v8i1.3256.p1-9.2020.

Arnone, R.D. and Walling, J.P. (2007). Waterborne pathogens in urban watersheds. *J. Water Health* 5: 149–162. https://doi.org/10.2166/wh.2006.001.

Bar-Or, I., Yaniv, K., Shagan, M. et al. (2020). Regressing SARS-CoV-2 sewage measurements onto COVID-19 burden in the population: a proof-of-concept for quantitative environmental surveillance. *medRxiv* https://doi.org/10.1101/2020.04.26.20073569.

Batt, C.A. (2014). Listeria: Listeria monocytogenes. In: *Encyclopedia of Food Microbiology*, 2e, 490–493. Elsevier Inc. https://doi.org/10.1016/B978-0-12-384730-0.00191-9.

Bedell, K., Buchaklian, A.H., and Perlman, S. (2016). Efficacy of an automated multiple emitter whole-room ultraviolet-C disinfection system against coronaviruses MHV and MERS-CoV. *Infect. Control Hosp. Epidemiol.* 37: 598–599. https://doi.org/10.1017/ice.2015.348.

Bintsis, T. and Bintsis, T. (2017). Foodborne pathogens. *AIMS Microbiol.* 3529 (3): 529–563. https://doi.org/10.3934/MICROBIOL.2017.3.529.

Blackburn, C.D.W. and Mcclure, P.J. (2002). *Foodborne Pathogens Hazards, Risk Analysis and Control.* Woodhead Publishing Limited.

Bond, T., Goslan, E.H., Parsons, S.A., and Jefferson, B. (2012). A critical review of trihalomethane and haloacetic acid formation from natural organic matter surrogates. *Environmental Technology Reviews* https://doi.org/10.1080/09593330.2012.705895 1: 93–113.

Bondad-Reantaso, M.G., Mackinnon, B., Bin, H. et al. (2020). Viewpoint: Sars-cov-2 (the cause of covid-19 in humans) is not known to infect aquatic food animals nor contaminate their products. *Asian Fish. Sci.* 33: 74–78. https://doi.org/10.33997/j.afs.2020.33.1.009.

Bosch, A., Pintó, R.M., and Guix, S. (2016). Foodborne viruses. *Curr. Opin. Food Sci.* 8: 110–119. https://doi.org/10.1016/J.COFS.2016.04.002.

Boslaugh, S. (2012). Disease eradication. In: *Encyclopedia of Epidemiology* (ed. S. Boslaugh). https://doi.org/10.4135/9781412953948.n115.

Brenna, H., Kutterolf, S., and Krüger, K. (2019). Global ozone depletion and increase of UV radiation caused by pre-industrial tropical volcanic eruptions. *Sci. Rep.* 91 (9): 1–14. https://doi.org/10.1038/s41598-019-45630-0.

Cabeça, T.K., Pizzolitto, A.C., and Pizzolitto, E.L. (2012). Activity of disinfectants against foodborne pathogens in suspension and adhered to stainless steel surfaces. *Braz. J. Microbiol.* 43: 3. https://doi.org/10.1590/S1517-838220120003000038.

Cabral, J.P.S. (2010). Water microbiology. bacterial pathogens and water. *Int. J. Environ. Res. Public Health* 7: 3657. https://doi.org/10.3390/IJERPH7103657.

Capita, R., Vicente-Velasco, M., Rodríguez-Melcón, C. et al. (2019). Effect of low doses of biocides on the antimicrobial resistance and the biofilms of *Cronobacter sakazakii* and *Yersinia enterocolitica*. *Sci. Rep.* 9: https://doi.org/10.1038/s41598-019-51907-1.

Carraturo, F., Del Giudice, C., Morelli, M. et al. (2020). Persistence of SARS-CoV-2 in the environment and COVID-19 transmission risk from environmental matrices and surfaces. *Environ. Pollut.* 265: https://doi.org/10.1016/J.ENVPOL.2020.115010.

CDC (2020). Food and Coronavirus disease 2019 (COVID-19). CDC [WWW Document]. Centers Dis. Control Prev. https://www.cdc.gov/coronavirus/2019-ncov/daily-life-coping/food-and-COVID-19.html (accessed 25 October 2021).

CDS (2021). CDS Interim guidelines [WWW Document]. https://www.cdc.gov/csels/dls/locs/2020/updated_interim_pui_guidelines_for_covid-19.html (accessed 14 July 2021).

Cervino, G., Fiorillo, L., Surace, G. et al. (2020). SARS-CoV-2 persistence: data summary up to Q2 2020. *Database* 5: 81. https://doi.org/10.3390/DATA5030081.

Chin, A.W.H., Chu, J.T.S., Perera, M.R.A. et al. (2020). Stability of SARS-CoV-2 in different environmental conditions. *The Lancet Microbe* 1: e10. https://doi.org/10.1016/S2666-5247(20)30003-3.

Damas, J., Hughes, G.M., Keough, K.C. et al. (2020). Broad host range of SARS-CoV-2 predicted by comparative and structural analysis of ACE2 in vertebrates. *Proc. Natl. Acad. Sci.* 117: 22311–22322. https://doi.org/10.1073/PNAS.2010146117.

Dellanno, C., Vega, Q., and Boesenberg, D. (2009). The antiviral action of common household disinfectants and antiseptics against murine hepatitis virus, a potential surrogate for SARS coronavirus. *Am. J. Infect. Control* 37: 649–652. https://doi.org/10.1016/j.ajic.2009.03.012.

Deng, L.Z., Mujumdar, A.S., Pan, Z. et al. (2019). Emerging chemical and physical disinfection technologies of fruits and vegetables: a comprehensive review. *Crit. Rev. Food Sci. Nutr.* 60: 2481–2508. https://doi.org/10.1080/10408398.2019.1649633.

Derraik, J.G.B., Anderson, W.A., Connelly, E.A., and Anderson, Y.C. (2020). Rapid evidence summary on SARS-CoV-2 survivorship and disinfection, and a reusable PPE protocol using a double-hit process. *medRxiv* https://doi.org/10.1101/2020.04.02.20051409.

Dev Kumar, G., Mishra, A., Dunn, L. et al. (2020). Biocides and novel antimicrobial agents for the mitigation of coronaviruses. *Front. Microbiol.* https://doi.org/10.3389/fmicb.2020.01351.

Duda-Chodak, A., Lukasiewicz, M., Zięć, G. et al. (2020). Covid-19 pandemic and food: present knowledge, risks, consumers fears and safety. *Trends Food Sci. Technol.* 105: 145–160. https://doi.org/10.1016/J.TIFS.2020.08.020.

DuPont, H.L. (1995). Diarrheal diseases in the developing world. *Infect. Dis. Clin. N. Am.* 9: 313–324.

Eggers, M., Eickmann, M., and Zorn, J. (2015). Rapid and effective Virucidal activity of povidone-iodine products against Middle East Respiratory Syndrome Coronavirus (MERS-CoV) and modified vaccinia virus Ankara (MVA). *Infect. Dis. Ther.* 4: 491–501. https://doi.org/10.1007/s40121-015-0091-9.

Egli, T., Köster, W., and Meile, L. (2002). Pathogenic microbes in water and food: changes and challenges. *FEMS Microbiol. Rev.* 26: 111–112. https://doi.org/10.1111/J.1574-6976.2002.TB00603.X.

Evans, D.J. and Evans, D.G. (1996). *Escherichia Coli in Diarrheal Disease, Medical Microbiology*. University of Texas Medical Branch at Galveston.

Facciolà, A., Riso, R., Avventuroso, E. et al. (2017). Campylobacter: from microbiology to prevention. *J. Prev. Med. Hyg.* https://doi.org/10.15167/2421-4248/jpmh2017.58.2.672.

Fan, Y., Zhao, K., Shi, Z.L., and Zhou, P. (2019). Bat coronaviruses in China. *Viruses* https://doi.org/10.3390/v11030210.

Faour-Klingbeil, D., Murtada, M., Kuri, V., and Todd, E. (2016). Understanding the routes of contamination of ready-to-eat vegetables in the Middle East. *Food Control.* 62: 125–133. https://doi.org/10.1016/J.FOODCONT.2015.10.024.

Fernández-Bravo, A. and Figueras, M.J. (2020). An update on the genus *Aeromonas*: taxonomy, epidemiology, and pathogenicity. *Microorganisms* https://doi.org/10.3390/microorganisms8010129.

Finkelstein, R.A. (1996). *Cholera, Vibrio cholerae O1 and O139, and Other Pathogenic Vibrios, Medical Microbiology*. University of Texas Medical Branch at Galveston.

Foegeding, P.M., Roberts, T., Bennett, J.M. et al. (1994). *Foodborne Pathogens: Risks and Consequences*. Elsevier.

Fung, T.S. and Liu, D.X. (2019). Human coronavirus: Host-pathogen interaction. *Annu. Rev. Microbiol.* https://doi.org/10.1146/annurev-micro-020518-115759.

García-Ávila, F., Valdiviezo-Gonzales, L., Cadme-Galabay, M. et al. (2020). Considerations on water quality and the use of chlorine in times of SARS-CoV-2 (COVID-19) pandemic in the community. *Case Stud. Chem. Environ. Eng.* 2: 100049. https://doi.org/10.1016/J.CSCEE.2020.100049.

Ghernaout, D., Elboughdiri, N., Ghernaout, D., and Elboughdiri, N. (2020). Disinfecting water: plasma discharge for removing coronaviruses. *Open Access Libr. J.* 7: 1–29. https://doi.org/10.4236/OALIB.1106314.

Giacobbo, A., Rodrigues, M.A.S., Zoppas Ferreira, J. et al. (2021). A critical review on SARS-CoV-2 infectivity in water and wastewater. What do we know? *Sci. Total Environ.* 774: 145721. https://doi.org/10.1016/J.SCITOTENV.2021.145721.

Giannella, R.A., 1996. Samuel Baron Medical Microbiology. 4 Chapter 21 *Salmonella*. University of Texas Medical Branch at Galveston.

Gillaspy, A.F., Iandolo, J.J., Tang, Y.W., Stratton, C.W., 2019. *Staphylococcus*, in: Thomas M.Schmidth Encyclopedia of Microbiology. Elsevier, pp. 309–320. https://doi.org/10.1016/B978-0-12-801238-3.02304-7

Godoy, M.G., Kibenge, M.J.T., and Kibenge, F.S.B. (2021). SARS-CoV-2 transmission via aquatic food animal species or their products: a review. *Aquaculture* 536: 736460. https://doi.org/10.1016/J.AQUACULTURE.2021.736460.

Goli, M. (2020). Review of novel human β-coronavirus (2019-nCoV or SARS-CoV-2) from the food industry perspective – appropriate approaches to food production technology. *Food Sci. Nutr.* https://doi.org/10.1002/fsn3.1892.

Guerrero-Latorre, L., Ballesteros, I., Villacrés-Granda, I. et al. (2020). SARS-CoV-2 in river water: implications in low sanitation countries. *Sci. Total Environ.* 743: 140832. https://doi.org/10.1016/J.SCITOTENV.2020.140832.

Han, J., Zhang, X., He, S., and Jia, P. (2020). Can the coronavirus disease be transmitted from food? A review of evidence, risks, policies and knowledge gaps. *Environ. Chem. Lett.* 191 (19): 5–16. https://doi.org/10.1007/S10311-020-01101-X.

Haramoto, E., Malla, B., Thakali, O., and Kitajima, M. (2020). First environmental surveillance for the presence of SARS-CoV-2 RNA in wastewater and river water in Japan. *Sci. Total Environ.* 737: 140405. https://doi.org/10.1016/J.SCITOTENV.2020.140405.

Hindawi, S.I., Hashem, A.M., Damanhouri, G.A. et al. (2018). Inactivation of Middle East respiratory syndrome-coronavirus in human plasma using amotosalen and ultraviolet A light. *Transfusion* 58: 52–59. https://doi.org/10.1111/trf.14422.

Jacobs, D.R., Mursu, J., and Meyer, K.A. (2012). The importance of food. *Arch. Pediatr. Adolesc. Med.* https://doi.org/10.1001/archpediatrics.2011.184.

Kakurinov, V. (2014). Food safety assurance systems: cleaning and disinfection. *Encycl. Food Saf.* 4: 211–225. https://doi.org/10.1016/B978-0-12-378612-8.00356-5.

Kangchuan, C., Chenshui, L., Gingxin, Q. et al. (1991). The epidemiology of diarrhoeal diseases in Southeastern China. *J. Diarrhoeal Diseases Res.* 9 (2): 94–99.

Kapikian, A.Z. and Shope, R.E. (1996). Rotaviruses, Reoviruses, Coltiviruses, and Orbiviruses. In: *Medical Microbiology* (ed. S. Baron).

Kariwa, H., Fujii, N., and Takashima, I. (2006). Inactivation of SARS coronavirus by means of povidone-iodine, physical conditions and chemical reagents. *Dermatology* 212: 119–123. https://doi.org/10.1159/000089211.

Kirby, R.M., Bartram, J., and Carr, R. (2003). Water in food production and processing: quantity and quality concerns. *Food Control* 14: 283–299. https://doi.org/10.1016/S0956-7135(02)00090-7.

KUCB (2021). *Crew of American Seafoods Vessel Tests Negative for COVID-19 in Unalaska*. KUCB.

Kumar, M., Patel, A.K., Shah, A.V. et al. (2020). First proof of the capability of wastewater surveillance for COVID-19 in India through detection of genetic material of SARS-CoV-2. *Sci. Total Environ.* 746: https://doi.org/10.1016/j.scitotenv.2020.141326.

La Rosa, G., Iaconelli, M., Mancini, P. et al. (2020). First detection of SARS-CoV-2 in untreated wastewaters in Italy. *Sci. Total Environ.* 736: https://doi.org/10.1016/j.scitotenv.2020.139652.

Langone, M., Petta, L., Cellamare, C.M. et al. (2021). SARS-CoV-2 in water services: presence and impacts. *Environ. Pollut.* 268: 115806. https://doi.org/10.1016/J.ENVPOL.2020.115806.

Leclercq, I., Batéjat, C., Burguière, A., and Manuguerra, J. (2014). Heat inactivation of the Middle East respiratory syndrome coronavirus. *Influenza Other Respir. Viruses* 8: 585. https://doi.org/10.1111/IRV.1226.

Leung, N.H.L., Chu, D.K.W., Shiu, E.Y.C. et al. (2020). Respiratory virus shedding in exhaled breath and efficacy of face masks. *Nat. Med.* 26: 676–680. https://doi.org/10.1038/s41591-020-0843-2.

Li, C., Xu, Y., Li, L. et al. (2019). Acid stress induces cross-protection for cadmium tolerance of multi-stress-tolerant *Pichia kudriavzevii* by regulating cadmium transport and antioxidant defense system. *J. Hazard. Mater.* 366: 151–159. https://doi.org/10.1016/j.jhazmat.2018.11.101.

Lin, L.T., Hsu, W.C., and Lin, C.C. (2014). Antiviral natural products and herbal medicines. *J. Tradit. Complement. Med.* 4: 24–35. https://doi.org/10.4103/2225-4110.124335.

Lin, S.-C., Ho, C.-T., Chuo, W.-H. et al. (2017). Effective inhibition of MERS-CoV infection by resveratrol. *BMC Infect. Dis.* 171 (17): 1–10. https://doi.org/10.1186/S12879-017-2253-8.

Mahlknecht, J., Padilla Reyes, D.A., Ramos, E. et al. (2021). The presence of SARS-CoV-2 RNA in different freshwater environments in urban settings determined by RT-qPCR: implications for water safety. *Sci. Total Environ.* 784: 147183. https://doi.org/10.1016/J.SCITOTENV.2021.147183.

Mandal, P., Gupta, A.K., and Dubey, B.K. (2020). A review on presence, survival, disinfection/removal methods of coronavirus in wastewater and progress of wastewater-based epidemiology. *J. Environ. Chem. Eng.* 8: 104317. https://doi.org/10.1016/j.jece.2020.104317.

Marriott, H. R., & Williams, M. D. (2018). Exploring consumers perceived risk and trust for mobile shopping: a theoretical framework and empirical study. *J. Retailing Consumer Services*, 42, 133–146. https://doi.org/https://doi.org/10.1016/J.JRETCONSER.2018.01.017.

Mead, P.S., Slutsker, L., Dietz, V., McCaig, L.F., Brese, J.S., Shapiro, C., Griffi, P.M., Tauxe, R.V., 1999. Food-releated illness and death in the United States. *Emerg. Infect. Dis.*, 5 (5): 607–25. https://doi.org/10.3201/eid0505.990502.

Medema, G., Heijnen, L., Elsinga, G. et al. (2020). Presence of SARS-Coronavirus-2 RNA in sewage and correlation with reported COVID-19 prevalence in the early stage of the epidemic in the Netherlands. *Environ. Sci. Technol. Lett.* 7: 511–516. https://doi.org/10.1021/ACS.ESTLETT.0C00357.

Mileto, D., Mancon, A., Staurenghi, F. et al. (2021). Inactivation of SARS-CoV-2 in the liquid phase: are aqueous hydrogen peroxide and sodium percarbonate efficient decontamination agents? *J. Chem. Health Saf.* 28: 260–267. https://doi.org/10.1021/acs.chas.0c00095.

Mpiana, P.T., Ngbolua, K.-T.-N., Tshibangu, D.S.T. et al. (2020). *Aloe vera* (L.) Burm. F. as a potential anti-COVID-19 plant: a mini-review of its antiviral activity. *European J. Med. Plants* 86–93. https://doi.org/10.9734/EJMP/2020/V31I830261.

Murphy, J.R. (1996). Corynebacterium Diphtheriae. *Zakażenia Corynebacterium Diphteriae Daw. i dziś* 69: 565–568.

Myers, J.H., Savoie, A., and Van Randen, E. (2003). Eradication and pest management. *Annu. Rev. Entomol.* https://doi.org/10.1146/annurev.ento.43.1.471 43: 471–491.

Nazarian, E.J., De Jesus, M., Musser, K.A., 2014. Legionella, in: Yi-Wei Tang, Max Sussman, Dongyou Liu, Joseph Schwartzman, Ian Poxton Molecular Medical Microbiology: 2nd. Elsevier Ltd, pp. 1611–1625. https://doi.org/10.1016/B978-0-12-397169-2.00090-1

Nemudryi, A., Nemudraia, A., Wiegand, T. et al. (2020). Temporal detection and phylogenetic assessment of SARS-CoV-2 in municipal wastewater. *Cell Reports Med.* 1: 100098. https://doi.org/10.1016/J.XCRM.2020.100098.

Nguyen-Viet, H. and Pham-Duc, P. (2019). Wastewater reuse in agriculture and health risk in Vietnam. In: *Water Sanit. 21st Century Heal. Microbiol. Asp. Excreta Wastewater Manag.* Global Water Pathog. Proj. https://doi.org/10.14321/WATERPATHOGENS.70.

Noorimotlagh, Z., Mirzaee, S.A., Jaafarzadeh, N. et al. (2020). A systematic review of emerging human coronavirus (SARS-CoV-2) outbreak: focus on disinfection methods, environmental survival, and control and prevention strategies. *Environ. Sci. Pollut. Res.* 281 (28): 1–15. https://doi.org/10.1007/S11356-020-11060-Z.

Noorimotlagh, Z., Mirzaee, S.A., Jaafarzadeh, N. et al. (2021). A systematic review of emerging human coronavirus (SARS-CoV-2) outbreak: focus on disinfection methods, environmental survival, and control and prevention strategies. *Environ. Sci. Pollut. Res.* https://doi.org/10.1007/s11356-020-11060-z.

Nwachcuku, N. and Gerba, C.P. (2004). Emerging waterborne pathogens: can we kill them all? *Curr. Opin. Biotechnol.* 15: 175. https://doi.org/10.1016/J.COPBIO.2004.04.010.

Oka, T., Wang, Q., Katayama, K., and Saif, L.J. (2015). Comprehensive review of human sapoviruses. *Clin. Microbiol. Rev.* 28: 32. https://doi.org/10.1128/CMR.00011-14.

Oliver, J.D. (2005). *Vibrio vulnificus, in: Oceans and Health: Pathogens in the Marine Environment*, 253–276. Springer US https://doi.org/10.1007/0-387-23709-7_10.

Organization, W.H., 2014. Guidelines for Drinking-Water Quality: Fourth Edition Incorporating the First Addendum.

O'Shea, H., Blacklaws, B.A., Collins, P.J. et al. (2019). *Viruses Associated with Foodborne Infections*. Ref. Modul. Life Sci https://doi.org/10.1016/B978-0-12-809633-8.90273-5.

Pan, T.M., Chiou, C.S., Hsu, S.Y. et al. (1996). Food-borne disease outbreaks in Taiwan, 1994. *J. Formos. Med. Assoc.* 95: 417–420.

Pascal, G. (2012). Food safety. *Arch. Pédiatrie* 19: H291. https://doi.org/10.1016/S0929-693X(12)71258-7.

Petrović, T. and D'Agostino, M. (2016). Viral contamination of food. In: *Antimicrobial Food Packaging*, 65–79. https://doi.org/10.1016/B978-0-12-800723-5.00005-X.

Pratelli, A. (2007). Action of disinfectants on canine coronavirus replication in vitro. *Zoonoses Public Health* 54: 383–386. https://doi.org/10.1111/j.1863-2378.2007.01079.x.

Pratelli, A. (2008). Canine coronavirus inactivation with physical and chemical agents. *Vet. J.* 177: 71–79. https://doi.org/10.1016/j.tvjl.2007.03.019.

Quevedo-León, R., Bastías-Montes, J., Espinoza-Tellez, T. et al. (2020). Inactivation of coronaviruses in food industry: the use of inorganic and organic disinfectants, ozone, and UV radiation. *Sci. Agropecu.* 11: 257–266. https://doi.org/10.17268/SCI.AGROPECU.2020.02.14.

Rabenau, H.F., Cinatl, J., Morgenstern, B. et al. (2005a). Stability and inactivation of SARS coronavirus. *Med. Microbiol. Immunol.* 194: 1–6. https://doi.org/10.1007/s00430-004-0219-0.

Rabenau, H.F., Kampf, G., Cinatl, J., and Doerr, H.W. (2005b). Efficacy of various disinfectants against SARS coronavirus. *J. Hosp. Infect.* 61: 107–111. https://doi.org/10.1016/j.jhin.2004.12.023.

Rai, N.K., Ashok, A., and Akondi, B.R. (2020). Consequences of chemical impact of disinfectants: safe preventive measures against COVID-19. *Crit. Rev. Toxicol.* https://doi.org/10.1080/10408444.2020.1790499.

Randazzo, W., Truchado, P., Cuevas-Ferrando, E. et al. (2020). SARS-CoV-2 RNA in wastewater anticipated COVID-19 occurrence in a low prevalence area. *Water Res.* 181: 115942. https://doi.org/10.1016/j.watres.2020.115942.

Rezny, B.R. and Evans, D.S. (2021). *Vibrio Parahaemolyticus, StatPearls*. StatPearls Publishing.

Richard Gorham, J. and Zurek, L. (2005). Filth and other foreign objects in food: a review of analytical methods and health significance. In: *Handbook of Food Science, Technology, and Engineering – 4 Volume Set* (ed. Y.H. Hui and F. Sherkat), 1439–1466. https://doi.org/10.1201/b15995-86.

Robertson, S., Li, J., and McClane, B.A. (2014). Bacteria: *Clostridium perfringens*. In: *Encyclopedia of Food Safety* (ed. Y. Motarjemi), 395–402. Elsevier https://doi.org/10.1016/B978-0-12-378612-8.00092-5.

Rusiñol, M., Hundesa, A., Cárdenas-Youngs, Y. et al. (2020). Microbiological contamination of conventional and reclaimed irrigation water: evaluation and management measures. *Sci. Total Environ.* 710: 136298. https://doi.org/10.1016/J.SCITOTENV.2019.136298.

Saikia, R.R., Deka, S., and Sarma, H. (2021). Biosurfactants from bacteria and fungi. In: *Biosurfactants for a Sustainable Future* (ed. H. Sarma and M.N.V. Prasad), 293–315. Wiley https://doi.org/10.1002/9781119671022.ch13.

Sandle, T. (2019). Assessing, controlling, and removing contamination risks from the process. In: *Biocontamination Control for Pharmaceuticals and Healthcare* (ed. T. Sandle), 287–314. Elsevier https://doi.org/10.1016/b978-0-12-814911-9.00017-1.

Sarkar, S. (2020). UHT processing – best technology for shelf - life extension of M. *Int. J. Food Sci. Nutr. Diet.* 1–2. https://doi.org/10.19070/2326-3350-200009e.

Sarma, H. and Prasad, M. (2021). *Biosurfactants for a Sustainable Future, Biosurfactants for a Sustainable Future*. Wiley https://doi.org/10.1002/9781119671022.

Sattar, S.A., Springthorpe, V.S., Karim, Y., and Loro, P. (1989). Chemical disinfection of non-porous inanimate surfaces experimentally contaminated with four human pathogenic viruses. *Epidemiol. Infect.* 102: 493–505. https://doi.org/10.1017/S0950268800030211.

Seyer, A. and Sanlidag, T. (2020). Solar ultraviolet radiation sensitivity of SARS-CoV-2. *The Lancet Microbe* 1: e8–e9. https://doi.org/10.1016/S2666-5247(20)30013-6.

Shenzhen Municipal Health Commission (2020). *Detection of SARS-CoV-2 on an Imported Chicken Wing Sample*. Shenzhen Municipal Health Commission.

Shereen, M.A., Khan, S., Kazmi, A. et al. (2020). COVID-19 infection: emergence, transmission, and characteristics of human coronaviruses. *J. Adv. Res.* 24: 91–98. https://doi.org/10.1016/J.JARE.2020.03.005.

Shuping, D.S.S. and Eloff, J.N. (2017). The use of plants to protect plants and food against fungal pathogens: a review. *African J. Tradit. Complement. Altern. Med. AJTCAM* 14: 120–127. https://doi.org/10.21010/AJTCAM.V14I4.14.

Sibanda, N., McKenna, A., Richmond, A. et al. (2018). A review of the effect of management practices on campylobacter prevalence in poultry farms. *Front. Microbiol.* https://doi.org/10.3389/fmicb.2018.02002.

Siddharta, A., Pfaender, S., Vielle, N.J. et al. (2017). Virucidal activity of world health organization-recommended formulations against enveloped viruses, including zika, ebola, and emerging coronaviruses. *J. Infect. Dis.* 215: 902–906. https://doi.org/10.1093/infdis/jix046.

Singh, V.P. (2018). Recent approaches in food bio-preservation – a review. *Open Vet. J.* 8: 104–111. https://doi.org/10.4314/ovj.v8i1.16.

Smith, M.L., Gandolfi, S., Coshall, P.M., and Rahman, P.K.S.M. (2020). Biosurfactants: a Covid-19 perspective. *Front. Microbiol.* 0: 1341. https://doi.org/10.3389/FMICB.2020.01341.

Subramaniam, M.D., Venkatesan, D., Iyer, M. et al. (2020). Biosurfactants and anti-inflammatory activity: a potential new approach towards COVID-19. *Curr. Opin. Environ. Sci. Heal.* 17: 72–81. https://doi.org/10.1016/J.COESH.2020.09.002.

Sunkari, E.D., Korboe, H.M., Abu, M., and Kizildeniz, T. (2021). Sources and routes of SARS-CoV-2 transmission in water systems in Africa: are there any sustainable remedies? *Sci. Total Environ.* 753: 142298. https://doi.org/10.1016/J.SCITOTENV.2020.142298.

Tiwari, A., Nagalli, S., 2021. *Clostridium Botulinum*. Salah Aboubakr, Amal Abu-Ghosh, Aninda B Acharya, Peyman Adibi Sedeh Food Microbiology Fundamentals and Frontiers 487–512 StatPearl.

Tyan, K., Kang, J., Jin, K., and Kyle, A.M. (2018). Evaluation of the antimicrobial efficacy and skin safety of a novel color additive in combination with chlorine disinfectants. *Am. J. Infect. Control* 46: 1254–1261. https://doi.org/10.1016/j.ajic.2018.04.223.

US Food and Drug Administration (2020). Food safety and the Coronavirus disease 2019 (COVID-19) [WWW Document]. *U.S. Food Drug*. https://www.fda.gov/food/food-safety-during-emergencies/food-safety-and-coronavirus-disease-2019-covid-19 (accessed 25 October 2021).

Vollenbroich, D., Özel, M., Vater, J. et al. (1997). Mechanism of inactivation of enveloped viruses by the biosurfactant Surfactin from *Bacillus subtilis*. *Biologicals* 25: 289–297. https://doi.org/10.1006/BIOL.1997.0099.

Waltenburg, M.A. (2020). Update: COVID-19 among workers in meat and poultry processing facilities – United States, April–May 2020. *MMWR Morb. Mortal. Wkly Rep.* 69: 887–892. https://doi.org/10.15585/MMWR.MM6927E2.

Wang, J., Shen, J., Ye, D. et al. (2020). Disinfection technology of hospital wastes and wastewater: suggestions for disinfection strategy during coronavirus disease 2019 (COVID-19) pandemic in China. *Environ. Pollut.* https://doi.org/10.1016/j.envpol.2020.114665.

Warren, B.R., Parish, M.E., and Schneider, K.R. (2006). Shigella as a foodborne pathogen and current methods for detection in food. *Crit. Rev. Food Sci. Nutr.* 46: 551–567. https://doi.org/10.1080/10408390500295458.

Wiktorczyk-Kapischke, N., Grudlewska-Buda, K., Wałecka-Zacharska, E. et al. (2021). SARS-CoV-2 in the environment – non-droplet spreading routes. *Sci. Total Environ.* 770: 85–94. https://doi.org/10.1016/j.scitotenv.2021.145260.

Willey, J.M., Sherwood, L., Woolverton, C.J., and Prescott, L.M. (2008). *Prescott, Harley, and Klein's Microbiology*. McGraw-Hill Higher Education.

Wood, A. and Payne, D. (1998). The action of three antiseptics/disinfectants against enveloped and non-enveloped viruses. *J. Hosp. Infect.* 38: 283–295. https://doi.org/10.1016/S0195-6701(98)90077-9.

Wurtzer, S., Marechal, V., Mouchel, J., and Moulin, L. (2020). Time course quantitative detection of SARS-CoV-2 in Parisian wastewaters correlates with COVID-19 confirmed cases. *medRxiv* https://doi.org/10.1101/2020.04.12.20062679.

Xiling, G., Yin, C., Ling, W. et al. (2021). in vitro inactivation of SARS-CoV-2 by commonly used disinfection products and methods. *Sci. Rep.* 111 (11): 1–9. https://doi.org/10.1038/s41598-021-82148-w.

Yaqub, T., Nawaz, M., Shabbir, M.Z. et al. (2020). A longitudinal survey for genome-based identification of SARS-CoV-2 in sewage water in selected lockdown areas of Lahore city, Pakistan; a potential approach for future smart lockdown strategy. *medRxiv* https://doi.org/10.1101/2020.07.31.20165126.

Ye, Y., Ellenberg, R.M., Graham, K.E., and Wigginton, K.R. (2016). Survivability, partitioning, and recovery of enveloped viruses in untreated municipal wastewater. *Environ. Sci. Technol.* 50: 5077–5085. https://doi.org/10.1021/ACS.EST.6B00876.

Yekta, R., Vahid-Dastjerdi, L., Norouzbeigi, S., and Mortazavian, A.M. (2021). Food products as potential carriers of SARS-CoV-2. *Food Control* https://doi.org/10.1016/j.foodcont.2020.107754.

Yuan, L., Zhang, S., Wang, Y. et al. (2018). Surfactin inhibits membrane fusion during invasion of epithelial cells by enveloped viruses. *J. Virol.* 92: https://doi.org/10.1128/JVI.00809-18.

Zambrano-Monserrate, M.A., Ruano, M.A., and Sanchez-Alcalde, L. (2020). Indirect effects of COVID-19 on the environment. *Sci. Total Environ.* 728: 138813. https://doi.org/10.1016/J.SCITOTENV.2020.138813.

Zhang, D., Zhang, X., Yang, Y. et al. (2021). SARS-CoV-2 spillover into hospital outdoor environments. *J. Hazardous Mater. Lett.* 2: 100027. https://doi.org/10.1016/j.hazl.2021.100027.

27

Modifying the Anthropocene Equation with One Health Concept

Nalika R. Dayananda

Department of Indigenous Medical Resources, Faculty of Indigenous Health Sciences and Technology, Gampaha Wickramarachchi University of Indigenous Medicine, Yakkala, Sri Lanka
Department of Chemistry, Faculty of Science, University of Kelaniya, Kelaniya, Sri Lanka

27.1 "A" for Anthropocene

The "Anthropocene" is now being used as a conceptual postulate in various contexts and communities to understand the evolving human–environment relationship. The Anthropocene is acclimated to narrate the time during which humans (*Homo sapiens*) have had a weighty impact on planet Earth. Whether or not we now inhabit the Anthropocene, a new geologic epoch, the age of humans (*Anthropos,* the ancient Greek word for humans) and humans are in the middle of a complex global system, the massive evidence now has been deposited and become apparent with the rapid global ecological consequences brought on by the humankind.

The concept of the Anthropocene can be described using a range of disciplines, such as geology, climate science, Earth system sciences, archaeology, history, philosophy, political economy, and social theory, as well as a range of timescales from deep Earth history to the modern era and the near and far future. Most importantly, the Anthropocene can be distinguished by a solidly interconnected community in several aspects, including the globalized food manufacturing and distribution system with supply and value chains, extensive trade with financial and capital markets, transport systems and widespread movements of people, mass expansion and exchange of technology, and widespread communication capacities (Helbing 2013). All these disciplines create challenges on different scales and make it an intriguing topic to address, with a deeper meaning in terms of the modern environmental challenges and the relationship between humans and the natural. The unbalance of the Earth's biological systems started when humans became a force of nature. It is a profound threat to human health and an existential threat to civilization since these natural systems comprise the most rudimentary ecological determinants of health (Crowley and Hyde 2008). While there has been a continuation of significant improvement in the health and well-being sector in many aspects, the current situation has come at an enormous and unsustainable stage with environmental degradation in the recent Anthropocene.

In the twenty-first century, the emergence of the Anthropocene, which is inversely proportionate to the Earth's geophysical processes, creates irreversible problems, including the degradation of ecosystem services/processors, the scarcity of essential resources, and the depletion of the planet's sinking ability, which are very difficult to deal with. The Holocene (before the Anthropocene) had an environment that was stable and adaptable, where complex human societies evolved, and it was the only current state of the Earth system that we know that can reliably support human existence plus ecological well-being. Since the Holocene was over, achieving effective planetary conservancy is urgent as we go to a great extent into the Anthropocene.

This new epoch has wise meaning for humanity, and humans need to be viewed as part of the biosphere, not separate from it. Depending on the collective actions of mankind, future circumstances may be beneficial or hostile to human life and the well-being of the Earth's biosphere. Awareness of both the current state of the planet and the effects of our actions is a critical factor in the Anthropocene. Instead, it seems quite apparent that sooner or later, the Earth will reach the end of the Anthropocene with humans or without humans. Therefore, humans should be active in this mission to take Earth into a new post-anthropocene period, and as humans, we have also never been better equipped with the tools to understand what is happening and what needs to be done.

One Health: Human, Animal, and Environment Triad, First Edition. Edited by Meththika Vithanage and Majeti Narasimha Vara Prasad.

27.2 The Inseparability of Human, Animal, and Environmental Health; One Health Concept

One Health is defined as a collaborative, multisectoral, and transdisciplinary approach – working at the local, regional, national, and global levels – to achieve optimal health outcomes by recognizing the interconnection between people, animals, plants, and their shared environment (CDC, GHSA 2018). The One Health paradigm emerged from the concept of interrelated and interdependent correlations of humans, animals, and ecosystems well-being.

There is a dynamic association between the Earth system and the live biosphere that consist of the atmosphere, the hydrosphere, the lithosphere, the cryosphere, and the climate system. The living biosphere is responsible for the global atmospheric circulations, water vapor and precipitation patterns, glacier spread, generating soils, upwelling currents of coastlines, ocean currents, ozone layer distribution, movements of the tectonic plates, and natural phenomena like earthquakes and volcanic eruptions (Figure 27.1). The hydrosphere or water serves as the bloodstream of the biosphere, and biogeochemical cycles are essential for all life on Earth (Falkenmark et al. 2019). The biosphere has existed for about 3.5 billion years. Modern humans (*H. sapiens*) have effectively been around in the biosphere for some 250,000 years (Mounier and Lahr 2019). Powered by the Sun, the biosphere and the Earth system coevolve with human actions as an integral part of this coevolution (Lenton et al. 2016). Therefore, the biosphere or the environment accommodates life-supporting ecosystems, facilitating essential ecosystem services supporting human well-being and socioeconomic development.

At its core, the One Health concept is established to understand the interdependence of human and environmental systems and promote multifaceted collaboration. There is a need for more systematic and multisectoral approaches to identifying public health emergencies and responding to health threats arising at the human–animal ecosystem interface globally. Therefore, the One Health concept is a planetary approach for expanding interdisciplinary collaborations at all levels, such as academia, research, government, policies, and industry, and communications in all aspects of health care for humans, animals, and the environment.

One Health addresses every sector that deals with planetary health such as agricultural production and land use; animals as sentinels for environmental agent and contaminants detection and response; antimicrobial resistance manipulation; biodiversity conservation; impacts of climate change on the health of animals, ecosystems, and

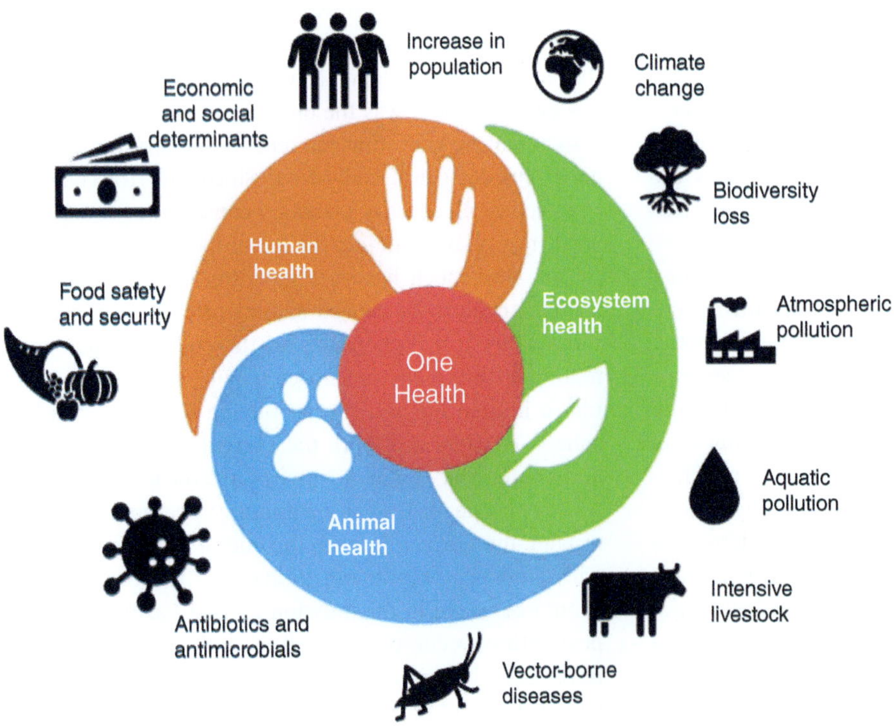

Figure 27.1 The One Health paradigm emerged from the concept of interrelated and interdependent correlations of humans, animals, and ecosystems well-being.

humans; clinical medicine and comparative medicine; disaster preparedness and response; disease surveillance, prevention, and response; economics; civil society; environmental health; food safety and security; global trade, commerce, and security; natural resources conservation; occupational health risks; plant–soil health; public policy and regulation; research and education; water safety and security; well-being of animals, humans, ecosystems, and planet. In addition, the social determinants of health (including education, neighborhood, built environment, social, and community context) play a critical role in health. Thus, there is a solid social and environmental justice aspect to One Health.

The synergism will advance health care for the twenty-first century and beyond by accelerating biomedical research discoveries, enhancing public health efficacy, expeditiously expanding the scientific knowledge base, and improving medical education and clinical care. It will help protect and save untold millions of human and animal lives in the present and future generations when adequately implemented.

27.3 Trends in Global Environmental Change in Recent Anthropocene

The artificial extensive "technosphere" emphasizes the significant role of humans in shaping global biosphere dynamics and has already left a deep imprint on the Earth system (Zalasiewicz et al. 2017), becoming a dominant force in regulating the evolution of all species on Earth. Human dominance is further reflected in the weight of the current human population, which is 10 times the weight of all wild mammals (Bar-On et al. 2018) (Figure 27.2). Humans have been in existence for only a tiny fraction of the Earth's history, but with the two episodes, the Earth has gone through extreme environmental changes, including near-complete freezing or much warmer periods, changes in atmospheric composition, rearrangement of land and ocean, and alterations to biodiversity.

The potent combination of the increase in global population, industrialization, urban development, and mass consumption trends directly impacts environmental functions, and it results in a lot of adverse hazards, more than just health issues. The ecological consequences create broader economic, social, and environmental problems. Most importantly, pollution and harmful changes in the biosphere can gradually destroy ecosystems and the existence of humans on Earth. This part of the chapter addresses the dangerous trends in global environmental changes due to anthropogenics.

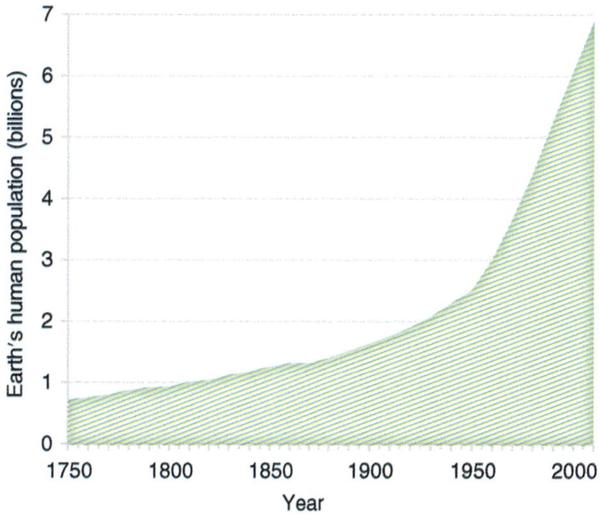

Figure 27.2 It has taken 4 million years to get to 1 billion people on the Earth and the global population is 7.9+ billion as of the year 2020. *Source:* Adapted from Steffen et al. (2015).

27.3.1 Climate Change and Global Warming

Earth has been oscillating between colder and warmer periods for over a million years. Still, the average mean temperature has never exceeded 2 °C (interglacial) above or 6 °C (deep ice age) below the pre-industrial temperature on Earth (14 °C), reflecting the importance of feedback from the living biosphere as part of regulating the temperature dynamics of the Earth (Whitlock et al. 2007). Anthropogenic climate change is now beyond dispute with the increase in the atmospheric concentration of carbon dioxide and radiative forcing. Atmospheric CO_2 concentrations have exceeded 300 ppm by volume (Figure 27.3), and radiative forcing has exceeded 1 watt per square meter above preindustrial levels at this moment, showing a considerable risk of irreversible climate change with global warming, which results in melting glaciers, accelerating the sea-level rise, and immediate shifts in forested and agricultural systems. This would endanger the ecological life-support systems and severely challenge the viability of the human community and animal life, resulting in unexpected events such as epidemics and pandemics.

27.3.2 Biodiversity Loss

Although species extinction is a natural process, biodiversity loss in the recent Anthropocene has accelerated extensively. Today, the species extinction rate is estimated to be 100–1000 times higher than what could be considered natural (Mece 2005). Changes in land use, mainly deforestation, exert the most significant effect due to converting

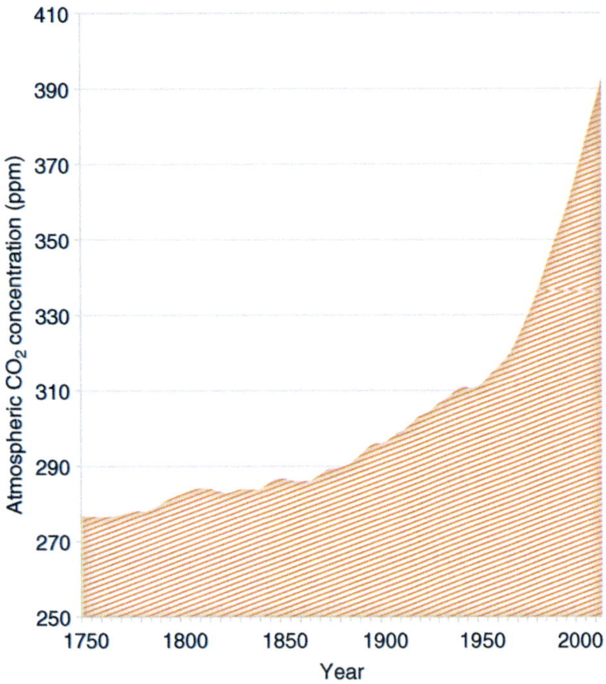

Figure 27.3 Carbon dioxide in the atmosphere far exceeds natural levels, which result in global warming and climate change. *Source:* Adapted from Steffen et al. (2015).

natural ecosystems into agriculture or urban areas and introducing new species (including invasive species) into both terrestrial and aquatic environments. However, Earth cannot sustain the current rate of biodiversity loss, which erodes ecosystem resilience.

27.3.3 Altering Biogeochemical Cycles; Nitrogen and Phosphorus Cycles

Biogeochemical cycles are the pathways by which elements like carbon, phosphorus, nitrogen, and sulfur, or compounds like water, flow between living organisms and the environment. Human activities can alter these cycles by producing or consuming in different quantities. For example, agricultural fertilizer and soil erosion have substantially increased biologically available nitrogen and phosphorous levels in natural systems. Human production of biologically available nitrogen, primarily driven by the synthetic production of nitrogen fertilizer, is now greater than all forms of crude output combined. The flow of phosphorous into the oceans, mainly caused by fertilizer from mines and livestock manure, is roughly three times the pre-industrial level. Excess nitrogen decreases plant diversity in terrestrial ecosystems, and the combination of excess nitrogen and phosphorous in water bodies leads to algal blooms and eutrophication.

27.3.4 Chemical Pollution

There are about 350,000 different types of artificial chemicals on the global market, from plastics to fertilizer/pesticides to industrial chemicals like flame retardants and insulators, excessively used in intensive agriculture, transportation, industries, and even households. Anthropogenic chemical pollution can pose one of the most significant environmental threats to humanity, animal life, and the environment, adversely affecting human communities' cognitive and physical health and food security. There are severe gaps in our understanding of the scale of the threat and the risks posed by the dispersal, mixture, and recombination of chemicals in the broader environment.

A large fraction of our population of nearly 7000 million people needs more access to food, water, and energy to improve their material standard of living, and the prospect of an additional 2000 million by 2050 intensifies the need for essential resources. These challenges come when the global environment shows clear signs of deterioration and, consequently, questions the continuing ability of the planet to provide the same accommodating environment that has facilitated human development over the past 10,000 years.

27.4 Challenges to One Health in the Recent Anthropocene

Anthropogenics to the Earth system are multiple, complex, interacting, often exponential in rate, and globally significant in magnitude and spatial scale (Lewis and Maslin 2015; Brondizio et al. 2019), and they affect every Earth system's components: land, water (fresh and marine), and atmosphere. There is no evidence that the Earth system has previously experienced these types, scales, and rates of change before what is increasingly referred to as a new epoch in Earth's geological history, the Anthropocene (Whitmee et al. 2015).

A significant increase in infectious agents' circulation was observed over the past few decades, and with the emergence and spread of epizootics, zoonoses, and epidemics, the risks of pandemics became more and more critical. The increasing occurrence of global health risks due to the emergence of new varieties of pathogens can be directly associated of the human-animal–ecosystem interface in the evolution. Human and animal health has also been threatened by antimicrobial resistance, environmental pollution, and the development of multifactorial and chronic diseases.

A broader understanding of ecosystem dynamics, which permeates the processes leading to the infectious agent's occurrence/recurrence, their dispersion, and their extinction in natural habitats, is essential in assessing the risk of infection. The emergence and re-emergence of infectious diseases are closely related to the biology and ecology of infectious agents, their hosts, and their vectors (Degeling et al. 2015). Processes such as mutation, recombination, horizontal transfer, and hybridization enhance the natural evolution of most parasitic organisms genetically, especially viruses, prokaryotes, and eukaryotes. Therefore, to predict the future threats associated with those pathogens, comprehensive studies on life cycles, transmission pathways, and transgression of species barriers of pathogens are needed, and further research is required. They could help explore pathogen dynamics in natural habitats and develop infection models close to environmental systems (Khan et al. 2018) to implement suitable health interventions.

Environmental pollution, climate change, biodiversity loss resulting from habitat destruction, and fragmentation have confirmed incentives for infectious diseases' occurrence and geographic distribution (Rabinowitz et al. 2018). The spread of bird flu, coronavirus, Ebola, chikungunya, dengue, and Zika diseases indicates altering the re-division of pathogens, their vectors, and their reservoirs due to global warming and other environmental alterations (Biermann et al. 2016). Environmental pollution is a planetary concern, and the risks can be expected in environments where the human population is very dense such as urbanized areas and coastal areas. Accumulating pollutants, such as micro- and nanoplastics, solid wastes, wastewater, and urban smokes, are linked to multiple anthropogenic releases nowadays (Sorrell et al. 2009). However, even remote areas are also contaminated, with many emerging organic and inorganic pollutants (Steffen et al. 2007). On the other hand, there is a threat to the survival and health of wildlife and domestic animals due to being exposed to hazardous levels of contamination. Reduction of their reproduction ability and capability to cope with pathogens can result in that, and it will be a direct threat to biodiversity loss and ecosystem malfunctioning (Taylor 2009).

Increased movement of humans, plants, and animals with their accompanying infectious agents has taken place in a short stretch of time with rapid and vast-scaled international trade and exchange of goods/services and the industrialization of agriculture, aquaculture, and agribusiness (Kates et al. 2001). Some industries with intensive breeding and farming practices have also brought out excessive stress on livestock, which has created the ideal environment for the spreading of unexpected infectious agents.

Intensive agriculture and livestock farming are also responsible for the overuse of fertilizers, pesticides, and especially antibiotics, which develop antibiotic resistance, and it is one of the most severe threats to food safety, security, and global health. Therefore, it is an urgent need to develop and implement novel approaches using a "One Health" concept to solve those adverse impacts through research and innovation and establish suitable policy frameworks covering the areas of public health, agriculture, and livestock farming.

Multifactorial diseases frequently appear in organisms with low immunity or defense capacities due to changes in nutrition, temperature, salinity, pH, exposure to pollutants, toxins, radiation, etc., due to various anthropogenic activities in the biosphere. Toxins contribute significantly to morbidity caused by both pathogens and other toxic substances through cumulative and chronic exposure. The immune system of organisms is the main target of these toxicants; they increase the risk of infectious disease occurrence; and it directly or indirectly affects the functioning of ecosystems. Therefore, the pollutant imposes a significant threat to biodiversity and interrupts the biotic interactions and processes in natural ecosystems. As a result, changes can happen in food web topology, which brings changes in the abundance of species in a particular environment, implying a massive threat to keystone species. On the other hand, it can result in biological invasion and increase resistant disease reservoir species.

The occurrence of some chronic noncommunicable diseases highlights the globalization of sanitary risks (Aguirre et al. 2016). Environmental changes mainly due to intensive agriculture, industrialization, urbanization, and particularly exposure to toxic substances are the possible reasons for chronic severe noninfectious diseases in humans, including respiratory, cardiovascular, neurological, and metabolic disorders, obesity, diabetes, and cancer. However, the prevention of these chronic diseases is a difficult challenge for the present and future generations because, in some cases, the exact root cause has been unidentified or questionable over the decades. Some of those diseases can have an animal origin that has been transmitted to humans. This indicates the importance of the man–animal–ecosystem interface in determining the evolution and emergence of chronic diseases in humans, just as in other species. Therefore, developing a bond between humans and veterinary medicine is necessary to identify the exact cause of these diseases, tackle such complex disease dynamics, and implement prevention and control strategies.

There is considerable potential for epidemics and pandemics with the increase in human populations and rapid and widespread long-distance travel. While viral in origin, the COVID-19 pandemic highlights the risks we face in a growingly interconnected world. The COVID-19 pandemic has exposed a connected and tightly coupled globalized world in rapid change. These situations provide scientific proof that people and nature are dynamically intertwined and embedded in the Earth's biosphere. Humans have transformed into the primary influence in adjusting the Earth system's future as a whole, placing extreme and unpredicted phenomena as part of these fluctuations, and those actions are quite challenging to the "One Health" of the biosphere when considering the prosperity of human civilizations, existence of animals, and also persistence of natural resources. Therefore, proper changes and adaptations toward sustainability are urgent in this Anthropocene with the help of modern technologies, social innovations, and cultural and indigenous knowledge to support the resilient ability of the biosphere through One Health concept.

27.5 From One Health Concept to Practice

These rapid environmental fluctuations due to human anthropogenics in the recent Anthropocene are linked with the emergence and reemergence of diseases, both infectious and noninfectious. Over recent years, some zoonoses and extreme events have shown the interdependence of human health, animal health, and ecosystem health. Therefore, initiating the "One Health" concept into practice constitutes a global holistic and transdisciplinary with multisector expertise and stakeholders in dealing with the health of mankind, animals, and ecosystems. It is not easy to adjust to current societal development pathways and guide humanity into sustainability, resulting in a stabilized Earth state. Stabilizing the Earth system or the biosphere into a safe-operating space will require transformative changes in many dimensions of human actions and relations. Defining the state of health of Earth's ecosystems is a huge challenge in the successful integration of the environment in conjunction with human and animal health, and inserting the "One Health" concept into action should initiate the collaboration of the research and development sector to establish the desired equilibrium or dynamics of multifunction ecosystems through decision-making on sustainable development, species conservation, and human, animal, and plant health (CDC, GHSA 2018).

Resilience is defined as the capacity of a socio-ecosystem to absorb disturbance and to maintain particular properties such as function, structure, identity, and feedback. Resilience should be treated dynamically, as it permits an ecosystem to shift among different steady states that possess different sets of processes that allow all the tasks to be sustained. On the one hand, it has been advocated that an integrated One Health approach addressing the potential health effects at the human/animal/environment interface will enhance the resilience of local communities through better disease prevention (Ruegg et al. 2017).

Besides, the concept of resilience is focused on system-based thinking and holistic approaches to enhance the diversity of organisms (from genes to species), redundancy, and adaptability of the socio-ecosystem to better face, which was expected from the One Health concept. Hence, the resilience of multifunctional ecosystems across space and time, and in both aquatic and terrestrial environments, depends on the contributions of many species and their distribution, redundancy, and richness at multitrophic levels performing critical functions in ecosystems and biosphere dynamics (Myers and Patz 2009). Health security must be addressed globally, integrating human health, animal health, plant health, ecosystem health, and biodiversity, considering ecological, evolutionary, and environmental sciences in understanding the emergence and re-emergence of infectious diseases.

Still, there is a need for vaccines and antibiotics to prevent early-occurred scourges, such as plague and tuberculosis, which are still infecting people and communities. Biodiversity builds, sustains, and keeps ecosystems resilient to changing environmental consequences, and biodiversity has the potential to control the spread of infectious agents with its dynamics and holobiont fitness, including predation, competition, and host–symbiont interactions. Moreover, biodiversity can dilute the disease transmission in both scale and content, but those processes are still poorly known. Identifying the functions of that side of the biosphere can be helpful to face upcoming epidemics and pandemics.

Eco-inspired innovative strategies can be developed to control infectious diseases using natural predators of bacteria, containing bacterial behavior and dynamics in the environment, antimicrobial peptides, effectors of innate immunity in metazoans, competition in prokaryotes, etc. These natural control mechanisms are authentic sources of inspiration for developing new anti-infectious strategies in an eco-friendly way. The responsible global platforms should develop international action plans based on One Health principle to overcome the health problems in the recent Anthropocene. For example, organizations like WHO promote and encourage research on finding new methods of fighting vector-borne transmission based on microbial symbiosis (Godlee and Waters 2018). Applying the "One Health" concept to noncommunicable chronic diseases should also be addressed, linked to exposure to multiple environmental stresses. An attentive interpretation of disease dynamics and implementing public policies to cover all the consequences of certain human activities, lifestyles, and behaviors in ecosystems should be searched for in order to get a better knowledge of causes for the occurrence of chronic diseases.

Promoting multidisciplinary integrative approaches that link expertise knowledge from all the related sectors is needed to develop a progressive health (human and animal) ecology and its ongoing evolutionary consequences (Figure 27.4). Long-term monitoring on multiannual demographic variations of organisms, landscape changes, practice changes, rearrangement of communities is required to investigate different spatial and temporal scales relevant to the pathogenic microorganisms and their disease transmission or exposure systems. These processes should facilitate the data handling facilities consisting of policies to collect, capitalize, and secure the data derived from ambitious research. It is necessary to implement a gradual reinforcement of biosecurity from a political point of view, including production, transport, and transformation of biological resources. In parallel, it is essential to break down the sectoral partitioning between public health, agronomy policy, and other sectors of activity.

To manage the health-related issues in the agricultural sector on both small and large scales, a strong partnership between scientists, farmers, and the vector control services should implement encouraging research and field trials to protect the crops/livestock while reducing the populations of vectors as much as possible by minimum usage of synthetic agrochemicals, which are toxic to the ecosystems. Therefore, it is clear that a comprehensive review of industrial agriculture and farming practices is vitally urgent. Overall, significant efficacy gains can be achieved through intersectoral cooperation in a "One Health" approach.

For the practical application of the One Health concept, existing barriers need to be removed by breaking down human and veterinary medicine from ecological, evolutionary, and environmental sciences. Integrative approaches should be promoted by linking factors underlying stress responses to their consequences on ecosystem functioning and evolution. Updated knowledge is required for the development of novel regulations inspired by environmental mechanisms leading to desired equilibrium and dynamics in healthy ecosystems and must provide in the near future a framework for more integrated operational initiatives to ensure human–animal–environmental health and its future.

27.6 Conclusion

The Anthropocene is a measure of the scale and tempo of human-caused change, including biodiversity loss, changes in the atmosphere and ocean chemistry, urbanization, and globalization. The recent Anthropocene has strongly modified and impoverished the biosphere and human-dominated landscapes. Addressing trends and changes in ecological, evolutionary, and environmental phenomena in the Anthropocene, a human-dominated geological epoch is crucial as they can severely impact the One Health of Earth's biosphere in many ways, including the emergence

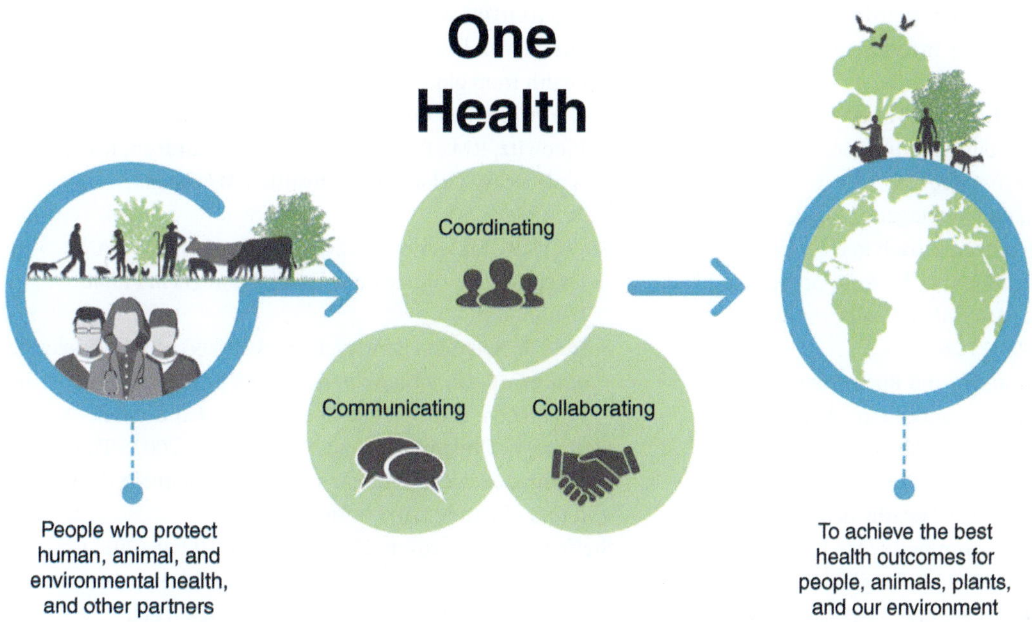

Figure 27.4 Foundation of One Health; coordination, collaboration, and communication. *Source:* https://www.cdc.gov/onehealth/images/multimedia/one-health-def.jpg.

and reemergence of infectious and noncommunicable chronic diseases, which create an immense threat to the environmental system as a whole. Implementing the "One Health" concept moves beyond science and impacts all the sectors covering health, agriculture, aquaculture, land management, urbanism, biological conservation, law, politics, and ethics. The planetary challenges confront humanity need governance that mobilizes the best that science offers with shared visions for sustainable futures and the will and competence to implement choices that will sustain humanity and the rest of the living world for the next millennium and beyond.

References

Aguirre, A.A., Beasley, V.R., Augspurger, T. et al. (2016). One health-transdisciplinary opportunities for SETAC leadership in integrating and improving the health of people, animals, and the environment. *Environmental Toxicology and Chemistry* 35: 2383–2391. https://doi.org/10.1002/etc.3557.

Bar-On, Y.M., Phillips, R., and Milo, R. (2018). The biomass distribution on Earth. *Proceedings of the National Academy of Sciences, USA* 115: 6506–6511.

Biermann, F., Bai, X., Bondre, N. et al. (2016). Down to earth: contextualizing the Anthropocene. *Global Environmental Change* 39: 341–350. https://doi.org/10.1016/j.gloenvcha.2015.11.004.

Brondizio, E., Settele, J., Díaz, S., and Ngo, H. (2019). *Global Assessment Report on Biodiversity and Ecosystem Services of the Intergovernmental Science-Policy Platform on Biodiversity and Ecosystem Services*. IPBES Secretariat 2019.

CDC Global Health Security Agenda (GHSA) (2018). Implementing the global health security agenda: progress and impact from U.S. Government investments. https://www.ghsagenda.org/docs/default-source/default-document-library/global-health-security-agenda-2017-progress-and-impact-from-u-s-investments.pdf (accessed 7 January 2023).

Crowley, T.J. and Hyde, W.T. (2008). Transient nature of late Pleistocene climate variability. *Nature* 456: 226–230. https://doi.org/10.1038/nature07365.

Degeling, C., Johnson, J., and Kerridge, I. (2015). Implementing a one health approach to emerging infectious disease: reflections on the socio-political, ethical and legal dimensions. *BMC Public Health* 15: 1307. https://doi.org/10.1186/s12889-015-261.

Falkenmark, L., Erlandsson, W., and Rockström, J. (2019). Understanding of water resilience in the Anthropocene. *Journal of Hydrology X* 2: https://doi.org/10.1016/j.hydroa.2018.100009.

Godlee, F. and Waters, A. (2018). Healthy people, healthy animals, and a healthy environment: One Health. *BMJ* 362: 3020. https://doi.org/10.1136/bmj.k3020.

Helbing, D. (2013). Globally networked risks and how to respond. *Nature* 497: 51–59.

Kates, R.W., Clark, W.C., Corell, R. et al. (2001). Sustainability science. *Science* 292: 641–642. https://doi.org/10.1126/science.1059386.

Khan, M.S., Rothman-Ostrow, P., and Spencer, J. (2018). The growth and strategic functioning of one health networks: a systematic analysis. *Lancet Planet Health* 2: 264–273. https://doi.org/10.1016/S2542-5196(18)30084-6.

Lenton, T.M., Dahl, T.W., Daines, S.J. et al. (2016). Earliest land plants created modern levels of atmospheric oxygen. *Proceedings of the National Academy of Sciences* 113 (35): 9704–9709.

Lewis, S.L. and Maslin, M.A. (2015). Defining the anthropocene. *Nature* 519: 171–180.

Mace, G. (2005). Biodiversity: millennium ecosystem assessment: current state and trends: findings of the condition and trends working group. In: *Ecosystems and Human Well-being* (ed. H. Hassan, R. Scholes and N. Ash) Ch. 4, 79–115. Island Press.

Mounier, A. and Lahr, M. (2019). Deciphering African late middle Pleistocene hominin diversity and the origin of our species. *Nature Communications* 10: 3406. https://doi.org/10.1038/s41467-019-11213-w.

Myers, S.S. and Patz, J. (2009). Emerging threats to human health from global environmental change. *Annual Review of Environment and Resources* 34: 223–252.

Rabinowitz, P.M., Pappaioanou, M., and Bardosh, K.L. (2018). A planetary vision for one health. *BMJ Global Health* 3: 1137.

Ruegg, S.R., McMahon, B.J., and Hasler, B. (2017). A blueprint to evaluate one health. *Frontiers in Public Health* 5: 20.

Sorrell, S., Speirs, J., Bentley, R. et al. (2009). *An Assessment of the Evidence for a Near-Term Peak in Global Oil Production*. London: UK Energy Research Centre.

Steffen, W., Crutzen, P.J., and McNeill, J.R. (2007). The Anthropocene: are humans now overwhelming the great forces of nature? *Ambio* 36: 614–621.

Steffen, W., Richardson, K., Rockström, J. et al. (2015). Planetary boundaries: guiding human development on a changing planet. *Science* 347: 6223. https://doi.org/10.1126/science.1259855.

Taylor, M.S. (2009). Innis lecture: environmental crises: past, present and future. *Canadian Journal of Economics* 42: 1240–1275. https://doi.org/10.1111/j.1540-5982.2009.01545.x.

Whitlock, C., Moreno, I., and Bartlein, P. (2007). Climatic controls of Holocene fire patterns in southern South America. *Quaternary Research* 68: 28–36. https://doi.org/10.1016/j.yqres.2007.01.012.

Whitmee, S., Haines, A., Beyrer, C. et al. (2015). Safeguarding human health in the Anthropocene epoch: report of The Rockefeller Foundation-Lancet Commission on planetary health. *Lancet* 386: 1973–2028.

Zalasiewicz, J., Steffen, W., Leinfelder, R. et al. (2017). Petrifying earth process: The stratigraphic imprint of key earth system parameters in the Anthropocene. *Theory, Culture & Society* 34 (2-3): 83–104.

28

Bioavailability of Trace Elements in Soils

G.A.H. Galahitigama and N.P.M. Abeysinghe

Department of Export Agriculture, Faculty of Agricultural Sciences, Sabaragamuwa University of Sri Lanka, Belihuloya, Sri Lanka

28.1 Introduction

With the industrial development throughout the world, the soil pollution from trace elements (TEs) has become one of the paramount environmental crises. Moreover, rapid urbanization and high-tech agricultural activities accelerated this issue to a severe level. The TEs accumulation in soil was caused by either natural or anthropogenic activities. As human activities, metal mining and smelting, sewage sludge application, pesticide application, electroplating, and fossil fuel burning were highly concerning (Yan et al. 2020). These anthropogenic activities have been considerably affecting TEs accumulation in soil for the last couple of decades (Sihlahla et al. 2020).

The main TEs in soils have been identified as Cr, As, Cd, Cu, Mo, Ni, Pd, Hg, and Ni. (Kumpiene et al. 2017). Nevertheless, numerous other metals, such as Ti and metalloids (e.g. Sn, Sd, and Se), are also found in TE-contaminated areas (Kumpiene et al. 2017). Several of these TEs (e.g. Cu, Zn, Mo, Zn, and Ni) are significant to complete the plant life cycle (Cempel and Nikel 2006), while some elements would become toxic when present in higher concentrations. For example, elements like Pd, As, Cd, and Hg severely impact the physiological development of crop growth and ultimately mitigate agricultural productivity (Clemens 2006). The accumulated TEs in soil can be adsorbed by plants, and consequently transferred to living organisms through the food chain and biomagnified in cells, resulting in serious health issues for both humans and other creatures (Rehman et al. 2017). In addition, humans can be exposed to deleterious TEs through inhalation of soil and dust or ingestion (Sakan et al. 2016). Thus, human health is largely determined by the quality of the soil.

Understanding mechanisms that affect soil quality and human health involves well defined of bioavailability and bioaccessibility processes (Petruzzelli et al. 2019). The bioaccumulation of metals depends on inherent solubility and soil characteristics as well as various soil physicochemical factors (Yan et al. 2020). Utilizing bioavailability perception for environmental risk estimation and management is becoming more popular right now. (Kumpiene et al. 2017). The implementation of phytotechnologies to reduce TE concentrations in a contaminated soil also has a link with bioavailability process (Kumpiene et al. 2017). Existing knowledge of the bioavailability process is widely used in several European countries (e.g. Germany, the Netherlands, and Switzerland) to assess the site-specific risk assessment and goal setting to develop guidelines to protect the environment as well as human health from TEs (Kumpiene et al. 2017).

Therefore, this chapter would discuss the key processes (bioavailability and bioaccessibility) involving bioaccumulation, soil physicochemical parameters affecting the bioavailability of TEs, assessment of methods for determining the bioavailability of TEs, and remedial methods to mitigate the bioavailability of metal(loid)s.

28.2 Bioavailability Process in Soil

The definition of bioavailability totally changes according to various disciplines, and there are over 20 diverse definitions found comprising relative bioavailability, absolute bioavailability, bioavailable fraction (US National Research Council-US NRC 2002). For instance, mammalian toxicologists define bioavailability as an element's capacity to pass a cell membrane and move inside a cell, whereas environmental experts define bioavailability as a chemical's availability for acclimation and potential toxicity (Kumpiene et al. 2017). Moreover, some researchers combined the two terms: bioavailability and bioaccessibility as a function of both biological and chemical possessions (Zhu et al. 2015).

One Health: Human, Animal, and Environment Triad, First Edition. Edited by Meththika Vithanage and Majeti Narasimha Vara Prasad.

However, according to the US NRC (2002), bioavailability mechanisms were defined as the specific physical, chemical, and biological interactions that affect how much exposure to chemicals in soil and sediments both plants and animals experience. These interactions can change in time and location and are quite dynamic (Kumpiene et al. 2017). Furthermore, TEs interact with living organisms; thus, the bioavailability process would elucidate more complexity.

As mentioned earlier, bioavailability process is accompanied by a sequence of complex mass transfer and sorption processes (Petruzzelli et al. 2019). The soil characteristics, properties of substances, and living organisms directly affect TEs concentration in a soil (Petruzzelli et al. 2019). Soil is composed of three phases, namely: solid, liquid, and gaseous, which are characterized by a significant number of reactions (e.g. adsorption, desorption, degradation, and moving between phases) and processes (Petruzzelli et al. 2019). Since the biological membrane might interact with TE and alter element uptake, the TEs present in the soil are difficult to pass through (Kumpiene et al. 2017). Therefore, each stage of the bioavailable process could be seen as a blockade to TE disclosure of living things (Kumpiene et al. 2017).

The key phases of the bioavailability process are shown in Figure 28.1. According to the figure, Phase A illustrates the presence of TEs in the solid phase, which is unavailable to most environmental processes, and should be transferred to the liquid phase or soil solution, and every element is potentially available for both micro- and macroorganisms in the soil (Petruzzelli et al. 2019). As described earlier, when pollutants/metals reach the soil, they form complex bonds with the solid phase through adsorption processes with mineral matrix (e.g. clays and oxides) and organic matrix (humic compounds), and contaminants/TEs are retained by the soil surfaces depending on the pollutant properties and the soil conditions (Petruzzelli et al. 2019).

The chemical environment of the soil solution would change frequently and facilitate metal release into the soil solution, allowing living organisms to absorb contaminants through different mechanisms like diffusion and dispersion (Petruzzelli et al. 2019). The trace metals also move through the cell membrane through the cell wall (Phase B, Figure 28.1). However, during the transferring stage, contaminants/metals might be exposed to further reactions such as hydrolysis, oxidation, photolysis, and degradation, which can modify the toxicity level and bioavailability of contaminants (Petruzzelli et al. 2019).

After contaminants arrive in a living cell (Phase C), the impact of the soil on the bioavailability process would become zero, unless only in the case of oral ingestion of soil, particularly by children (Petruzzelli et al. 2019). Then, absorbed contaminants further move to target sites of living organisms, known as the bioaccessibility process (Phase D), which measures the solubilized contaminants in the stomach and already absorbed substances in the intestine (Petruzzelli et al. 2019, Figure 28.1). Apart from general contamination pathway of soil-plant-food chain, other contamination routes exist, such as direct oral ingestion of soil, skin contact, and the inhalation of soil particles (Petruzzelli et al. 2019). The evaluation of health risks due to contaminated soils highly depends on the route of

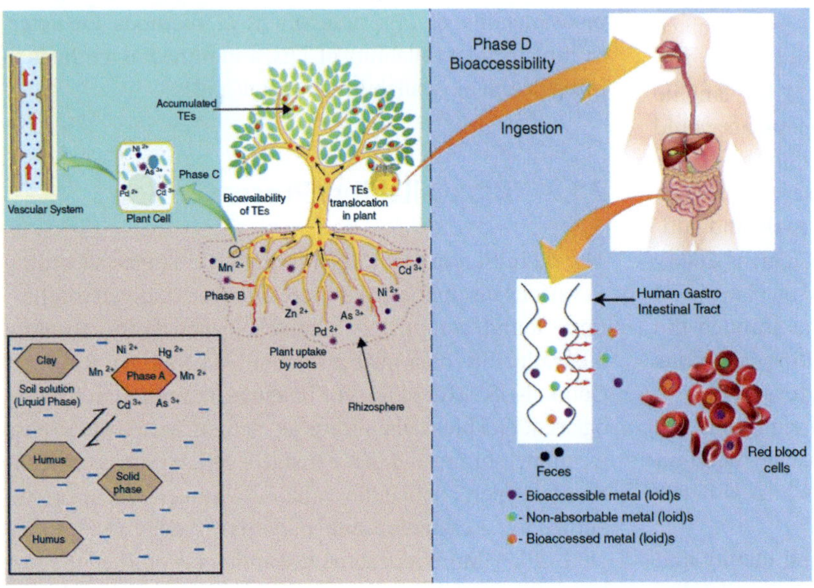

Figure 28.1 The process of trace metal(loid)s translocation from soil to plant (bioavailability) and then from plant to human body (bioaccessibility).

exposure to the soil and whether the digestive process releases contaminants from the soil itself (Petruzzelli et al. 2019).

The bioaccessibility process starts in the oral cavity and continues into stomach, with the intestine absorbing the most contaminants due to its large total surface area (Ng et al. 2015). Thus, the bioaccessibility of contaminants in soil is a significant factor to be considered, and the determination of bioaccessibility is also a crucial aspect of health risk assessment (Petruzzelli et al. 2019). Moreover, bioavailability and bioaccessibility are basically related to the characteristics of soil and contaminants, where the route of exposure is also important for the assessment process of contaminants (Petruzzelli et al. 2019).

28.3 Factors Affecting Bioavailability Process

When the plant is involved in the fundamental step of the TEs bioaccumulation process, contaminants should be dissolved in the soil solution (Petruzzelli et al. 2019). The bioavailability of metals to plants is mainly determined by sorption/desorption dynamics, which are primarily influenced by soil pH, soil minerals (e.g. clay, metal oxides, phosphates), redox potential/Eh, cation exchange capacity (CEC), plant factors, and time (Petruzzelli et al. 2019; Wang et al. 2020a).

28.3.1 pH

The mineralogical substrate of a particular soil from which the soil originated defines the soil pH, and it is the most significant parameter governing the elements in the soil (Petruzzelli et al. 2019). Numerous anthropogenic activities (e.g. wastewater irrigation for crops) also impact pH reduction in soil (Hou et al. 2020). Generally, the solubility of most TEs decreases as the soil pH increases (Petruzzelli et al. 2019). For instance, according to Wen et al. (2021), low pH range of soil enhances the Cd absorption rate of rice. Simultaneously, increased soil acidity speeds up the desorption of Cd from soil colloids, facilitating root absorption; thus, always the relationship between soil pH and Cd bioavailability is negative (Salam et al. 2019; Wen et al. 2021). Furthermore, alkaline conditions in soil would mitigate the mobilization of Cd ions, resulting in minimum Cd accretion in rice seeds (Gong et al. 2021).

28.3.2 Redox Potential

Numerous oxidation–reduction reactions that take place in soil solution are governed by the activity of free electrons in soil, indicated as the redox potential (Eh) of soil (Petruzzelli et al. 2019). Generally, submerged or organic matter-rich soils tend to have low Eh values, while dry and well-ventilated soils have higher Eh values (Petruzzelli et al. 2019). For example, in flooded paddy areas, soil Eh becomes extremely facilitated by oxidized sulfate, and nitrate, and additional ions can be used for respiration by soil microbes (Cui et al. 2020); concurrently, ions get electrons during the reduction reaction, which lowers the Eh (Lin et al. 2021). Thus, flooding leads to a decrease in the Eh, which facilitates the bioavailability of Cd through dissolving Cd in soil solution (Wu et al. 2019).

28.3.3 Organic Matter

Organic matter is a crucial factor that harmonizes the metal bioavailability of soil, since humic substances form complexes with elements that act as an adsorbent (Petruzzelli et al. 2019). The complexes formed with substances with a lower molecular weight are quite soluble in soil solutions, which enhance the metal concentration in the soil solution; on the other hand, higher molecular weight humic acids create stable complexes with elements and ultimately reduce the bioavailability potential of a particular element (Petruzzelli et al. 2019). For example, Cd accumulation in different compartments of the rice plant (e.g. roots, straw, and grains) become reduced after application of organic matter (Ali et al., 2020). However, sometimes dissolved humic substances might produce soluble complexes, enhancing the Cd bioavailability (Shahid et al. 2016). Furthermore, Hg also interacts with humic acids and produces highly stable complexes that reduce its bioavailability (Hou et al. 2020).

28.3.4 Clay

The clay fraction of soil is highly engaged in ion exchange reactions or adsorption processes. In this regard, clay particles form bonds with available elements existing in the soil through generating of hydroxyl ions (Reis et al. 2015). The adsorptive capacity of clay varies according to the clay type, and on most occasions, adsorption and retention processes are higher in expandable clays (Petruzzelli et al. 2019).

28.3.5 Cation Exchange Capacity

The CEC of a soil for TEs is strictly related to the specific surface area of the soil colloids (Petruzzelli et al. 2019). Basically, the humidity and clay fraction of the soil determine the Cation Exchange Capacity value; thus, negative charges of solid particles might be permanent or rely on the soil pH (Petruzzelli et al. 2019).

28.3.6 Oxides and Hydroxides

The hydroxides of Fe, Al, and Mn are distributed in coatings on soil particles, which have great sensitivity to the redox potential as well as to the metal concentration in soil solution (Petruzzelli et al. 2019). Several metal ions also get adsorbed with oxides and develop complex substances, which drastically reduce the bioavailability of specific metals (Petruzzelli et al. 2019).

28.3.7 Inherent Bioavailability Potential of Elements

The bioavailability and presence of metal(loid)s in soil varies considerably (Hou et al. 2020). According to O'Connor et al. (2019), though lead is more abundant in soil than other elements, lead accumulation is minimal as it forms insoluble compounds such as pyromorphite and manganese oxides. Moreover, the oxidation state of the metal(loid) s changes their bioavailability potential (Hou et al. 2020). For an example, *Atriplex atacamensis* only absorbs As(III) ions when compared to an As(V) oxidation state, which reduces the growth of plant (Vromman et al. 2018).

28.4 Soil–Plant Transfer of Trace Elements

The plant roots absorb the metal(loids) present in the soil solution and enter the vascular system mainly through two pathways, namely apoplastic and symplastic pathways (Yan et al. 2020). However, the most common pathway is symplastic path arbitrated by metallic ion transporters or carrier mediators (DalCorso et al. 2019). Soil–metal–plant relationship for the metal uptake of plants mainly depends on metal(loid)s concentration, numerous chelating compounds (e.g. organic acid), soil physicochemical properties, plant characteristics, etc. (Zhang et al. 2018, Figure 28.2). For instance, elevated concentrations of Zn(II) and Ca(II) ions act as competitors to Cd(II); thus, hindered cadmium uptakes and facilitates other essential mineral uptake (Murtaza et al. 2017). However, apart from root absorption, atmospheric deposition of metals (e.g.: Cd deposition in rice) also occurs especially in local-confined areas of emission (Feng et al. 2019); consequently, it penetrates to the vascular tissues through waxy layer of leaf (Zhou et al. 2020).

The metal(loid)s transfer through cell membrane basically by specialized transporters or channel proteins located in the plasma membrane (DalCorso et al. 2019). These metal transporters are further categorized into numerous groups such as ZIP, HMAs, MTPs, and NRAMPs (Yan et al. 2020, Figure 28.2). Transporters of ZIP family mainly transport Fe, Mn, and Zn cations from root to shoot (Yan et al. 2020), whereas HMAs transport Cd and Zn from roots to shoots over long distances. MTPs family translocates Zn and Ni cations toward extracellular space and internal compartments (Gustin et al. 2011). The naturally resistant associated macrophage proteins (NRAMPs) are localized in the plasma membrane and tonoplast, which mediate the translocation of Cu, Mn, Cd, and Fe ions (Bastow et al. 2018). For instance, in rice, OsNramp5 is important to Cd uptake and translocation to the root zone of the plant (Ma et al. 2021), while OsHMA3 is responsible for Cd movement to vacuole or sequestration process. Furthermore, Cd translocation from the root to the shoot is mainly governed by OsHMA2 (Ismael et al. 2019) and OsHMA3, a very recently discovered protein, also aids in the movement of Cd from the root to the shoot (Wiggenhauser et al. 2021). Apart from metal carriers, complexing agents, such as amino acids and organic acids, produce ligands for the chelation of metal ions (Yan et al. 2020).

28.4.1 Assessment of Bioavailability of Trace Metal(loid)s

28.4.1.1 Soil Metal Pollution Assessment

The level of trace metal contamination of a particular soil can be estimated through various mathematical models/pollution indices (Ramírez et al. 2021). Basically, these pollution indices are categorized into two parts: single pollution indices and total complex indices (Khan et al. 2021). As single pollution indices, Contamination Factor (CF), Enrichment Factor (EF), Pollution Index (PI), and Threshold Pollution Index (PI_T) are widely used in experiments (Shaheen et al. 2020). By using multi-element indices, total complex indices were developed. Modified Contamination Factor (mC_{deg}), Average Pollution Index (PI_{Avg}), Pollution Load Index (PLI), and New Pollution Index (PIN) are a few of the total complex indices used to determine the metal pollution of a contaminated soil (Weissmannov'a and Pavlovský 2017). In addition, numerous sequential extraction methods have been used to determine the potential movement of metal(loid)s in soil by using different extractions such as EDTA, KCl, KNO_3, HNO_3, HF, and NH_4NO_3 (Khan et al. 2021).

28.4.1.2 Plant Metal Remediation Assessment

Both the bioconcentration factor (BCF) and the translocation factor (TF) can be used to estimate the assimilation capacity of TEs from the soil (Azab and Hegazy 2020). Based on the metal(loid)s availability in soil and its uptake efficiency by plants, this indicates the phytoremediation

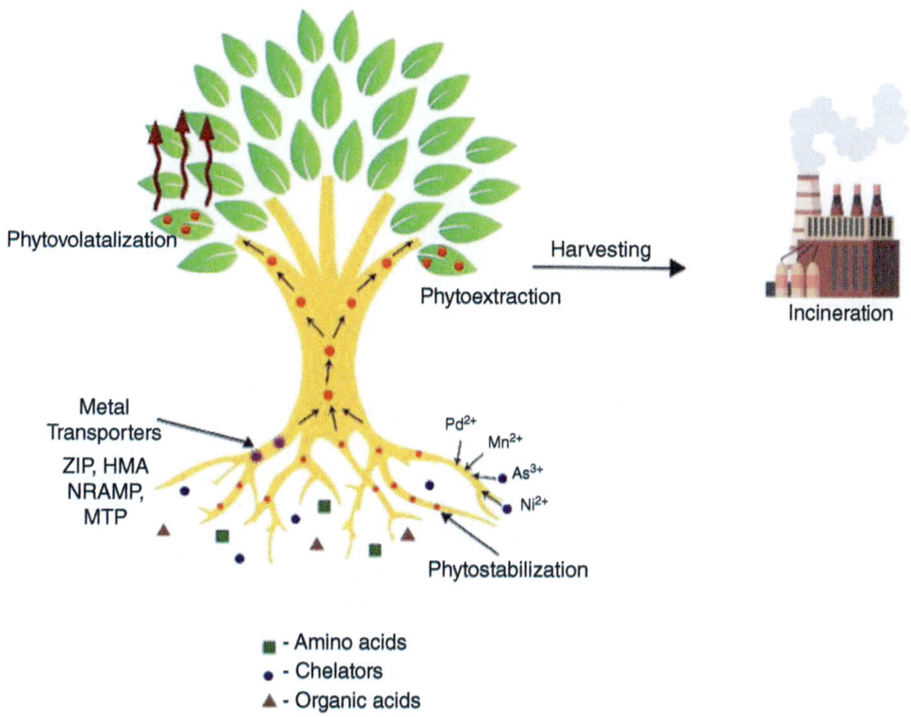

Figure 28.2 Soil–metal–plant relationship for the TEs uptake of and different phytoremediation strategies.

potential of the plant (Usman et al. 2019). As a formula, BCF can be expressed as follows:

$$BCF = C_{\text{plant part}} / C_{\text{soil}}$$

where C_{plant} part is the metal concentration in plant tissues such as roots, stems, or leaves, and C_{soil} is the metal concentration in the particular soil (Azab and Hegazy 2020). Generally, BCF is a highly descriptive value that designates the capability of plants to accumulate metal(loid)s in plant tissues. For instance, if $BCF_{root} > 1$, the plant has a strong metal(loid)s accumulation capacity root and is considered a phytostabilizer, whereas if $BCFs_{hoot} > 1$, the plant is suitable as a phytoextractor (Ramírez et al. 2021).

TF value gives the information about the translocation ability of the elements in the plant, thus providing information relevant to the accumulation mechanism of these metal(loid)s in shoots from the roots (Ramírez et al. 2021). The TF value would be calculated as follows:

$$TF = C_{\text{shoot}} / C_{\text{root}}$$

where the C_{shoot} is the metal(loid)s concentration of the plant issue (stem or leaves) and C_{root} is the metal(loid)s concentration in the root.

When TF value > 1 gives the idea of higher translocation ability of elements from root to shoot; which is a unique characteristic of a phytoextractor species (Ramírez et al. 2021). Furthermore, a plant with higher TF value (more than 1) and relatively higher $BCFs_{hoot}$ (more than 1) can be considered as an accumulator/phytoextractor, while $BCF_{root} > 1$ and $TF < 1$ would be identified as a phytostabilizer species (Sharma et al. 2020).

28.5 Strategies Used to Control the Bioavailability of TEs

Depending on available metal(loid)s, soil physicochemical properties, and available resources, one determine the suitable soil remediation technique to apply for the particular soil (Palansooriya et al. 2020). There are different types of remediation strategies available to minimize TEs bioavailability to plants as well as their bioaccessibility in animal body (Palansooriya et al. 2020).

28.5.1 Incorporation of Soil Amendments with Soil

Using the immobilization techniques, mobility of metal(loids)s would be reduced by incorporating various soil amendments, both organic (e.g. biochar, animal waste, biosolids, compost, and plant residues) and inorganic (e.g. clay minerals, metal oxides, phosphates, and liming ingredients). Besides improving metal immobilization, these amendments would improve the soil physicochemical characteristics and are concurrently considered as an environmentally friendly approach in sustainable agriculture (Palansooriya et al. 2020).

Use of soil amendments is considered an in situ remediation method that considered an inexpensive and less environmental disturbance method (Palansooriya et al. 2020). However, in some occasions, it has reported some contradictory results also (Shaheen et al. 2017).

28.5.1.1 Biochar

Biochar is produced through pyrolysis of several biological wastes, such as grasses, crop residues, sewage, wood, and animal waste (Shaheen et al. 2019). Biochar carries out the immobilization process basically through activation of electrostatic interactions, surface precipitation, and ion exchange mechanisms (Shaheen et al. 2019). However, according to recent research findings, novel modifications of biochar pyrolysis have been found, especially for enhancement of metal binding abilities such as ammonia-ambiance pyrolysis, steam activation, microwave-assisted pyrolysis, and clay mineral modifications (Wang et al. 2021). Besides metal immobilization, biochar application would improve rhizosphere microbial activities, soil fertility, and carbon sequestration and prevent soil acidification (Wang et al. 2021).

28.5.1.2 Industrial By-Products

Industrial waste-based products are largely available from different industries. For instance, in coal industry, "coal combustion fly ash" is a major by-product, and the presence of mineral compounds in the ash has the capability to immobilize metals with oxides (Palansooriya et al. 2020). Similarly, "red mud" derived from alumina industry contained oxides (e.g. Al_2O_3, SiO_2, CaO, Fe_2O_3) that had the potential to be used as an immobilizing mediator for contaminated soil (Wang et al. 2018).

28.5.1.3 Natural Minerals

Incorporation of minerals with soil is an excellent method to adsorb trace metals through activation of surface complexation and precipitation mechanisms (Wang et al. 2021). Especially, modified clay minerals application (e.g. modified montmorillonite with humic acid) is considered as a viable option to augment Hg and Cd stabilization (Wang et al. 2020c). Similarly, Liang et al. 2019 found mercapto-modified attapulgite for Cd immobilization in soil. In addition to clay, different other natural minerals are also being tested for sustainable remediation strategies (Wang et al. 2021).

28.5.1.4 Metal Oxides

Metal oxides are considered as immobilization mediators as they promote inner-sphere complexation and precipitation of metals (Wang et al. 2021). These oxides include hydroxides, oxyhydroxides, and hydrous oxides (Wang et al. 2021), where iron oxides, manganese oxides, aluminum oxides, and magnesium oxides are the major metal oxides used to stabilize heavy metals (Shen et al. 2019). Both cationic and anionic metal(loid)s can be stabilized utilizing metal oxides for long-term metal fixing (Hou et al. 2020). For instance, MgO-based binders stabilize Cd and Pd precipitation under alkaline soil condition (Shen et al. 2019).

28.5.2 Phytomining

Phytomining is an environmentally healthy method that could be used for metal mining compared to open-cast mining activities, and this method would effectively be used in lands that were contaminated with metal(loid)s (Wang et al. 2021). Plants response to metal(loid)s are highly diverse. However, excessive metal absorption by plants leads to harmful results. Therefore, plants have developed several tolerance and resistance strategies to mitigate the negative impact of toxic elements on plants' growth and development (Yan et al. 2020). Generally, the plants that accumulate toxic metals beyond the normally accepted level are termed as "hyperaccumulators" (Wang et al. 2021). In phytomining process, we mainly target these hyperaccumulator species and extract metals from contaminated soils such as mine tailings and metalliferous soils (Wang et al. 2021). After completion of the metal absorption process, the biomass produced from hyperaccumulator plant should be incinerated or well treated (Antoniadis et al. 2021).

Plant selection for the phytomining process is a crucial aspect. Vigorous growth, higher biomass production, and adaptation to the wild nature/environment are key characteristics of a hyperaccumulator plant; thus, native wild plants are more suitable for the phytomining process (Ramírez et al. 2021). Recently conducted research on suitability of wild plants for phytomining is shown in Table 28.1. However, metal bioavailability can be achieved through changing soil pH, adding chelating agents, applying organic amendments, cropping patterns, and harvesting strategies (Antoniadis et al. 2021; Wang et al. 2021).

Apart from metal removal, phytomining provides other benefits as well. The plant canopy reduces wind erosion and runoff while improving the rhizosphere environment (Wang et al. 2021). However, sometimes accuracy of remediation would reduce and require considerable time period for remediation process are major consequences of this strategy (Wang et al. 2021).

28.5.3 Phytoremediation

This approach is quite similar to phytomining, but phytoremediation mainly focuses on the pollutants removal or

Table 28.1 Phytoremediation capacities of terrestrial wild plants (relevant to latest research experiments).

No	Plant species	Plant type	Pot/field trial	Soil texture	Soil pH	Existing metals in soil	Initial metal concentration in soil (mg/Kg)	BCF (shoot)	TF	Phytoextractor/ phytostabilizer	Hyperaccumulator/ non-hyperaccumulator	Key findings	References
1	*Artemisia vulgaris*	Herbaceous perennial	Pot trial	Sand – 33% silt – 39% clay – 28%	5.8	Cd	9	7.53	1.48	Phytoextractor (Cd)phytostabilizer (Zn)	Non-hyperaccumulator	Most highly PTE absorbing especially Zn and Cd, lesser degree of Cu and Ni	Antoniadis et al. (2021)
						As	120.8	<1	3.05				
						Cr	145.3	<1	2.31				
						Pd	176	<1	1.65				
						Zn	880.1	6.855	<1				
	Stellaria holostea	Herbaceous perennial				Cr	145.3	<1	<1	Potential phytostabilizer (Zn)	Non-hyperaccumulator		
						Zn	880.1	3.538	<1				
						Cd	9	<1	2.4				
	Galium mollugo	Herbaceous annual				Cd	9	<1	<1	Potential phytostabilizer (Zn)	Non-hyperaccumulator		
						Zn	880.1	1.91	<1				
2	*Ailanthus glandulosa* L.	Deciduous tree	Field trial	Loamy soil (coarse fragments – 36.69%, sand – 39.5%, clay – 5.97%)	N/A	Pd	22 948.6	<1	8.03	Potential phytostabilizer of	Non-hyperaccumulator	*Verbascum thapsus* L. identified as a hyperaccumulator for Cd	Čudić et al. (2016)
						Cr	41.7	<1	1.67				
						Zn	85 301.7	<1	2.57				
	V. thapsus L.	Herbaceous biannual				Cd	11 613	<1	<1	Potential phytoextractor	Hyperaccumulator (Cd)		
						Pd	22 948.6	<1	<1				
						Cr	41.7	<1	1				
	Artemisia artemisiifolia L.	Annual herb				Cd	11 613	<1	1.308	Potential phytoextractor	Non-hyperaccumulator		
						Zn	101 220	<1	<1				
	Populus spp.	Deciduous tree				Pd	22 948.6	<1	<1	Potential phytoextractor	Non-hyperaccumulator		
3	*Acalypha alopecuroida*	Annual herb	Field trial	Clay loam luvic calcisols (WRB)	8.12	Pd	386.54	<1	1.4	Phytoextractor (Zn)	Non-hyperaccumulator	Any of these plants has the potential to phytoremediate Cr and Pd metals. However, bioaccumulation potential of Zn is higher than Pd and Cr	Ramírez et al. (2021)
						Zn	119.2	1.5	1.31				
						Cr	15.67	<1	1.21				
	Heliotropium angiospermum	Perennial Shrub				Pd	386.54	<1	<1	Phytoextractor (Zn)	Non-hyperaccumulator		
						Zn	119.2	1.84	1.59				
						Cr	15.67	<1	1.49				
	Sida rhombifolia	Shrub				Pd	386.54	<1	<1	Phytoextractor (Zn)	Non-hyperaccumulator		
						Zn	119.2	1.55	1.19				
						Cr	15.67	<1	1.2				
	Bidens pilosa	Annual weed				Zn	119.2	1.25	<1	Potential phytostabilizer	Non-hyperaccumulator		

(*Continued*)

Table 28.1 (Continued)

No	Plant species	Plant type	Pot/field trial	Soil texture	Soil pH	Existing metals in soil	Initial metal concentration in soil (mg/Kg)	BCF (shoot)	TF	Phytoextractor/ phytostabilizer	Hyperaccumulator/ non-hyperaccumulator	Key findings	References
4	*Conyza bonariensis*	Annual herb	Field trial	Silt loam	7.5	Pd	127	N/A	<1	—	Non-hyperaccumulator	None of the plants have been identified as hyper accumulators	Abou-Shanad et al. (2017)
	Lactuca serriola	Annual or Biennial herb			6.6	Cu	245	N/A	2.09	Potential phytoextractor	Non-hyperaccumulator		
	Amaranthus sp.	Herb			6.6	Pd	127	N/A	6.63	Potential phytoextractor	Non-hyperaccumulator		
	Anagallis sp.	Annual flowering plant			7.4	Pd	77	N/A	7.92	Potential phytoextractor	Non-hyperaccumulator		
	Malva parviflora	Annual herb			7.9	Cu	230	N/A	6.3	Potential phytoextractor	Non-hyperaccumulator		
	Chenopodium ambrosioides	Annual or Short-lived perennial herb			7.5	Zn	10	N/A	2.4	Potential phytoextractor	Non-hyperaccumulator		
5	*Rhazya stricta* L.	Shrub	Pot experiment	N/A	N/A	Cd	10	1.4	0.88	Phytostabilizer	Non-hyperaccumulator	*R. stricta* has exhibited mobility of heavy metals and potential to phytoremediator for lightly polluted soil	Azab and Hegazy (2020)
						Zn	50	1.2	0.88				
6	*Pteriduum aquilinum*	Fern	Field trial	N/A	N/A	Cd	0.8	28.55	1.26	Phytostabilizer	Non-hyperaccumulator	Plants showed positive correlation of translocation of heavy metals (Ex: Hg—Cd, Hg—Zn, Hg—Pd, Cd—Pd, Cd—Zn) as well as negative correlations (Cr—Hg, Cr—Cd, Cd—Hg)	Fu et al. (2019)
						Hg	1.72	<1	1.88	Phytoextractor			
						Cr	8.15	6.89	<1	Phytostabilizer			
	Fagopyrum dibotrys	Perennial plant				Cr	58.51	<1	12.39	Phytoextractor	Non-hyperaccumulator		
	Pteris vittata	Fern				Cd	10.07	16.27	2.06	Phytostabilizer	Non-hyperaccumulator		
						Cr	13.85	5.31	<1	Phytostabilizer			
						Zn	156	7.31	<1	Phytostabilizer			
	Dryopteris erythrosora	Fern				Cd	10.07	4.98	<1	Phytostabilizer	Non-hyperaccumulator		
						Zn	156	6.43	<1	Phytostabilizer			
	Rumex patientia	Herbaceous perennial				Cr	58.51	<1	3.44	Phytoextractor	Non-hyperaccumulator		
7	*Tetraena qataranse*	Dwarf shrub	Field trial	N/A	8.05	Cd	1	1.5	1.6	Phytoextractor (Cd)and phytostabilizer (Cr, Cu, Ni)	Non-hyperaccumulator	Cd bio availability become less with an increase pH level	Usman et al. (2019)
						Cr	24.2	1.5	<1				
						Cu	8	3.9	<1				
						Ni	7.2	12.2	<1				

immobilization capabilities of plants (Wang et al. 2021). The phytoremediation process is composed of a few strategies, namely phytoextraction, phytostabilization, and phytovolatalization; among these strategies, phytoextraction is widely used or well-studied approach for phytoremediation (Wang et al. 2021). In phytoextraction techniques, trace metal(loid)s are absorbed by roots, transmitted to stem or leaves, and accumulated in above ground parts/harvesting parts (Wang et al. 2021). Then, biomass should be harvested at the right stage and incinerated; the ash derived from the process is safely disposed of in landfills (Antoniadis et al. 2021). However, biomass combustion and disposal procedures of ashes should be carefully monitored, as they directly impact health and cause environmental pollution (Antoniadis et al. 2021). The phytostabilization technique totally differs from the phytoextraction process. In phytostabilization, plant root exudates would decrease the metal mobility in the rhizosphere, which ultimately reduces the bioavailability of metals (Yan et al. 2020, Figure 28.2). This can occur due to metal precipitation or physical adsorption by plants (Wang et al. 2021). Phytovolatalization involves remediation process through the transfer of volatilized contaminants (e.g. Hg) from soil to atmosphere (Awa and Hadibarata 2020, Figure 28.2). Generally, metallophytes or metal-tolerant plant species are the ideal candidates for phytoremediation, and numerous research have already been conducted to identify these species (Wang et al. 2021). According to plant physicochemical reactions to high metal concentrations in soil, metallophytes could be further divided into three categories, such as accumulators, indicators, and excluders (Lago-Vila et al. 2019). Accumulators absorb metal(loid)s from the soil and efficiently transfer them to the shoot; thus, these plants would use the phytoextraction process (Wang et al. 2021, Figure 28.2). Indicators bioaccumulate metals in plant tissues, while excluders avoid metal uptake as well as translocation, ensuing phytostabilization approach (Wang et al. 2021).

Phytoremediation is a nature-based remediation method and can be used effectively for large areas (Wang et al. 2021). Similar to phytomining, plant selection for phytoremediation is a critical step, which determines the effectiveness of the remediation process. Especially, the availability of the selected plant species and their survival ability under local climatic conditions are highly concerning (Yan et al. 2020). Therefore, native or indigenous plants are more suitable for remediation than exotic species (Ramírez et al. 2021). In addition, fast growing ability, high biomass production, and well-developed root system are other key characteristics of a phytoremediator species (Yan et al. 2020). Simultaneously, plant species extract relatively large quantities of metal(loid)s or hyperaccumulators, which are also effectively used for the remediation process, thus speed-up the metal removal from soil (Wang et al. 2021).

28.5.4 Microbial Bioremediation

Microbial intervention in metals removal process is quite interesting to study. Most of the microbes in the soil are genetically resistant to heavy metals or trace metal absorption, and some can survive in extreme metal concentrated soil (Hou et al. 2020). However, as a result of intensively conducted research, some of the microbial species have been identified that are useful for the microbial remediation process (Wang et al. 2021). Basically, microbial bioremediation depends on stabilization, bioaccumulation, or detoxification strategies (Wang et al. 2021). Microbial-based stabilization occurs through the production of carbonates or oxides (Wang et al. 2021). For instance, *Providencia* sp. produces biogenic manganese oxide by oxidizing Mn(II) ions, which is a highly binding or stabilizing compound (Li et al. 2020). Nevertheless, the long-term stabilizing capacity of these compounds should be further analyzed under different environmental conditions, as several factors directly impact binding stability (Wang et al. 2021).

The microbial-induced detoxification strategies would involve the remediation of several TEs such as Cr, Hg, and As through oxidation of toxic forms to nontoxic or relatively low-hazardous forms (Wang et al. 2021). For example, Hg(II) converted into Hg(0) is derived by some bacterial species via series of enzymatic reactions, reducing the toxicity of particular metal (Wang et al. 2020b). Simultaneously, detoxification of Cr(VI) is mainly done by *Bacillus*, *Pseudomonas*, and *Enterobacter* species (Tan et al. 2021), since *Acidovorax* and *Azoarcus* species are used to detoxify As(III) into less toxic As(V) (Zhang et al. 2017).

Though microbial-based remediation is an environmentally healthy process, it consists of several drawbacks. Especially, microbial detoxification process is highly sensitive to environmental changes; thus, sometimes detoxification reactions would reverse and lead to the formation of toxic compounds in the soil (Beckers et al. 2019). For instance, enhancement of Eh in soil would disturb the microbial detoxification process of Hg(II), leading more Hg to accumulate in soil (Beckers et al. 2019). Furthermore, Saran et al. 2020 reported that some plant-growth promoting bacteria (PGPB) are involved in the phytostabilization process and reduce the bioavailability of Cd and Pd to a considerable level (Saran et al. 2020). However, apart from the bioremediation process, most of other microorganisms (e.g. plant-growth promoting bacteria) are involved in plant growth and development, metal tolerance, and metal bioavailability (Alka et al. 2020).

28.5.5 Artificially Established Wetlands

Constructed wetlands are artificial systems that are generally used for waste water treatment (Wang et al. 2021). Metal retention in wetlands is mediated in a variety of ways. Among them, sorption is a major process focusing on chemisorption and physisorption as potential long- and short-term immobilization techniques (Hu et al. 2020). Some aquatic plants bioaccumulate metal(loid)s, but few of them are considered as hyperaccumulators (Lu et al. 2018). In addition to the sorption process, wetland biotransformation and detoxification processes resemble microbial-induced bioremediation, which was described earlier (Section 28.5.4).

28.5.6 Soil Washing

Soil washing is a metal-specific process that proceeds through a washing solution and extracts the toxic metals, thus keeping the soil below the threshold level (Wang et al. 2021). The particular washing solution leads to an elevation of metal mobility while keeping the soil physicochemical properties (Wang et al. 2021). The success of the soil washing process is mainly determined by the type of extractant and water; chelating agents, surfactants, bases, and acids are prominent extractants used in the cleaning process (Liu et al. 2020). However, some washing solutions would results in some negative impacts. For example, after soil washing through EDTA chelates, remaining EDTA might cause harmful effects to soil microorganisms as well as groundwater pollution (Duo et al. 2019). Thus, natural organic solvents (Meng et al. 2017), biosurfactants, and biodegradable chelants (Guo et al. 2018) should be introduced after conducting both laboratory and field trials (Wang et al. 2021).

28.5.7 Bio-Electrokinetic Remediation

A unique technique called "electrokinetic remediation" uses an external electric field to remove harmful metals from soil that has been contaminated (López Vizcaíno et al. 2018). Nevertheless, it is difficult to practice this process practically due to high energy consumption; thus, microbial fuel cells (MFCs) have emerged very recently as an innovative bio-electrochemical system (Aarthy et al. 2019). The whole process ensues under anaerobic conditions, and both anode and cathode reactions result in metal removal through the microbial oxidation process (Wang et al. 2021). Compared to phytoremediation, this technique requires relatively less duration for the remediation process, and microbial activities/density would accelerate the process; thus, the application of organic matter is a significant practice to enhance the microbial activities in the area (Zhang et al. 2019).

Metal(loid)s movement of soil highly depend on geochemical nature of soil, and mostly liable forms of metals migrate more easily compared to less-liable forms; therefore, several auxiliary regents such as acetic or citric acid might useful to mobilize the elements through acidification of soil (Zhang et al. 2020). However, this method has not yet become famous in the field as environmental factors and soil heterogeneity characteristics directly influence the process (Wang et al. 2021).

28.5.8 Low-Temperature Thermal Desorption

This strategy is more effective for remediation of volatile metal(loid)s in polluted soil, especially Hg (Wang et al. 2021). According to research findings, incorporation of chemical agents such as citric and $FeCl_3$ would reduce the heating temperature around 400 °C and accelerate the Hg removal competency (Wang et al. 2021). Hg volatilization at low temperature might be due to the low pH environment supplied by the incorporated acids or due to the production of volatile Hg compounds such as $HgCl_2$ or Hg_2Cl_2 (Wang et al. 2021).

Similar to other remediation strategies, this method also consists of a few drawbacks such as time consuming, reduce the soil sustainability as a result of addition of acids, less feasibility, etc. (Wang et al. 2021).

28.6 Remarks

The accumulation of TEs in the soil is directly impacted by both human and natural activity. Among them, most of toxic trace metals accumulate in the soil owing to human activities. Considerable portion of the accumulated trace metal(loid)s would be taken up by plants and leads to bioaccumulate in plant tissues, which ultimately deposit in human body through oral ingestion and cause crucial health hazards for humans. The bioavailability of TEs depends mostly on soil physicochemical properties as well as inherent metal(loid)s characteristics. With the objective of mitigating TEs plant absorption, numerous remediation strategies have been used. Basically, to lessen the mobility of metal(loid)s, various types of soil amendments are being applied. Simultaneously, phytoremediation, microbial remediation, establishment of wetlands, and energy-based remediation measures are also widely used in the current scenario. However, it is important to investigate novel technologies to eliminate the exciting consequences of current methods. In addition, introducing plants with highly efficient metal uptake and translocate capacities (transgenic plants) through genetic engineering is a viable option for phytoremediation. Similarly, identification of suitable microorganisms that could be used in the bioremediation process and further understanding of microbial activities on metal(loid)s would be essential. Finally, identifying the drawbacks of energy-based remediation measures and introducing sustainable mechanisms to mitigate the trace metal(loid)s accumulation as well as remediate polluted soils are timely needed prerequisites.

References

Aarthy, M., Rajesh, T., and Thirunavoukkarasu, M. (2019). Critical review on microbial fuel cells for concomitant reduction of hexavalent chromium and bioelectricity generation. *J. Chem. Technol. Biotechnol.* 95 (5): https://doi.org/10.1002/jctb.6257.

Abou-Shanad, R.A.I., Amel, A.T., Weam, H.E., and Mahmound, M.M. (2017). Phytoremediation potential of wild plants collected from heavy metals contaminated soils. *Int. J. Geol. Agric. Environ. Sci.* 5 (4): 15–19.

Ali, W., Mao, K., Zhang, H. et al. (2020). Comprehensive review of the basic chemical behaviours, sources, processes, and endpoints of trace element contamination in paddy soil-rice systems in rice-growing countries. *J. Hazard. Mater.* 397: 122720. https://doi.org/10.1016/j.jhazmat.2020.122720.

Alka, S., Shahir, S., Ibrahim, N. et al. (2020). The role of plant growth promoting bacteria on arsenic removal: a review of existing perspectives. *Environ. Technol. Innov.* 17: 100602. https://doi.org/10.1016/j.eti.2020.100602.

Antoniadis, V., Shaheen, S.M., Stark, H.J. et al. (2021). Phytoremediation potential of twelve wild plant species for toxic elements in a contaminated soil. *Environ. Int.* 146: https://doi.org/10.1016/j.envint.2020.106233.

Awa, S.H. and Hadibarata, T. (2020). Removal of heavy metals in contaminated soil by phytoremediation mechanism: a review. *Water Air Soil Pollut.* 231: 47. https://doi.org/10.1007/s11270-020-4426-0.

Azab, E. and Hegazy, A.K. (2020). Monitoring the efficiency of *Rhazya stricta* L. plants in phytoremediation of heavy metal-contaminated soil. *Plan. Theory* 9 (9): 1057. https://doi.org/10.3390/plants9091057.

Bastow, E.L., Garcia De La Torre, V.S., Maclean, A.E. et al. (2018). Vacuolar iron stores gated by NRAMP3 and NRAMP4 are the primary source of iron in germinating seeds. *Plant Physiol.* 177: 1267–1276. https://doi.org/10.1104/pp.18.00478.

Beckers, F., Awad, Y.M., Beiyuan, J. et al. (2019). Impact of biochar on mobilization, methylation, and ethylation of mercury under dynamic redox conditions in a contaminated floodplain soil. *Environ. Int.* 127: 276–290. https://doi.org/10.1016/j.envint.2019.03.040.

Cempel, M. and Nikel, G. (2006). Nickel: a review of its sources and environmental toxicology. *Pol. J. Environ. Stud.* 15: 375–382.

Clemens, S. (2006). Toxic metal accumulation, responses to exposure and mechanisms of tolerance in plants. *Biochimie* 88: 1707–1719. https://doi.org/10.1016/j.biochi.2006.07.003.

Čudić, V., Stojiljković, D., and Jovović, A. (2016). Phytoremediation potential of wild plants growing on soil contaminated with heavy metals. *Arh. Hig. Rada Toksikol.* 67 (229–239): https://doi.org/10.1515/aiht-2016-67-2829.

Cui, H., Zhang, X., Wu, Q. et al. (2020). Hematite enhances the immobilization of copper, cadmium and phosphorus in soil amended with hydroxyapatite under flooded conditions. *Sci. Total Environ.* 708: 134590. https://doi.org/10.1016/j.scitotenv.2019.134590.

DalCorso, G., Fasani, E., Manara, A. et al. (2019). Heavy metal pollutions: state of the art and innovation in phytoremediation. *Int. J. Mol. Sci.* 20: 3412. https://doi.org/10.3390/ijms20143412.

Duo, L., Yin, L., Zhang, C., and Zhao, S. (2019). Ecotoxicological responses of the earthworm *Eisenia fetida* to EDTA addition under turfgrass growing conditions. *Chemosphere* 220: 56–60. https://doi.org/10.1016/j.chemosphere.2018.12.106.

Feng, W., Guo, Z., Xiao, X. et al. (2019). Atmospheric deposition as a source of cadmium and lead to soil-rice system and associated risk assessment. *Ecotoxicol. Environ. Saf.* 180: 160–167. https://doi.org/10.1016/j.ecoenv.2019.04.090.

Fu, S., Wei, C., Xiao, Y. et al. (2019). Heavy metals uptake and transport by native wild plants: implications for phytoremediation and restoration. *Environ. Earth Sci.* 78: 103. https://doi.org/10.1007/s12665-019-8103-9.

Gong, L., Wang, J., Abbas, T. et al. (2021). Immobilization of exchangeable Cd in soil using mixed amendment and its effect on soil microbial communities under paddy upland rotation system. *Chemosphere* 262: 127828. https://doi.org/10.1016/j.chemosphere.2020.127828.

Guo, X., Zhang, G., Wei, Z. et al. (2018). Mixed chelators of EDTA, GLDA, and citric acid as washing agent effectively remove Cd, Zn, Pb, and Cu from soils. *J. Soils Sediments* 18: 835–844. https://doi.org/10.1007/s11368-017-1781-6.

Gustin, J.L., Zanis, M.J., and Salt, D.E. (2011). Structure and evolution of the plantcation diffusion facilitator family of ion transporters. *BMC Evol. Biol.* 11: 76. https://doi.org/10.1186/1471-2148-11-76.

Hou, D., O'Connor, D., Igalavithana, A.D. et al. (2020). Metal contamination and bioremediation of agricultural soils for food safety and sustainability. *Nat. Rev. Earth Environ.* 1 (7): 366–381. https://doi.org/10.1038/s43017-020-0061-y.

Hu, Z., Chu, Y., and Ma, Y. (2020). Design of a combined constructed wetland system and its application on swine wastewater treatment. *Int. J. Environ. Eng. (U. S.).* 146: 1602. https://doi.org/10.1061/(ASCE)EE.1943-7870.0001602.

Ismael, M.A., Elyamine, A.M., Moussa, M.G. et al. (2019). Cadmium in plants: uptake, toxicity, and its interactions with selenium fertilizers. *Metallomics* 11: 255–277. https://doi.org/10.1039/c8mt00247a.

Khan, S., Naushad, M., Lima, E.C. et al. (2021). Global soil pollution by toxic elements: current status and future perspectives on the risk assessment and remediation strategies – a review. *J. Hazard. Mater.* 417: 126039. https://doi.org/10.1016/j.jhazmat.2021.126039.

Kumpiene, J., Giagnoni, L., Marschner, B. et al. (2017). Assessment of methods for determining bioavailability of trace elements in soils: a review. *Pedosphere* 27: 389–406. https://doi.org/10.1016/S1002-0160(17)60337-0.

Lago-Vila, M., Arenas-Lago, D., Rodríguez-Seijo, A. et al. (2019). Ability of *Cytisus scoparius* for phytoremediation of soils from a Pb/Zn mine: assessment of metal bioavailability and bioaccumulation. *J. Environ. Manag.* 235: 152–160. https://doi.org/10.1016/j.jenvman.2019.01.058.

Li, D., Li, R., Ding, Z. et al. (2020). Discovery of a novel native bacterium of *Providencia* sp. with high biosorption and oxidation ability of manganese for bioleaching of heavy metal contaminated soils. *Chemosphere* 241 (125039): https://doi.org/10.1016/j.chemosphere.2019.125039.

Liang, X.F., Li, N., He, L.Z. et al. (2019). Inhibition of Cd accumulation in winter wheat (*Triticum aestivum* L.) grown in alkaline soil using mercapto-modified attapulgite. *Sci. Total Environ.* 688: 818–826. https://doi.org/10.1016/j.scitotenv.2019.06.335.

Lin, J., He, F., Owens, G., and Chen, Z. (2021). How do phytogenic iron oxide nanoparticles drive redox reactions to reduce cadmium availability in a flooded paddy soil? *J. Hazard. Mater.* 403: 123736. https://doi.org/10.1016/j.jhazmat.2020.123736.

Liu, J., Xue, J., Yuan, D. et al. (2020). Surfactant washing to remove heavy metal pollution in soil: a review. *Recent Innov. Chem. Eng.* 13: 3–16. https://doi.org/10.2174/24055 20412666190912151737.

López Vizcaíno, R., Yustres, A., Asensio, L. et al. (2018). Enhanced electrokinetic remediation of polluted soils by anolyte pH conditioning. *Chemosphere* 199: 477–485. https://doi.org/10.1016/j.chemosphere.2018.02.038.

Lu, G., Wang, B., Zhang, C. et al. (2018). Heavy metals contamination and accumulation in submerged macrophytes in an urban river in China. *Int. J. Phytoremediation* 20: 839–846. https://doi.org/10.1080/15226514.2018.1438354.

Ma, J.F., Shen, R.F., and Shao, J.F. (2021). Transport of cadmium from soil to grain in cereal crops: a review. *Pedosphere* 31: 3–10. https://doi.org/10.1016/S1002-0160(20)60015-7.

Meng, F., Yuan, G., Wei, J. et al. (2017). Humic substances as a washing agent for Cd-contaminated soils. *Chemosphere* 181: 461–467. https://doi.org/10.1016/j.chemosphere.2017.04.127.

Murtaza, G., Javed, W., Hussain, A. et al. (2017). Soil-applied zinc and copper suppress cadmium uptake and improve the performance of cereals and legumes. *Int. J. Phytoremediat.* 19: 199–206. https://doi.org/10.1080/15226514.2016.1207605.

Ng, J.C., Juhasz, A., and Smith, E. (2015). Assessing the bioavailability and bioaccessibility of metals and metalloids. *Environ. Sci. Pollut. Res.* 22: 8802–8825. https://doi.org/10.1007/s11356-013-1820-9.

O'Connor, D., Hou, D., Ok, Y.S. et al. (2019). Mercury speciation, transformation, and transportation in soils, atmospheric flux, and implications for risk management: a critical review. *Environ. Int.* 126: 747–761. https://doi.org/10.1016/j.envint.2019.03.019.

Palansooriya, K.N., Shaheen, S.M., Chen, S.S. et al. (2020). Soil amendments for immobilization of potentially toxic elements in contaminated soils: a critical review. *Environ. Int.* 134: https://doi.org/10.1016/j.envint.2019.105046.

Petruzzelli, G., Pedron, F., and Rosellin, I. (2019). Bioavailability and bioaccessibility in soil: a short review and a case study. *AIMS Environ. Sci.* 7: 208–225. https://doi.org/10.3934/environsci.2020013.

Ramírez, A., García, G., Werner, O. et al. (2021). Implications of the phytoremediation of heavy metal contamination of soils and wild plants in the industrial area of Haina, Dominican Republic. *Sustainability* 13: 1403. https://doi.org/10.3390/su13031403.

Rehman, M.Z., Rizwan, M., Ali, S. et al. (2017). Remediation of heavy metal contaminated soils by using Solanum nigrum: a review. *Ecotoxicol. Environ. Saf.* 143: 236–248. https://doi.org/10.1016/j.ecoenv.2017.05.038.

Reis, A.T., Lopes, C.B., Davidson, C.M. et al. (2015). Extraction of available and labile fractions of mercury from contaminated soils: the role of operational parameters. *Geoderma* 259: 213–223. https://doi.org/10.1016/j.geoderma.2015.06.004.

Sakan, S., Popović, A., Škrivanj, S. et al. (2016). Comparison of single extraction procedures and the application of an index for the assessment of heavy metal bioavailability in river sediments. *Environ. Sci. Pollut. Res.* 23: 485–500. https://doi.org/10.1007/s11356-016-7341-6.

Salam, A., Bashir, S., Khan, I. et al. (2019). Biochar induced Pb and Cu immobilization, phytoavailability attenuation in Chinese cabbage, and improved biochemical properties in naturally co-contaminated soil. *J. Soils Sediments* 19: 2381–2392. https://doi.org/10.1007/s11368-019-02250-5.

Saran, A., Imperato, V., Fernandez, L. et al. (2020). Phytostabilization of polluted military soil supported by bioaugmentation with PGP trace element tolerant bacteria isolated from helianthus petiolaris. *Agronomy* 10: 204. https://doi.org/10.3390/agronomy10020204.

Shaheen, S.M., Shams, M.S., Khalifa, M.R. et al. (2017). Various soil amendments and environmental wastes affect the (im)mobilization and phytoavailability of potentially toxic elements in a sewage effluent irrigated sandy soil. *Ecotoxicol. Environ. Saf.* 142: 375–387. https://doi.org/10.1016/j.ecoenv.2017.04.026.

Shaheen, S.M., Niazi, N.K., Hassan, N.E.E. et al. (2019). Wood-based biochar for the removal of potentially toxic elements in water and wastewater: a critical review. *Int. Mater. Rev.* 64: 216–247. https://doi.org/10.1080/09506608.2018.1473096.

Shaheen, S.M., Antoniadis, V., Kwon, E. et al. (2020). Soil contamination by potentially toxic elements and the associated human health risk in geo-and anthropogenic contaminated soils: a case study from the temperate region (Germany) and the arid region (Egypt). *Environ. Pollut.* 262: 114312. https://doi.org/10.1016/j.envpol.2020.114312.

Shahid, M., Dumat, C., Khalid, S., Niazi, N. K., Antunes, P. M. C. (2016). Cadmium bioavailability, uptake, toxicity and detoxification in soil-plant system. Reviews of Environmental Contamination and Toxicology (eds Gunther, F. A. and De Voogt, P.), Springer.73–137

Sharma, P., Tripathi, S., and Chandra, R. (2020). Phytoremediation potential of heavy metal accumulator plants for waste management in the pulp and paper industry. *Heliyon* 6 (7): https://doi.org/10.1016/j.heliyon.2020.e04559.

Shen, Z., Pan, S., Hou, D. et al. (2019). Temporal effect of MgO reactivity on the stabilization of lead contaminated soil. *Environ. Int.* 131: 104990. https://doi.org/10.1016/j.envint.2019.104990.

Sihlahla, M., Mouri, H., and Nomngongo, P.N. (2020). Assessment of bioavailability and mobility of major and trace elements in agricultural soils collected in Port St Johns, Eastern Cape, South Africa using single extraction procedures and pseudo-total digestion. *J. Environ. Health Sci. Eng.* 18: 1615–1628. https://doi.org/10.1007/s40201-020-00581-x.

Tang, X., Huang, Y., Li, Y. et al. (2021). Study on detoxification and removal mechanisms of hexavalent chromium by microorganisms. *Ecotoxicol. Environ. Saf.* 208: 111699. https://doi.org/10.1016/j.ecoenv.2020.111699.

US National Research Council-US NRC (2002). *Bioavailability of Contaminants in Soils and Sediments: Processes, Tools, and Applications*. Washington: National Academies Press.

Usman, K., Al-Ghouti, M.A., and Abu-Dieyeh, M.H. (2019). The assessment of cadmium, chromium, copper, and nickel tolerance and bioaccumulation by shrub plant *Tetraena qataranse*. *Sci. Rep.* 9: 5658. https://doi.org/10.1038/s41598-019-42029-9.

Vromman, D., Martínez, J.P., Kumar, M. et al. (2018). Comparative effects of arsenite (As(III)) and arsenate (As(V)) on whole plants and cell lines of the arsenic-resistant halophyte plant species *Atriplex atacamensis*. *Environ. Sci. Pollut. Res.* 25: 34473–34486. https://doi.org/10.1007/s11356-018-3351-x.

Wang, Y., Li, F., Song, J. et al. (2018). Stabilization of Cd, Pb, Cu and Zn contaminated calcareous agricultural soil using red mud: a field experiment. *Environ. Geochem. Health* 40: 2143–2153. https://doi.org/10.1007/s10653-018-0089-9.

Wang, P., Peng, H., Liu, J. et al. (2020a). Effects of exogenous dissolved organic matter on the adsorption–desorption behaviors and bioavailabilities of Cd and Hg in a plant–soil system. *Sci. Total Environ.* 728: 138252. https://doi.org/10.1016/j.scitotenv.2020.138252.

Wang, L., Hou, D., Cao, Y. et al. (2020b). Remediation of mercury contaminated soil, water, and air: a review of emerging materials and innovative technologies. *Environ. Int.* 134: 105281. https://doi.org/10.1016/j.envint.2019.10528.

Wang, L., Li, X., Tsang, D.C.W. et al. (2020c). Green remediation of Cd and Hg contaminated soil using humic acid modified montmorillonite: immobilization performance under accelerated ageing conditions. *J. Hazard. Mater.* 387: 122005. https://doi.org/10.1016/j.jhazmat.2019.122005.

Wang, L., Rinklebe, J., Tack, F.M.G., and Hou, D.A. (2021). Review of green remediation strategies for heavy metal contaminated soil. *Soil Use Manag.* 1–28. https://doi.org/10.1111/sum.12717.

Weissmannov'a, H.D. and Pavlovský, J. (2017). Indices of soil contamination by heavy metals– methodology of calculation for pollution assessment (minireview). *Environ. Monit. Assess.* 189: 616. https://doi.org/10.1007/s10661-017-6340-5.

Wen, E., Yang, X., Chen, H. et al. (2021). Iron-modified biochar and water management regime induced changes in plant growth, enzyme activities, and phytoavailability of arsenic, cadmium and lead in a paddy soil. *J. Hazard.*

Mater. 407: 124344. https://doi.org/10.1016/j.jhazmat.2020.124344.

Wiggenhauser, M., Aucour, A.M., Bureau, S. et al. (2021). Cadmium transfer in contaminated soil-rice systems: insights from solid-state speciation analysis and stable isotope fractionation. *Environ. Pollut.* 269: 115934. https://doi.org/10.1016/j.envpol.2020.115934.

Wu, C., Shi, L., Xue, S. et al. (2019). Effect of sulfuriron modified biochar on the available cadmium and bacterial community structure in contaminated soils. *Sci. Total Environ.* 647: 1158–1168. https://doi.org/10.1016/j.scitotenv.2018.08.087.

Yan, A., Wang, Y., Tan, S.N. et al. (2020). Phytoremediation: a promising approach for revegetation of heavy metal-polluted land. *Front. Plant Sci.* 11: 359. https://doi.org/10.3389/fpls.2020.00359.

Zhang, J., Zhao, S., Xu, Y. et al. (2017). Nitrate stimulates anaerobic microbial arsenite oxidation in Paddy soils. *Environ. Sci. Technol.* 51: 4377–4386. https://doi.org/10.1021/acs.est.6b06255.

Zhang, L., Rylott, E.L., Bruce, N.C., and Strand, S.E. (2018). Genetic modification of western wheat grass (*Pascopyrum smithii)* for the phytoremediation of RDX and TNT. *Planta* 249: 1007–1015. https://doi.org/10.1007/s00425-018-3057-9.

Zhang, T., Hu, L., Zhang, M. et al. (2019). Cr(VI) removal from soils and groundwater using an integrated adsorption and microbial fuel cell (A-MFC) technology. *Environ. Pollut.* 252: 1399–1405. https://doi.org/10.1016/j.envpol.2019.06.051.

Zhang, J., Cao, X., Wang, H. et al. (2020). Simultaneous enhancement of heavy metal removal and electricity generation in soil microbial fuel cell. *Ecotoxicol. Environ. Saf.* 192: 110314. https://doi.org/10.1016/j.ecoenv.2020.110314.

Zhou, J., Du, B., Liu, H. et al. (2020). The bioavailability and contribution of the newly deposited heavy metals (copper and lead) from atmosphere to rice (*Oryza sativa* L.). *J. Hazard. Mater.* 384: 121285. https://doi.org/10.1016/j.jhazmat.2019.121285.

Zhu, X., Yang, F., and Wei, C. (2015). Factors influencing the heavy metal bioaccessibility in soils were site dependent from different geographical locations. *Environ. Sci Pollut R.* 18: 13939–13949. https://doi.org/10.1007/s11356-015-4617-1.

29

"Light" as an Environmental Factor for the Well-Being of the "Plant, Animal, and Human Triad"

Prasada Rao Allu[1], Lakshmi Badrinarayanan[2], and Sailaja V. Elchuri[2]

[1] *Department of Horticulture, Sikkim Central University, Gangtok, Sikkim, India*
[2] *Department of Nanobiotechnology, Vision Research Foundation, Sankara Nethralaya, Chennai, Tamil Nadu, India*

29.1 Introduction

Sunlight is the principal source of energy for the planet Earth. The wave theory of light was popular in the nineteenth century, and this could explain the phenomenon of reflection, refraction, polarization interference, and diffraction of light (Thomson et al. 2010). The important features of the wave theory of light are:

1) Wavelength: different colors of the white light spectrum have different wavelengths: blue light 4.510^{-5} cm, green light 5.4×10^{-5} cm, and red light 6.6×10^{-5} cm.
2) The velocity of light was determined by Romer in 1676 as 3×10^{8} m.
3) Polarization of light: When light passes through a crystal it can split. However, at the beginning of the twentieth century, Einstein proposed photoelectric theory emphasizing the particle theory of light and proposed discrete energy particles called photons. Plank proposed a unit called quantum. Energy E is proportional to frequency. The particle and wave theory of lights were integrated to form quantum mechanics in the latter part of the century (Ditchburn 1952).

There are several phenomena in which light activates living and non-living objects on the Earth (Gudkov et al. 2017). Some important effects are *phototropism, photosynthesis, circadian rhythms, heliotropism, vision, phototherapy, synthesis of metabolites, and photocatalysis* (Figure 29.1). This chapter describes some aspects of light effects on plants, animals, and humans. However, the effect of light on chemical reactions is not covered here.

29.2 Phototropic Movements in Retina and Visual Function

Light is the primary source for performing numerous functions in living beings. The principal light mediated response is vision in humans and animals. Visual organs in humans play a critical role in finding/identification of objects around them to better survive in their place of living and do routine activities. Light perceived through an eye in humans specially the iris controls the amount of light that enters the eye by dilation process that facilitates to process sharp and clear vision due to the presence of photoreceptors. These are specialized neurons positioned in the retina, which convert light into electrical signals and send via optic nerve to the brain for performing the process of vision. Primarily, there are two types of photoreceptors present in human eye: rods and cones. Cone photoreceptors detect color through bright light and have specialized function to process blue (short-wavelength), green (medium-wavelength), and red (long-wavelength) light. Whereas the rod photoreceptors are sensitive to low-light levels. The photoreception in the receptor cells relies on the chemical response of a light-sensitive pigment rhodopsin in the retina of the eye.

In humans, light mediated movements are established in rods of the retina where the growth of the photoreceptors takes place in the direction of the light. This was first studied in 1937 and is called the Stiles Crawford effect (Stiles 1937). Due to diurnal variation and availability of light in different environmental conditions, the image formation on the retina may not be always same. In addition,

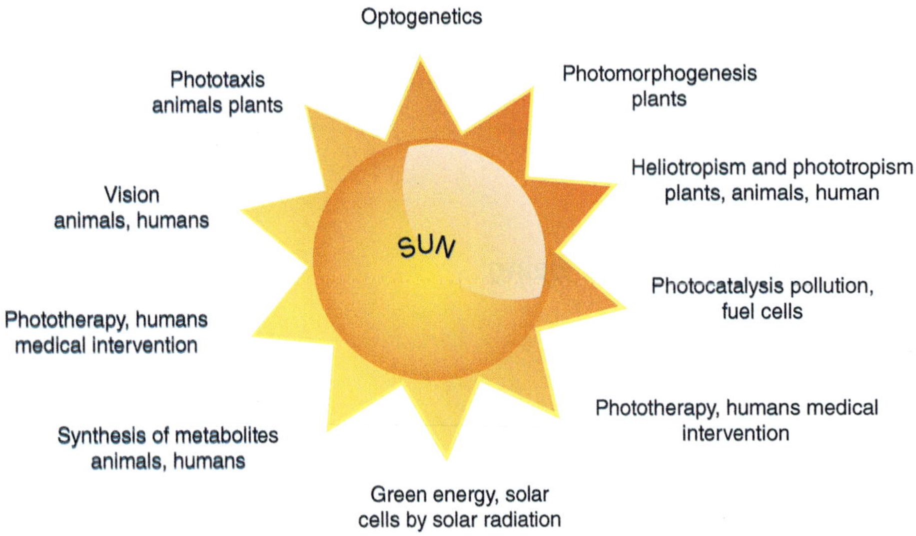

Figure 29.1 Effects of light on organisms and processes.

dysfunction in the eye due to age and other health conditions also affects the vision of humans and other animals. Normally, light passes in straight lines through the center of the pupil, and it is slanting in the periphery. This phenomenon is thought to occur due to the inner and the outer segments of the photoreceptors for guiding the light waves. Moreover, the photoreceptors are upright in the center of the retina, whereas they are tilted in the periphery. Studies revealed that the growth of photoreceptors is mostly associated with the direction of the light, and the degree of tilting is due to phototropism. Further, it is stated that this is not due to the developmental processes in the retina but is a phototropic response. Smallman et al. (2001) proposed that numerous external processes such as cataract surgery and pupil displacement can change the orientation of the photoreceptor cells. Several modeling studies with light gradients and directions were done to understand the phenomenon. Recently, this phenomenon is explained in primate retinas using classical immunohistochemistry and expansion microscopy that can visualize structures in three dimensions (Verschueren et al. 2022). The study proposed that the cone photoreceptor architecture is responsible for the Stiles Crawford effect. The actin and other cytoskeletal proteins arrangements lead to cell polarity in cone cells enabling the tilting of these cells toward the direction of the light. This phenomenon helps with phototransduction in the receptor cells and response to spectral quality of light. The oblique light reduces aberrations and glare when greater light intensity enters the eye. Additionally, the phototropic behavior by cones reduces the role of unwanted light that can influence the quality of image, contrast, and sharpness. The pupils may be widened or narrowed depending on the intensity of the light. If the pupils are wide (in general in low light condition) angular light is beneficial compared to straight light. The phototropism and its aid in vision is also observed in the retina of frogs and primates.

29.3 Phototropism in Plants

Tropic movements facilitate realignment of leaves and petioles that are associated with hormonal activity and/or voltage mediated response at the sites of action mediated through spectral quality/direction/intensity of light. Movements in plants were observed by classic studies of Darwin (1888). The movements are a result of light sensing through blue light and UV light receptors, aligning the photosynthetic tissue toward the light followed by the formation of gradients in the auxin hormone, which leads to the formation of asymmetric growth (Hohm et al. 2013). The spectral quality of (red, UV, and blue) light mediated phototropic responses were proposed in plants. The influence of light response curves includes the first positive and negative curve, the second positive and negative curve, and a possible third positive curve (du Buy and Nuernbergk 1934; Briggs 1960). However, the first and second positive curves were observed in many monocots and dicots by several researchers that are mediated by photoreceptors like phytochromes, phototropins, and cryptochromes. The blue light receptors phototropin I and II were proposed to mediate the positive curves, and the first negative curve could be the dark relaxation of the photoreceptors, which can be again activated due to the light gradient present in the tissue. Red light potentiated the blue light response and phytochrome enabled the first positive fluence curve.

The involvement of phototropins and phytochromes was shown by Jaedicke et al. (2012). They used protonema of *Physcomitrella patens* to understand the interactions between the two photoreceptors on the plasma membrane. When these two photoreceptors were put in *Arabidopsis thaliana,* the plant could show phototropic response. Recently, the signaling and phosphorylation events mediated through Phototropin 1 are elucidated in *Zea mays*. The low fluence blue light increased phosphorylation of serine at positions 291 and 376 of the protein accounting for the fluence response of the receptor. The phosphorylated protein affected the first positive curve of the phototropism (Suzuki et al. 2019). However, several unanswered questions persist as the fluency is several order magnitudes compared to the receptor phosphorylation (Briggs 2014). Several signaling intermediates for the blue light mediated response and the fluencies are under investigations. The phototropic response by this receptor is under low fluence rates and shuts off in high fluence rates by operating a molecular modification (phosphorylation) of phytochrome kinase substrate 4 (PKS4) (Schumacher et al. 2018).

The role of auxin receptors in the phototropic response is well studied (Briggs 2014). The auxin mediated growth response is shown to be mediated through annexin 1 (also known as *AtANN1*) and annexin 2 (*AtANN2*). These proteins perform the functions of calcium mediated responses, metabolism, and vesicle trafficking. Presence of these two genes that encode annexin proteins in *A. thaliana* could elicit blue light mediated phototropic response. However, when these genes are mutated, the mutated proteins in the plants could not respond well to blue light (Wang et al. 2022). There are several signaling intermediates that are identified in plants in addition to annexins that can mediate blue light mediated responses in plants. Nonphototropic hypocotyl 3 (NPH3) protein is one such protein that can mediate the light response by phosphorylation and dephosphorylation of the protein. It acts as a scaffold protein that can bring interaction with NPH1 protein that is a serine threonine kinase. This kinase senses blue light and performs downstream signaling causing phototropic changes. The role of NPH3 protein in the blue light mediated signaling cascade is studied recently. The blue light can cause alterations in the C-terminal domain of this protein, dissociate from membrane, and the dephosphorylation happens in cytosol. The dynamic membrane and cytosol localization mediated by light is found necessary for the growth mediated response by light. If localization of the protein is restricted either to the membrane or to the cytosol, the function of the protein is abolished resulting in the absence of phototropism. These studies emphasize a molecular signaling mechanism that can mediate phototropism (Reuter et al. 2021). Several key signaling players are still under investigation, and several key mediating partners for phototropin mediated morphogenesis are identified recently. These are Adinosine triphosphate (ATP)-binding cassette transporter (ABCB19) and Calcineurin B-like (CBL)-interacting protein kinase 23 (CIPK23) (Inoue et al. 2020; Jenness et al. 2020). In the presence of low blue light, phytochrome interacting factors (PIFs) will be induced by cryptochrome1 (Cry1) receptor to mediate phototropic response in *A. thaliana.* The protein expression is repressed in the presence of high fluence light. The interaction of red and blue lights by phytochrome and cryptochromes has regulated the expression of PIFs and mediates auxin signaling leading to phototropic response (Boccaccini et al. 2020). The directional light mediates leaf blade expansion through phototropin signaling leading to the formation of flat thin leaf blade. The directional light elicits different proteins on the adaxial and abaxial leaf surfaces as a part of signaling cascade to promote growth of leaf blade. Non Phototropic Hypocotyl 3 (NPH3) expressed specifically on the adaxial surface enabling the growth of leaf blade. Another protein termed "phytochrome kinase substrate 3" was a downstream regulating protein for leaf blade growth and expansion that is mediated through blue light photoreceptor (Legris et al. 2021). Plants possess plasticity to respond to environmental cues such as light intensity, temperature variations, and drought stress through light signaling and modulating downstream players through transcription and post-translation events such as phosphorylation (Pierik et al. 2021).

29.4 Phototropisms and Phototaxis in Animals

The phototropism in animals is demonstrated in several animal species by researchers in the early twentieth century (Hartline 1923). Recent study in the holobiont *Exaiptasia pallida* (Aiptasia) established that blue light favored both phototropism and phototactic movements (whole organism toward light) and the symbiotic algae were responsible for the coral reef to perform these functions. This organism could not respond to blue light if the symbiotic algae were absent due to the increase in calcium deposits by the blue light in the corals (Foo et al. 2020). Further, blue light stimulated higher calcification in coral reefs through the activation of calcium channels and symport of calcium (Enríquez et al. 2016). In the coral larvae of *Pocillopora verrucose* organisms, light can enable the upright position paving way for greater dispersal and survival of the species (Mulla et al. 2021). Phototaxis is observed in animals that have symbiotic relationship (kleptoplasty) with *Paramecium bursaria* (Iwatsuki and

Naitoh 1981), worm *Symsagittifera roscoffensis* (Serôdio et al. 2011), and sea slugs (Miyamoto et al. 2015). Interestingly, light quantity regulated the phototactic movements in the symbiotic sea anemone *Aiptasia* (Strumpen et al. 2022).

Light induced reduction in cannibalistic behavior of animals such as prawn (*Penaeus japonicus*), rockfish (*Sebastes schlegelii*), and *Clarias gariepinus*. In dark conditions, the animals tend to aggregate with each other increasing the chance of cannibalism and reduction in the animal numbers. The phototropic/phototaxis behavior in these animals enabled dispersal of the animals reducing cannibalism (Su et al. 2020). Phototropism in female sand flies played a significant role in enabling them to move toward light and the researchers used the light traps to collect the flies. These flies are vectors for *Leishmania* parasites, and the parasites were found in roe deer, humans, hare, and cow. The research showed that natural reservoirs were present for *Leishmania* that causes kala-azar disease in humans (Calzolari et al. 2022).

29.5 Photomorphogenesis

Light mediated development of organs is photomorphogenesis. The process is predominantly mediated by phytochromes. These photopigments were discovered about 50 years ago and are well-studied plant photoreceptors. The crystal structure is worked out, and there are numerous classes of phytochromes, phyA to phyE. These function in seedling development (de-etiolation). Additionally, they help in the processes of senescence, flower development, and avoiding shade in plants. However, photomorphogenesis is mediated by not only phytochromes but also cryptochromes and UV receptors.

The well studied phytochrome photoreceptors consists of apoprotein and billin chromophore. They respond to red light. The inactive form is called Pr form that absorbs light in the red region of the spectrum and gets converted into active Pfr form by changing photoreceptor confirmation. The inactive Pr form is present in the cytosol, and after it gets converted into active form the receptor goes into the nucleus and performs changes in transcriptomic signature of the cell followed by protein synthesis resulting in photomorphogenesis. The regulation of active Pfr signaling is facilitated by a protein with ubiquitin ligase function termed "constitutive photomorphogenic 1" (COP1). This protein is known to play a role in photomorphogenesis. In dark this can ubiquitinate the phytochrome proteins and degrade them. When light signal is perceived by photoreceptors, they regulate the COP1 activity and promote photomorphogenesis (Ponnu and Hoecker 2021). Alternatively, other downstream proteins can mediate phytochrome regulation. These are PIF3 and PIF1 transcription factors that can bind to elongated hypocotyl 5 (Hy5) transcription factor that in turn is regulated through B-box transcription factors (BBXs) and regulate photomorphogenesis (Zhang et al. 2017).

29.6 Photosynthesis

Sunlight is the main source of energy on the Earth. Light energy is converted to chemical energy by the process of photosynthesis. The generalized equation for photosynthesis is

$$6CO_2 + 12H_2O + \text{Light energy} \rightarrow C_6H_{12}O_6 + 6O_2 + 6H_2O$$

The equation is proposed to emphasize that oxygen is produced by splitting of water (Stirbet et al. 2020). However, photosynthetic bacteria can use hydrogen sulfide instead of water as electron donor and utilize light energy to convert into chemical energy. Briefly in the thylakoids of chloroplasts, there are two photosystems – PS I and PS II reaction centers that can absorb light energy and through series of electron transport processes convert this energy into chemical energy. A small portion is given out as heat energy and 1–2% as chlorophyll fluorescence. Another main feature is oxidation of water and production of nicotinamide adenine dinucleotide hydrogen phosphate ($NADPH_2$) and ATP. The CO_2 is fixed by ribulose-1,5-bisphosphate carboxylase-oxygenase (RuBisCo) and converted to glucose through cyclic process (Calvin 1989; Stirbet et al. 2020). Mathematical modeling is applied recently to study the process of photosynthesis wherein the main features of light reactions and carbon metabolism have been integrated (Matuszyńska et al. 2019). However, there are several alternative cycles in the autotrophs living in oceans (Berg 2011; Hügler and Sievert 2011). The example of alternate pathway is found in archaea. Recent studies elucidated the genes involved in ammonia oxidation and carbon fixation by autotrophic hydroxy propionate/hydroxybutyrate cycle in the phylum Thaumarchaeota (Könneke et al. 2014). A reverse tricarboxylic acid cycle (TCA cycle) is identified after CO_2 fixation that could have arisen as the probable mechanism due to the elevated CO_2 levels on primitive Earth in *Hippea maritima* (Steffens et al. 2021). Another predominant carbon fixation is through C_4 cycle termed Hatch–Slack cycle (Hatch and Slack 1966; Furbank 2017). Later several plant species were identified as intermediate CO_2 photosynthetic behavior between C_3 and C_4 plant species (Rajendrudu and Das 1990).

In recent times, research is focused on improving C_3 metabolism by various modeling approaches and introducing energy-efficient C_4 pumps into these plants (Jurić et al. 2019). Modeling studies are also extended to explain C_3–C_4 phenomenon in response to environmental factors such as light, temperature, and CO_2 intensities. Computational simulations identified that light saturation in mesophyll and light-limiting conditions in the bundle sheath are the prominent features of C_3–C_4 intermediate plant *Flaveria chloraefolia*. The plant adjusted to varying light intensities by varying the pigment protein complexes and regulating glycine shuttle (Johnson et al. 2021). Recently, advances in synthetic biology have enabled reduction in energy consuming toxic byproduct of photorespiration of RUBP carboxylase by introducing β-hydroxy aspartate cycle from bacteria in *A. thaliana* peroxisomes. Here the introduction and production of C_4 metabolites by the bypass shunt have effectively demonstrated lowered carbon and nitrogen losses under photorespiration processes (Roell et al. 2021). Presently, the genomic and evolutionary aspect of C_4 photosynthesis enzymes and introducing C_4 pumps into rice plants to increase productivity are intense areas of research to improve photosynthesis and yield in crop plants.

29.7 Heliotropic Movements in Animals, Humans, and Plants

Positive or negative heliotropic movements were observed in animals like *Hydra*, *Porthesia chrysorrhce*, *Sphinx euphorbiw*, *Tenebrio molitor* and *Melolontha vulgaris*, frogs, white mice, *Gammarus locust*, *Cuma rathkii*, slugs, planarians, earthworms, leeches, and other worms such as *Spirographis spcllanzanii* (Andrews 1892). The heliotropic movements were explained by light stimulus resulting in movement of hands and legs. In humans a phenomenon of latent heliotropism is present, where the eye movements are present in response to light stimulus; this results in sending the signal for performing muscular movements of the body/neck. The latent heliotropism is present in patients with hereditary disorder or trauma. They possess abnormal tilting of head in response to light visual fields and are unaware of the head movements (Brodsky 2002).

The efficiency with which utilization of light energy takes place by diverse photosynthetic types of plant species is remarkably variable, and it depends on various physiological and biochemical factors. An important strategy of ecophysiological natural phenomenon evolved by plants is leaf heliotropism, which facilitates the leaves to maximize or minimize the solar perception by orienting their leaves perpendicular or parallel to solar beam. Heliotropism is of two types: when leaf lamina remains perpendicular to solar beam throughout the day it is named as "diaheliotropism," while the position of lamina parallel to direction of solar beam is called "paraheliotropism" (Koller 1990). Solar tracking behavior of leaves has been previously documented in a wide variety of dicotyledonous plants from more than 20 families (Sailaja and Das 1996; Nilsen and Forseth 2018). The leaf azimuth and inclination angles vary in a canopy from plant to plant. These change with respect to time of the day. A diaheliotropic plant is known to maximize solar interception compared to horizontal (static) leaved plant (Sailaja and Das 1996). The leaf azimuth and inclination angles are important parameters used in remote sensing to find canopy light interception. The contribution from leaf movements can be estimated using these techniques (Huemmrich 2013). These movements play a pivotal role in increasing photosynthetic performance of plants and help the plants to respond to environmental clues (Nilsen and Forseth 2018). Several 3D models are developed to understand the contribution of heliotropism for maximizing photosynthetic efficiency and be beneficial for plant growth under abiotic stresses such as drought stress. Recently, an abiotic stress gene *DREB/CBF* that codes for transcription factor was introduced into soybean plants because of its ability to regulate stress response genes. The transgenic strain could achieve higher grain yield in drought-stressed condition by increasing diaheliotropic and paraheliotropic movements, which increased water use efficiency and lowered transpiration rates (Rakocevic et al. 2018). Heliotropic movements work synergistically with temperature sensing movements to understand environmental clues, adapt, and increase growth and survival of the plants. Heliotropic movements in plants grown in University of Hyderabad as case study and their response to blue light is presented next.

29.8 Heliotropic Movements in Plants – Case Study of Plants Grown at University of Hyderabad

C_4 plants show higher rates of net CO_2 assimilation, photosynthetic radiation use efficiency, and water use efficiency over C_3 the species. However, in diaheliotropic and paraheliotropic plants, the photosynthetic radiation use and water use efficiency were inhibited 4–12% and 11–31% at 12 noon, respectively. Whereas photosynthetic radiation use efficiency and water use efficiency for non-trackers were substantially inhibited at 12.00 noon and were 27.8% and 43%, respectively (Table 29.1). Heliotropic plants have maximized photosynthetic and water use efficiencies by increasing the quantum efficiency of PSII measured as Fv/Fm and did not alter in heliotropic plants throughout the day (Table 29.2). However, in static leaved plants midday

Table 29.1 Net photosynthetic rate and transpiration rates of heliotropic plants measured at 09:00 and 12:00 hours.

Plant species	Photosynthetic rate (μ mol quanta.m^{-2} s^{-1})		Transpiration rates	
	9 a.m.	12 Noon	9 a.m.	12 Noon
Leguminous plants				
Cyamopsis tetragonoloba	27.39	26.21	5.16	6.70
Cajanus cajan	22.01	21.00	4.37	5.73
Canavalia ensiformis	17.14	18.66	3.91	6.02
Vigna unguiculata	23.45	22.20	4.75	5.72
Dolichos lablab	21.14	18.18	4.78	6.37
Phaseolus mungo	22.26	21.49	4.39	6.20
Phaseolus radiatus	24.69	25.77	4.95	6.46
Non-leguminous plants				
Amaranthus viridis	40.66	40.28	5.13	6.12
Cleome gynandra	41.63	41.79	5.15	5.42
Ricinus communis	25.74	25.83	5.66	7.02
Hibiscus cannabinus	23.75	22.13	5.28	6.75
Physalis minima	23.36	22.83	5.84	7.16
Waltheria indica	26.02	24.77	6.73	7.63
Static leaves				
Morus alba	13.36	10.60	3.83	5.65
Lycopersicon esculentum	20.06	15.47	4.95	7.47

Values are average of five independent measurements made on different plants.

Table 29.2 Diurnal variation in quantum efficiency of PSII.

Species	Fv/Fm		
	9 a.m.	12 Noon	3 p.m.
Leguminous plants			
Cyamopsis tetragonoloba	0.74a	0.73a	0.71a
Cajanus cajan	0.72a	0.69a	0.70a
Canavalia ensiformis	0.71a	0.70a	0.71a
Vigna unguiculata	0.72a	0.58b	0.65b, c
Dolichos lablab	0.70a	0.57b	0.64b, c
Phaseolus mungo	0.73a	0.56b	0.67b, c
Phaseolus radiatus	0.71a	0.57b	0.66b, c
Non-leguminous plants			
Amaranthus viridis	0.76a	0.79a	0.76a
Cleome gynandra	0.79a	0.80a	0.78a
Ricinus communis	0.74a	0.72a	0.71a
Hibiscus cannabinus	0.73a	0.69a	0.70a
Physalis minima	0.76a	0.75a	0.74a
Waltheria indica	0.73a	0.69a	0.70a
Static leaves			
Morus alba	0.70a	0.51b	0.58b, c
Lycopersicon esculentum	0.71a	0.53b	0.59b, c

Values are means of 10 independent measurements per trial and three trials in a day. 09:00 hour values followed by the letter "a" are not different from those at 12:00 and 15:00 hours; 12:00 and 15:00 hours values followed by "b" are significantly ($P \leq 0.01$) lower than those at 09:00 hour values followed by "c" are significantly ($P \leq 0.01$) higher than those at 12:00 hour.

depression of photosynthesis is due to the increase in closed PSII reaction centers (Sailaja and Das 1996). Thus, heliotropic movements can maximize photosynthetic performance of the plant under low water and dry regions and during high light incidence during midday improving the photosynthesis of the plants.

The leaves of *Ricinus communis* were facing east in the morning and west by the evening indicating diaheliotropism (Figure 29.2a,b). Higher *Cos I* values during the entire day were observed for both non-pulvinar *R. communis* and pulvinar *Cicer arietinum* (0.9 ± 0.20) compared to static leaved plants (0.7 ± 0.34). The pulvinus is the site of heliotropic movements and the motor organ is known to respond to spectral quality of light by increasing turgidity mediated by increased potassium ion concentration through the opening of potassium ion channels coupled to sodium potassium pump present on plasma membrane due to altered membrane potential. The pulvinus is responsible for leaf movements by performance of rhythmic volume changes in opposite cells of the pulvinus (Moran 2015). These cells are called flexor and extensor cells that are present on the adaxial and abaxial surface of the leaf, respectively. In a study using *A. thaliana,* it was demonstrated that blue light induced the leaf surface into a perpendicular position similar to solar tracking behavior resulting in increased light interception indicating the role of blue light (Inoue et al. 2005). Measuring the *Cos I* of leaf surface is considered as a method to track leaf movements in heliotropic plants. Blue light increased *Cos I* measurements in *R. communis* plants indicating role of blue light in pulvinar *C. arietinum and non-pulvinar R. communis* plants. (Figure 29.2c). The blue light induced *Cos I* was inhibited by using inhibitor for H^+/ATPase on the leaf surface (Figure 29.2d), indicating a prominent role of proton pump localized on plasma membrane to regulate *R. communis* leaf movements. In order to understand the region in the petiole where leaf movements occur, protoplasts from bending region (1 cm distance from leaf base) and non-bending region (6 cm away from leaf base) were isolated to study the physiological response of blue light in these cells. An increase in blue light mediated K^+ ions and protoplast volume in the bending region of petiole

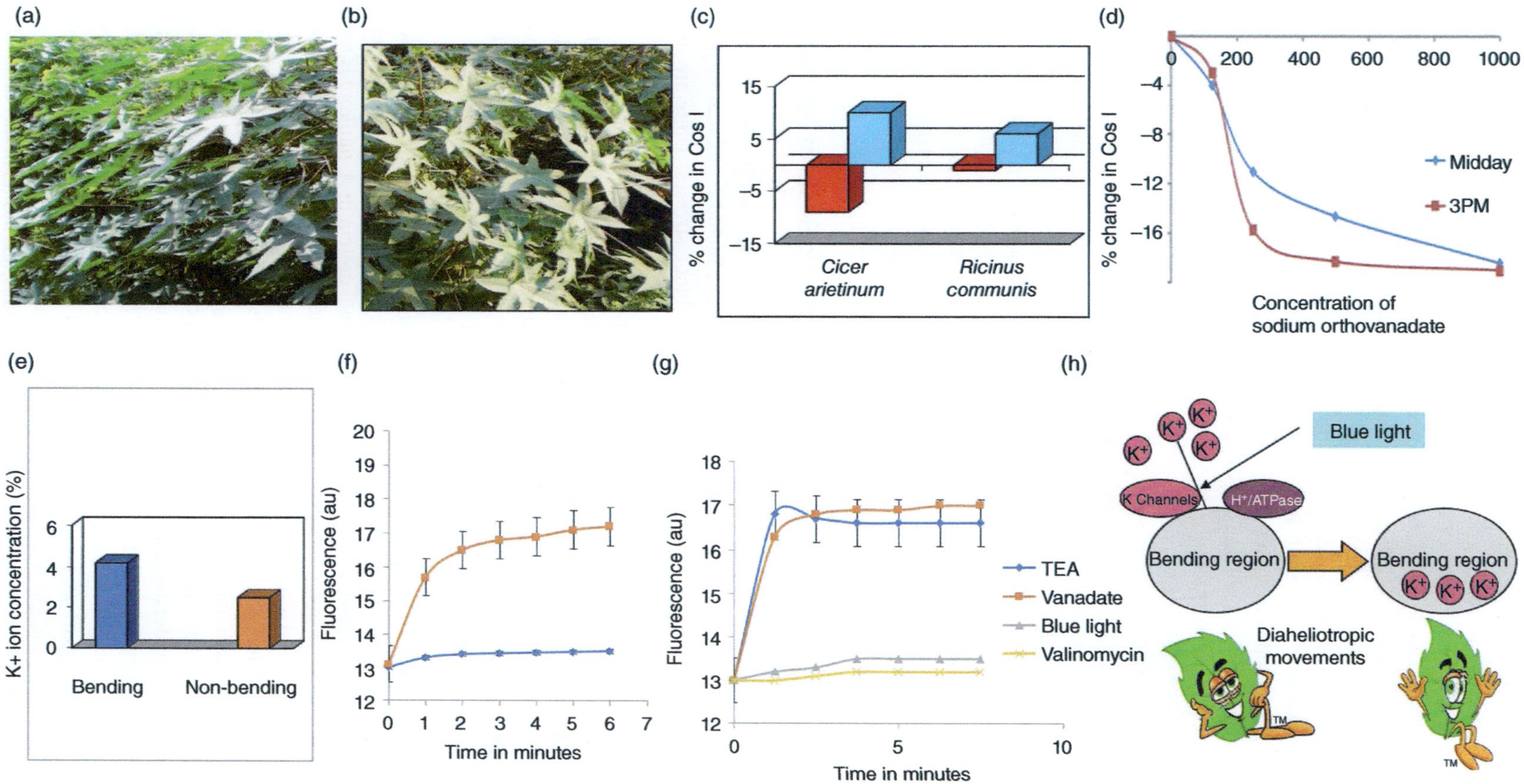

Figure 29.2 Blue light regulates leaf movements through membrane depolarization. (a) Leaves facing east in the morning. (b) Leaves facing west in the evening. (c) Blue light increases Cos I in pulvinar plant *C. arietinum* and non-pulvinar plant *R. communis L.* (d) Blue light induced increase in Cos I is through H+/ATPase. (e) Protoplasts isolated from bending region (less than 1 cm from leaf base) and non-bending region (6–7 cm) from leaf base exhibited increased K^+ concentration. (f) Blue light increases depolarization in the protoplasts isolated from bending region of *R. communis*. (g) Blue light response is by regulating K^+ channels. (h) Cartoon picture showing effect of blue light on leaf movements.

compared to non-bending region facilitated turgor-related leaf movements (Figure 29.2e). A blue light mediated increase in membrane depolarization was also clearly demonstrated in the bending region of petiole (Figure 29.2f). When vanadate, an inhibitor of H+/ATPase is added, blue light mediated membrane depolarization is inhibited (Figure 29.2g), indicating metabolic energy mediated extrusion of H^+ is essential for the uptake of K^+ that causes increase in turgor and cellular volume facilitating leaf movements in the bending zone. Blue light induced regulation of protoplast volume was observed from pulvinus of *Phaseolus vulgaris* (Wang et al. 2001)˙ In the presence of ionophore valinomycin at high (200 mM) external K^+ concentration, membrane depolarization was observed without blue light effect indicates that the K^+ channels are open (Figure 29.2g). In the absence of valinomycin, blue light treatment alone resulted in the opening of K^+ channels. When tetraethylammonium (TEA) a K^+ channel blocker was used, blue light mediated membrane potential changes were absent implicating channel mediated movement of K^+. The K^+ channels were present in the bending region of *R. communis* that are regulated by light, while light regulated channels are absent in non-bending region of the petiole that could aid the plant in heliotropic movement. This is an interesting and novel case study of a non-pulvinar plant able to perform solar tracking movements in the absence of specialized motor organ pulvinus. The pictorial representation of leaf movements is given in the *R. communis* in the Figure 29.2h.

29.9 Solar Tracking can be Modeled by Quantum Mechanics

The external environment can enable plant systems to design their own methods and strategies to process the cues and come up with responses for adaptations. The mathematical understanding of the cues and response is proposed recently, and the biological entities are made up of atoms. Therefore, these particles are present in open environment and respond to the cues. The signal processing can be described by quantum theory and wave function governed by stochastic Schrödinger equation (Brody 2022). The author proposes that the whole system operates as an aggregation of quantum particles, thereby enabling the wave function theory to be useful in understanding the dynamic nature of light response on plants and their adaptations. The author used signal processing in continuous open environment by employing the equations proposed by Diósi (1988). The plant response to sunlight is considered as a response of a system in open environment, and the signal processing could also be described by stochastic Schrödinger equation. The model uses this continuous signal processing and then erasing the signal accompanied by energy utilization and heat production. It also uses Brownian motion of particles in open environments. According to the model they proposed that a daisy plant may use 10^{-2} eV of energy in the night to enable the plant to track the Sun again in the morning. A model for solar tracking in open environment using signal processing used quantum-mechanical models (Brody 2022). In the model the important constituents are Hamiltonian and the Lindblad operators. In quantum mechanics the Hamiltonian operator is the sum of total energy (potential and kinetic energies) of a system. In the solar tracking of a plant, the Hamiltonian operator changes as the Sun's location is not constant. The Lindblad operator is the effect in an open system in quantum mechanics. A solar tracking plant is the effect due to changing position of the Sun and therefore can be described by Lindblad operator. The quantum theory of solar tracking predicts that the movement should be slow in response to the sun. If they are rapid, they may be detrimental to plants. This agrees with slow movements in plants in response to the Sun's position.

29.10 Genetic Basis of Movements

The potassium ion (K^+ ion) channels regulate several functions in the plant including ionic transport in xylem and phloem and abiotic stresses. There are different kinds of channels, namely (i) voltage gated channels and (ii) voltage independent channels. The voltage gated channels can be inward or outward rectifying channels and weak and silent rectifying channels (Dreyer et al. 2019). The K^+ ions transport plays a prominent role in turgor related tissues such as stomata and pulvinus. Several genes regulate the coding of the channel proteins. In some cases the genes arose by the phenomenon of gene duplications and mutations (Schachtman et al. 1992). They code for series of channel pore-forming proteins that regulate the uptake of K^+ ions, e.g. the channel protein in *A. thaliana* is termed potassium channel protein (KAT1). This protein belongs to Shaker family of proteins. Further, several channel proteins are present in the plant. Tandem-pore K^+ channels (TPK1, TPK2, TPK3, TPK4, and TPK5) perform the function as voltage independent channels. These are located on plasma membrane and facilitate K^+ ions transport across the membrane. *OsAKTs* and *OsKATs* genes are identified in rice plants that can regulate these channels and regulate drought and salinity stress (Obata et al. 2007; Moon et al. 2017). Recently, using genomic analysis and bioinformatic techniques, additional family of *OsAKTs* and *OsKATs* was identified that coded for K^+ ion channel proteins

(Musavizadeh et al. 2021). A novel channel (VvK3.1) was identified by using voltage gated channels and molecular biological techniques such as *in situ* hybridizations in grapevine. The gene functioned in regulation of K^+ ions in the tissue. In the absence of this gene, the pulvinus organ could not perform para heliotropic leaf movements. This channel protein is found to form a network with VvCIPK03–VvCBL04 proteins that can synergistically regulate K^+ ions (Nieves-Cordones et al. 2019). Several genes such as *ELP1* and its orthologs *APULVINIC* (*APU*) and *SLEEPLESS* (*SLP*) can regulate pulvinus formation. If these genes are mutated, a petiole-like structure was formed in the plants instead of pulvinus, and then the leaf movements were totally abolished (Chen et al. 2012; Zhou et al. 2012). These genes are belong to *LATERAL ORGAN BOUNDARIES* domain (LBD) family of genes that code for transcription factors that can regulate the genes encoding pulvinus development. In a non-pulvinus forming species *A. thaliana*, the *Lateral Organ Boundaries (LOB)* gene that code for transcription factor that controls the plant organ boundaries. The LOB protein forms a feedback loop and can regulate brassinosteroids (BR), which are phytohormones involved in several signaling events that regulate formation of organ boundaries. The key players that can recognize the BR molecule are leucine-rich repeat (LRR) receptor-like kinase, *brassinosteroid insensitive 1* (*BRI1*), *BRI1-LIKE1* (*BRL1*), *BRL3*, and the coreceptor *BRI1-associated kinase 1* (*BAK1*). The *petiolule-like pulvinus* (*PLP*) gene plays a key role in pulvinus architecture due to the regulation of BR phytohormones. It has regulated another gene *MtBAS1* that is responsible for pulvinus structure and function. The absence of these genes in the pulvinus resulted in changed motor cell architecture and defective plant movements (Kong et al. 2021). The *mini organ 1* (*MIO1*) gene encodes F-box protein small leaf, and bushy 1 (*SLB1*) is known to affect the pulvinus growth and differentiation. This gene affects the cellular proliferation of pulvinus. The *Mio1* mutant plant exhibited abnormal pulvinus structure, and in these mutants, scanning electron microscopy (SEM) measurements reveal that decrease in the number of motor cells. After restoration of the gene by complementation experiments, the pulvinus structure and leaf movements were restored in *Medicago truncatula* (R108) pulvinus motor organ (Zhou et al. 2021).

There are several receptors in plants that can absorb photons and regulate light response in plants. These receptors channelized for sensing UV light, blue light, and red light. UVR8 is principal photoreceptor that mediates UV light mediated phototropic movements. Cryptochromes are known to respond to blue light and mediate several plant and animal responses (Wang and Lin 2020). There are two cryptochrome receptors, cryptochrome 1 and cryptochrome 2 (*CRY1* and *CRY2*), that are identified in plants, insects, and mammals including humans. These receptors might have evolved from bacterial photolyase and have two domains: photolyase homology region that can bind to FAD and a C-terminal CRY region. The cryptochromes act as light receptors, regulate transcription of interacting proteins, and mediate circadian rhythms. In animals they regulate many processes, e.g. sleep, temperature, and metabolism, in a single day. The *Cry*1 and *Cry2* genes could be activated by transcription factor called circadian locomotor output cycles kaput (CLOCK). The transcription factor consists of a basic helix loop helix structure. Additionally, it has a Per-Arnt-Sim (PAS) domain that acts as a molecular sensing function that aids in the recognition of molecular clues. This transcription factor can modulate the cryptochromes transcription by attaching to their genes. Further another core transcription regulator is called aryl hydrocarbon receptor nuclear translocator like (ARNTL/BMAL1). This also contains PAS domain and can regulate cryptochrome expression. These two form a heterodimer and regulate period (*PER*) and cryptochrome (Cry1 and Cry2) gene transcription (Takahashi 2016). The circadian clocks consist of central clock that is present in the suprachiasmatic nucleus region of the brain, and peripheral clocks that operate in all organs of humans and several diseases are known to exist when the biological clock is disrupted. Light enters the body through eyes and then reaches the brain that initiates the diurnal cycles. Then the brain sends signals to other body parts enabling the circadian clock related behavior and processes in humans. Studies on the effect of circadian clock in humans revealed that several genes (about 43% of the transcriptome) are regulated at the transcription level by the diurnal rhythms (Zhang et al. 2014). Further, post-translation regulation, actin, and chromatin remodeling are known to regulate circadian clock in humans. There are several diseases associated with single nucleotide polymorphisms (SNPs)/mutations in circadian clock regulating genes in humans. Mutations in cryptochromes, *CLOCK, PER*, and *BMAL1* lead to sleep disorders. Genome-wide association studies were performed to identify novel genes controlling circadian clock in humans (Gottlieb et al. 2015). Mutations in HCRTR2 receptor is associated with a sleep disorder called narcolepsy in dogs and humans (Chabas et al. 2003). Interestingly, the cryptochromes regulate fat cell function (Miller et al. 2020), diabetes, and gluconeogenesis (Lamia et al. 2011). These receptors play a role in several metabolic functions. Therefore, the receptor small molecule interactions should help in identifying novel small molecules for metabolic and sleep disorder therapies.

Blue light mediated growth was proposed by phototropins that absorb UVA/blue light in *A. thaliana*. Phototropins work with cryptochromes to respond differentially under increased incidence of blue light. Phototropins are encoded by *Phot1* and *Phot2* genes that are evolved by gene duplication (Li et al. 2015). The copy number varies between the species. There are seven gene copies in moss *P. patens,* three copies in fern *Adiantum capillus-veneris*, and one copy in liverworts *Marchantia polymorpha and Apopellia endiviifolia* (Yong et al. 2021). The phototropin blue light sensing receptor tyrosine kinases are known to mediate phototropism, chloroplast movements, stomatal opening, and leaf expansion (Ishishita et al. 2020). The phototropins and their signaling partners can be regulated using light treatments. These can effectively improve plant growth and photosynthesis under various abiotic stresses and aid in designing plants with high performance (Sharma et al. 2021). The blue light receptor phototropin 2 structure and blue light response have been studied by small angle X-ray scattering (Nakasako et al. 2020). This receptor consists of light activating domains termed light-oxygen-voltage sensing domains (LOV1 and LOV2) and kinase domain. By using absorption measurements, mutations in the core active sites, and scattering experiments, researchers have elucidated that blue light can elicit structural change in the domains of the receptor and activate kinase function that forms basis for downstream signaling when the whole receptor is studied. However, if the domains were studied independently, blue light elicited response is found only in tyrosine domains (Nakasako et al. 2020). It is established that LOV2 domain undergoes structural changes to activate kinase function (Hart and Gardner 2021). There are phototropin-like proteins across the plant and animal kingdoms that respond to environmental stimuli. In *Chlamydomonas reinhardtii,* there is one phototropin and it has higher sequence similarity to phototropin 2 of higher plants. Similarly, there is another kinase (histidine kinase) in bacteria that is regulated by blue light. It has one LOV and kinase domain. A recent study in *Erythrobacter litoralis* (*HTCC2594*, EL34) by crystallography showed interaction between the domains to sense blue light and then undergo series of confirmational changes resulting in autophosphorylation of the kinase domain, leading to downstream signaling (Dikiy et al. 2019). Additionally, the light-activated domains have been identified in fungi and animals. They help the organisms to respond to environmental cues. The phenomenon of heliotropism in developing sunflower plant is documented before (Briggs 2014). However, the role of photoreceptors in flower head movement in *A. thaliana* in response to light is described recently (Serrano et al. 2021).

29.11 Vision in Animals, Unicellular to Multicellular Organism, and Rhodopsin Cycle

Diurnal and nocturnal insects have developed different visual strategies to navigate. Nocturnal insects can absorb very few photons and can navigate in stellar light (Somanathan et al. 2007; Narendra and Ramirez-Esquivel 2017). The compound eye of the insects can maximize visual response. Additionally, light signal response is slow, with spatial and temporal summation and a good contrast in optic lobes that helps in vision (Warrant 2017). The vertebrates possess retina, and it is first observed in chordates. The visual structure is optimized in various species to survive in various environments. Zebra fish emerged as a model to study visual system development (Dell'Orco et al. 2021).

The retina is the innermost layer of the eye, made up of photoreceptor cells such as rods, cones, retinal pigment epithelial cells (RPE), and retinal ganglion cells (RGC). Rods are the elongated structure made up of specialized neurons that convert electrical stimuli from the light photons into chemical stimuli that are processed in the central nervous system as vision. Rods receive the light from the retina and help in maintaining the size, shape, and brightness of the image, but they cannot perceive its color and fine details, wherein the cone comes into action. Rod is composed of four parts, namely, the outer and the inner segment, the cell body, and the synaptic region. This synaptic region is the retinal neuronal transmission that connects to the RGC's axons and the optic nerve, where the image is being processed. Rod cells are present in the retinal region, whereas only one-third of the cones are present in the retina layer. Cones are chiefly present in the fovea and centralis regions.

The outermost layer of the rod has rhodopsin, a light-sensitive G-protein coupled receptor biological sensory protein. Rhodopsin is a conjugate of a protein moiety (scotopsin) and carotene derivative (*11-cis retinal*), that is majorly involved in visual phototransduction (PTD). PTD involves cyclic decomposition and reconstitution of rhodopsin. When the light source hits the rods, the electrons in the rod's *11-cis-retinaldehyde* are excited and get converted into *all-trans-retinal*. As a result, the scotopsin moiety disintegrates from the rhodopsin (absorption: 500 nm) with the release of many byproducts, which changes the rhodopsin configuration by isomerization. The major byproducts of this process include an unstable *Bathorhodopsin* (absorption: 543 nm) that decays into *Lumirhodopsin* (absorption: 497 nm), which further decays into *Metarhodopsin I* (absorption: 480 nm) and *Metarhodopsin II* (*activated rhodopsin*) (absorption: 380 nm) and *free all-trans-retinal* (absorption: 380 nm). The entire decay process happens in less than a few seconds and completely releases the scopoletin and *11-all-trans-retinal* components. *Metarhodopsin II* further activates transducing and rod-resistant phosphodiesterase, which in turn affects cyclic guanosine monophosphate (cGMP) action (holding sodium ion balance in the rod cells). Consequently, cGMP is destroyed, sodium channels are closed, and sodium flux into the rod outer segment is slowed, causing hyperpolarization, leading to its decomposition. However, this process will be reactivated when the rhodopsin kinase gets into action, which converts the *11-trans retinal*, that is reconverted into an *11-cis retinal* that regenerates new rhodopsin (reconstitution). This cyclic visual process (Figure 29.3a) is important, as its failure will initially lead to night blindness that further worsens to complete blindness. Night blindness majorly occurs via the mutation in the *RHO* gene. Several diseases such as age-related macular degeneration, congenital stationary night blindness, and Leger congenital amaurosis are caused due to defective phototransduction and retinoid cycle enzymes (Kiser et al. 2012).

Cones contain two components, namely photopsins and retinal. The photopsins are responsible for the color vision that comprises blue-, red-, and green-sensitive pigment. The cone photobiology is studied recently using zebra fish as a model. This is used to elucidate the visual cycle as retina, the visual process is closer to humans, and vast mutations in the process are available for genetic studies (Zhang et al. 2011). Human cone cells are known to possess three types of opsins to see colors in the visible spectrum (red, green, and blue). Several diurnal mammals possess these three types of opsins. However, certain birds and insects have a fourth opsin that functions in UV light. Interestingly, advances in genomics have identified multiple opsin genes in insects and fishes. There are 8–11 genes in fishes, 27 in daphnia for visual perception, and 15–23 genes in dragonflies. The environmental cues are responsible for evolution of these genes by gene duplication and mutations (Colbourne et al. 2011; Thoen 2016). The opsin lineages are well studied in vertebrates. However, such studies including genotype–phenotype correlations are absent in insects. Recently, the insect opsins were cloned in

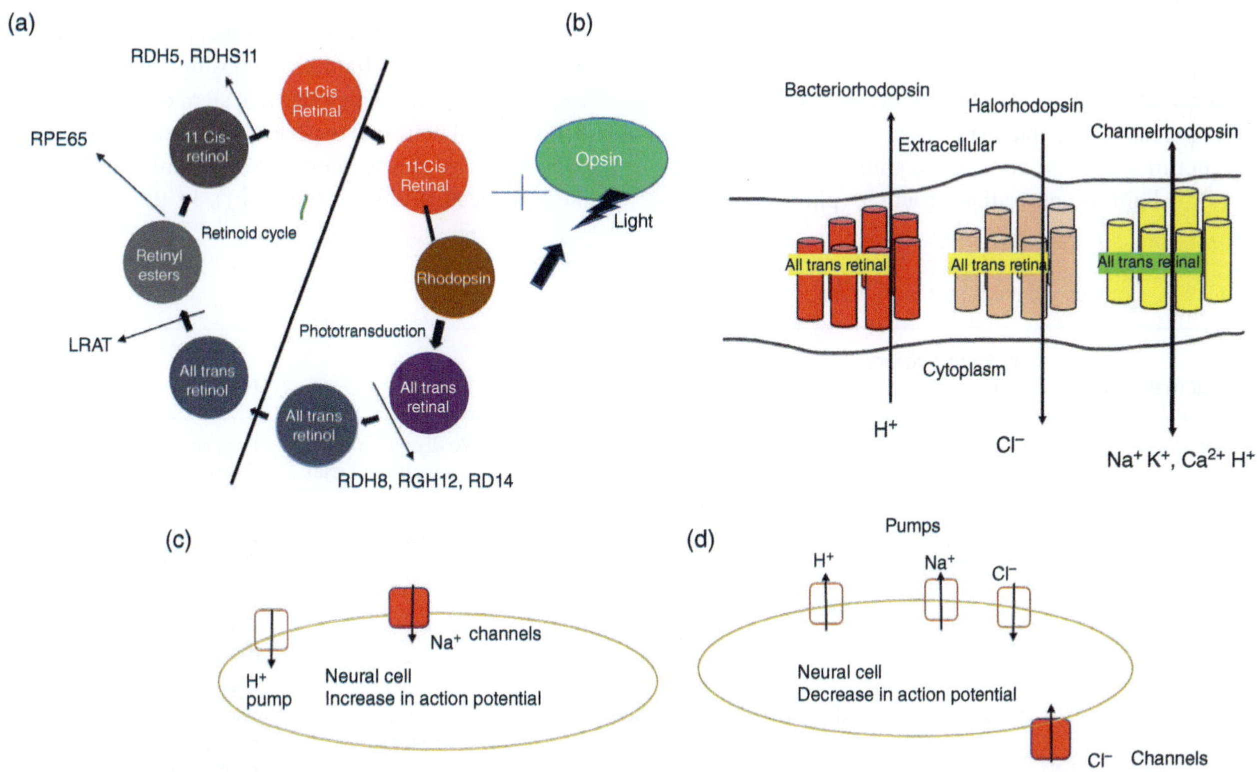

Figure 29.3 (a) Rhodopsin cycle: Phototransduction takes place in rod cells, and the visual cycle takes place in rod cells and retinal pigment epithelium cells. After absorbing photons 11-cis retinal combines with opsin to form rhodopsin. A series of enzymes such as retinol dehydrogenases (RDH8, RGH12, RD14), lecithin: retinol acyltransferase (encoded by LRAT), retinal pigment epithelium specific 65 kDa (RPE65), and retinol dehydrogenases (RDH8, RGH12, RD14) mediate the cycle. (b) Ancient rhodopsins that are used in optogenetics: Bacteriorhodopsin can pump protons. Halorhodopsin chloride ions and channelrhodopsin pumps cations. They all cause hyperpolarization. (c, d) Use of microbial rhodopsin for depolarization/hyperpolarization of nerve cells thereby mediating action potential and nerve impulses in nerve cells.

human embryonic kidney cells with T receptor (HEK293T) cells, purified, and spectral characteristics were studied. The researchers showed that there are adaptations in insect color vision that give them evolutionary benefit to survive, find mate, etc. (Liénard et al. 2021).

29.12 Optogenetics: Photoreceptors, Neural Circuits, and Light-Induced Channels

The new field of optogenetics gained importance in the past decade. It has three elements: (i) microbial opsins. These proteins can induce electric current in a membrane after absorbing light. (ii) General gene expression techniques that can target gene expression of opsin in the brain. (iii) The light is guided to brain cells to perform desired work (Deisseroth 2015). The primitive rhodopsins used in optogenetics are bacteriorhodopsin, halorhodopsin, and channelrhodopsin. The channelrhodopsin I and II are from *Clamydomonas*. These are transmembrane proteins, which act as ionic pumps that function to generate electrochemical gradients and in phototaxis movements (Figure 29.3b) (Boyden et al. 2005). These were used to study light mediated neuronal response by mediating ionic channels. These microbial rhodopsins are used in optogenetics because (i) the pigment 11-cis retinal concentration is higher in microbes compared to animals. (ii) In animals after the light isomerization reaction (photobleaching), 11-cis retinal gets converted to all trans-retinal. However, the back conversion is by rhodopsin cycle (Figure 29.3a) series of chemical reactions mediated by enzymes. In microbes the conversion of all trans-retinal into 11-cis retinal is thermal reaction and does not need series of steps. (iii) The voltage gated channels can perform depolarization and hyperpolarization thereby exciting nerve cell and bringing back to its non-excited state. Thus, they are valuable tools in the optogenetics field (Figure 29.3c, d). The light-activated domains (LOVs) of opsins are the key proteins and are known to be activated by blue light (Losi et al. 2018). Mutations in the domains are engineered by site-directed mutagenesis to suit and improve the light excitable property in these domains (Kawano et al. 2015). The possibilities of using these rhodopsins are huge in neuroscience and in retinal disorders. For example, initially embryonic stem cells are differentiated into gamma-aminobutyric acid (GABA)-releasing interneurons (GI). These types of neurons are important in epilepsy disease as these become dysfunctional or reduced in number. Therefore, adding more of these cells that can work and generate neuron excitation is important. If this can be controlled by just shining light on the cells, then it is a valuable therapy. For achieving this, researchers have introduced blue light responsive channelrhodopsin 2 receptor (from *Clamydomonas*) into the embryonic stem cells (that could later become GI neurons) to perform the function and mitigate seizures in mouse models and in human research studies (Gonzalez-Ramos et al. 2021). In this work, only

Table 29.3 Optogenetic drugs in clinical trials for retinal degeneration.

Clinical trial number	Sponsoring agency/ company	Drug	Trial	Features
NCT05294978	University Hospital, Basel, Switzerland	To find out dormant cone cells that can be activated by light (for optogenetic drugs)	No drugs observational trial	For people with retinal dystrophies
NCT04945772	Nanoscope Therapeutics Inc.	Optogenetic drug vMCO-010	Phase 2	For people with retinal dystrophies/retinitis pigmentosa
NCT04919473	Nanoscope Therapeutics Inc.	Optogenetic drug vMCO-010	Phase 1	For people with retinal dystrophies/retinitis pigmentosa (completed)
NCT02556736	Allegran clinical trial	Drug: RST-001 Optogenetic drug	Phase 1/2 (completed)	For people with retinal dystrophies/retinitis pigmentosa
NCT03326336	GenSight Biologics	Combination product: gene therapy: GS030-DP and medical device: GS030-MD GS030-drug product (GS030-DP)	Phase 1	For people with retinal dystrophies/retinitis pigmentosa

Source: Taken from Clinicaltrials.gov.

one type of rhodopsin that can be activated by only blue light is used. Red light does not mediate this response. Recently, simultaneously two opsin receptors were engineered to respond to different spectral lights (Li et al. 2022). Different spectral light intensities were used to regulate neuronal function. Optogenetics using microbial rhodopsins could effectively modulate visual field in monkeys by modulating brain function (Jazayeri et al. 2012). A red light specific opsin was engineered from *Haloarcula salinarum* (stark strain) and the researchers called this jaws. This functioned as red light regulated chloride pump. It could effectively function in mouse model of cone degenerative disease, retinitis pigmentosa (Chuong et al. 2014). Optogenetics has made it's way into the clinic to cure retinal degeneration. A patient was treated with adenovirus mediated delivery of Chrimson R receptors into the retina. The photoreceptors were stimulated with light using goggles. A partial restoration of sight was observed in the retinitis pigmentosa patient (Sahel et al. 2021). Several channelrhodopsins were developed and are in trials for retinitis pigmentosa (Table 29.3). There is a trial first to see if there are dormant cone cells in low vision patients due to retinal degeneration in multiple hospitals. These patients can be benefited by optogenetic treatments by shining light to stimulate cone cells. There are three drugs that are adenovirus derived containing channelrhodopsins controlled by universal promoters to work in the cone cells. Once the channelrhodopsins express and perform the role of light induced depolarization/hyperpolarization in cone cells, they can perform the photoreceptor function facilitated by channelrhodopsins.

The brain function was previously studied using electrical impulses. Clinically, this is useful to understand brain disorders. Further, brain can emit weak photons and ultraweak photon emissions (UPE). The photon amplitude was measured between left and right side of the brain. The emitted light was found to be 10^{-12} w/m^2 (Costa et al. 2016). The photon amplitude varied between 2 and 3 Hz between the two halves of the brain. The energy of 10^{-14} j/s was calculated from the neurons, and the number of neurons that can emit the photons was found to be $10^6/10^7$ by using quantum mechanics. These photons are measured to understand the brain function (Salari et al. 2015). UPE was observed in animal brain slices and metabolism and glutamate regulated this behavior. Additionally, redox reactions and ATP are known to regulate this phenomenon. Schwartz et al. (2005) explained the brain function in physical and mathematical models by integrating quantum mechanics. This approach was further proposed and explained the role of metabolism in the UPE (Salari et al. 2021). The classic equation discovered by Plank states that energy is proportional to wavelength. It can be obtained by multiplying frequency with Plank's constant. This theory can explain the UPE in the brain, and the energy can be converted into light that can be measured by various devices. Human beings are considered as higher order animals due to their thinking and consciousness. Several researchers tried to answer the superior nature of human brain among the animals in the world. The UPE from brain sections of bull frog, mouse, chicken, pig, monkey, and human brains is different. There is a gradual increase from 691 nm wavelength of light to 895 nm. Interestingly, different regions of human brain such as frontal cortex, hippocampus, motor cortex, primary occipital cortex, sensory cortex, and temporal cortex exhibited variation in the wavelength of light emitted. The researchers proposed that longer wavelength photon emission in humans indicates lower energy needed to communicate between neurons in more efficient way, and this could account for more superior human brain function (Wang et al. 2016). In future, advances in CHIP designing should enable the UPE measurements in diseased state and could become a standard care in the clinic (Salari et al. 2021). The measuring of UPE has been used to predict UV damage in skin (Tsuchida and Kobayashi 2020).

29.13 Metabolites, Circadian Clock, and Sleep Pattern in Humans Under Altered Light Conditions

Ultraviolet light in the normal sunlight is responsible for the synthesis of vitamin D. It is synthesized by skin in normal light/UVB. The isomerization of 7-dehydrocholesterol takes place to get converted to provitamin and then vitamin. This is further converted into 1,25-dihydroxyvitamin D (1,25D) by activation process, and this molecule possesses hormonal activity (DeLuca 2016). This is responsible for several metabolic functions in the cell. Recently, the role of vitamin D binding protein (DBP) in the formation of activated hormone is elucidated. The mice that lack this protein could not make active 1,25D. Interestingly, the weather and vitamin D levels played a prominent role in COVID-19 infections. The analysis of UV radiation using weather data in European countries and COVID-19 infections revealed that the exposure to this radiation reduced the viral infections (Mukherjee et al. 2022). The severity of the disease is associated with reduced vitamin D levels. The vitamin is known to affect immune response through TLR2 signaling (Peng et al. 2021). The lockdown that was imposed to control the spread of COVID-19 made people stay indoors and receive less daily light including UV rays needed to fight infection. Increased death rate (about 11%) was observed in human subjects using modeling studies. Authors predicted an exposure to light, in addition to lockdowns as effective measures to stop infections (Moozhipurath and Kraft 2021). Additionally, vitamin D status varies across different regions of people in various continents. People living in high latitudes such as Alaska have low vitamin D levels due to the presence of low light and prolonged dark winters (Lips et al. 2021). A study in children from Bangladesh identified 43% children have low vitamin D levels. Sunlight exposure, UVB index, and mutations in vitamin D pathway genes were measured, and they found correlations between sunlight exposure and vitamin D levels in the cohorts. Similarly, elderly population who have limited exposure to light experience lower vitamin D levels and need fortification in food/supplements (Brouwer-Brolsma et al. 2016). Thus, adequate Vitamin D levels are needed for normal body functioning and to fight infections and diseases. The exposure to sunlight is most efficient means of getting Vitamin D in humans.

A 24-hour biological clock involving day light and night dark period is present in plants, animals, and humans that is termed "circadian rhythm" (Schibler and Sassone-Corsi 2002). In humans the light signal is received by the retina and then passed on to hypothalamus of the brain. There is a region called suprachiasmatic nucleus in the hypothalamus that is a master clock regulator, and then the signal is communicated to other organs such as heart, liver, muscle, pancreas, and adrenal system. These organs act as peripheral clocks. The circadian clocks are modulated due to environmental factors, genetic makeup of a person, behavior of a person, and food habits (Stenvers et al. 2019). However, the principal zeitgeber (time giver) that controls the circadian clock is light. The disruption in the clock is a leading cause of diabetes and Alzheimer's disease. Additionally, the disruption of circadian clock causes metabolic disorders and increased risk for cardiac problems and cancer. The molecular regulation of the rhythms is controlled by several genes. Two transcription factors termed circadian locomotor output cycles kaput (CLOCK) protein and aryl hydrocarbon receptor nuclear translocator like (ARNTL)/BMAL1. These are transcription factors and they control the positive regulation of the clock through transcription/translation feedback loop (TTFL). They recognize E-box elements 5′-CACGTG in the circadian regulated genes. These two proteins form heterodimer and regulate several genes that are regulated periodically in various organs. They also drive the expression of period (*PER*)*1/2* genes and cryptochrome *Cry* () genes. These genes are transcription repressors that form negative feedback loop to regulate the rhythms. Genome-wide association studies have identified mutations in the TTFL components in several sleep neurological and metabolic disorders (Jagannath et al. 2017).

The low light exposure is known to cause depression, insomnia, and mood disorders in people. A study of 502,000 people in the United Kingdom showed that a median of 2.5 hours should be spent outdoors. Additional hours spent outside decreased the odds of getting depressive disorders and increased happiness (Burns et al. 2021). The study also stressed the need for maintaining circadian rhythms for maintaining adequate sleep time for reduced depression and mood disorders. In a large cohort study in the United Kingdom, deviation from day/night circadian rhythms have been correlated with mood disorders, bipolar disorder, lowered happiness, slow reaction times, and lowered health satisfaction. These findings were not dependent on economic status, education, lifestyle, and demographic factors (Lyall et al. 2018). The duration of sunlight exposure per day was a governing factor for dementia progress, especially in people over 60. A large cohort of people surveyed in UK Biobank revealed that exposure to sunlight for two hours compared to an hour reduced the risk of dementia progress (Ma et al. 2022). Similarly, irregular sleep habits in the pandemic had increased incidence of mental disorders (Czeisler et al. 2022).

29.14 Light Therapy for Human Diseases

Phototherapy has been in clinical practice and research and clinical trials are ongoing to bring the therapy to cure several diseases. The therapy is widely available in diseases/disorders like dermatology, neurological, mood, sleep, pediatric, neonatal, ocular, and oncology (Lim et al. 2013; Dogra and Mahajan 2015; Abraha et al. 2017). Several clinical trials are in progress that are studying phototherapy for various diseases. There are about 2000 entries at http://clinicaltrials.gov.website. Out of these, about 270 trials are still recruiting patients. A representative 31 trials are presented in Table 29.4. However, for the full list the website could be consulted. A wide variety of diseases including cancer, mental, neurological, and metabolic disorders are key constituents for phototherapy. The mechanisms to understand the effect of light are under investigations. A mechanism where light elevates depression is proposed recently. Light operates through the retina and lateral habenula circuit through retina-vLGN/IGL-LHb pathway (Huang et al. 2019). This circadian clock is known to regulate habenula of the epithalamus region and control neuronal and mental health disorders (Son et al. 2021). Recently, an innovative strategy of blue light therapy was proposed for Chagas disease caused by *Trypanosoma cruzi*.

Table 29.4 Clinical trials that are recruiting patients for various diseases using phototherapy.

No.	Study title	Conditions	Interventions
1	Effect of phototherapy on serum calcium	Phototherapy Side effects	None
2	Cycled phototherapy	Hyper bilirubinemia Premature infant	Device: phototherapy lights
3	Molecular responses caused by UV exposure of human skin	Ultraviolet light burn	Other: ultraviolet light exposure
4	Broadband emission LED phototherapy source versus narrow band	Neonatal hyperbilirubinemia Jaundice, neonatal	Device: Blue-green LED phototherapy
5	Combined intense pulsed light (IPL) with fractional erbium:YAG laser ablation in scar prevention	Intense pulsed light Erbium-yttrium aluminum Garnet laser Scar prevention	Device: fractional Er:YAG laser Device: intense pulse light
6	A trial of the irradiance level of phototherapy for neonatal jaundice	Neonatal jaundice	Other: high irradiance level of phototherapy Other: low irradiance level of phototherapy
7	Using early time-restricted feeding and timed light therapy to improve glycemic control in adults with type 2 diabetes	Diabetes mellitus type 2 Time-restricted feeding Light therapy, complications	Behavioral: no change in meal timing Behavioral: timed light therapy
8	BUBOLight®, a new phototherapy device for the treatment of the newborn's jaundice	Neonatal jaundice	Device: BUBOLight device
9	Low level laser (LLL) phototherapy in oral lesions resulting from anti-neoplastic prevention	Oral mucositis Osteoradionecrosis Osteonecrosis, bisphosphonate	Device: preventive, LLL phototherapy and topical vitamin E
10	Blue light phototherapy	Grover's disease Psoriasis vulgaris	Device: blue light phototherapy
11	Phototherapy versus pregabalin in treatment of refractory uremic pruritis	Refractory uremic pruritis	Device: Narrow band (NB) UVB phototherapy Drug: pregabalin
12	Phase II study – trial of a phototherapy light device to improve sleep health	Sleep	Device: phototherapy device
13	Evaluating mental health improvements after using home phototherapy device with UVB LEDs	Usability Quality of life	Device: MySOLIUS
14	Broadband vs. narrowband phototherapy for eczema trial nested in the CACTI cohort	Atopic dermatitis Skin diseases Eczema	Device: narrowband UVB phototherapy Device: broadband UVB phototherapy
15	Efficacy of osteopathic manipulative medicine (OMM) and phototherapy for patients with chronic lower back pain	Chronic lower back pain	Procedure: osteopathic manipulative medicine Procedure: phototherapy
16	Efficacy of light therapy device LUMINETTE® in major depressive disorder	Major depressive disorder Unipolar depression	Device: active light therapy (LUMINETTE®) Device: placebo light therapy
17	Light intensity physical activity trial	Diabetes mellitus Physical exercise Light intensity physical activity	Device: wrist-worn feedback physical activity monitor
18	Light therapy for Parkinson disease (PD) – dose selection	Parkinson's disease Sleep disorder Fatigue	Device: SunRay light boxes

(*Continued*)

Table 29.4 (Continued)

No.	Study title	Conditions	Interventions
19	Morning bright light to improve sleep quality in veterans	Brain injuries, traumatic Post-traumatic stress disorder	Other: morning bright light therapy
20	Bright light therapy as possible treatment option for multiple sclerosis (MS)-fatigue	Multiple sclerosis Fatigue	Device: bright light therapy Device: dim red light
21	The effect of cycled light on premature infants and mothers	Preterm infant development Retinopathy of prematurity Sleep quality Quality of life	Behavioral: cycled light experimental
22	Pulsed dye laser and intense pulsed light configured with different wavelength bands in improving erythematotelangiectatic rosacea	Erythematotelangiectatic rosacea	Device:
23	Use of blue light emitting diode in the treatment of women with bacterial vaginosis: a clinical trial	Vaginosis, bacterial	Device: blue light emitting diode (LED) 401 ±5 nm
24	Morning light treatment for traumatic stress: the role of amygdala reactivity	Stress	Device: light therapy A via the Re-Timer®
25	Red light treatment in peripheral artery disease	Peripheral artery disease Claudication, intermittent Vasodilation	Device: red light (670 nm energy) Drug: Octafluoropropane
26	A wearable morning light treatment for postpartum depression	Postpartum depression	Device: bright light therapy
27	Use of 405 nm blue light emitting diode in the treatment of women with vulvovaginal candidiasis: a clinical trial	Candidiasis, vulvovaginal	Device: blue LED 405 nm Other: questionnaire of anamnesis
28	Myopia control using bright light therapy and myopic defocus	Myopia	Other: a high intensity light box and myopic defocus
29	Effects of green light exposure on epileptic spikes in patients with refractory epilepsy	Epilepsy Epilepsy intractable	Device: green light exposure
30	Green light effect on anxiety	Anxiety	Device
31	Near-infrared light photo biomodulation treatment for retinal vein occlusion macular edema	Retinal vein occlusion Macular edema	Device: Ellex Integ NIR laser

Source: Taken from Clinicaltrials.gov on 8 June 2022.

29.15 Conclusion and Prospects

In conclusion, light is the guiding force for the existence of life and several processes in plants, animals, and humans. Optimum light levels are needed for proper functioning of the three organisms on the planet Earth. In humans several light therapies and light mediated gene expressions that can regenerate dead neurons and photoreceptor cells are in clinical trials. These new therapy options can come from bench to bedside shortly, paving the way for personalized medicine.

Acknowledgments

The chapter is dedicated to Late Prof. V.S. Rama Das (VSR) under whose guidance Prasad Rao Allu and Sailaja V. Elchuri worked as postdoctoral fellows at the University of Hyderabad, Hyderabad, India. This work is a part of the grant on "Heliotropic plants" ref 21(0325/95/EMR-II, dated 8-3-1995 funded to VSR. Indian Council for Medical Research SRF to LB and Science and Engineering Research Board grant (EMR/2015/000607) to SVE are gratefully acknowledged.

References

Abraha, I., Rimland, J.M., Trotta, F.M. et al. (2017). Systematic review of systematic reviews of non-pharmacological interventions to treat behavioural disturbances in older patients with dementia. The SENATOR-OnTop series. *BMJ Open* 7 (3): 1–30.

Andrews, E.A. (1892). Heliotropic animals. *Am. Nat.* 26 (305): 400–407.

Berg, I.A. (2011). Ecological aspects of the distribution of different autotrophic CO_2 fixation pathways. *Appl. Environ. Microbiol.* 77 (6): 1925–1936.

Boccaccini, A., Legris, M., Krahmer, J. et al. (2020). Low blue light enhances phototropism by releasing cryptochrome1-mediated inhibition of PIF4 expression. *Plant Physiol.* 183 (4): 1780–1793.

Boyden, E.S., Zhang, F., Bamberg, E. et al. (2005). Millisecond-timescale, genetically targeted optical control of neural activity. *Nat. Neurosci.* 200 (9): 1263–1268.

Briggs, W.R. (1960). Light dosage and phototropic responses of corn and oat coleoptiles. *Plant Physiol.* 35 (6): 951–962.

Briggs, W.R. (2014). Phototropism: some history, some puzzles, and a look ahead. *Plant Physiol.* 164 (1): 13–23.

Brodsky, M.C. (2002). Latent heliotropism. *Br. J. Ophthalmol.* 86 (12): 1327–1328.

Brody, D.C. (2022). Open quantum dynamics for plant motions. *Sci. Rep.* 12 (3042): 1–10.

Brouwer-Brolsma, E.M., Vaes, A.M.M., van der Zwaluw, N.L. et al. (2016). Relative importance of summer sun exposure, vitamin D intake, and genes to vitamin D status in Dutch older adults: the B-PROOF study. *J. Steroid Biochem. Mol. Biol.* 164: 168–176.

Burns, A.C., Saxena, R., Vetter, C. et al. (2021). Time spent in outdoor light is associated with mood, sleep, and circadian rhythm-related outcomes: a cross-sectional and longitudinal study in over 400,000 UK biobank participants. *J. Affect. Disord.* 295: 347–352.

du Buy, H.G. and Nuernbergk, E. (1934). Phototropismus und Wachstum der Pflanzen. *Erg. Biol.* 207–322.

Calvin, M. (1989). Forty years of photosynthesis and related activities. *Photosynth. Res.* 21: 3–16.

Calzolari, M., Romeo, G., Bergamini, F. et al. (2022). Host preference and Leishmania infantum natural infection of the sand fly Phlebotomus perfiliewi in northern Italy. *Acta Trop.* 226: 106246.

Chabas, D., Taheri, S., Renier, C., and Mignot, E. (2003). The genetics of narcolepsy. *Annu. Rev. Genomics Hum. Genet.* 4: 459–483.

Chen, J., Moreau, C., Liu, Y. et al. (2012). Conserved genetic determinant of motor organ identity in *Medicago truncatula* and related legumes. *Proc. Natl. Acad. Sci. U. S. A.* 109 (29): 11723–11728.

Chuong, A.S., Miri, M.L., Busskamp, V. et al. (2014). Noninvasive optical inhibition with a red-shifted microbial rhodopsin. *Nat. Neurosci.* 17 (8): 1123–1129.

Colbourne, J.K., Pfrender, M.E., Gilbert, D. et al. (2011). The ecoresponsive genome of *Daphnia pulex. Science* 331 (6017): 555–561.

Costa, J.N., Dotta, B.T., Persinger, M.A. et al. (2016). Lagged coherence of photon emissions and spectral power densities between the cerebral hemispheres of human subjects during rest conditions: phase shift and quantum possibilities. *World J. Neurosci.* 6 (2): 119–125.

Czeisler, M.É., Capodilupo, E.R., Weaver, M.D. et al. (2022). Prior sleep-wake behaviors are associated with mental health outcomes during the COVID-19 pandemic among adult users of a wearable device in the United States. *Sleep Heal.* 8 (3): 311.

Darwin, C.R. (1888). *Power of Movement in Plants.* London: John Murray.

Deisseroth, K. (2015). Optogenetics: 10 years of microbial opsins in neuroscience. *Nat. Neurosci.* 18 (9): 1225.

Dell'Orco, D., Koch, K.W., and Rispoli, G. (2021). Where vision begins. *Pflugers Arch. Eur. J. Physiol.* 473 (9): 1333–1337.

DeLuca, H.F. (2016). Vitamin D: historical overview. *Vitam. Horm.* 100: 1–20.

Dikiy, I., Edupuganti, U.R., Abzalimov, R.R. et al. (2019). Insights into histidine kinase activation mechanisms from the monomeric blue light sensor EL346. *Proc. Natl. Acad. Sci. U. S. A.* 116 (11): 4963–4972.

Diósi, L. (1988). Continuous quantum measurement and Itô formalism. *Phys. Lett. A* 129 (8–9): 419–423.

Ditchburn, R.W. (1952). *Light.* London: Blackie and Son, Ltd.

Dogra, S. and Mahajan, R. (2015). Phototherapy for mycosis fungoides. *Indian J. Dermatol. Venereol. Leprol.* 81 (2): 124–135.

Dreyer, I., Vergara-Jaque, A., Riedelsberger, J., and González, W. (2019). Exploring the fundamental role of potassium channels in novel model plants. *J. Exp. Bot.* 70 (21): 5985–5989.

Enríquez, S., Suggett, D., Allemand, D. et al. (2016). Light enhanced calcification in hermatypic corals: new insights from light spectral responses. *Front. Mar. Sci.* 1: 122.

Foo, S.A., Liddell, L., Grossman, A., and Caldeira, K. (2020). Photo-movement in the sea anemone Aiptasia influenced by light quality and symbiotic association. *Coral Reefs* 39: 47–54.

Furbank, R.T. (2017). Walking the C_4 pathway: past, present, and future. *J. Exp. Bot.* 68 (2): e1–e10.

Gonzalez-Ramos, A., Waloschková, E., Mikroulis, A. et al. (2021). Human stem cell-derived GABAergic neurons functionally integrate into human neuronal networks. *Sci. Rep.* 11 (1): 1–16.

Gottlieb, D.J., Hek, K., Chen, T.H. et al. (2015). Novel loci associated with usual sleep duration: the CHARGE consortium genome-wide association study. *Mol. Psychiatry* 20 (10): 1232–1239.

Gudkov, S.V., Andreev, S.N., Barmina, E.V. et al. (2017). Effect of visible light on biological objects: physiological and pathophysiological aspects. *Phys. Wave Phenom.* 25 (3): 207–213.

Hart, J.E. and Gardner, K.H. (2021). Lighting the way: recent insights into the structure and regulation of phototropin blue light receptors. *J. Biol. Chem.* 296 (100594): 1–9.

Hartline, H.K. (1923). Influence of light of very low intensity on phototropic reactions of animals. *J. Gen. Physiol.* 6 (2): 137–152.

Hatch, M.D. and Slack, C.R. (1966). Photosynthesis by sugar-cane leaves. A new carboxylation reaction and the pathway of sugar formation. *Biochem. J.* 101 (1): 103–111.

Hohm, T., Preuten, T., and Fankhauser, C. (2013). Phototropism: translating light into directional growth. *Am. J. Bot.* 100 (1): 47–59.

Huang, L., Xi, Y., Peng, Y. et al. (2019). A visual circuit related to habenula underlies the antidepressive effects of light therapy. *Neuron* 102 (1): 128–142. e8.

Huemmrich, K.F. (2013). Simulations of seasonal and latitudinal variations in leaf inclination angle distribution: implications for remote sensing. *Adv. Remote Sens.* 02: 93–101.

Hügler, M. and Sievert, S.M. (2011). Beyond the Calvin cycle: autotrophic carbon fixation in the ocean. *Annu. Rev. Mar. Sci.* 3 (1): 261–289.

Inoue, S.I., Kinoshita, T., and Shimazaki, K.I. (2005). Possible involvement of phototropins in leaf movement of kidney bean in response to blue light. *Plant Physiol.* 138 (4): 2004.

Inoue, S.I., Kaiserli, E., Zhao, X. et al. (2020). CIPK23 regulates blue light-dependent stomatal opening in *Arabidopsis thaliana*. *Plant J.* 104 (3): 679–692.

Ishishita, K., Higa, T., Tanaka, H. et al. (2020). Phototropin2 contributes to the chloroplast avoidance response at the chloroplast-plasma membrane interface. *Plant Physiol.* 183 (1): 304–316.

Iwatsuki, K. and Naitoh, Y. (1981). The role of symbiotic Chlorella in photoresponses of Paramecium bursaria. *Proc. Japan Acad. Ser. B* 57 (8): 318–323.

Jaedicke, K., Lichtenthäler, A.L., Meyberg, R. et al. (2012). A phytochrome-phototropin light signaling complex at the plasma membrane. *Proc. Natl. Acad. Sci. U. S. A.* 109 (30): 12231–12236.

Jagannath, A., Taylor, L., Wakaf, Z. et al. (2017). The genetics of circadian rhythms, sleep and health. *Hum. Mol. Genet.* 26 (R2): R128–R138.

Jazayeri, M., Lindbloom-Brown, Z., and Horwitz, G.D. (2012). Saccadic eye movements evoked by optogenetic activation of primate V1. *Nat. Neurosci.* 15 (10): 1368–1370.

Jenness, M.K., Tayengwa, R., and Murphy, A.S. (2020). An ATP-binding cassette transporter, ABCB19, regulates leaf position and morphology during Phototropin1-mediated blue light responses. *Plant Physiol.* 184 (3): 1601–1612.

Johnson, J.E., Field, C.B., and Berry, J.A. (2021). The limiting factors and regulatory processes that control the environmental responses of C_3, C_3–C_4 intermediate, and C_4 photosynthesis. *Oecologia* 197 (4): 841–866.

Jurić, I., Hibberd, J.M., Blatt, M., and Burroughs, N.J. (2019). Computational modelling predicts substantial carbon assimilation gains for C_3 plants with a single-celled C_4 biochemical pump. *PLoS Comput. Biol.* 15 (9): e1007373.

Kawano, F., Suzuki, H., Furuya, A., and Sato, M. (2015). Engineered pairs of distinct photoswitches for optogenetic control of cellular proteins. *Nat. Commun.* 6 (6256): 1–8.

Kiser, P.D., Golczak, M., Maeda, A., and Palczewski, K. (2012). Key enzymes of the retinoid (visual) cycle in vertebrate retina. *Biochim. Biophys. Acta* 1821 (1): 137–151.

Koller, D. (1990). Light-driven leaf movements. *Plant Cell Environ.* 13 (7): 615–632.

Kong, Y., Meng, Z., Wang, H. et al. (2021). Brassinosteroid homeostasis is critical for the functionality of the *Medicago truncatula* pulvinus. *Plant Physiol.* 185 (4): 1745–1763.

Könneke, M., Schubert, D.M., Brown, P.C. et al. (2014). Ammonia-oxidizing archaea use the most energy-efficient aerobic pathway for CO_2 fixation. *Proc. Natl. Acad. Sci. U. S. A.* 111 (22): 8239–8244.

Lamia, K.A., Papp, S.J., Yu, R.T. et al. (2011). Cryptochromes mediate rhythmic repression of the glucocorticoid receptor. *Nature* 480 (7378): 552–556.

Legris, M., Szarzynska-Erden, B.M., Trevisan, M. et al. (2021). Phototropin-mediated perception of light direction in leaves regulates blade flattening. *Plant Physiol.* 187 (1): 1235–1249.

Li, F.W., Rothfels, C.J., Melkonian, M. et al. (2015). The origin and evolution of phototropins. *Front. Plant Sci.* 6: 637.

Li, L., Lu, L., Ren, Y. et al. (2022). Xie Y Colocalized, bidirectional optogenetic modulations in freely behaving mice with a wireless dual-color optoelectronic probe. *Nat. Commun.* 13 (1): 1–14.

Liénard, M.A., Bernard, G.D., Allen, A. et al. (2021). The evolution of red color vision is linked to coordinated rhodopsin tuning in lycaenid butterflies. *Proc. Natl. Acad. Sci. U. S. A.* 118 (6): e2008986118.

Lim, S.H., Tran-Viet, K.N., Yanovitch, T.L. et al. (2013). CYP1B1, MYOC, and LTBP2 mutations in primary congenital glaucoma patients in the United States. *Am J. Ophthalmol.* 155 (3): 508–517. e5.

Lips, P., de Jongh, R.T., and van Schoor, N.M. (2021). Trends in vitamin D status around the world. *JBMR Plus* 5 (12): 1–6.

Losi, A., Gardner, K.H., and Möglich, A. (2018). Blue-light receptors for optogenetics. *Chem. Rev.* 118 (21): 10659–10709.

Lyall, L.M., Wyse, C.A., Graham, N. et al. (2018). Association of disrupted circadian rhythmicity with mood disorders, subjective wellbeing, and cognitive function: a cross-sectional study of 91 105 participants from the UK biobank. *The LANCET Psychiat.* 5 (6): 507–514.

Ma, L.Z., Ma, Y.H., Ou, Y.N. et al. (2022). Time spent in outdoor light is associated with the risk of dementia: a prospective cohort study of 362094 participants. *BMC Med.* 20 (1): 1–10.

Matuszyńska, A., Saadat, N.P., and Ebenhöh, O. (2019). Balancing energy supply during photosynthesis – a theoretical perspective. *Physiol. Plant.* 166 (1): 392–402.

Miller, S., Son, Y.L., Aikawa, Y. et al. (2020). Isoform-selective regulation of mammalian cryptochromes. *Nat. Chem. Biol.* 16 (6): 676–685.

Miyamoto, A., Sakai, A., Nakano, R., and Yusa, Y. (2015). Phototaxis of sacoglossan sea slugs with different photosynthetic abilities: a test of the 'crawling leaves' hypothesis. *Mar. Biol.* 162 (6): 1343–1349.

Moon, S.J., Kim, H.Y., Hwang, H. et al. (2017). A dominant negative OsKAT2 mutant delays light-induced stomatal opening and improves drought tolerance without yield penalty in rice. *Front. Plant Sci.* 8 (772): 1–9.

Moozhipurath, R.K. and Kraft, L. (2021). Association of lockdowns with the protective role of ultraviolet-B (UVB) radiation in reducing COVID-19 deaths. *Sci. Rep.* 11 (1): 1–9.

Moran, N. (2015). *Rhythmic Leaf Movements: Physiological and Molecular Aspects. Rhythms in Plants: Dynamic Responses in a Dynamic Environment*, 57–95. Springer International Publishing.

Mukherjee, S.B., Gorohovski, A., Merzon, E. et al. (2022). Seasonal UV exposure and vitamin D: association with the dynamics of COVID-19 transmission in Europe. *FEBS Open Bio.* 12 (1): 106–117.

Mulla, A.J., Lin, C.H., Takahashi, S., and Nozawa, Y. (2021). Photo-movement of coral larvae influences vertical positioning in the ocean. *Coral Reefs* 40 (4): 1297–1306.

Musavizadeh, Z., Najafi-Zarrini, H., Kazemitabar, S.K. et al. (2021). Genome-wide analysis of potassium channel genes in rice: expression of the OsAKT and OsKAT genes under salt stress. *Genes* 12 (5): 784.

Nakasako, M., Oide, M., Takayama, Y. et al. (2020). Domain organization in plant blue-light receptor phototropin2 of *Arabidopsis thaliana* studied by small-angle X-ray scattering. *Int. J. Mol. Sci.* 21 (18): 1–21.

Narendra, A. and Ramirez-Esquivel, F. (2017). Subtle changes in the landmark panorama disrupt visual navigation in a nocturnal bull ant. *Phil. Trans. R. Soc. B Biol Sci.* 372 (1717): 20160068.

Nieves-Cordones, M., Andrianteranagna, M., Cuéllar, T. et al. (2019). Characterization of the grapevine shaker K+ channel VvK3.1 supports its function in massive potassium fluxes necessary for berry potassium loading and pulvinus-actuated leaf movements. *New Phytol.* 222 (1): 286–300.

Nilsen, E.T. and Forseth, I.N. (2018). The role of leaf movements for optimizing photosynthesis in relation to environmental variation. In: *The Leaf: A Platform for Performing Photosynthesis* (ed. W.W. Adams and I. Terashima), 401–423. Cham: Springer.

Obata, T., Kitamoto, H.K., Nakamura, A. et al. (2007). Rice shaker potassium channel OsKAT1 confers tolerance to salinity stress on yeast and rice cells. *Plant Physiol.* 144 (4): 1985.

Peng, M.Y., Liu, W.C., Zheng, J.Q. et al. (2021). Immunological aspects of SARS-CoV-2 infection and the putative beneficial role of vitamin-D. *Int. J. Mol. Sci.* 22 (10): 5251.

Pierik, R., Fankhauser, C., Strader, L.C., and Sinha, N. (2021). Architecture and plasticity: optimizing plant performance in dynamic environments. *Plant Physiol.* 187 (3): 1029–1032.

Ponnu, J. and Hoecker, U. (2021). Illuminating the COP1/SPA ubiquitin ligase: fresh insights into its structure and functions during plant photomorphogenesis. *Front. Plant Sci.* 12: 662793.

Rajendrudu, G. and Das, V.S.R. (1990). C_3 -like carbon isotope discrimination in C_3 –C_4 intermediate *Alternanthera* and *Parthenium* species. *Curr. Sci.* 59 (7): 377–379.

Rakocevic, M., Müller, M., Matsunaga, F.T. et al. (2018). Daily heliotropic movements assist gas exchange and productive responses in DREB1A soybean plants under drought stress in the greenhouse. *Plant J.* 96 (4): 801–814.

Reuter, L., Schmidt, T., Manishankar, P. et al. (2021). Light-triggered and phosphorylation-dependent 14-3-3 association with NON-PHOTOTROPIC HYPOCOTYL 3 is required for hypocotyl phototropism. *Nat. Commun.* 12 (1): 1–15.

Roell, M.S., von Borzykowski, L.S., Westhoff, P. et al. (2021). A synthetic C_4 shuttle via the β-hydroxyaspartate cycle in C_3 plants. *Proc. Natl. Acad. Sci. U. S. A.* 118 (21): 1–9.

Sahel, J.A., Boulanger-Scemama, E., Pagot, C. et al. (2021). Partial recovery of visual function in a blind patient after optogenetic therapy. *Nat. Med.* 27 (7): 1223–1229.

Sailaja, M.V. and Das, V.S.R. (1996). Leaf solar tracking response exhibits diurnal constancy in photosystem II efficiency. *Environ. Exp. Bot.* 36 (4): 431–438.

Salari, V., Valian, H., Bassereh, H. et al. (2015). Ultraweak photon emission in the brain. *J. Integr. Neurosci.* 14 (3): 419–429.

Salari, V., Rodrigues, S., Saglamyurek, E. et al. (2021). Are brain–computer interfaces feasible with integrated photonic chips? *Front. Neurosci.* 15: 1–17.

Schachtman, D.P., Schroeder, J.I., Lucas, W.J. et al. (1992). Expression of an inward-rectifying potassium channel by the *Arabidopsis* KAT1 cDNA. *Science* 258 (5088): 1654–1658.

Schibler, U. and Sassone-Corsi, P. (2002). A web of circadian pacemakers. *Cell* 111 (7): 919–922.

Schumacher, P., Demarsy, E., Waridel, P. et al. (2018). A phosphorylation switch turns a positive regulator of phototropism into an inhibitor of the process. *Nat. Commun.* 9 (2403): 1–9.

Schwartz, J.M., Stapp, H.P., and Beauregard, M. (2005). Quantum physics in neuroscience and psychology: a neurophysical model of mind–brain interaction. *Philos. Trans. R. Soc. B Biol. Sci.* 360 (1458): 1327.

Serôdio, J., Silva, R., Ezequiel, J., and Calado, R. (2011). Photobiology of the symbiotic acoel flatworm *Symsagittifera roscoffensis*: algal symbiont photoacclimation and host photobehaviour. *J. Mar. Biol. Assoc. UK* 91 (1): 163–171.

Serrano, A.M., Vanhaelewyn, L., Vandenbussche, F. et al. (2021). Cryptochromes are the dominant photoreceptors mediating heliotropic responses of *Arabidopsis* inflorescences. *Plant Cell Environ.* 44 (10): 3246–3256.

Sharma, S., Sanyal, S.K., Sushmita, K. et al. (2021). Modulation of phototropin signalosome with artificial illumination holds great potential in the development of climate-smart crops. *Curr. Genomics* 22 (3): 181.

Smallman, H.S., MacLeod, D.I.A., and Doyle, P. (2001). Realignment of cones after cataract removal. *Nature* 412 (6847): 604–605.

Somanathan, H., Borges, R.M., Warrant, E.J., and Kelber, A. (2007). Visual ecology of Indian carpenter bees I: light intensities and flight activity. *J. Comp. Physiol. A.* 194 (1): 97–107.

Son, J.Y., Sabath, M.B., Lane, K.J. et al. (2021). Long-term exposure to PM2.5 and mortality for the older population: effect modification by residential greenness. *Epidemiology* 32 (4): 477–486.

Steffens, L., Pettinato, E., Steiner, T.M. et al. (2021). High CO_2 levels drive the TCA cycle backwards towards autotrophy. *Nature* 592: 784–788.

Stenvers, D.J., Scheer, F.A.J.L., Schrauwen, P. et al. (2019). Circadian clocks and insulin resistance. *Nat. Rev. Endocrinol.* 15 (2): 75–89.

Stiles, W.S. (1937). The luminous efficiency of monochromatic rays entering the eye pupil at different points and a new colour effect. *Proc. R. Soc. Lond. Ser. B Biol. Sci.* 123 (830): 90–118.

Stirbet, A., Lazár, D., Guo, Y., and Govindjee, G. (2020). Photosynthesis: basics, history and modelling. *Ann. Bot.* 126 (4): 511–537.

Strumpen, N.F., Rädecker, N., Pogoreutz, C. et al. (2022). High light quantity suppresses locomotion in symbiotic Aiptasia. *Symbiosis* 86 (3): 293–304.

Su, Z., Xu, W., Shi, H., and He, J. (2020). eVols at University of Hawaii at Manoa: research progress on the cannibalistic behavior of aquatic animals and the screening of cannibalism-preventing shelters. *Isr. J. Aquac. Bamidgeh* 72 (1): 1–16.

Suzuki, H., Koshiba, T., Fujita, C. et al. (2019). Low-fluence blue light-induced phosphorylation of Zmphot1 mediates the first positive phototropism. *J. Exp. Bot.* 70 (20): 5929–5941.

Takahashi, J.S. (2016). Transcriptional architecture of the mammalian circadian clock. *Nat. Rev. Genet.* 18 (3): 164–179.

Thoen, M.P. (2016) Host-plant resistance to western flower thrips in *Arabidopsis*. Doctoral dissertation. Wageningen University and Research.

Thomson, B.K., Kelvin, B., and Thomson, W. (2010). *Baltimore Lectures on Molecular Dynamics and the Wave Theory of Light*. Cambridge University Press.

Tsuchida, K. and Kobayashi, M. (2020). Ultraviolet A irradiation induces ultraweak photon emission with characteristic spectral patterns from biomolecules present in human skin. *Sci. Rep.* 10 (21667): 1–8.

Verschueren, A., Boucherit, L., Ferrari, U. et al. (2022). Planar polarity in primate cone photoreceptors: a potential role in Stiles Crawford effect phototropism. *Commun. Biol.* 5 (89): 1–13.

Wang, Q. and Lin, C. (2020). Mechanisms of cryptochrome-mediated photoresponses in plants. *Annu. Rev. Plant Biol.* 71: 103.

Wang, X., Haga, K., Nishizaki, Y., and Iino, M. (2001). Blue-light-dependent osmoregulation in protoplasts of *Phaseolus vulgaris* Pulvini. *Plant Cell Physiol.* 42 (12): 1363–1372.

Wang, Z., Wang, N., Li, Z. et al. (2016). Human high intelligence is involved in spectral redshift of biophotonic activities in the brain. *Proc. Natl. Acad. Sci. U. S. A.* 113 (31): 8753–8758.

Wang, X., Han, L., Yin, H. et al. (2022). AtANN1 and AtANN2 are involved in phototropism of etiolated hypocotyls of *Arabidopsis* by regulating auxin distribution. *AoB Plants* 14 (1): plab075.

Warrant, E.J. (2017). The remarkable visual capacities of nocturnal insects: vision at the limits with small eyes and tiny brains. *Phil. Trans. R. Soc. B Biol. Sci.* 372 (1717): 20160063.

Yong, L.K., Tsuboyama, S., Kitamura, R. et al. (2021). Chloroplast relocation movement in the liverwort *Apopellia endiviifolia*. *Physiol. Plant.* 173 (3): 775–787.

Zhang, F., Vierock, J., Yizhar, O. et al. (2011). The microbial opsin family of optogenetic tools. *Cell* 147 (7): 1446–1457.

Zhang, R., Lahens, N.F., Ballance, H.I. et al. (2014). A circadian gene expression atlas in mammals: implications for biology and medicine. *Proc. Natl. Acad. Sci. U. S. A.* 111 (45): 16219–16224.

Zhang, X., Huai, J., Shang, F. et al. (2017). A PIF1/PIF3-HY5-BBX23 transcription factor cascade affects photomorphogenesis. *Plant Physiol.* 174 (4): 2487–2500.

Zhou, C., Han, L., Fu, C. et al. (2012). Identification and characterization of petiolule-like pulvinus mutants with abolished nyctinastic leaf movement in the model legume *Medicago truncatula*. *New Phytol.* 196 (1): 92–100.

Zhou, S., Yang, T., Mao, Y. et al. (2021). The F-box protein MIO1/SLB1 regulates organ size and leaf movement in *Medicago truncatula*. *J. Exp. Bot.* 72 (8): 2995–3011.

Index

One Health: Human, Animal, and Environment Triad, First Edition. Edited by Meththika Vithanage and Majeti Narasimha Vara Prasad.

f

g

h